Environmental Factors, Genes, and the Development of Human Cancers

Deodutta Roy · M. Tevfik Dorak
Editors

Environmental Factors, Genes, and the Development of Human Cancers

Springer

Editors
Deodutta Roy
Department of Environmental and Occupational Health
Robert Stempel College of Public Health & Social Work
Florida International University
Miami, FL 33199-0001, USA
droy@fiu.edu

M. Tevfik Dorak
Department of Environmental and Occupational Health
Robert Stempel College of Public Health & Social Work
Florida International University
Miami, FL 33199-0001, USA
mdorak@fiu.edu

ISBN 978-1-4419-6751-0 e-ISBN 978-1-4419-6752-7
DOI 10.1007/978-1-4419-6752-7
Springer New York Dordrecht Heidelberg London

Library of Congress Control Number: 2010933752

Printed on acid-free paper

Springer is part of Springer Science+Business Media (www.springer.com)

Preface

Cancer is a complex disease. Only 5–10% of human cancers are hereditary in nature. Many of us think of environmental agents when we think of carcinogens. The environment includes all that surrounds us, and environmental influences include not only chemical, physical and biological toxicants, but also diet and lifestyle. In this broadest sense, the environment contributes substantially in the development of human cancer. Now everyone accepts the role of the environment in causation of cancer but there seems to be an unnecessary struggle to divide the roles of genes and environment as if they are distinct contributors. The ongoing "nature versus nurture" argument is unproductive. Genes and environmental factors work in concert to protect from or to cause cancer and there is no need to worry about the proportion of their relative contribution. There are lessons to be learned from the classic example of phenylketonuria (PKU). In this monogenic disorder, no harm is possible unless the environmental element is involved. One other aspect missing in the current discussions is the spatial and temporal continuity and variability of environmental exposures, and exposure at critical windows. While exposure assessment at a time point and correlations with follow up data is a common research design and the results obtained are still valuable, there is certainly room for improvement.

The overall goal of this book is to comprehensively present conceptual and methodological aspects of the environment and cancer relationship, and to describe the gaps in knowledge. To do so, we invited eminent investigators from around the world to share their expertise. We were fortunate to put together this book, thanks to the generosity of contributors. Thus, this book contain chapters from the world's experts focused on the current knowledge that supports the role of environment in the cancer etiology and in the growth of malignant lesions, and discuss who may be susceptible to environmental influences. There is a comprehensive coverage of most relevant aspects of the cancer and environment relationship incorporating interactions with genetics. Gene–environment interactions are discussed through each specific cancer-based approach to address the question of how genetic variations can influence susceptibility to the individual type of cancer. It also highlights and summarizes epigenetic changes that increase the risk for susceptibility to a particular type of cancer, particularly in the presence of specific environmental factors.

This book is divided into three parts. The first part highlights basic principles of the environment and gene–environment interactions in cancer susceptibility, tools for analysis, and discusses epigenetic changes that increase the risk for susceptibility to a particular type of cancer, particularly in the presence of specific environmental factors. Additionally, it includes chapters on the statistical and epidemiological methodology for study designs and on different modeling approaches to uncover the complexity of cancer pathology that involves the interaction of genes and the environment.

In the second part of the book, gene and environment interactions are discussed for specific cancers to address the question of how genetic variations can modify susceptibility to the effects of environmental factors. In the last part, case studies are presented on specific environmental factors that interact with genes to cause specific types of cancer. Thus, the book encompasses from general to specific approaches to understanding the joint roles played by genes and environment in cancer development and provides statistical and epidemiologic background for analysis of association studies. It is our hope that the readers will be encouraged to design more comprehensive studies for combined analysis of genetic and environmental determinants of cancer susceptibility and for their interactions to fill the gaps in our knowledge.

Miami, FL Deodutta Roy
Miami, FL M. Tevfik Dorak

Acknowledgments

Besides our gratitude to all contributors, the editors would like to thank Rachel Waren, Todd Dillard and Jenny Wolkowicki of Springer US, and Vignesh Kumar of Integra Software Services Pvt Ltd, India for the editorial assistance and excellent coordination to produce this important monograph. The support of our families and their never ending sacrifice especially during the preparation of this book are greatly acknowledged.

Contents

Contributors

Melissa L. Armas Department of Anatomy and Cell Biology, UF Shands Cancer Center, University of Florida, Gainesville, FL 32610, USA

Nadia Barahmani Section of Hematology-Oncology, Department of Pediatrics, Childhood Cancer Epidemiology and Prevention Center, Texas Children's Cancer Centre, Baylor College of Medicine, Houston, TX 77030, USA, nxbarahm@txccc.org

Paolo Boffetta Lifestyle Environment and Cancer Group, International Agency for Research on Cancer (IARC), F-69008 Lyon, France, cap6@columbia.edu

Yashmin Choudhury Radiation and Molecular Biology Unit, Department of Biochemistry, North-Eastern Hill University, Shillong 793 022, India

John B. Colerangle Sanofi-Aventis Pharmaceuticals, Regulatory Pharmacology and Toxicology – US, Bridgewater, NJ 08807, USA, john.colerangle@sanofi-aventis.com

Shahnjayla K. Connors Department of Anatomy and Cell Biology, UF Shands Cancer Center, University of Florida, Gainesville, FL 32610, USA

Charronne F. Davis Genomic Immunoepidemiology Laboratory, HUMIGEN, The Institute for Genetic Immunology, Hamilton, NJ 08690, USA

Alok Deoraj Department of Environmental and Occupational Health, Florida International University, Miami, FL 33199, USA, adeoraj@fiu.edu

M. Tevfik Dorak Department of Environmental and Occupational Health, Robert Stempel College of Public Health & Social Work, Florida International University, Miami, FL 33199-0001, USA, mdorak@fiu.edu

Quentin Felty Department of Environmental and Occupational Health, FIU Stempel School of Public Health, Florida International University, Miami, FL 33199, USA, feltyq@fiu.edu

Zdenko Herceg Epigenetics Group, International Agency for Research on Cancer (IARC), F-69008 Lyon, France, herceg@iarc.fr

Aruna S. Jaiswal Department of Anatomy and Cell Biology, UF Shands Cancer Center, University of Florida, Gainesville, FL 32610, USA

Prasanna Jayakar Department of Neurological Surgery, School of Medicine, Miami Children's Hospital, University of Miami, Miami, FL 33155, USA

Brian Kunkle Department of Environmental and Occupational Health, Robert Stempel School of Public Health, Florida International University, Miami, FL 33199, USA

Richard J.Q. McNally Institute of Health and Society, Newcastle University, Newcastle upon Tyne, UK, richard.mcnally@ncl.ac.uk

Satya Narayan Department of Anatomy and Cell Biology, UF Shands Cancer Center, University of Florida, Gainesville, FL 32610, USA, snarayan@ufl.edu

M. Fatih Okcu Section of Hematology-Oncology, Department of Pediatrics, Childhood Cancer Epidemiology and Prevention Center, Texas Children's Cancer Centre, Baylor College of Medicine, Houston, TX 77030, USA, mfokcu@txccc.org

Kenneth Olden Laboratory of Molecular Carcinogenesis, Department of Health and Human Services, National Institute of Environmental Health Sciences, National Institutes of Health, Research Triangle Park, NC 27709, USA, olden@niehs.nih.gov

Tuya Pal Department of Cancer Epidemiology and Genetics, Moffitt Cancer Center, Tampa, FL, USA, tuya.pal@moffitt.org

Harekrushna Panda Department of Anatomy and Cell Biology, UF Shands Cancer Center, University of Florida, Gainesville, FL, 32610, USA

Sue K. Park Department of Preventive Medicine and Cancer Research Institute, Seoul National University, College of Medicine, Seoul, Korea

Rosemarie G. Ramos Laboratory of Molecular Carcinogenesis, Department of Health and Human Services, National Institute of Environmental Health Sciences, National Institutes of Health, Research Triangle Park, NC 27709, USA, ramosr@niehs.nih.gov

Deodutta Roy Department of Environmental and Occupational Health, Robert Stempel College of Public Health & Social Work, Florida International University, Miami, FL 33199-0001, USA, droy@fiu.edu

David Sandberg Department of Neurological Surgery, School of Medicine, Miami Children's Hospital, University of Miami, Miami, FL 33155, USA

Thomas A. Sellers Department of Cancer Epidemiology and Genetics, Moffitt Cancer Center, Tampa, FL, USA

Rajesh N. Sharan Radiation and Molecular Biology Unit, Department of Biochemistry, North-Eastern Hill University, Shillong 793 022, India, rnsharan@nehu.ac.in; rnsharan@gmail.com

Aesun Shin Cancer Epidemiology Branch, Research Institute, National Cancer Center, Goyang-si, Korea

Esma Ucisik-Akkaya Graduate Program in Molecular Genetics and Microbiology, Stony Brook University, Stony Brook, NY 11794-5222, USA, eucisikakkay@ic.sunysb.edu

Jenny Permuth Wey Department of Cancer Epidemiology and Genetics, Moffitt Cancer Center, Tampa, FL, USA

Xuesen Wu Department of Epidemiology and Statistics, Bengbu Medical College, Bengbu, Anhui 233030, China, xuesenwu@gmail.com

Momiao Xiong School of Public Health, Human Genetics Center, The University of Texas Health Science Center at Houston, Houston, TX 77225, USA, momiao@gmail.com

Keun-Young Yoo Department of Preventive Medicine, Seoul National University College of Medicine, Seoul, Korea, kyyoo@plaza.snu.ac.kr

Changwon Yoo Department of Epidemiology and Biostatistics, Robert Stempel School of Public Health, Florida International University, Miami, FL 33199-0001, USA, cyoo@fiu.edu

Part I
General Principles

Chapter 1
Introduction

Deodutta Roy and M. Tevfik Dorak

Abstract The interplay between genetic variants and environmental factors determines the phenotype, and therefore, their joint consideration is more likely to yield the true estimate of the cancer risk. This chapter attempts to introduce some of the fundamental challenges-related to the basic principles of the environment and gene–environment interactions in cancer susceptibility. The comprehensive understanding of the environment and interaction between genes and environment for development of each specific type of human cancer is needed for better assessing risk factors and prevention of the cancers.

Keywords Gene–environment interactions · Cancer susceptibility

Cancer has a complex etiology. Cancer is often described as a genetic disorder, but this refers to acquired somatic genetic alterations that give a single cell growth advantage. There are rare cancers due to inherited germline mutations that tend to show familial aggregation. Such mutations alone account for 5–10% of human cancers (Lynch et al., 2004). Most human cancers are non-hereditary or sporadic. Somatic mutations that give rise to cancer can be caused by sun (which can lead to skin cancer), exposure to radiation or toxic chemicals, or even random events within the cells, especially when they are under proliferative stress. While the sequencing of the entire human genome has made it easy to identify variation in genes, genes alone do not wholly explain individual susceptibility to cancer. It has been recognized that cancer is caused by multiple interacting factors, including genes, hormones, and broader environment whose components interact across the lifespan (Le Marchand, 2005; Hemminki et al., 2006). We are learning slowly about possible links between environmental factors, genetics, and development of each type of human cancers. Genes and environmental factors that trigger the development of

D. Roy (✉)
Department of Environmental and Occupational Health, Robert Stempel College of Public Health & Social Work, Florida International University, Miami, FL 33199-0001, USA
e-mail: droy@fiu.edu

D. Roy, M.T. Dorak (eds.), *Environmental Factors, Genes, and the Development of Human Cancers*, DOI 10.1007/978-1-4419-6752-7_1,

cancer are not necessarily the same as those that contribute to its progression and metastasis. We have tools available to identify genetic variants, but it is more difficult to define an individual's environment and agents that the individual has been exposed. However sophisticated, exclusively genetic approaches have not been able to unravel a sizeable portion of heritability in complex disorders (Maher, 2008). Genome-wide association studies have yielded unsuspected associations but even cumulative results fail to explain susceptibility to lead to preventive measures (Offit, 2009). Among the possible reasons cited for this failure, the most prominent one may be the lack of consideration of interactions between genes and environment (Hunter, 2005; Murcray et al., 2009). In even broader terms, gene–gene interactions and interactions among environmental factors are equally important. It remains a challenge to understand how genes and the environment interact to affect the risk of developing cancer. Various innovative genetic approaches are being used to understand cancer susceptibility and a consensus is emerging that genetic variants are effect modifiers for environmental agents (Kelada et al., 2003; Kraft and Hunter, 2005; Le Marchand, 2005). A paradigm shift in our scientific strategies for studying risk factors for cancer is imminent. Our understanding of the environment and interaction between genes and environment needs to adapt to the better understanding of cancer development.

1.1 Environment and Cancer

When we think of non-hereditary factors as environmental factors, many of us think of toxic chemical carcinogens. The environmental health determinants, however, include all that surrounds us, and environmental influences include not only chemical, physical and biological agents, but also hormones, diet and lifestyle. Environmental factors are complex, variable, interactive and dynamic. Multiple exposures to the same or different factors may occur with some temporal or spatial relationship and their order, time-to-exposure, e.g., whether it occurs at a critical window, co-existing exposures may all vary among individuals who are exposed to the same factors. In this broadest sense, the contribution of environment to the development of human cancer is substantial.

One of the best studied cancers is breast cancer. Its conventional risk factors are well-established (Fig. 1.1). Exposure to some of these multiple endogenous and exogenous environmental factors can occur at different periods of a lifespan. Alcohol, smoking and obesity are known to influence estrogen metabolism and exogenous estrogen enhances radiation-induced breast carcinogenesis. These environmental factors are likely to have a complex interaction pattern that will influence breast cancer. Once we are able to design studies with a comprehensive approach to examination of complex and interactive environmental exposures across the lifespan in the context of genetically-mediated susceptibility, the results are likely to be more informative.

Most molecular epidemiological and statistical genetic studies have examined the effects of limited number of environmental factors alone for their main effects, not considering their interaction, their impacts on physiology of a target organ of

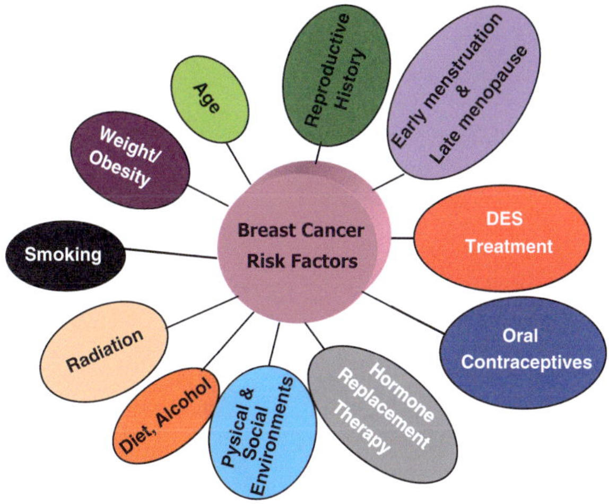

Fig. 1.1 Conventional risk factors for breast cancer

cancer, and mechanism by which these environmental factors contribute to carcinogenic steps (Le Marchand, 2005). Additionally, statistical models to analyze complex environment–environment, gene–gene, and gene–environment interactions are still being developed (Kelada et al., 2003; Kraft et al., 2007; Khoury and Wacholder, 2009; Murcray et al., 2009). Common statistical approaches currently in use have greater power to detect main effects rather than interactions. Exposure to environmental carcinogens can have different effects in different individuals depending on their age, gender, ethnic background, psychosocial stress level, and behavior and lifestyle choices, such as smoking, alcohol consumption, diet and amount of sleep and exercise. While gene–gene and gene–environment interactions are recognized, different environmental factors are seen as independent, not interacting. Better recognition of each and every environmental factor in terms of their relationship to cancer susceptibility should lead to broader consideration of them in future studies. Some subsets of the population are inherently more susceptible to cellular and genetic damage for a number of reasons, including genetic susceptibility, nutritional status, other social or cultural influences, or in the case of children, the vulnerability of developing systems to environmental insult. Thus, not just the dosage of a single exposure, co-existing exposures, their timing and pattern of exposure (one-off, continuous, repeated) need to be taken into account in cancer association studies (Fig. 1.2).

1.2 Interactions Between Genes and Environment, and Risk of Cancer

The term "gene and environment interaction" is often used to emphasize that both genes and environment are important. Such a situation can be better described as gene and environment "coaction" or "joint action" rather than interaction (Dempfle

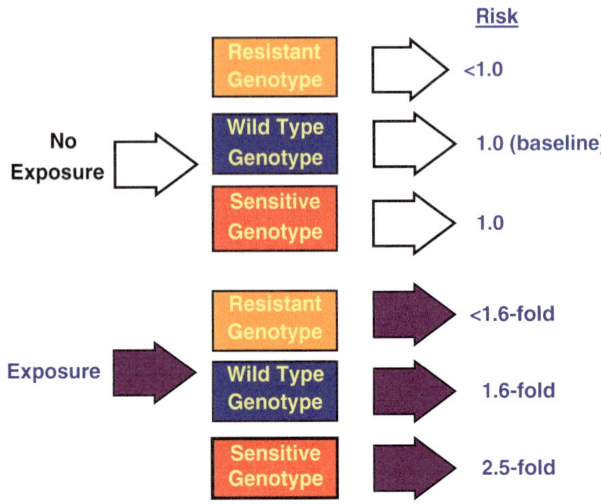

Fig. 1.2 A hypothetical illustration of influence of genetic make up and exposure of environmental factors on the cancer risk

et al., 2008). Interaction refers to modification of the effect of the environment on the phenotype by gene variants, or vice versa. It is also important to keep in the mind that (1) each individual originates from a single cell, which turns into trillions of cells by birth. Each cell contains approximately 30,000 genes that code for 1.5 million alternative forms of proteins. The gene, which is a piece of DNA, is like an empty gun, because it cannot perform any function unless transcribed to an mRNA and translated to a protein. The protein product of the gene is like a bullet, because it impacts cellular functions. Formation and function of a protein are influenced by intra- and extra-cellular environment within a tissue. (2) A large number of genes are considered to be involved in the development of cancer. A minimum of 6–8 gene mutations and gene activation by genetic/epigenetic mechanisms is needed for the development of a particular type of cancer. (3) From the single cell throughout the life span, an individual is exposed to numerous environmental factors. As indicated above, environment constitutes everything that surrounds us both internally and externally, including toxicants, hormones, diet, psychosocial behaviors and life styles (Fig. 1.3). Like genes, environmental factors also interact. From the initial transformation event, it takes 5–15 years to develop clinically recognized cancers. (4) A single exposure to an internal or external environmental factor alone can not explain the development of a malignant tumor, rather it appears that exposure to multiple environmental factors across the lifespan and their sequence and interaction matter. Based on our current knowledge we know that (i) a gene may be genetically/and or epigenetically turned on or off to make mRNA or protein by the environment, which include physical and social components; (ii) the genes modify the cellular response to an environmental stimulus, and (iii) the environmental modulation of the normal cell phenotypic expression leads to the development of a particular type of a cancer. In the realm of gene–environment interactions that

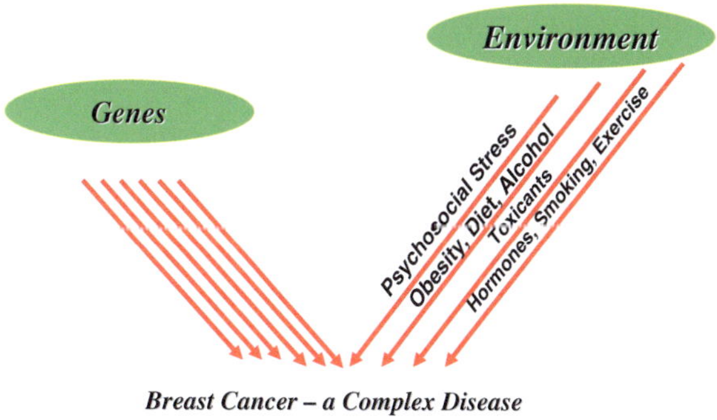

Fig. 1.3 Interactions between environment and genes, and breast cancer

affect cancer phenotype, toxicants such as tobacco smoke and alcohol, redox state, hormones and diet are the best-studied environmental factors.

1.3 Biological and Statistical Interaction

There is some confusion concerning the interpretation of interactions from biological versus statistical points of view. Biological interaction is the result of physical interactions among molecules in biochemical pathways so that the effect of a gene on a phenotype depends on other gene(s). Statistical interaction is defined as deviation from an additive scale if incidence rate differences are used as the effect size or deviation from multiplicative scale if relative risks or odds ratios are used (Clayton and McKeigue, 2001; Hunter, 2005) (Fig. 1.4). In fact, any interaction can be interpreted as a deviation from additive or multiplicative scale depending on the context (Ottman, 1996). Alternative terms to describe the same statistical observation include non-additivity, effect measure modification or heterogeneity of effects (Dempfle et al., 2008). Statistical evidence of interaction does not necessarily imply biomolecular interactions in the etiology of a disease nor provides any

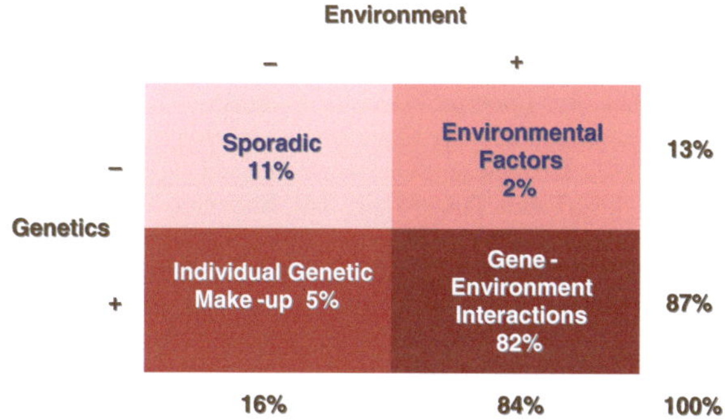

Fig. 1.4 A hypothetical example of gene–environment interaction and cancer

inference about biological modes of joint action. Like any other statistical finding, which may well be a spurious finding, it is also important to replicate any such observation for validity. Also important is the need to consider interactions among environmental factors as well as among genetic markers, and between gene and environment. The least popular of these is the interaction among environmental factors. An example exists in breast cancer. The risk of breast cancer is increased 3.9-fold in premenopausal smokers, 2.4-fold if endogenous estradiol levels are high but 10-fold by smoking and estradiol levels jointly.

1.4 Benefits of Considering the Environment in Genetic Association Studies

Since it is the interplay between genetic variants and environmental factors that determines the phenotype, their joint consideration is more likely to yield the true estimate of the risk. More importantly, if the environment is overlooked and if indeed there is an interaction that has not been explored, an association that is exclusive to one stratum may be obscured in the overall (main effect) analysis (Kraft et al., 2007). An interaction analysis however would yield a stronger association and such associations are more likely to be reproducible in different studies. Missing environmental component in genetic association may well be a major factor in inconsistencies across multiple studies in different populations. The inclusion of data about environmental health determinants in the design of genetic association studies in cancer is crucial given the substantial role played by the environment (Le Marchand, 2005; Hemminki et al., 2006). The temporal trends in the incidence of common cancers and in fact other complex disorders such as asthma are the best indicators of the involvement of the environment in their etiology since the genetic constitution of the population cannot have changed in such short time periods.

References

Clayton, D., McKeigue, P.M., 2001. Epidemiological methods for studying genes and environmental factors in complex diseases. Lancet 358, 1356–1360.

Dempfle, A., Scherag, A., Hein, R., Beckmann, L., Chang-Claude, J., Schafer, H., 2008. Gene-environment interactions for complex traits: definitions, methodological requirements and challenges. Eur J Hum Genet 16, 1164–1172.

Hemminki, K., Lorenzo Bermejo, J., Forsti, A., 2006. The balance between heritable and environmental etiology of human disease. Nat Rev Genet 7, 958–965.

Hunter, D.J., 2005. Gene–environment interactions in human diseases. Nat Rev Genet 6, 287–298.

Kelada, S.N., Eaton, D.L., Wang, S.S., Rothman, N.R., Khoury, M.J., 2003. The role of genetic polymorphisms in environmental health. Environ Health Perspect 111, 1055–1064.

Khoury, M.J., Wacholder, S., 2009. Invited commentary: from genome-wide association studies to gene-environment-wide interaction studies – challenges and opportunities. Am J Epidemiol 169, 227–230; discussion 234–225.

Kraft, P., Hunter, D., 2005. Integrating epidemiology and genetic association: the challenge of gene–environment interaction. Philos Trans R Soc Lond B Biol Sci 360, 1609–1616.

Kraft, P., Yen, Y.C., Stram, D.O., Morrison, J., Gauderman, W.J., 2007. Exploiting gene–environment interaction to detect genetic associations. Hum Hered 63, 111–119.

Le Marchand, L., 2005. The predominance of the environment over genes in cancer causation: implications for genetic epidemiology. Cancer Epidemiol Biomarkers Prev 14, 1037–1039.

Lynch, H.T., Shaw, T.G., Lynch, J.F., 2004. Inherited predisposition to cancer: a historical overview. Am J Med Genet C Semin Med Genet 129, 5–22.

Maher, B., 2008. Personal genomes: the case of the missing heritability. Nature 456, 18–21.

Murcray, C.E., Lewinger, J.P., Gauderman, W.J., 2009. Gene–environment interaction in genome-wide association studies. Am J Epidemiol 169, 219–226.

Offit, K., 2009. Breast cancer single-nucleotide polymorphisms: statistical significance and clinical utility. J Natl Cancer Inst 101, 973–975.

Ottman, R., 1996. Gene–environment interaction: definitions and study designs. Prev Med 25, 764–770.

Chapter 2
Gene–Environment Interactions, Phenotypic Changes, and Human Health

Rosemarie G. Ramos and Kenneth Olden

Abstract The contribution of the environment to the development of chronic disease has historically been documented. As early as 1775, scrotal and nasal cancer was observed among chimney sweepers in London, England by British physician, Percival Potts. His hypothesis was that these cancers were induced by cumulative environmental exposure to chimney soot as they worked. The discipline of cancer epidemiology has continued in the tradition of Dr. Potts. The purpose of this discipline has not been to prove a cause-effect relationship between exposure and development of disease but to identify the "common thread" of exposures. Today, cancer epidemiology incorporates various scientific disciplines (i.e., risk assessment, toxicology, cellular and molecular biology) to quantify the dose-response relationship between an individual and suspect environmental factor. With the completion of the Human Genome Project in 2003, we now know that individual genetic variability plays a significant role in modifying the effect of environmental exposures on disease development. Additionally, the utility of assessing the individual's genetic variability is invaluable in estimating the degree of severity at time of diagnosis as well as the risk of metastasis and other complications. This chapter explores the relationship of gene–environment interactions in cancer from an environmental epidemiology and public health perspective.

Keywords Gene–environment interactions · Cancer · Environmental epidemiology · Public health perspective

R.G. Ramos (✉)
Laboratory of Molecular Carcinogenesis, Department of Health and Human Services, National Institute of Environmental Health Sciences, National Institutes of Health, Research Triangle Park, NC 27709, USA
e-mail: ramosr@niehs.nih.gov

D. Roy, M.T. Dorak (eds.), *Environmental Factors, Genes, and the Development of Human Cancers*, DOI 10.1007/978-1-4419-6752-7_2,

2.1 History of the Relationship Between Genes, Environment, and Human Disease

The belief that the environment plays a critical role in human disease development dates back to the 1700s. As early as 1775, Dr. Percival Potts reported that the incidence of scrotal cancer among chimney sweeps was linked to their occupational exposure to soot (Harrison, 2004). In 1854, Dr. John Snow documented that a cholera outbreak in the Soho area of London, England could be traced to a specific public water source; the Broad Street Pump (Newsom, 2006). Through the use of statistics and geographical maps (i.e., geographic epidemiology) showing the neighborhood-specific distribution of disease incidence, he was able to convince public officials to remove this environmental hazard and eventually the incidence of cholera diminished. In more modern times, environmental exposures that are associated with human disease include poor air quality, hazardous chemicals in the occupational setting, agricultural pesticides, and personal lifestyle choices (i.e., smoking, alcohol use, diet). However, it has become apparent that not every individual who is exposed to a particular environmental factor (i.e., cigarettes, heavy drinking, a high-fat diet) will develop the associated disease (i.e., lung, liver, or pancreatic cancer, respectively). Furthermore, diseases with an environmentally-related etiology are no longer restricted to cancer and now include asthma, cardiovascular disease, and obesity (Bernal-Pacheco and Roman, 2007; Grarup and Andersen, 2007, Newbold et al., 2007; Rundle et al., 2007; Heinrich et al., 2008).

The variability of an individual's response to environmental stimuli was originally thought to have been a function of the dose of the environmental stimuli and the route of exposure. More recently, these risk assessments have expanded the definition of "environmental stimuli" to include social and economic risk factors (i.e., educational attainment, housing characteristics). In addition to disease development being the "response", researchers now examine the incidence of health complications and reduction in quality of life. With the evolution of genomics, individual variability in response to environmental stimuli is better understood. The completion of the Human Genome Project has resulted in considering one's genotype as an additional risk factor in dose-response risk assessments. Additionally, the Human Genome Project has given rise to two emerging and exciting fields; molecular epidemiology and bioinformatics.

Molecular epidemiology is a multi-disciplinary field that seeks to characterize the prevalence of functional biomarkers among diseased and non-diseased populations (Khoury et al., 2004, 2005). With the emergence of this discipline, the ability to quantify the relationship between environmental exposures and disease-specific mechanisms is now possible. Thus, molecular epidemiology allows a novel approach to improve population health by identifying the patterns of variability that increase the risk for disease morbidity and mortality. Bioinformatics is a field that was developed in response to the need of molecular biologists who required the creation and management of large datasets containing nucleotide and amino sequences as well as protein domains and structures that could be queried and one where updates could be routinely performed (National Center for Biotechnology Information, 2004). Thus, the field of bioinformatics was well-suited to assume the task of merging the information from molecular biology and epidemiology studies. Ultimately, the powerful analytical tools of molecular epidemiology and bioinformatics will enable biomedical researchers to assess the contribution from multiple sources of risk (i.e., genes, social/physical environment) towards normal and "not-so-normal" physiological processes.

2.2 Health Disparities and Genetics

Historically, disproportionate rates of disease and mortality have been attributed to the lack of adequate economic and social "safety nets". The aforementioned Broad Street Pump event in 1850s London, England was highly influenced by the concentration of inadequate housing and the poor in the Pump's immediate vicinity (Newsom, 2006). When the pump was closed, the cholera epidemic virtually disappeared. Other significant advances in controlling the spread of infectious disease were possible due to the development of vaccines during the twentieth century. Although the overall vaccination rates for the US population are approximately 90%, lower rates among subgroups (i.e., minorities, poor, elderly) continue to persist due to barriers to health care and lack of health information (Szilagyi et al., 2002). Community-based strategies that target these barriers and improve vaccination rates have become working models for vaccine programs, especially within the medically underserved areas in the US. More recently, preventive care (i.e., screening for cancer, hypertension, diabetes) has emerged as a leading public health issue. Studies examining the effect of promoting preventive care have shown that mortality rates due to cardiovascular disease and colon, prostate, and breast cancer have steadily decreased for most groups since the 1990s. However, these studies have also shown that females, the poor, and ethnic/racial minorities still experience higher rates of morbidity due to preventable chronic diseases (Lander et al., 2001; CDC National Office of Public Health Genomics, 2004; Chien et al., 2005; Chlebowski et al., 2005; Doty and Holmgren, 2005, Commonwealth Fund, 2006; Harris et al., 2006; Blendon et al., 2007; Graham et al., 2007). These studies suggest that underlying societal, institutional, and economic factors continue to influence the persistence of health disparities even with increased public health strategies. Thus, it has become obvious that the issue of health disparities in the US is complex and multi-factorial for which there is no "magic bullet" solution.

The role of individual genetic variability in response to common environmental stimuli has long been suspected as being a significant contributor to the prevalence of health disparities. Many in the biomedical research community had envisioned that the Human Genome Project would finally provide the tools to quantify the genetic contribution to health disparities. It was soon apparent that genetics explained only a fraction of disparities in chronic disease. However, the

Human Genome Project has helped biomedical researchers identify trends in functional genomic variability (i.e., gene–protein interactions) among populations who experience greater disease morbidity and mortality (i.e., the disease phenotype). Often the inciting event for these disparate trends is the environmental exposure to one or more agents. An example of such is the exposure to cigarette smoking and asbestos. Individually, asbestos exposure and cigarette smoking confer a degree of risk for cancer development. However, together these environmental agents act synergistically to influence the resulting cancer phenotype (i.e., stage of invasiveness at diagnosis) (Liddell, 2001; Berry and Liddell, 2004). Additionally, if these exposures occur in an individual who is genetically predisposed to reduced bioavailability to detoxifying enzymes, such as cytochrome P-450 or glutathione-S-transferase, the risk for cancer is significantly higher (Christiani, 2000).

An emerging interest of molecular epidemiologists is the characterization of common, functional haplotypes among diseased individuals. Haplotypes are defined as a set of single nucleotide polymorphisms (SNPs) on a chromatid whose association is statistically significant (National Human Genome Research Institute, 2007). Thus, the identification of functional haplotypes among those who are experiencing greater morbidity due to a chronic disease would be invaluable. Furthermore, haplotype studies of various SNPs that demonstrate significant association with disease would provide further insight to explain disparities of disease severity.

2.3 Studying Gene–Environment Interactions and Disease

The current environment of risk-exposure assessments is one of great opportunity. Improving population health using newer and more powerful predictive models to quantify the cumulative contribution from multiple sources of risk (i.e., exposure, age, gender, genes) continue to be developed. The movement of modern biomedical research to a collaborative, multidisciplinary effort exemplifies the complexity of the genomic contribution to human health and disease. Table 2.1 lists some of the largest initiatives that will likely have an impact on global health in the near future.

The National Institutes of Health (NIH) recently launched the Genetic Association Information Network (GAIN) which is a public-private partnership that will fund studies which aim to examine genome-wide associations in diseases such as depression, and certain autoimmune disorders (National Human Genome Research Institute, 2006). The Genes, Environment, and Health (GEI) Initiative is another NIH program that seeks to further our understanding of gene–environment interactions by identifying new pathways of interaction and developing newer measurements of an individual's response to environmental stimuli including genomics, proteomics, and metabolomics (National Institutes of Health, 2007). Building on their prior successes with the Framingham Heart Study, the National Heart, Lung, and Blood Institute (NHLBI) of the NIH has retained 9,000 of the original Framingham Study participants and their family members for the Framingham

Table 2.1 Summary of the largest gene by environment initiatives that will affect global public health

	Objective(s)	Citations
The NIH Long Life Family Study http://www.longlifefamilystudy.org/	1. Identify characteristics of exceptional families that protect them from disease and disability, including lifestyle and genes 2. Identify positive factors that influence their longevity is also of interest	1. *In the genes: Searching for Methuselah.* NIH Medline Plus Winter 2007 2. *Live long? Die young? Answer isn't just in genes.* New York Times, Aug. 31, 2006
The NIH Road Map Initiative http://nihroadmap.nih.gov/	1. To identify major opportunities and gaps in biomedical research 2. Lays out a vision for a more efficient and productive system of medical research 3. Identifies the most compelling opportunities in three main areas: new pathways to discovery, research teams of the future, and re-engineering the clinical research enterprise	*The NIH roadmap*. Science, Vol. 302, 3 Oct. 2003
National Center for Toxicogenomics	To determine how disease may be influenced by environmental factors using bioinformatics combined with microarray-based strategies	*National Center for Toxicogenomics: An intoduction.* Environmental Health Perspectives Vol. 111, No. 1T, Jan. 2003
Chemical Effects in Biological Systems Knowledgebase (CEBS) http://cebs.niehs.nih.gov/cebs	Integrates study design, clinical pathology, and histopathology data from all studies to enable discrimination of critical study factors	*Systems toxicology and the chemical effects in biological systems (CEBS) knowledge Base.* Environmental Health Perspectives Toxicogenomics, Vol. 111, IT, Jan. 2003
The SNP Consortium http://snp.cshl.org	Identified and mapped 1.5 million individual single nucleotide polymorphisms (SNPs) which are genetic markers (sequence "landmarks" in the genome) used to create genetic maps. These data have been made publicly available to researchers over the internet	*The SNP consortium* website: past, present and future. Nucleic Acids Research, Vol. 31, No. 1, pp. 124–127, 2003

Table 2.1 (continued)

	Objective(s)	Citations
HapMap Project http://www.hapmap.org/	Aims to map the patterns of common SNP variation across the globe and to examine at combinations of SNPs that are inherited together, known as haplotypes	*A second generation human haplotype map of over 3.1 million SNPs*. Nature, Vol. 449, pp. 851–861, 2007
International Cancer Genome Consortium	The project aims to avoid duplication and waste by coordinating the cancer types studied and by establishing common standards of data collection and analysis	*International consortium to tackle cancer genomes*. Published online 30 April 2008, Nature, doi:10.1038/453015a
NIH Cancer Genome Atlas Project	Co-funded by the National Cancer Institute and the National Human Genome Research Institute, this project seeks to the prevention, diagnosis, and treatment of cancer through genome surveillance—monitoring the genome for subtle changes that are suspected of contributing to cancer morbidity and mortality	*NIH Institutes launch joint venture to map cancer genome*. Journal of the National Cancer Institute, Vol. 98, No. 3, February 1, 2006
The NIEHS Sister Study	A landmark study that seeks to untangle the link between the environment and breast cancer. This study envisions the enrollment of 50,000 female volunteers who have has a sister diagnosed with breast cancer	*Sister study hopes to answer breast cancer questions*. Environmental Health Perspectives, Vol. 109, No. 8, August 2001

Genetic Research Study. This study aims to identify genes that may underlie diseases, such as heart disease and stroke, across three generations of family members (National Heart Lung and Blood Institute, 2006). Using the aforementioned model, genome-wide association studies are being planned using pooled DNA samples obtained from the cohorts of the NIH's Women's Health Study and the Women's Health Initiative.

Twin studies have provided great insight to the familial or inherited contribution to disease development. In Finland, a landmark study of like- and opposite-sexed monozygotic (MZ) and dizygotic (DZ) twins has continued to examine the concordance and discordance of genetic traits with respect to cancer, obesity, osteoarthritis, asthma, and cardiovascular disease (Verkasalo et al., 1999; Lichtenstein et al., 2000). However, an exclusive genetic contribution to disease development in the study group ($n > 3{,}000$) has been less than 20%. Other twin studies have provided the evidence supporting the contribution of environmental factors, including the social and parental environment, to disease development among MZ and DZ twins such as depression and addiction disorders. More recently, it has been suggested that differential environmental exposures induce epigenetic changes in cells and this could be the mechanism that explains discordance for disease development among MZ twins (Poulsen et al., 2007).

The contribution of race or ethnicity towards the development of environmentally-related disease has been studied extensively amongst Ashkenazi Jews (i.e., of medieval German origin). Such studies have found a disproportionately higher incidence of breast and ovarian cancer among this population when compared to other populations. One explanation for this trend is provided by a recent study that found a higher prevalence (8%) of abnormal breast cancer (BRCA 1) genes among Ashkenazi Jew females diagnosed with breast cancer (John et al., 2007). In the same study, the authors found a lower prevalence (2%) of this risk factor for breast and ovarian cancer among white Anglo females. However, most cancer studies that have sought a race-ethnic basis for cancer disparities have had contradictory results. Most of the contradiction is due to differential environmental exposures which are now recognized as powerful confounding factors.

2.4 The Environment, Genes, and Cancer

The contribution of the environment to the incidence of cancer is not a new hypothesis. In fact, decades of epidemiological studies have revealed that risk conferred environmental factors is significant for 80–90% of newly-diagnosed cancers. However, many of these studies state that environmental exposures alone are not sufficient to incite the development of cancer. This suggests that an individual's genotype confers some degree of susceptibility to the ill-effects of environmental exposures such as tobacco smoke, alcohol use and exposure to industrial and agricultural chemicals. Additionally, the definition of environmental risk factors for cancer has expanded to include one's diet, the "built environment" and physical activity. This section will discuss the current evidence for a gene–environment interaction in the risk for diagnosis of cancer as well as the increased risk of death due to cancer. To ease the reading of the following section, a glossary of frequently used terms is provided in Table 2.2 and a list of candidate genes, including their abbreviations, and their functions, is provided in Table 2.3. A summary of the evidence presented in this section supporting the relationship between genes, environmental exposures and cancer is found in Table 2.4.

2.4.1 Bladder Cancer

The National Cancer Institute (NCI) estimated that for the year 2008, there were 68,810 new cases of bladder cancer and an additional 14,100 lives lost (National Cancer Institute, 2007a). Gender disparities have been observed in the risk for bladder cancer among male smokers (OR = 7.1) when compared to female smokers (OR = 5.1). However, this disparity is reversed among non-smokers as the effect cumulative exposure to environmental tobacco smoke on bladder cancer incidence appears to affect more women than men (Anton-Culver et al., 1993). Studies have shown that although the frequency of bladder cancer diagnosis is 50% higher in Whites, the mortality rate among Whites and African-Americans is comparable (Prout et al., 2000). This suggests that bladder cancer in African-Americans is either diagnosed at a later stage of disease or this group is more susceptible to an aggressive form of this disease.

The altered expression of carcinogen detoxifying genes (i.e., NAT2, GSTM1) and the DNA repair enzymes (i.e., NER enzymes) have been shown to confer an increased risk of bladder cancer. A 2006 study of the role NER genes plays in bladder cancer found that possessing one of the 22 SNPs that are found in seven NER genes significantly predicted the incidence of bladder cancer risk ($p = 0.04$) (Garcia-Closas et al., 2006). Further pair-wise association analysis found that the risk of bladder cancer increased 1.5–2-fold when the variants were carried in both copies of four of the seven genes being studied.

The risk of bladder cancer from the decreased production of enzymes responsible for detoxification or DNA repair is further increased among cigarette smokers. A gene–environment interaction is biologically plausible since NAT2 and GSTM1 are responsible for detoxifying the cigarette-containing compounds, aromatic amines and polycyclic aromatic hydrocarbons. These compounds are also known to induce DNA damage. In 2005, a meta-analysis conducted by Garcia-Closas et al. found an increased risk of bladder cancer among smokers with SNPs in either NAT2 gene ($p = 0.008$) or the GSTM1 gene ($p < 0.0001$) (García-Closas et al., 2005). An examination by this same group of investigators found that the risk for bladder cancer among individuals with a SNP in one of the NER enzyme genes conferred a significant risk ($p = 0.02$) but SNPs in two genes conferred a much more substantial risk ($p < 0.001$) (Garcia-Closas et al., 2006).

The distribution of the NAT2 and GSTM1 alleles has been estimated to be 40 and 50%, respectively, in the European and the US White populations (Vineis, 2004).

Table 2.2 Glossary of terms used in this chapter

Genotype	The genetic constitution of an individual
Phenotype	The observable properties of an organism that are produced by the interaction of the genotype and the environment
Bioavailability	The degree and rate at which a substance, such as an endogenous protein, is made available at the site of physiological activity
Healthy people	A set of health objectives for the Nation to achieve over the prescribed decade. Healthy People 2010 outlined the objectives for the decade 2000–2010; Healthy People 2020 will outline the objectives for the decade 2010–2020. It can be used by many different people, States, communities, professional organizations, and others to help them develop programs to improve health
Single nucleotide polymorphisms (SNPs)	Sites in the DNA sequence where individuals differ at a single DNA base
Haplotype	Defined as a set of proximal single nucleotide polymorphisms (SNPs) on a chromatid that are inherited together in a "block" and whose association is statistically significant. The block of SNPs that characterize the haplotype are referred to as "tag SNPs"
Framingham heart study	The objective of the Framingham Heart Study was to identify the common factors or characteristics that contribute to cardiovascular disease by following its development over a long period of time in a large group of participants who had not yet developed overt symptoms of CVD or suffered a heart attack or stroke. To date, the study has expanded to three generations of related participants
Women's Health Initiative (WHI)	is a long-term national health study that focuses on strategies for preventing heart disease, breast and colorectal cancer and fracture in postmenopausal women. This 15-year project involves over 161,000 women ages 50–79, and is one of the most definitive, far reaching programs of research on women's health ever undertaken in the US
Odds ratio (OR)	The unit of measure used to compare the presence of a risk factor for disease in a sample of diseased subjects vs. non diseased controls. An odds ratio = 1 indicates no risk; an odds ratio < 1 = a protective factor; an odds ratio > 1 = a risk factor. Additionally, the odds ratio is accompanied by a 95% confidence interval (i.e. that there is < a 5% likelihood that the risk is attributed to chance). When the confidence interval includes 1, the odds ration is considered "not statistically significant"
Oncogene	A gene that normally directs cell growth. When mutated, an oncogene can promote and/or allow the uncontrolled growth of cancer. Mutations to oncogenes occur via environmental exposures or hereditary factors
Tumor suppressor gene (also known as anti-oncogene)	Responsible for producing the protein that controls cell growth. When mutated, aberrant cell growth and subsequently cancer, may occur. As with oncogene, mutations to tumor suppressor genes can occur via environmental exposures or hereditary factors

Table 2.3 Dictionary of genes cited in this chapter

Gene	Abbreviation	Category	Function
Alcohol dehydrogenase	ADH	Detoxification of ethanol	ADH is a group of enzymes that function to metabolize ingested alcohols which could otherwise be toxic. The production of this enzyme is lower in females when compared to males and its genetic expression is higher among those of European ancestry when compared to those of Asian ancestry
Aldehyde dehydrogenase	ALDH	Detoxification of ethanol	ALDH is a group of enzymes that function to metabolize aldehydes, the intermediate products of alcohol degradation
Ataxia-telangiectasia	ATM	DNA repair	ATM controls cell growth by coordinating DNA repair via activation of other proteins
Breast cancer Type 1 or Type 2 susceptibility gene	BRCA1 BRCA2	Tumor suppressor gene	BRCA genes participate in repairing cells with breaks in double-stranded DNA
Cell-cycle checkpoint kinase	CHEK2	Cell cycle regulation	CHEK2 is an enzyme is critical for cell cycle regulation via apoptosis and DNA repair via cell cycle arrest
Cytochrome p450	CYP1A1 CYP1B1 CYP2E1	Phase 1 detoxification	CYP450 enzymes are primarily tasked with the Phase 1 detoxification and biotransformation of xenobiotics. Specifically, CYP450 is a family of heme proteins tasked with the breakdown of exogenous substances (i.e., drugs and toxic compounds) as well as endogenous metabolic products (i.e., bilirubin, the breakdown product of hemoglobin)
Epoxide hydrolase	EPHX	Phase 2 detoxification	An enzyme that functions in detoxification during drug metabolism. This enzyme is critical in the conversion of intermediate metabolites (epoxides) to compounds that can be excreted from the body. These metabolites, which are generated as a result of cytochrome P450 break-down of aromatic compounds, are also mutagenic
Glypican 3	GPC3	Organ and tissue development	GPC 3 is an oncofetal protein. An oncofetal protein is one that is expressed during embryogenesis and is involved in organogenesis. The exact biological function of GPC3 is not known. However, GPC3 has been observed to be over-expressed in liver and skin cancer tumors

Table 2.3 (continued)

Gene	Abbreviation	Category	Function
Glutathione-S-transferase M, T, P variants	GSTM1 GSTT1 GSTP1	Phase 2 detoxification	GST enzymes play a critical role in the detoxification of various intermediate metabolites. These metabolites are often reactive inducing DNA damage and damage to DNA repair processes thus increasing the risk of carcinogenesis
Human epidermal growth factor receptor 2	HER2/neu	Growth factor	HER2 is known to regulates cell growth and differentiation. The expression of HER2 on tumors is a critical for chemotherapy. Tumors that are negative for HER2 have poor response to chemotherapy
Midkine	MDK	Growth factor	Several cancers report an over-expression of MDK and is a pre-operative predictor of prognosis, including metastases. However, the exact mechanism by which it influences cancer prognosis is not known
Myeloperoxidase	MPO	Phase 1 detoxification	MPO plays a role in the metabolic activation of pro-carcinogens found in cigarettes. Thus, differential expression of this enzyme has been hypothesized to influence the risk of lung cancer among smokers
Methylenetetrahydrofolate reductase	MTHFR	Conversion of ingested folic acid to bioactive form	MTHFR catalyzes the bioconversion of folic acid or vitamin B9. This is significant since dietary sources of methyl donors (i.e., folic acid) are hypothesized to decrease the risk of cancers of the digestive system
N-acetyl transferase	NAT2	Phase 2 detoxification	This family of enzymes facilitates the biotransformation of intermediate metabolites from Phase 1 detoxification via acetylation. These metabolites include polycyclic hydrocarbons that are found in cigarettes and cigarette smoke
Nucleotide excision repair	NER	DNA repair	NER enzymes are critical for DNA repair in damaged cells, specifically that which occurs as a result of oxidative damage

Table 2.3 (continued)

Gene	Abbreviation	Category	Function
NAD(P)H:quinone acceptor xidoreductase	NQO	Phase 2 detoxification	NQO enzymes are a family of enzymes that detoxify endogenous and exogenous substances via reduction of the intermediate metabolite, quinones, via electron reduction reactions. This enzymatic activity protects cells against oxidative stress; a risk factor for carcinogenesis
Tumor protein 53	TP53	Cell cycle regulation	This gene regulates the cell cycle via cell cycle arrest when damage to DNA occurs and if necessary, induction of apoptosis. Because of this function, it is often referred to as the guardian of the genome especially since it is a key player in the anti-cancer activities of many cells
Progression elevated gene	PEG10	Tumor progression	The expression of this gene is elevated in the presence of DNA damage and during cancer cell progression. Its expression also correlates with genomic stability
Phosphatase and tensin homolog deleted on chromosometen	PTEN	Tumor suppressor gene	Cell cycle regulation via signaling to damaged cells to stop dividing and undergo apoptosis
Thymidylate synthase	TS		
Excision repair cross-complementing group 2	XDP (also known as ERCC2)	DNA repair	Transcription-coupled nucleotide excision repair
X-ray repair cross-complementing group	XRCC	DNA repair	Base excision repair
V-raf murine sarcoma viral oncogene homolog B1	BRAF	Oncogene	A mutated form of the normal, cellular genes, known as proto-oncogenes, that contributes to the production of a cancer. Since they direct cell growth, the mutated oncogenes are hypothesized to increase the growth and spread of cancer cells

Table 2.3 (continued)

Gene	Abbreviation	Category	Function
Melanocortin-1-recpetor	MC1R	Production of melanin	A key protein that regulates skin and hair color. It is found at the surface of cells that produce melanin called melanocytes. In the 1990s variants of the MC1R gene were found in 30% of humans who have red hair and fair skin. Individuals with skin cancer also have a higher frequency of mutations in this gene although the exact mechanism responsible remains unknown
8q24		Region (locus) on chromosome 8	Polymorphisms in the region of this locus on chromosome 8 have been shown to be significantly associated with prostate and breast cancer
Insulin growth factor	IGF1	Cell cycle regulation	Through binding on various cells in various tissues, IGF stimulates cell growth and plays a critical role in anti-apoptotic activity
Estrogen receptor beta	ESR2	Nuclear receptor	This protein plays a key role in DNA binding and subsequent gene transcription. It is normally expressed in the nucleus of normal epithelial and blood cells as well as their malignant counterparts
Androgen receptor	AR	Nuclear receptor	This protein plays a key role in DNA binding and subsequent gene transcription. Genes that are regulated by the androgen receptor are critical for the development and maintenance of the male sexual phenotype
Serine peptidase inhibitor, Kazal type 1	SPINK1	Trypsin inhibitor	Mutations of this protein are found to correlate with risk for acute and chronic pancreatitis

Table 2.4 Summary of the risk for cancer posed gene by environment interactions cited in this chapter

Cancer	Candidate gene(s)	Environmental exposure(s)	Phenotypic change due to interaction between genes and environment
Bladder	NAT2 GSTM1 NER	Smoking confers higher risk in males	Substantial increase in risk for smokers with SNPs in these genes
		Exposure to environmental tobacco smoke (ETS) confers higher risk for females	Effect of ETS on those with SNPs not known
Breast	CYP1B1 NAT2	Smoking	2.6–5.1× increase in risk for breast cancer among smokers 2.5× increase in risk among smokers
Colorectal	CYP2E1	Frequent red meat or processed meat consumption	2×–3× increase in risk for rectal cancer among heavy meat eaters
	XRCC	Smoking	2.5× risk among "ever-smokers"
	XDP	Alcohol consumption	2.9× risk among "ever-drinkers"
Esophageal	ADH ALDH	Alcohol consumption	2× increase in risk amongst regular drinkers 2× risk among moderate drinkers 4.5× risk among heavy drinkers
Leukemia	CYP1A1	Chemicals	CYP1A1 variants carriers: *In-utero* exposure to pesticides confers 5x increases risk of ALL; same exposure in childhood confers 3.6× increase in risk
	MTHFR TS	Diet	Increased bioavailability of folate reduces risk for cancer
	CYP450 GST		Gene–gene interactions among Phase I and Phase II enzyme genes (i.e., CYP450 and GST, respectively) with SNPs confer 2–10× risk for ALL

Table 2.4 (continued)

Cancer	Candidate gene(s)	Environmental exposure(s)	Phenotypic change due to interaction between genes and environment
Liver	NAT2	Smoking Alcohol-related cirrhosis	The risk for liver cancer increases 2× for smokers with liver disease (from OR = 1.23 to OR =2.67)
	GSTM1	Hepatitis infection	Risk from null GSTM1 genotype doubles from OR = 1.18 to OR = 1.26 in HepA infected patients
	EPHX	Heavy peanut butter consumption	Risk from heterozygous EPHX genotype increases from OR = 2.75 to OR = 3.63 among those with heavy peanut butter consumption
Lung	CYP1A1	Smoking	2× risk among light smokers (< 30 pack years)
	EPHX	Western lifestyle	7× risk among young Mexican Americans
	GSTM1 and GSTP1	Environmental tobacco smoke Smoking	2× risk among those with GSTM1 null genotype 4.5× risk among those with both GSTM1 null genotype and mutation in one or both GSTP1 alleles
	MPO		0.25 reduction in risk for lung cancer
	NAT2		1.9× risk among smokers and non-smokers
Melanoma	BRAF2 and BRAF 4	Male gender	Exact risk still not known
Mesothelioma	GSTM1 NAT2	Asbestos-occupational exposure	1.9× risk among carriers of NAT2 fast-acetylator genotype 2.4× risk among carriers of *BOTH* NAT2 fast acetylator and GSTM1-null genotypes
Pancreatic	NQO1	Smoking	NQO1 levels were 6× greater
	GSTT1		GSTT-null genotype conferred a 5.0× increased risk among White female "ever" smokers and 3.2× risk among White male "ever" smokers
Prostate	GSTM	Smoking	3.8× increased risk among smokers (> 30 pack years)
	GSTP	Diet rich in cruciferous vegetables	Protective relationship has been established in-vitro
	NAT2	Smoking	2× risk among smokers

However, the global distribution of the NER genes is harder to quantify since they are numerous and have overlapping functions. Genome screening projects, such as the HapMap project, continue to identify the NER gene variants that confer the most risk individually or in tandem with SNPs of other detoxifying or DNA repair genes. The knowledge generated from studies, such as the HapMap project, will have a substantial impact on how human health risk assessments are conducted in the future.

2.4.2 Breast Cancer

Breast cancer has long been a threat to women's health. In 2008, the NCI estimated that 182,460 women were be diagnosed with breast cancer and claimed the lives of 40,480 (National Cancer Institute, 2007b). In spite of this grim statistic, it is encouraging that both breast cancer incidence and mortality have shown a downward trend over the past 20 years. This is likely a result of improved public health outreach and communication strategies that seek to increase awareness of screening and knowledge of risk factors among women and their health care providers.

As with other chronic diseases, higher rates of breast cancer mortality are observed for African-American females when compared to the national average (i.e., 33.5/100,000 and 25.0/100,000, respectively). Even more disturbing is the fact that this disparity exists even as the diagnostic rate of breast cancer is lower among African-American females (i.e., 117.5/100,000) when compared to national rate (i.e., 126.1/100,000) (Ries et al., 2008). Studies have shown that African-American women are less likely to be screened for breast cancer even though there is substantial evidence that this group suffers from a disproportionate burden of breast cancer mortality (Sassi et al., 2006). Additionally, they are more likely to be diagnosed with breast cancer that has progressed to a more advanced stage and is clinically characterized by poor prognostic markers (i.e., estrogen receptor-negative) (Chlebowski et al., 2005; Acharya et al., 2008).

Environmental risk factors for breast cancer include lifestyle choices such as smoking, alcohol use, obesity, reduced or no physical activity, high-red meat diet, hormone replacement therapy, and parity (Mustacchi, 1961; MacMahon et al., 1970; Cerhan et al., 1998; Cho et al., 2006; Sillanpaa et al., 2007; Vona-Davis et al., 2007; Zhang et al., 2007). With respect to environmental exposures, animal studies conducted by the National Toxicology Program have found an association between exposure to 48 different chemicals and the development of mammary tumors (National Toxicology Program, 2007a). However, studies demonstrating a causal relationship between chemicals and breast cancer in humans have been contradictory. Additionally, identifying the critical periods of exposure to chemicals which are hypothesized to confer the greatest risks for cancer has been challenging. To date, the majority of the evidence associating chemical exposure to human breast cancer has been obtained from occupational studies (Brody and Rudel, 2003). A 2001 study by Davis et al. found that night shift workers of having an increased risk of breast cancer which has led to a suggested role for melatonin;

the naturally-occurring hormone that serves as a critical antioxidant and provides protection against DNA damage (Davis et al., 2001; Schernhammer et al., 2001).

Familial history of breast or any other type of cancer confers a risk for cancer diagnosis. Females who carry mutations in the BRCA1 and BRCA2 genes have a 20% increase in risk of developing breast cancer during their early 30s to 63% after age 70 (Claus et al., 1998). In this same study, by Claus 66% of BRCA mutation carriers reported a family history of breast cancer. However, it is estimated that 8 out of 9 women who develop breast cancer do not have an affected first-degree relative (Collaborative Group on Hormonal Factors in Breast Cancer, 2001). This suggests a potent role of the environment or gene–environment interactions in the majority of breast cancer cases.

The genotype of the breast cancer patient affects not only their susceptibility to environmental insults but their response to treatments. Genetic mutations in the PTEN gene have been shown to increase the risk of resistance to trastuzumab (i.e., Herceptin) therapy which counters the aberrant cell proliferation activity of the HER2/neu protein that is seen in 15–22% of early stage breast cancers (Berns et al., 2007). Assessments of mutations in the tumor suppressor gene, p53, are considered powerful prognostic markers for poor outcomes among "node-negative" breast cancer patients (Silvestrini et al., 1993). A 2007 study found that mutations in 2 different alleles of the cell-cycle checkpoint kinase (CHEK2) gene conferred an elevated risk of breast cancer (Bell et al., 2007). Among female breast cancer patients, the P85L variant was more frequent among African–Americans and Ashkenazi Jews while the 1100delC was observed more frequently only among African–Americans. Female relatives of patients with the disease ataxia-telangiectasia are often carriers of mutations in the ataxia-telangiectasia (ATM) gene (i.e., the gene responsible for the disease) and consequently are at significant risk for breast cancer before the age of 60 (OR = 2.9) and after (OR = 6.4) (Athma et al., 1996; Thompson et al., 2005).

With respect to a gene-environment role in breast cancer, the NAT2, and cytochrome-p450 (CYP) genes each play a critical role in the production of enzymes necessary for detoxification of the compounds found in tobacco smoke and the metabolites of alcohol (Klaassen, 2001). Sillanpaa et al. found that among women smokers, the risk for breast cancer was increased by the presence of a SNP in the CYP1B1 gene or the combination of SNPs in both the NAT2 and CYP1A1 genes (Sillanpaa et al., 2007). In 2004, a study found that among Connecticut women exposed to environmental polychlorinated biphenyls (PCBs), a known endocrine disruptor, the risk for breast cancer was marginally increased (OR = 1.5) (Zhang et al., 2004). Additionally, Zhang et al. found that among women who were exposed to PCBs and who also possessed a specific SNP in the CYP1A1 gene m2 variant, the risk for breast cancer doubled (OR = 2.1) with the risk quadrupling (OR = 4.1) among post-menopausal women. This finding is significant since the CYP1A1 m2 variant is believed to be present in approximately 12% of the White female population. Studies such as these have a substantial public health impact since many endocrine disruptors are known to persist for long periods of time in the environment. This is complicated by the fact that the global distribution of the variant alleles in candidate genes for breast cancer is not yet known.

2.4.3 Colorectal Cancer

Currently, death due to colorectal cancer is the third leading cause of cancer-related mortality in the Western world (National Cancer Institute, 2007c). The occurrence of this cancer before the age of 50 is about equal between men and women. However, after age 50 men become increasingly vulnerable. Colorectal cancer incidence and mortality has steadily decreased for most groups, except American Indians and Alaskan Natives, while rates among Whites and African–Americans remain the highest. Recent studies have found significant variation among race and ethnic groups with respect to stage of diagnosis and risk for mortality (Chien et al., 2005; Alexander et al., 2007). The primary contributing factors to these disparities are patient education and access to preventive screening.

The environmental risk factors for colorectal cancer are reflective of the "Western lifestyle". These risk factors include diet, alcohol consumption, smoking, physical activity, and obesity. Moore et al. found that among subjects enrolled in the Framingham cohort, obesity defined by a BMI > 30 conferred a 1.5-fold risk among those 30–54 years of age and 2.4-fold risk among subjects age 55–79 (Moore et al., 2004). Additionally, the risk conferred by a high BMI was greater among males when compared to females. These authors also found that a large waist circumference (> 39 inches) conferred at least a 2-fold risk for colorectal cancer with the greatest risk observed among sedentary older and younger adults (relative risks = 3.0–4.4, respectively). More recently, Chia et al. found that an elevated serum level of the obesity biomarker, leptin, was associated with a 3.3-fold risk for colorectal among men (Chia et al., 2007). A 2005 multinational European cancer study found that both male and female who frequently consumed red meat were at an increased risk for colorectal cancer (OR = 1.35) with the risk increasing after the age of 50 (OR = 1.71) (Norat et al., 2005). Conversely, a diet rich in fish conferred a reduced risk of cancer before the age of 50 (OR = 0.69 vs. 1.5) and after the age of 50 (OR = 1.28 vs. 2.4).

In a study among Finnish men 42–61 years of age at baseline, heavy weekly consumption of alcohol (14 servings of beer or 16 servings of liquor) conferred a 3.5-fold lifetime risk for diagnosis of colorectal cancer (Toriola et al., 2008). A recent longitudinal study among adults 50–71 years of age at baseline observed an inverse linear correlation between exercise frequency ($\geq$ 5 times a week) and colon cancer (OR = 0.79) among (Howard et al., 2008) men. Additionally, men who were sedentary ($\geq$ 9 h a day watching television or videos) were at a 1.6-fold increased risk for colon cancer. This risk is further increased by smoking status and affects not only the incidence but the aggressiveness of the tumor (Botteri et al., 2008).

In addition to the evidence identifying elements of the "Western lifestyle" as independent risk factors for colorectal cancer, recent studies have found that this risk is further modified by an individual's genotype. The evidence supporting a role for the interaction between diet and SNPs in the CYP2E1 gene was published in 2002 (Le Marchand et al., 2002). The authors found that individuals who were carriers of a functional SNP in the CYP2E1 gene had a baseline elevated risk for developing rectal cancer. This risk was increased 2- to 3-fold among those who consumed a diet that was rich in either red meat or processed meats or ate pickled products. These findings are significant since the pro-carcinogenic *N*-nitrosamine compounds, which are found in both types of meats, are bio-activated by the CYP450 enzymes resulting in DNA adduct formation. Thus, it is biologically plausible that a SNP which results in an increased induction of these CYP450 enzymes accompanied by a diet rich in *N*-nitrosamine compounds would result in a significant risk of developing colorectal cancer. The evidence supporting the risk imposed by cigarette smoking and alcohol consumption suggests a significant role of SNPs in the DNA repair genes XRCC1 and XDP. In 2005, Stern et al. found that among patients diagnosed with colorectal cancer and functional SNPs in the XRCC1 genes, a history of "ever smoking" conferred a significant risk for colorectal cancer (OR = 2.9) (Stern et al., 2006). Additionally, among individuals with SNPs in the XDP gene, a statistically significant contribution (OR = 2.5) from alcohol consumption among "ever drinkers" when compared to "never drinkers" was observed.

In an environment of robust cell cycle activity, such as the digestive system, there are many factors that contribute to the homeostasis that averts neoplastic growth. There is growing evidence of the role that methyl-donor nutrients (i.e., folic acid-containing foods) play in chemoprevention thus a diet that is rich in grains, fruits, and vegetables should be intuitive. Additionally, reduced intake of red meats and other foodstuffs which are known to induce the generation of DNA adducts or free radicals is currently advocated by public health professionals especially since the population distribution of functional SNPs in DNA repair genes is not yet known.

2.4.4 Esophageal Cancer

Since the 1970s, the growth in the incidence and mortality rate of esophageal cancer has exceeded the annual growth rate of every other cancer (Brown and Devesa, 2002; Pickens and Orringer, 2003). In the US, the increase in the incidence of esophageal cancer has been greatest among White males but the mortality rates among African–American males remains higher even though the diagnosis among this group has declined steadily over the last 15 years (Blot and McLaughlin, 1999; National Cancer Institute, 2007d). There has been some question about the contribution of improved diagnostics to the increase in esophageal cancer. However, a 2005 study found that when adjusted for the increased use of endoscopies, the incident rate and the primary site of diagnosis (the lower third of the esophagus) has remained steady since 1975 (Pohl and Welch, 2005). Risk factors for esophageal cancer include reflux disease (Barrett's esophagus), obesity, extremely low weight, and low fruit and vegetable consumption (Morris Brown et al., 1995; Engel et al., 2003; Samanic et al., 2006; Corley et al., 2008). More recently, the risk conferred role by alcohol consumption has come under greater scrutiny.

The association between esophageal cancer and alcohol consumption has been studied extensively in Japanese men (Miyazaki et al., 2002; Sakata et al., 2005; Ishikawa et al., 2006). It has been reported that heavy alcohol consumption and death due to alcohol-associated diseases has increased dramatically among Japanese males (Makimoto et al., 2000). Adding to the increased prevalence of this risk factor is the identification of SNPs, amongst Japanese men, in the genes encoding for two enzymes that are critical for detoxifying ethanol; alcohol dehydrogenase (ADH) and aldehyde dehydrogenase (ALDH) (Tanaka et al., 1996, 1997). Researchers have examined the association between the polymorphisms in the ADH and ALDH genes among Eastern Asian men and the risk of being diagnosed with esophageal cancer (Yang et al., 2005; Chen et al., 2006). Yang et al. found an increased risk of esophageal cancer among Japanese men who possessed an ALDH polymorphism and were either moderate drinkers (OR = 1.88) or heavy drinkers (OR = 4.62). Chen et al. also found that the risk of esophageal cancer was further modified by the lifetime drinking (i.e., > 300–350 cc. of beer for 20 consecutive years) resulting in a 20-fold increase among those with an ADH gene polymorphism and 30-fold increase among those with an ALDH gene polymorphism.

Although the majority of gene–environment interaction studies, with respect to esophageal cancer, have been conducted among "frequent/heavy drinkers" (i.e., 2 six packs of beer/day), the risk conferred from a susceptible genotypes among other categories of drinkers is not known. These include "binge-drinkers", younger vs. older drinkers and those who drink alcoholic beverages with higher alcohol content (i.e., 12% ethanol in hard liquor vs. 5% ethanol in beer). Furthermore, the degree of penetrance or the population distribution of the candidate genes for esophageal cancer remains unknown. Such information could have a dramatic effect population health since the 5-year survival rate of this cancer is 20–25%.

2.4.5 Leukemia

Leukemia is a cancer that originates in the bone marrow and results in a large number of blood cells to be produced. Although this cancer occurs more often in adults than in children (10 to 1), is the most common pediatric cancer and is the leading cause of mortality among children < 14 years of age. This cancer is most likely to be diagnosed in White males although the mortality rates between Whites and African-Americans are comparable. Leukemia is also divided into four types; acute lymphocytic leukemia (ALL), chronic lymphocytic leukemia (CLL), acute myelogenous leukemia (AML), and chronic myelogenous leukemia (CML). ALL is the most common type of leukemia in children while AML, primarily found in older adults, is the most common among adults. Epidemiologic surveillance studies have reported geographic variation in the incidence of leukemia (i.e., higher incidence in wealthier, developed countries) but the identification of population-attributable factors is lacking.

Environmental exposures that have been identified as risk factors for leukemia include ionizing radiation and benzene. Benzene is used a solvent in the production of many chemicals and is found in gasoline due to its natural occurrence in crude oil. The current classification of benzene as a known carcinogen has existed since 1980 and is based on various human studies (Savitz and Andrews, 1997; National Toxicology Program, 2005b). Additionally, the potential human health threat of benzene exposure (i.e., inhalation or ingestion) has been recognized by several federal agencies including the Department of Health and Human Services, the Environmental Protection Agency, the Department of Transportation, and the Occupational and Safety Hazard Administration. At the cellular level, toxicity is caused by the production of reactive oxygen species as benzene is being metabolized by CYP450 enzymes (Agency for Toxic Substances and Disease Registry, 2005). Tissue-specific targets of the reactive oxygen species appear to be the hematopoietic cells and the bone marrow tissue (Ross et al., 1996).

Environmental exposure to ionizing radiation occurs in everyday life. Although in small amounts, sources of environmental radiation include those which are naturally-occurring such as radon which is found in granite and coal and those from man-made sources such as TVs, X-rays, and cigarette smoke (National Institutes of Health, 2000). As with benzene, a significant portion of the scientific data that established a relationship between radiation exposure and leukemia has been obtained from human studies (Lewis, 1957; Lewis et al., 1957). Since ionizing radiation is known to induce DNA damage, it is logical to assume that any health effects would be a function of the duration of the dose. However, for an individual whose DNA repair machinery is compromised (i.e., SNPs in essential detoxifying and/or DNA repair genes), the risk of developing leukemia due to environmental exposures to ionizing radiation would be expected to be higher.

Recent studies have identified candidate genes that confer an increased risk for developing acute myeloid leukemia. Majumdar et al. reported a significant risk of developing AML among individuals who were carriers of the GSTM1 null genotype (OR = 3.25), or were homozygous for polymorphisms in the NAT2 (OR = 3.19) or CYP1A1 2A (OR = 4.88) (Majumdar et al., 2008). Smith et al. found that the frequency of diminished or no NQO was higher among their cohort of patients who had been diagnosed with leukemia (OR = 1.49) when compared to matched controls who did not have leukemia (Smith et al., 2001). Polymorphisms in the folate metabolizing genes, 5,10-methylenetetrahydrofolate reductase, serine hydroxymethyltransferase, and thymidylate synthase have been reported to confer protection against developing ALL in adults (Skibola et al., 1999, 2002). Since the cells involved in leukemia are characterized by a high turnover rate, the reduced bioavailability of folate which results in an increased risk of DNA damage due to an accumulation of uracil in the DNA is significant.

The interest in fetal or *in-utero* programming for adult diseases has included studies interested in assessing the relationship of maternal exposure to radiation or benzene during pregnancy and the development of ALL in the offspring. Most of these investigations have focused on exposures incurred within the occupational setting. Infante-Rivard et al. found that high occupational exposure to extremely low frequency magnetic fields (i.e., sewing machine and electronic factories), was associated with a two-fold increase in risk of ALL, the most common type of pediatric leukemia, in the offspring (Infante-Rivard and Deadman, 2003). An earlier study by this same group found an increased risk of developing ALL among children who possessed SNPs in the CYP1A1, CYP2D6, GSTT1, and GSTM1 genes and had been exposed to insecticides, rodenticides, or pesticides *in-utero* or during infancy (Infante-Rivard et al., 1999). During this study, the researchers found that the incidence of ALL was significantly related to *in-utero* or early childhood exposure to multiple products and SNPs in the CYP1A1 gene. When examining the risk for ALL conferred from the child's genotype, they observed a significant interaction between outdoor skin repellents exposures, *in-utero* (OR = 5.5) or in childhood (OR = 3.6), possessing the CYP1A1 ml variant, and ALL. When examining the influence of the CYP1A1 m2 variant, a significant risk for ALL was found among those possessing this allele who had been exposed *in-utero* to ant, roach, or wasp pesticides. However, even with such evidence, the mechanisms that would explain the effects from *in-utero* exposures radiation or chemicals on fetal development of biotransformation and DNA repair enzymes remains unknown.

Different studies have found a gene–gene interaction in the risk for ALL which highlights the importance of the interactions between SNPs at various loci. In their study, Canalle et al. examined the risk conferred by polymorphisms in the genes that encode for both Phase I (CYP1A1, and CYP2E1) and Phase II (GSTM1, GSTT1, GSTP1) detoxifying and metabolizing enzymes (Canalle et al., 2004). Initially, they observed an increase in risk conferred by a solo and rare SNP in the GSTP1 gene (OR = 2.7). However, a synergistic effect on the risk for developing ALL was observed among individuals whose possessed multiple variants in the CYP1A1, CYP2E1, GSTM1, and GSTP1 genes (OR = 10.2). Gene–gene interaction in the risk for ALL has also been found in studies examining the relationship between ALL and SNPs in the CYP2E1, MPO and NQO1 genes. A synergistic effect on the risk of ALL was found amongst individuals who carried the wild-type MPO allele and the CYP2E1 and NQO1 variants (OR = 5.4) (Krajinovic et al., 2002). Sinnett et al. have also examined the interaction between the genes involved in the Phase I (i.e., CYP1A1, CYP2D6) and Phase II (i.e., GSTM1, GSTT1, NAT1 and NAT2) xenobiotic biotransformation pathways (Sinnett et al., 2000). Although an elevated risk was conferred by the individual variants (OR = 1.6–1.7), the risk increased with the simultaneous presence of SNPs in CYP450 and GST genes (OR = 2.6). Additionally, the risk increased in slow acetylators who also possessed SNPs in the NAT genes (OR = 3.3).

With the unknown population distribution of genes critical for protection against oxidative stress and repair of DNA damage coupled with the ubiquitous presence of benzene in our environment (i.e., gasoline, environmental tobacco smoke), the effect on cancer-related population health risk may yet to be realized.

2.4.6 Liver Cancer

Hepatocellular carcinoma (HCC) or liver cancer is an aggressive cancer with a poor 5-year survival rate. This statistic may explain why HCC is the third leading cause of cancer-specific mortality across the globe (Parkin et al., 2005). In the US, the incidence and mortality rate of liver cancer is higher among men when compared to women and among Hispanics, Asian–Americans and Pacific Islanders when compared to African–Americans and Whites (National Cancer Institute, 2007e). Global population studies have also found a higher prevalence of liver cancer among Asian and sub-Saharan African populations which is consistent with the geographic region's high prevalence of Hepatitis B and C (Raza et al., 2007). Individuals who have been diagnosed with heritable hemochromatosis, a metabolic disorder resulting in "iron-overload", are also at an increased risk of developing liver cancer.

Population-attributable risk factors such as chronic liver infections (i.e., Hepatitis A, B, or C), heavy alcohol consumption, and regular ingestion of aflatoxin (a compound found in nuts) explain the majority of new cases of liver cancer around the world. Alfatoxin, a naturally-occurring mycotoxin produced by certain *Aspergillus* species, is found in crops such as nuts, oilseeds, and cereals which are main diet staples in many Asian and African countries. The risk conferred from Hepatitis B virus (HBV), Hepatitis C virus (HCV), or aflatoxin ingestion is due to their effects on the genes involved in DNA damage repair (Pang et al., 2008). The HBV, a DNA virus, is characterized by the production of the viral protein, HBx, which subsequently reduces the bioavailability of p53. The HCV, an RNA virus, also inhibits cellular apoptosis via the production of the HCV core proteins, NS3 and NS5A (Ghosh et al., 1999; Marusawa et al., 1999; Kwun et al., 2001). NS3 and NS5A promote aberrant cell growth by inhibiting the activity of other proteins involved in apoptosis such as p21 (WAF), Fas, and TNF-α. The ingestion of alflatoxin also induces mutations in the p53 gene (Shen and Ong, 1996; Liu et al., 2008). This may explain the disproportionate burden of liver cancer in Asian populations where HBV is endemic and daily nut consumption is high.

The lack of a diagnostic biomarker for liver cancer contributes to the poor 5-year survival rate (Parkin et al., 2005). Since the 1970s, diagnosis of liver cancer has relied on the serological detection of α-fetoprotein (AFP), a non-specific liver protein that has a high false-positive rate since its is also observed in those with cirrhosis and hepatitis (Taketa, 1990). To date, the identification of preventive biomarkers for use in the screening of "at-risk" individuals for liver cancer has progressed slowly. However, research that seeks to identify predictive biomarkers (i.e., cytokine profiles) that characterize the chronic inflammation seen in liver cancer (especially in the presence of cirrhosis or infection) has made significant strides in recent years. This is significant since persistent inflammation is also characterized by a high turnover of cells which in turn increases the risk of malignant transformation and would explain why in the absence of surgical resection or a liver transplant, a poor prognosis accompanies a diagnosis of liver cancer (Moss and Blaser,

2005; Mazzanti et al., 2008). Recent studies at the National Cancer Institute have discovered a unique cytokine profile of the T-helper lymphocyte cells found in the cancerous liver microenvironment (Jia et al., 2007). Wang et al. identified the GPC3 gene that encodes for extracellular protein glypican 3 which is detectable in serum and elevated in patients with liver cancer. Other studies have found elevated levels of PEG10 and MDK in the sera of liver cancer patients (Kato et al., 2000). Future studies that seek to identify individuals who are genetically predisposed to the overproduction of these critical proteins (i.e., polymorphisms in the GPC3, PEG10, and/or MDK genes) would have a significant impact on global morbidity and mortality rates that are attributed to liver cancer.

As with other cancers, there has been an increased focus on the synergy between cigarette smoking and polymorphisms in the NAT2 gene among individuals who have chronic liver disease (i.e., cirrhosis, Hepatitis infection). Tobacco use has been shown to act synergistically with alcohol use in the development of liver cancer (Marrero et al., 2005). Polymorphisms in the NAT2 gene have been found to increase the risk of liver cancer among smokers and smokers with Hepatitis B (Yu et al., 2000; Farker et al., 2003). With respect to aflatoxin ingestion, the environmental insult is induced by the metabolite, aflatoxin 8,9 epoxide, which is detoxified by epoxide hydrolase (EPHX) and GSTM1 (Tiemersma et al., 2001). Tiemersa et al. has reported that among populations who consume high daily levels of peanut butter and who also report high rates of Hepatitis B infection, there is a significant contribution from the GSTM1 null or EPHX heterozygous genotype towards the risk of liver cancer.

Liver cancer is unique in that its incidence is primarily attributed to lifestyle factors. With the increase of other population-attributable factors such as obesity and consumption of processed foods and the continued lack of an early diagnostic or prognostic biomarker, liver cancer will likely be categorized an emerging public health threat within the next decade.

2.4.7 Lung Cancer

Lung cancer continues to be the leading cause of cancer-related deaths among men and women in the US. Although the mortality rate for males has declined, the mortality rate for females has remained steady (National Cancer Institute, 2007f). Lung cancer is characterized by a lengthy, asymptomatic latent period (i.e. >10 years) and poor prognosis. The lack of an early diagnostic tool is an additional factor for lung cancer mortality (Godley et al., 2003). Although regularly CT scans have been suggested for those "at risk", it is believed that the benefit of such would be overshadowed by the cost of these services and the increased risk for other cancers conferred from radiation exposure (Bach et al., 2007).

Environmental risk factors for lung cancer include a family history of lung cancer, smoking, second-hand tobacco smoke, exposure to naturally-occurring radon gas, and occupational exposure to asbestos, silica, and chromium (Alberg and Samet, 2003; Etzel et al., 2003; Alberg et al., 2007). Interestingly, public and occupational health has made tremendous strides in increasing awareness of and reducing exposures to environmental risk factors. However, lung cancer incidence and associated mortality continues to be a significant health issue in the US. Furthermore, the differential lung cancer incidence among those who are equally exposed to environmental risk factors strongly suggests a key role for individual genomic variability.

Genes in which functional SNPs have been identified to confer risk for lung cancer include the following; CYP450, EPHX, MPO, NQO, and GST. In studies where no smoking history was available or subjects were never smokers, a genetic contribution was observed from the CYP1A1 alone or GSTM1 variants in the presence of the CYP1A1 SNP (Taioli et al., 1998; Hung et al., 2003; Taioli et al., 2003; Raimondi et al., 2005). Two separate studies have described a relationship between SNPs in the EPHX gene and lung cancer risk in non-smokers. One study found an increased risk for lung cancer among non-smokers conferred from a SNP in the EPHX gene but another observed a protective effect from the interaction of SNPs in both the EPHX and GSTM1 genes (Zhou et al., 2001, 2002). Studies have found elevated levels of NQO in cancer lung cancer tissue of non-smokers as well as the increased, but statistically insignificant, prevalence of SNPs in the NQO gene (Schlager and Powis, 1990; Alexandrie et al., 2004). The findings presented in this paragraph are especially relevant since these candidate genes play key roles in detoxifying chemicals, including polycyclic aromatic hydrocarbons (a primary component of cigarette smoke and air pollution). Additionally, these findings suggest that SNPs in these genes affect the stoichiometric balance that is required to efficiently metabolize and detoxify numerous toxicants.

Of all the cancer risk factors identified to date, cigarette smoking continues to be the most frequently cited. A history of cigarette smoking is indicated in 85–90% of all lung cancers. However, the evidence demonstrating an increased risk conferred by polymorphisms in the genes that detoxify carcinogens found in cigarettes has been inconsistent. In a study to examine the effect of mutations in the CYP1A1 gene, Ishibe et al. only observed a significant effect among light smokers (<30 pack years), no effect amongst heavy smokers and no modification on these effects by race (i.e., African–American) (Ishibe et al., 1997). Another study found a higher expression of CYP1A1 in lung tissue of ex-smokers when compared to current and non-smokers ($p < 0.007$) (Kim et al., 2004). The enzyme EPHX has a critical detoxifying role with respect to carcinogens found in cigarettes but its effect on lung cancer has been examined in only few studies. In an interesting study examining the effect of SNPs in the EPHX gene among Mexican-Americans, Wu et al. found an increase risk of lung cancer among Mexican-Americans (OR = 3.6) with an even higher risk in the group < 65 years of age (OR = 7.4) (Wu et al., 2001). Although Hispanics have lower rates of lung cancer, this study suggests the contribution from a non-traditional source of environmental exposures; that from ethnic acculturation (i.e., the Western lifestyle). Wenzlaff et al. found that among their cohort of non-smokers who reported heavy exposure to environmental tobacco smoke (i.e., > 20 years of ETS), those possessing the GSTM1 null genotype had more than a two-fold risk for lung cancer. Furthermore, this genotype acted synergistically with mutations in one or both alleles of the GSTP1 conferred a four-fold lung cancer risk (Wenzlaff et al., 2005). This is significant since the majority of non-smoking lung cancer patients report being exposed to ETS. A puzzling aspect of the relationship between smoking and lung cancer is the fact that not all smokers develop lung cancer. Prior to the knowledge of genomic risk factors, variability in response to carcinogens was suspected of being a function of the variability of population-attributable risk factors (i.e., diet, use of hormones, alcohol consumption). However, studies examining the differential expression of MPO have found that individuals, especially smokers, who possess a SNP in this gene are actually protected from developing lung cancer (Schabath et al., 2002; Taioli et al., 2007). However, caution must be exercised in interpreting these results as a "license to smoke" since this observation has only been observed in lung cancer studies while smoking is well-established as an independent risk factor for cancer and other chronic diseases. The NAT1 "fast" genotype has been observed to confer an increased risk of lung cancer (OR = 1.92) but not the NAT2 "slow" genotype (Wikman et al., 2001). However, when this study group was stratified by smoking status, the NAT1 "fast" genotype was observed more frequently among individuals diagnosed with small cell carcinoma and among those > 60 years of age. Since mutations in the enzyme, NQO, result in reduced bioavailability of this enzyme, researchers have been interested in whether this reduction in enzyme activity results in reduced bio-activation of carcinogens thus reducing the risk for lung cancer. However, the results from such hypothesis-driven studies have been contradictory. Xu et al. found that former smokers possessing the NQO1 C/T genotype had almost a four-fold risk of lung cancer (Wikman et al., 2001). However, Lawson et al. found no relationship between smoking, the NQO1 C/T genotype, and lung cancer (Lawson et al., 2005). Interestingly, a small cohort study found that the wild-type NQO1 (i.e., normal NQO carcinogen-activating activity) was more prevalent in African Americans who had been diagnosed with lung cancer suggesting that mutations in this gene may explain the increased incidence of cancer among African-Americans (Wiencke et al., 1997).

Contrary to the gene–environment interactions cited in other cancers, the role of exposure to tobacco smoke appears to be the primary determinant of lung cancer development. Even more discouraging is the fact that the genes of interest have a very wide applicability in the metabolism and biotransformation of toxicants (i.e., they act on a wide variety of agents). As the results of the HapMap project are incorporated into prevention and practice, it is likely that haplotype characterization, in combination with environmental exposure assessment, will provide the tools for predicting and reducing lung cancer morbidity and mortality.

2.4.8 Melanoma

The skin is the largest organ in the human body. Melanoma is the cancer that forms in the skin cells (melanocytes) which produces melanin, the pigment that gives skin its color (National Cancer Institute, 2008a). Melanoma is the deadliest form of skin cancer even though there is a favorable prognosis when diagnosed early. Since the 1980s, the rate of melanoma diagnosis among Whites, the most susceptible group in the US, has increased from about 13/100,000–24.6/100,000 in 2005 (National Cancer Institute, 2008b). However, the mortality rate among all races and ethnicities has remained steady. The incidence of melanoma occurs more frequently in males when compared to females and more frequently among individuals > 50 years of age although it can occur at any age. Among individuals who are newly diagnosed with melanoma, only 10% report having a family history (American Cancer Society, 2008). Therefore, a majority of melanoma cases are likely attributed to other risk factors such as UV exposure, immuno-suppression, and seemingly benign skin conditions such as moles and freckles.

Heritability is a primary risk factor for melanoma. It is estimated that individuals with a mutations in any of the three highly penetrant genes, p16, ARF, or CDK4, will incur a 67% lifetime risk of developing melanoma (Pho et al., 2006). However, carriers of these mutations account for less than ½ of all melanoma cases. Recent studies suggest that low penetrant genes may interact to modify the risk of melanoma. Two such genes are the BRAF and the MC1R. Mutations in the oncogene BRAF have been reported more frequently among males with a family history of melanoma (Meyer et al., 2003). This may partially explain why melanoma occurs more frequently in males than females. Other studies have found an increased frequency of BRAF mutations among melanoma patients who had intermittent sun exposure suggesting risk factors other than UV rays from sunlight may be involved in the development of this cancer (Maldonado et al., 2003). Another candidate gene is the MC1R gene which is responsible for skin pigmentation. The MC1R, a receptor found on the surface of melanocytes, is responsive alpha-melanocyte stimulating hormone (α-MSH) which is secreted during exposure to ultraviolet rays such as those found in direct sunlight. Some of the MC1R variants result in reduced or blunted expression of α-MSH and confer an increased risk for melanoma (Valverde et al., 1996). A recent report found that among individuals with no evidence of excessive sun exposure, and whose melanoma tumors developed in areas that were not continuously exposed to the sun (i.e., the trunk), the likelihood of mutations in both BRAF and MC1R were significantly greater (Landi et al., 2006). Additionally, this study found that the risk for melanoma conferred by a mutation in BRAF increased incrementally with the concomitant presence of one or two variant MC1R genes (OR for one copy = 2.8; OR for two copies = 5.7). Although the majority of study subjects were younger, the interaction of age with melanoma risk was not statistically significant ($p = 0.22$).

Although studies to date suggest divergent pathways in the development of melanoma, proactive measures to reduce exposure to environmental factors, such as direct sunlight, is encouraged. Furthermore, since the UV rays of sunlight induce DNA damage, risk factors that reduce DNA damage repair capability (i.e., cigarette smoking) should be avoided. Finally, since research on this cancer is still in its early stages, the "window of vulnerability" is not known. Thus, protection of young children from prolonged exposure to direct sunlight should always be avoided.

2.4.9 Occupational-Related Cancer

Occupational settings have historically been the "gold standard" for confirming an environmental contribution to disease. A landmark study published in 1979 set the current standard for occupational exposure assessments which must now consider the contribution of individual genomic variability to the risk occupationally-related disease (Lower et al., 1979). Furthermore, understanding the contribution of an individual's genotype during the risk assessment process is crucial especially when estimating what amount of risk from occupational exposures that employers, regulators, and society are willing to accept in this risk/benefit "trade-off". The best example of a current dichotomy is the occupational exposure to asbestos.

Asbestosis is an occupationally-related disease attributed to the environmental exposure to asbestos. Asbestos, now recognized as a human carcinogen, had been used in the US since the 1800s in a variety of occupational settings ranging from insulation in houses and buildings to pads in vehicle brakes and clutches (National Toxicology Program, 2005a; Agency for Toxic Substances and Disease Registry, 2007). In 1970, the use of asbestos began to be phased out culminating in an EPA ban on all new uses in 1989. However, its established uses were allowed to continue which includes many buildings and homes built before 1970 and many vehicles on the road today. A growing public health concern is the use of personal protective equipment among the workforce that may be regularly exposed to asbestos, especially demolition workers in older, urban cities. More recently, protecting disaster, recovery, and first-responder teams from asbestos exposure has become an emerging occupational public health issue, especially after the attacks on September 11, 2001 (Landrigan et al., 2004; Johnson et al., 2005).

As with other diseases, polymorphisms in the GSTM1 and NAT2 genes have been cited as risk factors for asbestosis (Hirvonen et al., 1996). This is significant since these enzymes modulate the cellular response to oxidative stress that occurs in the lung upon asbestos exposure. In the absence of such critical detoxifying enzymes, lung-scarring inflammation occurs with the subsequent replacement of viable lung tissue with fibrous tissue. Additionally, asbestosis has been firmly established as the leading risk factor for mesothelioma; a malignant cancer of the mesothelium. This cancer of the membranes lining the chest and abdominal cavities and surrounding internal organs is often asymptomatic for many years but once diagnosed, is difficult to control. A recent study conducted in Europe found that among Italian workers, NAT2 fast-acetylator genotype were significantly associated with malignant mesothelioma risk (OR = 1.9) (Neri et al., 2006). Additionally, the combination of a GSTM1-null and NAT2 fast-acetylator genotype further increased the risk of this aggressive cancer (OR = 2.4). It should be mentioned that in this same study, no effect was found among Finnish workers but this observation is hypothesized to be attributed to the source of asbestos. With respect to the contribution of smoking to asbestos-related cancer, the EPA's official risk advisory states a conferred risk from smoking and asbestos exposure towards lung cancer but not towards mesothelioma (Environmental Protection Agency, 2008).

As previously mentioned, the individuals at the most risk of exposure to asbestos are those in the construction and demolition trades. Although the US Occupational and Safety Hazard Administration has strict occupational standards regarding maximum personal exposure limits under normal circumstances, exposures are much harder to control during extraordinary situations, such as building collapses and fires. In spite of the evidence, the global use of asbestos in developing continues today even though studies have confirmed a relationship between its use the incidence of asbestosis, mesothelioma and lung cancer.

2.4.10 Pancreatic Cancer

Currently in the US, pancreatic cancer is the fourth leading cause of cancer-related deaths. Both the incidence and mortality rate is about 50% higher in African–American males when compared to White males and it more frequently affects males of all races when compared to females (National Cancer Institute, 2007g). However, a recent study has reported that this disparity is explained by racial differences in cigarette smoking and prevalence of diabetes mellitus (Silverman et al., 2003). Trend analysis over the past two decades has shown very little improvement in either incidence or mortality rates in this cancer which has a poor prognosis since it is usually diagnosed at an advanced stage.

The evidence linking individual genetic variability and pancreatic cancer is sparse. The primary genetic risk factor for pancreatic cancer is hereditary pancreatitis. Chronic pancreatitis is a confirmed independent risk factor for pancreatic cancer. In 1996, a mutation in the cationic trypsinogen gene (PRSS1) was found to be common among individuals who suffered from a severe form of pancreatitis that onset during early adulthood (Whitcomb et al., 1996). More recently, this same group reported that through a multi-city linkage analysis, the frequency of this mutation in families affected by chronic pancreatitis was geo-specific in the US (i.e., more common in Minnesota, New York, Central Mid-Atlantic States, Kentucky, Ohio) (Applebaum-Shapiro et al., 2001). This study is a prime example of how genomics, in combination with the residential environment, may be able to address regional disparities in disease prevalence and severity. In addition to mutations in the PRSS1 gene, carriers of mutations in the BRCA genes are also at an increased risk of pancreatic cancer (Murphy et al., 2002; Hahn et al., 2003).

Cigarette smoking, some cigars, and heavy use of smokeless tobacco have been identified as leading environmental risk factors for pancreatic cancer (Silverman, 2001; Alguacil and Silverman, 2004). Additionally, smoking has been found to increase the risk conferred by other factors (i.e., family history, diabetes mellitus) for pancreatic cancer in women (Hassan et al., 2007). A study released by the National Cancer Institute found that among male smokers, the risk for pancreatic cancer was twice as high in those in the highest quartile of serum insulin levels when compared to those in the lowest quartile (Stolzenberg-Solomon et al., 2005). Although the "Western" diet and alcohol use have been shown to be significant risk factors for some cancers of the digestive system, this is not the case for pancreatic cancer

(Michaud et al., 2005). However, obesity in women (as measured by body mass index) has been identified as a significant risk factor for many cancers, including pancreatic (OR = 1.24) (Reeves et al., 2007). In 2002, an NIH-sponsored symposium on the risk factors for pancreatic cancer concluded that heavy alcohol use (> 15 g of alcohol/day or 10–11 drinks) was a leading cause of both chronic and acute pancreatitis, which are major risk factors for pancreatic cancer (American Pancreatic Association, 2003).

A recent study examined the utility of using NQO1 expression as a biomarker for pancreatic cancer among smokers (Lyn-Cook et al., 2006). NQO1 has been shown to be elevated in different types of cancer tissues. Thus, the investigators in this study were interested in the interaction of NQO1 expression and smoking among individuals with respect to pancreatic cancer. When compared to the NQO1 level in normal pancreatic tissue obtained from non-smokers, the NQO1 level in tissue from pancreatic cancer patients, who were also smokers, was six times higher. Although there are various mutations in this gene, there was no correlation between genotype and disease incidence. These findings suggest that although NQO1 normally protects cells from oxidative stress, in large quantities this enzyme may also be deleterious to the human body. Another candidate gene was examined for its interaction with heavy smoking (i.e., > 41 pack years) in conferring risk for pancreatic cancer (Duell et al., 2002). This study found that deletions in the GSTT1 gene increased the risk for pancreatic cancer five-fold in females and three-fold in males when compared "never" smokers with pancreatic cancer and this genotype. Interestingly, the risk of pancreatic cancer among carriers of this genotype was not significant in either never smokers or light smokers (i.e. < 40 pack years) demonstrating the powerful influence that cigarette smoking has on cancer risk.

2.4.11 Prostate Cancer

Prostate cancer is currently the most frequent occurring cancer and the second leading cause of cancer-related mortality among men (National Cancer Institute, 2007h). Although overall rates of incidence and deaths have decreased due to increased screening for prostate cancer, these rates remain significantly higher among African–American men when compared to all other ethnic and race groups in the US (Godley et al., 2003; Cohen et al., 2006; Talcott et al., 2007). Additionally, this group of men is more likely to be diagnosed, via the prostate-specific antigen (PSA) test, at a later stage of disease development. This suggests disparities in both the quality of health care delivery to and health-seeking behavior among African-American men. Globally, geographic disparities have also been reported with rates higher among countries with high-fat diets and second-generation immigrants from developing countries to developed countries (Whittemore et al., 1995; Hayes, 2001). Therefore, the identification of relevant environmental risk factors has become increasingly urgent as the incidence of this preventable but deadly disease continues to rise.

To date, few studies have been able to determine a significant genetic contribution to disparities in prostate cancer incidence and mortality. With the evolution of genome-wide association studies, patterns of mutations at specific loci among patients diagnosed with prostate cancer have become evident but the clinical relevance of these biomarkers has yet to be determined (Xu et al., 2005; Thomas et al., 2008). A decade ago, shorter repeat lengths in one or both of the CAG and GGN sequences within the androgen receptor (AR) were found to confer a 1.5–2.0 times increased risk for developing prostate cancer among men 44–64 years of age (Stanford et al., 1997). At the time this finding was proposed to be a novel biomarker to predict the risk for prostate cancer, especially among African–Americans for whom the incidence is disproportionately higher when compared to other races and ethnicities. Despite numerous investigations, the most recent publication regarding this hypothesis found no association between shorter lengths between CAG and GGN repeats and the increased risk of prostate cancer among African-American men when compared to White men (Lange et al., 2008). Mutations in the BRCA genes are established risk factors for breast cancer. Interestingly, a recent study examining the risk conferred by BRCA for prostate cancer reported that males who are carriers of BRCA mutations are an increased risk ($p = 0.01$) for developing prostate cancer as well as having tumor histopathology (i.e., tumor grade) that is indicative of poor prognosis (Mitra et al., 2008). In 2006, a multi-city prostate cancer research group found that a mutation in a DNA segment on chromosome 8 found among men with African ancestry increased the risk of prostate cancer especially before the age of 70 years (Freedman et al., 2006). However, this variation only explained a fraction of early-onset cancer cases. Other studies have examined the risk conferred by SNPs in the PTEN, IGF-1, and ER-β genes which are observed in other cancers (Cheng et al., 2006; Haiman et al., 2006; Chen et al., 2007) but have been inconclusive in establishing a significant association with prostate cancer risk.

Although many studies have explored various risk factors for prostate cancer, scientific evidence has confirmed the significant contributions from the consumption of smoked meats, a diet high in animal fat and cigarette smoking (Hayes et al., 1999; Plaskon et al., 2003; Tang et al., 2007). These risk factors are also significant for other cancers such as pancreatic and liver. Among middle-aged men who smoke and who are carriers of the GSTM1-null genotype, the risk for developing prostate cancer increased linearly with the individual's pack years ($p < 0.007$) with the greatest risk observed for those with > 30 pack years (Agalliu et al., 2006). Another study found that sulforaphane, which is found in cruciferous vegetables, induces intracellular glutathione synthesis (a critical detoxification and anticarcinogenic process) in human prostate cancer cell lines. This finding provides a plausible mechanism by which a diet rich in leafy green vegetables is a protective factor against prostate cancer especially since prostate cancer cells are characterized by the loss of glutathione expression (Brooks et al., 2001). Polymorphisms in the NAT2 can result in either a slow- or fast-acetylator genotype. With respect to prostate cancer, the NAT2 slow acetylator genotype has been found to be more prevalent among these cancer patients (OR = 2.21) with the greatest prevalence among the patients who were smokers (OR = 3.8) (Hamasaki et al., 2003). Furthermore, the NAT2 slow-acetylator genotype was more frequent among patients with advanced stage of disease, metastasis, and high tumor grade. As a result of the accumulating evidence supporting a gene–environment interaction in the incidence and severity of prostate cancer, public health campaigns promoting prostate cancer screening and avoidance of the above-mentioned risk factors has increased substantially in recent years.

2.5 Summary

With the advent of molecular epidemiology and bioinformatics, biomedical researchers are now able to associate the presence of a quantifiable biomarker (i.e., genetic variants) with the risk of developing a specific disease. Furthermore, scientists can now characterize "genomic trends" (i.e., functional genomic variant frequencies) among diseased populations. Soon researchers will be able to translate these discoveries into improving population health and identify targets for disease prevention while furthering our understanding of the interactions of various physiological mechanisms.

The objective of this chapter was to discuss a select group of cancers for which there exists published evidence demonstrating a significant contribution from the environment towards cancer incidence, morbidity, and mortality. Here we have presented the evidence supporting the contribution to cancer development from several genes that play key roles in DNA damage repair or xenobiotic biotransformation. Additionally, we have presented a summary of evidence that for some cancers, the interaction between genetic polymorphisms (i.e., gene–gene interactions) confers an added risk as well. As initiatives such as the HapMap project progress, we may soon be able to estimate the global distribution of the critical polymorphisms thus "fine-tuning" the contribution of environmental exposures towards the development of cancer.

References

Acharya, C. R., D. S. Hsu, et al. (2008). "Gene expression signatures, clinicopathological features, and individualized therapy in breast cancer." JAMA **299**(13): 1574–1587.

Agalliu, I., W. J. Langeberg, et al. (2006). "Glutathione S-transferase M1, T1, and P1 polymorphisms and prostate cancer risk in middle-aged men." Prostate **66**(2): 146–56.

Agency for Toxic Substances and Disease Registry (2005). "Interaction profile for: Benzene, Toluene, Ethylbenzene, and Xylenes (BTEX)." Retrieved May 14, 2008.

Agency for Toxic Substances and Disease Registry (2007). "Asbestos Toxicity: Who Is at Risk of Exposure to Asbestos?" Retrieved June 20, 2008, from http://www.atsdr.cdc.gov/csem/asbestos/risk2.html

Alberg, A. J., A. Kouzis, et al. (2007). "A prospective cohort study of bladder cancer risk in relation to active cigarette smoking and household exposure to secondhand cigarette smoke." Am J Epidemiol **165**(6): 660–6.

Alberg, A. J. and J. M. Samet (2003). "Epidemiology of lung cancer." Chest **123**(90010): 21S–49.

Alexander, D. D., J. Waterbor, et al. (2007). "African–American and Caucasian disparities in colorectal cancer mortality and survival by data source: an epidemiologic review." Cancer Biomark **3**(6): 301–13.
Alexandrie, A.-K., F. Nyberg, et al. (2004). "Influence of CYP1A1, GSTM1, GSTT1, and NQO1 genotypes and cumulative smoking dose on lung cancer risk in a Swedish population." Cancer Epidemiol Biomarkers Prev **13**(6): 908–14.
Alguacil, J. and D. T. Silverman (2004). "Smokeless and other noncigarette tobacco use and pancreatic cancer: a case-control study based on direct interviews." Cancer Epidemiol Biomarkers Prev **13**(1): 55–8.
American Cancer Society (2008). "What Are The Risk Factors for Melanoma?" Retrieved June 16, 2008, from http://www.cancer.org/docroot/CRI/content/CRI_2_2_2X_What_causes_melanoma_skin_cancer_50.asp?sitearea=
American Pancreatic Association (2003). "Mechanisms of alcoholic pancreatitis. Proceedings of the conference, Chicago, Illinois, USA, November 2002." Pancreas **27**(4): 281–355.
Anton-Culver, H., A. Lee-Feldstein, et al. (1993). "The association of bladder cancer risk with ethnicity, gender, and smoking." Ann Epidemiol **3**(4): 429–33.
Applebaum-Shapiro, S. E., R. Finch, et al. (2001). "Hereditary pancreatitis in North America: the Pittsburgh-Midwest Multi-Center Pancreatic Study Group Study." Pancreatology **1**(5): 439–43.
Athma, P., R. Rappaport, et al. (1996). "Molecular genotyping shows that ataxia-telangiectasia heterozygotes are predisposed to breast cancer." Cancer Genet Cytogenet **92**(2): 130–4.
Bach, P. B., J. R. Jett, et al. (2007). "Computed tomography screening and lung cancer outcomes." JAMA **297**(9): 953–61.
Bell, D., S. H. Kim, et al. (2007). "Genetic and functional analysis of CHEK2 (CHK2) variants in multiethnic cohorts." Int J Cancer **121**(12): 2661–7.
Bernal-Pacheco, O. and G. C. Roman (2007). "Environmental vascular risk factors: new perspectives for stroke prevention." J Neurol Sci **262**(1–2): 60–70.
Berns, K., H. M. Horlings, et al. (2007). "A functional genetic approach identifies the PI3K pathway as a major determinant of trastuzumab resistance in breast cancer." Cancer Cell **12**(4): 395–402.
Berry, G. and F. D. Liddell (2004). "The interaction of asbestos and smoking in lung cancer: a modified measure of effect." Ann Occup Hyg **48**(5): 459–62.
Blendon, R. J., T. Buhr, et al. (2007). "Disparities in health: perspectives of a multi-ethnic, multi-racial America." Health Aff **26**(5): 1437–47.
Blot, W. J. and J. K. McLaughlin (1999). "The changing epidemiology of esophageal cancer." Semin Oncol **26**(5 Suppl 15): 2–8.
Botteri, E., S. Iodice, et al. (2008). "Cigarette smoking and adenomatous polyps: a meta-analysis." Gastroenterology **134**(2): 388–95.
Brody, J. G. and R. A. Rudel (2003). "Environmental pollutants and breast cancer." Environ Health Perspect **111**(8): 1007–19.
Brooks, J. D., V. G. Paton, et al. (2001). "Potent induction of phase 2 enzymes in human prostate cells by sulforaphane." Cancer Epidemiol Biomarkers Prev **10**(9): 949–54.
Brown, L. M. and S. S. Devesa (2002). "Epidemiologic trends in esophageal and gastric cancer in the United States." Surg Oncol Clin N Am **11**(2): 235–56.
CDC National Office of Public Health Genomics (2004, September 2007). "Public Health Genomics at CDC-Accomplishments and Priorities 2004." Retrieved Jan 14, 2008, from http://www.cdc.gov/genomics/activities/ogdp/2004/niosh.htm
Canalle, R., R. V. Burim, et al. (2004). "Genetic polymorphisms and susceptibility to childhood acute lymphoblastic leukemia." Environ Mol Mutagen **43**(2): 100–9.
Cerhan, J. R., B. C. Chiu, et al. (1998). "Physical activity, physical function, and the risk of breast cancer in a prospective study among elderly women." J Gerontol A Biol Sci Med Sci **53**(4): M251–6.
Chen, Y. J., C. Chen, et al. (2006). "Interactive effects of lifetime alcohol consumption and alcohol and aldehyde dehydrogenase polymorphisms on esophageal cancer risks." Int J Cancer **119**(12): 2827–31.

Chen, Y. C., P. Kraft, et al. (2007). "Sequence variants of estrogen receptor beta and risk of prostate cancer in the National Cancer Institute Breast and Prostate Cancer Cohort Consortium." Cancer Epidemiol Biomarkers Prev **16**(10): 1973–81.

Cheng, I., D. O. Stram, et al. (2006). "Common genetic variation in IGF1 and prostate cancer risk in the Multiethnic Cohort." J Natl Cancer Inst **98**(2): 123–34.

Chia, V. M., P. A. Newcomb, et al. (2007). "Leptin concentrations, leptin receptor polymorphisms, and colorectal adenoma risk." Cancer Epidemiol Biomarkers Prev **16**(12): 2697–703.

Chien, C., L. M. Morimoto, et al. (2005). "Differences in colorectal carcinoma stage and survival by race and ethnicity." Cancer **104**(3): 629–39.

Chlebowski, R. T., Z. Chen, et al. (2005). "Ethnicity and breast cancer: factors influencing differences in incidence and outcome." J Natl Cancer Inst **97**(6): 439–48.

Cho, E., W. Y. Chen, et al. (2006). "Red meat intake and risk of breast cancer among premenopausal women." Arch Intern Med **166**(20): 2253–9.

Christiani, D. C. (2000). "Smoking and the molecular epidemiology of lung cancer." Clin Chest Med **21**(1): 87–93.

Claus, E. B., J. Schildkraut, et al. (1998). "Effect of BRCA1 and BRCA2 on the association between breast cancer risk and family history." J Natl Cancer Inst **90**(23): 1824–9.

Cohen, J. H., V. J. Schoenbach, et al. (2006). "Racial differences in clinical progression among Medicare recipients after treatment for localized prostate cancer (United States)." Cancer Causes Control **17**(6): 803–11.

Collaborative Group on Hormonal Factors in Breast Cancer (2001). "Familial breast cancer: collaborative reanalysis of individual data from 52 epidemiological studies including 58,209 women with breast cancer and 101,986 women without the disease." Lancet **358**(9291): 1389–99.

Commonwealth Fund (2006). "Hispanic and African American Adults Are Uninsured at Rates One-and-a Half to Three Times Higher Than White Adults." Retrieved Jan 08, 2008, from http://www.commonwealthfund.org/usr_doc/DisparitiesReleaseFINAL7-26-06.pdf?section=4059

Corley, D. A., A. Kubo, et al. (2008). "Abdominal obesity and the risk of esophageal and gastric cardia carcinomas." Cancer Epidemiol Biomarkers Prev **17**(2): 352–8.

Davis, S., D. K. Mirick, et al. (2001). "Night shift work, light at night, and risk of breast cancer." J Natl Cancer Inst **93**(20): 1557–62.

Doty, M. M. and A. L. Holmgren (2005). "Health Care Disconnect: Gaps in Coverage and Care for Minority Adults." Commonwealth Fund pub. 941, Vol. 21. Retrieved Jan 08, 2008, from http://www.commonwealthfund.org/publications/publications_show.htm?doc_id=386220#areaCitation

Duell, E. J., E. A. Holly, et al. (2002). "A population-based, case-control study of polymorphisms in carcinogen-metabolizing genes, smoking, and pancreatic adenocarcinoma risk." J Natl Cancer Inst **94**(4): 297–306.

Engel, L. S., W. H. Chow, et al. (2003). "Population attributable risks of esophageal and gastric cancers." J Natl Cancer Inst **95**(18): 1404–13.

Environmental Protection Agency (2008). "Asbestos (CASRN 1332-21-4)." Integrated Risk Information System. Retrieved June 25, 2008, from Asbestos (CASRN 1332-21–4).

Etzel, C. J., C. I. Amos, et al. (2003). "Risk for smoking-related cancer among relatives of lung cancer patients." Cancer Res **63**(23): 8531–5.

Farker, K., U. Schotte, et al. (2003). "Impact of N-acetyltransferase polymorphism (NAT2) in hepatocellular carcinoma (HCC) – an investigation in a department of surgical medicine." Exp Toxicol Pathol **54**(5–6): 387–91.

Freedman, M. L., C. A. Haiman, et al. (2006). "Admixture mapping identifies 8q24 as a prostate cancer risk locus in African–American men." Proc Natl Acad Sci USA **103**(38): 14068–73.

Garcia-Closas, M., N. Malats, et al. (2006). "Genetic variation in the nucleotide excision repair pathway and bladder cancer risk." Cancer Epidemiol Biomarkers Prev **15**(3): 536–42.

García-Closas, M., N. Malats, et al. (2005). "NAT2 slow acetylation, GSTM1 null genotype, and risk of bladder cancer: results from the Spanish Bladder Cancer Study and meta-analyses." The Lancet **366**(9486): 649–59.

Ghosh, A. K., R. Steele, et al. (1999). "Hepatitis C virus NS5A protein modulates cell cycle regulatory genes and promotes cell growth." J Gen Virol **80**(**Pt 5**): 1179–83.

Godley, P. A., A. P. Schenck, et al. (2003). "Racial differences in mortality among Medicare recipients after treatment for localized prostate cancer." J Natl Cancer Inst **95**(22): 1702–10.

Graham, R. R., W. Ortmann, et al. (2007). "Specific combinations of HLA-DR2 and DR3 class II haplotypes contribute graded risk for disease susceptibility and autoantibodies in human SLE." Eur J Hum Genet **15**(8): 823–30.

Grarup, N. and G. Andersen (2007). "Gene–environment interactions in the pathogenesis of type 2 diabetes and metabolism." Curr Opin Clin Nutr Metab Care **10**(4): 420–6.

Hahn, S. A., B. Greenhalf, et al. (2003). "BRCA2 germline mutations in familial pancreatic carcinoma." J Natl Cancer Inst **95**(3): 214–21.

Haiman, C. A., D. O. Stram, et al. (2006). "Common genetic variation at PTEN and risk of sporadic breast and prostate cancer." Cancer Epidemiol Biomarkers Prev **15**(5): 1021–5.

Hamasaki, T., H. Inatomi, et al. (2003). "N-acetyltransferase-2 gene polymorphism as a possible biomarker for prostate cancer in Japanese men." Int J Urol **10**(3): 167–73.

Harris, K. M., P. Gordon-Larsen, et al. (2006). "Longitudinal trends in race/ethnic disparities in leading health indicators from adolescence to young adulthood." Arch Pediatr Adolesc Med **160**(1): 74–81.

Harrison, R. (2004). Polycyclic aromatic hydrocarbons. In Current Occupational and Environmental Medicine. New York, NY, McGraw-Hill.

Hassan, M. M., M. L. Bondy, et al. (2007). "Risk factors for pancreatic cancer: case-control study." Am J Gastroenterol **102**(12): 2696–707.

Hayes, R. B. (2001). "Gene–environment interrelations in prostate cancer." Epidemiol Rev **23**(1): 163–7.

Hayes, R. B., R. G. Ziegler, et al. (1999). "Dietary factors and risks for prostate cancer among blacks and whites in the United States." Cancer Epidemiol Biomarkers Prev **8**(1): 25–34.

Heinrich, K. M., R. E. Lee, et al. (2008). "How does the built environment relate to body mass index and obesity prevalence among public housing residents?" Am J Health Promot **22**(3): 187–94.

Hirvonen, A., S. T. Saarikoski, et al. (1996). "Glutathione S-transferase and N-acetyltransferase genotypes and asbestos-associated pulmonary disorders." J Natl Cancer Inst **88**(24): 1853–6.

Howard, R. A., D. M. Freedman, et al. (2008). "Physical activity, sedentary behavior, and the risk of colon and rectal cancer in the NIH-AARP Diet and Health Study." Cancer Causes Control Nov;**19**(9): 939–53.

Hung, R. J., P. Boffetta, et al. (2003). "CYP1A1 and GSTM1 genetic polymorphisms and lung cancer risk in Caucasian non-smokers: a pooled analysis." Carcinogenesis **24**(5): 875–82.

Infante-Rivard, C. and J. E. Deadman (2003). "Maternal occupational exposure to extremely low frequency magnetic fields during pregnancy and childhood leukemia." Epidemiology **14**(4): 437–41.

Infante-Rivard, C., D. Labuda, et al. (1999). "Risk of childhood leukemia associated with exposure to pesticides and with gene polymorphisms." Epidemiology **10**(5): 481–7.

Ishibe, N., J. K. Wiencke, et al. (1997). "Susceptibility to lung cancer in light smokers associated with CYP1A1 polymorphisms in Mexican- and African–Americans." Cancer Epidemiol Biomarkers Prev **6**(12): 1075–80.

Ishikawa, A., S. Kuriyama, et al. (2006). "Smoking, alcohol drinking, green tea consumption and the risk of esophageal cancer in Japanese men." J Epidemiol **16**(5): 185–92.

Jia, H.-L., Q.-H. Ye, et al. (2007). "Gene expression profiling reveals potential biomarkers of human hepatocellular carcinoma." Clin Cancer Res **13**(4): 1133–9.

John, E. M., A. Miron, et al. (2007). "Prevalence of pathogenic BRCA1 mutation carriers in 5 US racial/ethnic groups." JAMA **298**(24): 2869–76.

Johnson, S. B., A. M. Langlieb, et al. (2005). "Rethinking first response: effects of the clean up and recovery effort on workers at the world trade center disaster site." J Occup Environ Med **47**(4): 386–91.

Kato, M., T. Shinozawa, et al. (2000). "Increased midkine expression in hepatocellular carcinoma." Arch Pathol Lab Med **124**(6): 848–52.

Khoury, M. J., R. Davis, et al. (2005). "Do we need genomic research for the prevention of common diseases with environmental causes?" Am J Epidemiol **161**(9): 799–805.

Khoury, M. J., R. Millikan, et al. (2004). "The emergence of epidemiology in the genomics age." Int J Epidemiol **33**(5): 936–44.

Kim, J. H., M. E. Sherman, et al. (2004). "Expression of cytochromes P450 1A1 and 1B1 in human lung from smokers, non-smokers, and ex-smokers." Toxicol Appl Pharmacol **199**(3): 210–19.

Klaassen, C. (2001). Casarett & Doull's Toxicology: The Basic Science of Poisons. New York, NY, McGraw-Hill.

Krajinovic, M., H. Sinnett, et al. (2002). "Role of NQO1, MPO and CYP2E1 genetic polymorphisms in the susceptibility to childhood acute lymphoblastic leukemia." Int J Cancer **97**(2): 230–6.

Kwun, H. J., E. Y. Jung, et al. (2001). "p53-dependent transcriptional repression of p21(waf1) by hepatitis C virus NS3." J Gen Virol **82**(Pt 9): 2235–41.

Lander, E. S., L. M. Linton, et al. (2001). "Initial sequencing and analysis of the human genome." Nature **409**(6822): 860–921.

Landi, M. T., J. Bauer, et al. (2006). "MC1R germline variants confer risk for BRAF-mutant melanoma." Science **313**(5786): 521–2.

Landrigan, P. J., P. J. Lioy, et al. (2004). "Health and environmental consequences of the world trade center disaster." Environ Health Perspect **112**(6): 731–9.

Lange, E. M., A. V. Sarma, et al. (2008). "The androgen receptor CAG and GGN repeat polymorphisms and prostate cancer susceptibility in African–American men: results from the Flint Men's Health Study." J Hum Genet **53**(3): 220–6.

Lawson, K. A., K. Woodson, et al. (2005). "Association of the NAD(P)H:quinone oxidoreductase (NQO1) 609C->T polymorphism with lung cancer risk among male smokers." Cancer Epidemiol Biomarkers Prev **14**(9): 2275–6.

Le Marchand, L., T. Donlon, et al. (2002). "Red meat intake, CYP2E1 genetic polymorphisms, and colorectal cancer risk." Cancer Epidemiol Biomarkers Prev **11**(10 Pt 1): 1019–24.

Lewis, E. B. (1957). "Leukemia and ionizing radiation." Science **125**(3255): 965–72.

Lewis, J. H., J. H. Burchenal, et al. (1957). "Studies of hemostatic mechanisms in leukemia and thrombocytopenia." Am J Clin Pathol **28**(5): 433–46.

Lichtenstein, P., N. V. Holm, et al. (2000). "Environmental and heritable factors in the causation of cancer – analyses of cohorts of twins from Sweden, Denmark, and Finland." N Engl J Med **343**(2): 78–85.

Liddell, F. D. (2001). "The interaction of asbestos and smoking in lung cancer." Ann Occup Hyg **45**(5): 341–56.

Liu, Z. M., L. Q. Li, et al. (2008). "Hepatitis B virus infection contributes to oxidative stress in a population exposed to aflatoxin B1 and high-risk for hepatocellular carcinoma." Cancer Lett **263**(2): 212–22.

Lower, G. M., Jr., T. Nilsson, et al. (1979). "N-acetyltransferase phenotype and risk in urinary bladder cancer: approaches in molecular epidemiology. Preliminary results in Sweden and Denmark." Environ Health Perspect **29**: 71–9.

Lyn-Cook, B. D., Y. Yan-Sanders, et al. (2006). "Increased levels of NAD(P)H:quinone oxidoreductase 1 (NQO1) in pancreatic tissues from smokers and pancreatic adenocarcinomas: a potential biomarker of early damage in the pancreas." Cell Biol Toxicol **22**(2): 73–80.

MacMahon, B., P. Cole, et al. (1970). "Age at first birth and breast cancer risk." Bull World Health Organ **43**(2): 209–21.
Majumdar, S., B. C. Mondal, et al. (2008). "Association of cytochrome P450, glutathione S-transferase and N-acetyl transferase 2 gene polymorphisms with incidence of acute myeloid leukemia." Eur J Cancer Prev **17**(2): 125–32.
Makimoto, K., H. Oda, et al. (2000). "Is heavy alcohol consumption an attributable factor for cancer-related deaths among Japanese men?" Alcohol Clin Exp Res **24**(3): 382–5.
Maldonado, J. L., J. Fridlyand, et al. (2003). "Determinants of BRAF mutations in primary melanomas." J Natl Cancer Inst **95**(24): 1878–90.
Marrero, J. A., R. J. Fontana, et al. (2005). "Alcohol, tobacco and obesity are synergistic risk factors for hepatocellular carcinoma." J Hepatol **42**(2): 218–24.
Marusawa, H., M. Hijikata, et al. (1999). "Hepatitis C virus core protein inhibits Fas- and tumor necrosis factor alpha-mediated apoptosis via NF-kappaB activation." J Virol **73**(6): 4713–20.
Mazzanti, R., L. Gramantieri, et al. (2008). "Hepatocellular carcinoma: epidemiology and clinical aspects." Mol Aspects Med **29**(1–2): 130–43.
Meyer, P., C. Sergi, et al. (2003). "Polymorphisms of the BRAF gene predispose males to malignant melanoma." J Carcinog **2**(1): 7.
Michaud, D. S., H. G. Skinner, et al. (2005). "Dietary patterns and pancreatic cancer risk in men and women." J Natl Cancer Inst **97**(7): 518–24.
Mitra, A., C. Fisher, et al. (2008). "Prostate cancer in male BRCA1 and BRCA2 mutation carriers has a more aggressive phenotype." Br J Cancer **98**(2): 502–7.
Miyazaki, M., S. Ohno, et al. (2002). "The relation of alcohol consumption and cigarette smoking to the multiple occurrence of esophageal dysplasia and squamous cell carcinoma." Surgery **131**(1 Suppl): S7–S13.
Moore, L. L., M. L. Bradlee, et al. (2004). "BMI and waist circumference as predictors of lifetime colon cancer risk in Framingham Study adults." Int J Obes Relat Metab Disord **28**(4): 559–67.
Morris Brown, L., C. A. Swanson, et al. (1995). "Adenocarcinoma of the esophagus: role of obesity and diet." J Natl Cancer Inst **87**(2): 104–109.
Moss, S. F. and M. J. Blaser (2005). "Mechanisms of disease: inflammation and the origins of cancer." Nat Clin Pract Oncol **2**(2): 90–7; quiz 1 p following 113.
Murphy, K. M., K. A. Brune, et al. (2002). "Evaluation of candidate genes MAP2K4, MADH4, ACVR1B, and BRCA2 in familial pancreatic cancer: deleterious BRCA2 mutations in 17%." Cancer Res **62**(13): 3789–93.
Mustacchi, P. (1961). "Ramazzini and Rigoni-Stern on parity and breast cancer. Clinical impression and statistical corroboration." Arch Intern Med **108**: 639–42.
National Cancer Institute (2007a). "A snapshot of bladder cancer." Retrieved May 09, 2008, from http://www.cancer.gov/aboutnci/servingpeople/snapshots/bladder.pdf
National Cancer Institute (2007b). "A snapshot of breast cancer." Retrieved May 09, 2008, from http://www.cancer.gov/aboutnci/servingpeople/snapshots/breast.pdf
National Cancer Institute (2007c). "A snapshot of colorectal cancer." Retrieved June 03, 2008, from http://www.cancer.gov/aboutnci/servingpeople/snapshots/colorectal.pdf
National Cancer Institute (2007d). "A snapshot of esophageal cancer." Retrieved May 9, 2008, from http://www.cancer.gov/aboutnci/servingpeople/snapshots/esophageal.pdf
National Cancer Institute (2007e). "A snapshot of liver and bile duct cancers." Retrieved May 09, 2008, from http://www.cancer.gov/aboutnci/servingpeople/snapshots/liver.pdf
National Cancer Institute (2007f). "A snapshot of lung cancer." Retrieved May 18, 2008, from http://www.cancer.gov/aboutnci/servingpeople/snapshots/lung.pdf
National Cancer Institute (2007g). "A snapshot of pancreatic cancer." Retrieved June 24, 2008, from http://www.cancer.gov/aboutnci/servingpeople/snapshots/Pancreatic.pdf
National Cancer Institute (2007h). "A snapshot of prostate cancer." Retrieved June 26, 2008, from http://www.cancer.gov/aboutnci/servingpeople/snapshots/prostate.pdf

National Cancer Institute (2008a). "Skin Cancer." Retrieved June 17, 2008, from http://www.cancer.gov/cancertopics/types/skin/
National Cancer Institute (2008b). "Melanoma." Retrieved June 16, 2008, from http://www.cancer.gov/aboutnci/servingpeople/snapshots/melanoma.pdf
National Center for Biotechnology Information (2004). "Just the Facts: A Basic Introduction to the Science Underlying NCBI Resources." Retrieved May 20, 2008, from http://www.ncbi.nlm.nih.gov/About/primer/bioinformatics.html
National Heart Lung and Blood Institute (2006). "NHLBI to Launch Framingham Genetic Research Study." Retrieved June 09, 2008, from http://www.nhlbi.nih.gov/new/press/06-02-06.htm
National Human Genome Research Institute (2006). "Genetic Association Information Network Launched: Novel Public-Private Partnership Created to Unravel the Genetics Of Common Disease Through Whole Genome Association Studies." Retrieved June 09, 2008, from http://www.genome.gov/17516722
National Human Genome Research Institute (2007). "International HapMap Project." Retrieved June 03, 2008, from http://www.genome.gov/10001688
National Institutes of Health (2000). "What We know About Radiation-Fact Sheet." Retrieved May 14, 2008, from http://www.nih.gov/health/chip/od/radiation/
National Institutes of Health (2007). "The Genes, Environment and Health Initiative (GEI)." Retrieved June 10, 2008, from http://www.gei.nih.gov/
National Toxicology Program (2005a). "11th Report on Carcinogens." Eleventh Edition. From http://ntp.niehs.nih.gov/index.cfm?objectid=32BA9724-F1F6-975E-7FCE50709CB4C932
National Toxicology Program (2005b). "Benzene CAS No. 71-43-2." Report on Carcinogens Retrieved May 14, 2008 from http://ntp.niehs.nih.gov/ntp/roc/eleventh/profiles/s019benz.pdf
National Toxicology Program. (2007). "Chemicals Associated with Site-Specific Tumor Induction in Mammary Gland." Retrieved May 09, 2008, from http://ntp.niehs.nih.gov/index.cfm?objectid=E1D18034-123F-7908-7B2C2AE41B1F3778
Neri, M., E. Taioli, et al. (2006). "Metabolic genotypes as modulators of asbestos-related pleural malignant mesothelioma risk: a comparison of Finnish and Italian populations." Int J Hyg Environ Health **209**(4): 393–8.
Newbold, R. R., E. Padilla-Banks, et al. (2007). "Perinatal exposure to environmental estrogens and the development of obesity." Mol Nutr Food Res **51**(7): 912–17.
Newsom, S. W. (2006). "Pioneers in infection control: John Snow, Henry Whitehead, the Broad Street pump, and the beginnings of geographical epidemiology." J Hosp Infect **64**(3): 210–16.
Norat, T., S. Bingham, et al. (2005). "Meat, fish, and colorectal cancer risk: the European Prospective Investigation into cancer and nutrition." J Natl Cancer Inst **97**(12): 906–16.
Pang, R. W., J. W. Joh, et al. (2008). "Biology of hepatocellular carcinoma." Ann Surg Oncol **15**(4): 962–71.
Parkin, D. M., F. Bray, et al. (2005). "Global cancer statistics, 2002." CA Cancer J Clin **55**(2): 74–108.
Pho, L., D. Grossman, et al. (2006). "Melanoma genetics: a review of genetic factors and clinical phenotypes in familial melanoma." Curr Opin Oncol **18**(2): 173–9.
Pickens, A. and M. B. Orringer (2003). "Geographical distribution and racial disparity in esophageal cancer." Ann Thorac Surg **76**(4): S1367–9.
Plaskon, L. A., D. F. Penson, et al. (2003). "Cigarette smoking and risk of prostate cancer in middle-aged men." Cancer Epidemiol Biomarkers Prev **12**(7): 604–9.
Pohl, H. and H. G. Welch (2005). "The role of overdiagnosis and reclassification in the marked increase of esophageal adenocarcinoma incidence." J Natl Cancer Inst **97**(2): 142–6.
Poulsen, P., M. Esteller, et al. (2007). "The epigenetic basis of twin discordance in age-related diseases." Pediatr Res **61**(5 Pt 2): 38R–42R.
Prout, G. R., Jr., M. N. Wesley, et al. (2000). "Bladder cancer: race differences in extent of disease at diagnosis." Cancer **89**(6): 1349–58.

Raimondi, S., P. Boffetta, et al. (2005). "Metabolic gene polymorphisms and lung cancer risk in non-smokers. an update of the GSEC study." Mutat Res **592**(1–2): 45–57.
Raza, S. A., G. M. Clifford, et al. (2007). "Worldwide variation in the relative importance of hepatitis B and hepatitis C viruses in hepatocellular carcinoma: a systematic review." Br J Cancer **96**(7): 1127–34.
Reeves, G. K., K. Pirie, et al. (2007). "Cancer incidence and mortality in relation to body mass index in the Million Women Study: cohort study." BMJ **335**(7630): 1134.
Ries, L., D. Melbert , et al. (2008). "SEER Cancer Statistics Review, 1975–2005." Retrieved June 13, 2008, from http://seer.cancer.gov/csr/1975_2005/
Ross, D., D. Siegel, et al. (1996). "Cell-specific activation and detoxification of benzene metabolites in mouse and human bone marrow: identification of target cells and a potential role for modulation of apoptosis in benzene toxicity." Environ Health Perspect **104**(**Suppl 6**): 1177–82.
Rundle, A., A. V. Roux, et al. (2007). "The urban built environment and obesity in New York City: a multilevel analysis." Am J Health Promot **21**(4 Suppl): 326–34.
Sakata, K., Y. Hoshiyama, et al. (2005). "Smoking, alcohol drinking and esophageal cancer: findings from the JACC Study." J Epidemiol **15**(**Suppl 2**): S212–19.
Samanic, C., W. H. Chow, et al. (2006). "Relation of body mass index to cancer risk in 362,552 Swedish men." Cancer Causes Control **17**(7): 901–19.
Sassi, F., H. S. Luft, et al. (2006). "Reducing racial/ethnic disparities in female breast cancer: screening rates and stage at diagnosis." Am J Public Health **96**(12): 2165–72.
Savitz, D. A. and K. W. Andrews (1997). "Review of epidemiologic evidence on benzene and lymphatic and hematopoietic cancers." Am J Ind Med **31**(3): 287–95.
Schabath, M. B., M. R. Spitz, et al. (2002). "A myeloperoxidase polymorphism associated with reduced risk of lung cancer." Lung Cancer **37**(1): 35–40.
Schernhammer, E. S., F. Laden, et al. (2001). "Rotating night shifts and risk of breast cancer in women participating in the nurses' health study." J Natl Cancer Inst **93**(20): 1563–8.
Schlager, J. J. and G. Powis (1990). "Cytosolic NAD(P)H:(quinone-acceptor)oxidoreductase in human normal and tumor tissue: effects of cigarette smoking and alcohol." Int J Cancer **45**(3): 403–9.
Shen, H. M. and C. N. Ong (1996). "Mutations of the p53 tumor suppressor gene and ras oncogenes in aflatoxin hepatocarcinogenesis." Mutat Res **366**(1): 23–44.
Sillanpaa, P., L. Heikinheimo, et al. (2007). "CYP1A1 and CYP1B1 genetic polymorphisms, smoking and breast cancer risk in a Finnish Caucasian population." Breast Cancer Res Treat **104**(3): 287–97.
Silverman, D. T. (2001). "Risk factors for pancreatic cancer: a case-control study based on direct interviews." Teratog Carcinog Mutagen **21**(1): 7–25.
Silverman, D. T., R. N. Hoover, et al. (2003). "Why do Black Americans have a higher risk of pancreatic cancer than White Americans?" Epidemiology **14**(1): 45–54.
Silvestrini, R., E. Benini, et al. (1993). "p53 as an independent prognostic marker in lymph node-negative breast cancer patients." J Natl Cancer Inst **85**(12): 965–70.
Sinnett, D., M. Krajinovic, et al. (2000). "Genetic susceptibility to childhood acute lymphoblastic leukemia." Leuk Lymphoma **38**(5–6): 447–62.
Skibola, C. F., M. T. Smith, et al. (1999). "Polymorphisms in the methylenetetrahydrofolate reductase gene are associated with susceptibility to acute leukemia in adults." Proc Natl Acad Sci USA **96**(22): 12810–15.
Skibola, C. F., M. T. Smith, et al. (2002). "Polymorphisms in the thymidylate synthase and serine hydroxymethyltransferase genes and risk of adult acute lymphocytic leukemia." Blood **99**(10): 3786–91.
Smith, M. T., Y. Wang, et al. (2001). "Low NAD(P)H:quinone oxidoreductase 1 activity is associated with increased risk of acute leukemia in adults." Blood **97**(5): 1422–6.
Stanford, J. L., J. J. Just, et al. (1997). "Polymorphic repeats in the androgen receptor gene: molecular markers of prostate cancer risk." Cancer Res **57**(6): 1194–8.

Stern, M. C., K. D. Siegmund, et al. (2006). "XRCC1, XRCC3, and XPD polymorphisms as modifiers of the effect of smoking and alcohol on colorectal adenoma risk." Cancer Epidemiol Biomarkers Prev **15**(12): 2384–90.

Stolzenberg-Solomon, R. Z., B. I. Graubard, et al. (2005). "Insulin, glucose, insulin resistance, and pancreatic cancer in male smokers." JAMA **294**(22): 2872–8.

Szilagyi, P. G., S. Schaffer, et al. (2002). "Reducing geographic, racial, and ethnic disparities in childhood immunization rates by using reminder/recall interventions in urban primary care practices." Pediatrics **110**(5): e58.

Taioli, E., S. Benhamou, et al. (2007). "Myeloperoxidase G-463A polymorphism and lung cancer: a HuGE genetic susceptibility to environmental carcinogens pooled analysis." Genet Med **9**(2): 67–73.

Taioli, E., J. Ford, et al. (1998). "Lung cancer risk and CYP1A1 genotype in African Americans." Carcinogenesis **19**(5): 813–17.

Taioli, E., L. Gaspari, et al. (2003). "Polymorphisms in CYP1A1, GSTM1, GSTT1 and lung cancer below the age of 45 years." Int J Epidemiol **32**(1): 60–3.

Taketa, K. (1990). "Alpha-fetoprotein: reevaluation in hepatology." Hepatology **12**(6): 1420–32.

Talcott, J. A., P. Spain, et al. (2007). "Hidden barriers between knowledge and behavior: the North Carolina prostate cancer screening and treatment experience." Cancer **109**(8): 1599–606.

Tanaka, F., Y. Shiratori, et al. (1996). "High incidence of ADH2*1/ALDH2*1 genes among Japanese alcohol dependents and patients with alcoholic liver disease." Hepatology **23**(2): 234–9.

Tanaka, F., Y. Shiratori, et al. (1997). "Polymorphism of alcohol-metabolizing genes affects drinking behavior and alcoholic liver disease in Japanese men." Alcohol Clin Exp Res **21**(4): 596–601.

Tang, D., J. J. Liu, et al. (2007). "Grilled meat consumption and PhIP-DNA adducts in prostate carcinogenesis." Cancer Epidemiol Biomarkers Prev **16**(4): 803–8.

Thomas, G., K. B. Jacobs, et al. (2008). "Multiple loci identified in a genome-wide association study of prostate cancer." Nat Genet **40**(3): 310–5.

Thompson, D., A. C. Antoniou, et al. (2005). "Two ATM variants and breast cancer risk." Hum Mutat **25**(6): 594–5.

Tiemersma, E. W., R. E. Omer, et al. (2001). "Role of genetic polymorphism of glutathione-S-transferase T1 and microsomal epoxide hydrolase in aflatoxin-associated hepatocellular carcinoma." Cancer Epidemiol Biomarkers Prev **10**(7): 785–91.

Toriola, A. T., S. Kurl, et al. (2008). "Alcohol consumption and risk of colorectal cancer: the Findrink study." Eur J Epidemiol **23**(6): 395–401.

Valverde, P., E. Healy, et al. (1996). "The Asp84Glu variant of the melanocortin 1 receptor (MC1R) is associated with melanoma." Hum Mol Genet **5**(10): 1663–6.

Verkasalo, P. K., J. Kaprio, et al. (1999). "Genetic predisposition, environment and cancer incidence: a nationwide twin study in Finland, 1976–1995." Int J Cancer **83**(6): 743–9.

Vineis, P. (2004). "Individual susceptibility to carcinogens." Oncogene **23**(38): 6477–83.

Vona-Davis, L., M. Howard-McNatt, et al. (2007). "Adiposity, type 2 diabetes and the metabolic syndrome in breast cancer." Obes Rev **8**(5): 395–408.

Wenzlaff, A. S., M. L. Cote, et al. (2005). "GSTM1, GSTT1 and GSTP1 polymorphisms, environmental tobacco smoke exposure and risk of lung cancer among never smokers: a population-based study." Carcinogenesis **26**(2): 395–401.

Whitcomb, D. C., M. C. Gorry, et al. (1996). "Hereditary pancreatitis is caused by a mutation in the cationic trypsinogen gene." Nat Genet **14**(2): 141–5.

Whittemore, A. S., L. N. Kolonel, et al. (1995). "Prostate cancer in relation to diet, physical activity, and body size in blacks, whites, and Asians in the United States and Canada." J Natl Cancer Inst **87**(9): 652–61.

Wiencke, J. K., M. R. Spitz, et al. (1997). "Lung cancer in Mexican–Americans and African–Americans is associated with the wild-type genotype of the NAD(P)H:quinone oxidoreductase polymorphism." Cancer Epidemiol Biomarkers Prev **6**(2): 87–92.

Wikman, H., S. Thiel, et al. (2001). "Relevance of N-acetyltransferase 1 and 2 (NAT1, NAT2) genetic polymorphisms in non-small cell lung cancer susceptibility." Pharmacogenetics **11**(2): 157–68.

Wu, X., K. Gwyn, et al. (2001). "The association of microsomal epoxide hydrolase polymorphisms and lung cancer risk in African–Americans and Mexican–Americans." Carcinogenesis **22**(6): 923–8.

Xu, J., L. Dimitrov, et al. (2005). "A combined genomewide linkage scan of 1,233 families for prostate cancer-susceptibility genes conducted by the international consortium for prostate cancer genetics." Am J Hum Genet **77**(2): 219–29.

Yang, C. X., K. Matsuo, et al. (2005). "Esophageal cancer risk by ALDH2 and ADH2 polymorphisms and alcohol consumption: exploration of gene–environment and gene–gene interactions." Asian Pac J Cancer Prev **6**(3): 256–62.

Yu, M. W., C. I. Pai, et al. (2000). "Role of N-acetyltransferase polymorphisms in hepatitis B related hepatocellular carcinoma: impact of smoking on risk." Gut **47**(5): 703–9.

Zhang, S. M., I. M. Lee, et al. (2007). "Alcohol consumption and breast cancer risk in the Women's Health Study." Am J Epidemiol **165**(6): 667–76.

Zhang, Y., J. P. Wise, et al. (2004). "Serum polychlorinated biphenyls, cytochrome P-450 1A1 polymorphisms, and risk of breast cancer in Connecticut Women." Am J Epidemiol **160**(12): 1177–83.

Zhou, W., G. Liu, et al. (2002). "Genetic polymorphisms in N-acetyltransferase-2 and microsomal epoxide hydrolase, cumulative cigarette smoking, and lung cancer." Cancer Epidemiol Biomarkers Prev **11**(1): 15–21.

Zhou, W., S. W. Thurston, et al. (2001). "The interaction between microsomal epoxide hydrolase polymorphisms and cumulative cigarette smoking in different histological subtypes of lung cancer." Cancer Epidemiol Biomarkers Prev **10**(5): 461–6.

Chapter 3
Statistics for Testing Gene–Environment Interaction

Momiao Xiong and Xuesen Wu

Abstract This chapter introduces a number of new gene–environment interaction measures and develop novel statistics that are based on these new gene–environment interaction measures. These new statistics are simple, less computationally intensive and easy to implement. It is hoped that these developments may open a new avenue for large-scale genome-wide gene–environment interaction analysis, deciphering the genetic and physiological meaning of gene–environment interactions and developing sophisticated statistical methods for unraveling gene–gene and gene–environment interactions leading to the development of human cancers.

Keywords Statistics · Testing interaction between gene and binary or continuous environment · Cancer

3.1 Introduction

In the past 3 years, more than 305 genome-wide association studies (GWAS) that focused largely on individually testing association of single polymorphisms with diseases have been conducted (http://www.hgvbaseg2p.org/studies). These studies have identified more than 531 single nucleotide polymorphisms (SNPs) associated with the traits or diseases (Hindorff et al., 2009). These results provide substantial information for understanding the mechanisms of the diseases. Although great progress in GWAS has been made, the significant SNP associations identified by GWAS account for only a few percent of the genetic variance (Frazer et al., 2009, Altshuler et al., 2008). Searching for remaining genetic variance is a great challenge (Wang, 2008).

M. Xiong (✉)
School of Public Health, Human Genetics Center, The University of Texas Health Science Center at Houston, Houston, TX 77225, USA
e-mail: momiao@gmail.com

D. Roy, M.T. Dorak (eds.), *Environmental Factors, Genes, and the Development of Human Cancers*, DOI 10.1007/978-1-4419-6752-7_3,

One way to discover additional genetic variants is to study gene–gene and gene–environment interaction. Complex diseases are the consequence of the interplay of genetic and environmental factors. Development of disease is a dynamic process of gene–gene and gene–environment interactions within a complex biological system which is organized into complicated interacting networks (Ay, 2002). Modern complex theory assumes that the complexity is attributed to the interactions among the components of the system, therefore, interaction has been considered as a sensible measure of complexity of the biological systems. The more interactions between the components, the more complex system. The presence of gene–gene and gene–environment interaction can greatly obscure the main effects in GWAS. Gene–gene and gene–environment interactions are ubiquitous. Screening for only main effects might miss the vast majority of the genetic variants that interact with environment to cause diseases (Murcray et al., 2009; Phillips, 2008). We argue that the interactions hold a key for dissecting the genetic structure of complex diseases and elucidating the biological and biochemical pathway underlying the diseases (Cordell, 2009). Ignoring gene–environment interactions will likely mask the detection of a genetic effect and may lead to inconsistent association results across studies (Andrieu and Goldstein, 1998; Manolio et al., 2006).

Despite current enthusiasm for investigation of gene–environment interactions, published results that document these interactions in humans are limited, and the essential issue of how to define and detect gene–environment interactions remains unresolved. There are several serious obstacles in detection of gene–environment interaction. First, unlike genetic variants that can be precisely measured, environments including behavioral, chemical, physical and social factors (Khoury and Wacholder, 2009), are difficult to accurately measure. Gene–environment interaction is a dynamic process. Variation in the timing of exposure and the timing of subsequent risk will have large impact on gene–environment interaction and make replication of the results of significant gene–environment interaction extremely difficult. Third, the concept of gene–environment interactions is often used, but rarely specified with precision (Jakulin, 2005).

Over the last three decades, epidemiologists have debated intensely about how to define and measure interaction in epidemiologic studies (Ottman, 1996). Many researchers indicated the importance of distinguishing biological interaction and statistical interaction (Rothman et al., 1980; Cheverud and Routman, 1995; Hansen and Wagner, 2001; Puniyani et al., 2004; Liberman et al., 2007). Biological interaction between the gene and environment is often defined as the interdependent operation of genetic and environmental factors that cause diseases. In contrast, statistical interaction between the gene and environment is defined as the interdependence between the effects of genetic and environmental risk factors in the context of a statistical model. The effects of disease risk factors are often measured by relative risks and odds ratios and interaction is defined as departure from additive or multiplicative joint effects (Khoury and Wacholder, 2009). The classical definition of statistical interaction has the following limitations. First, both relative risks and odds ratios are mainly defined for binary variables. Their extensions to multiple categorical risk factors (for example, three genotypes and multiple categorical environments) are cumbersome. Second, statistical interactions are essentially model dependent. Linear models and generalized linear models (logistic regressions and log-linear models) of the genetic effects of the risk factors are often used to define statistical interactions. In the classical logistic regressions and log-linear models of the gene–environment interactions, the genetic effects of the risk factors are decomposed into main effects and interaction effects (or product term) in the model. But, such decomposition may not reflect the true nonlinear interaction between the gene and environment. In addition, in these models, the major part of the true biological interactions between the gene and environment is often partitioned into the marginal effects. The remaining part of the gene–environment interactions which is treated as a departure (or residual) from the logistic regression and log-lineal models is small and hard to detect. Third, the classical interaction models can hardly be applied to study interactions (including pair-wise and high-order interactions) among the components of the biological systems, and their complexity.

To overcome the limitations of the classical definition of the statistical interaction, various new definitions of interaction that are based on interdependence among the risk factors causing disease can be proposed. Interactions between genes and the environment can generally be defined as a stochastic dependence between genetic and environmental risk factors in causing phenotypic variation among individuals. This definition does not require specifying the statistical models of the risks, and is similar, although not exactly identical, to the definition of biological interaction.

One such definition of gene–environment interaction is based on disequilibrium between gene and environment. Similar to linkage disequilibrium (LD), the dependence between the gene and environment can be described by introducing the new concept of the disequilibrium between gene and environment. Gene–environment interaction will create disequilibrium between them. We can use the disequilibrium between gene and environment to measure interaction between gene and environment. Another quantity to characterizing dependence between gene and environment is mutual information. Mutual information between gene and environment is to measure departure of the joint distribution of gene and environment from their independent distribution and can be used to quantify the gene–environment interaction.

The current genetic studies of complex diseases are mainly based on the common disease common variant hypothesis. However, in addition to SNPs that are defined as genetic variants with a minor allele frequency (MAF) greater than 1%, there are other classes of human genetic variation: (a) rare variants that are defined as mutations with a MAF of less than 1% and (b) structural variants that can also be classified as common and rare structural variants. Common disease can also be caused by multiple rare mutations, each with a low marginal genetic effect. A more realistic model for common disease is that the entire spectrum of genetic variants ranging from rare to common makes contribution to disease. Next-generation DNA sequencing platforms including 4D4 Life Sciences (Roche), Illumina 1G Genome Analysis System, Applied Biosystems SOLiD sequencing and Helicos GSS Sequencing can effectively detect the entire spectrum of genomic variation and provide a powerful tool for systematic exploration of the universe of variants and interactions in the entire genome, and hence largely improve our ability to explore the remaining genetic variance which has not been identified by GWAS (Shendure and Ji, 2008). New sequencing technologies will detect millions of rare variants. It is important to know that rare variants have several inherent features that are largely different from the common genetic variants. First, rare variants are infrequent and irregularly spaced in the studied genomic region. Second, massive sequencing strategies result in the unbalanced sampling of parental alleles and produce large number of errors (Chaisson et al., 2009; Johnson and Slatkin, 2007).

Most traditional statistical methods for testing gene–environment interaction were originally designed for testing the interaction between common allele and environment. These methods are well suited for detection of interaction between common variant and environment, but are difficult to be applied to rare variants for the following reasons. First, multiple rare variants that jointly have significant risk effects, but individually make only a small contribution. In the presence of allelic heterogeneity, the power of current variant-by-variant tests for interaction between rare variant and environment will vanish. Second, new sequence technologies are highly error prone (Chaisson et al., 2009). Due to their large genotyping errors and low frequencies, the signal of rare alleles may be compatible with genotyping errors. Unless genotyping errors are properly taken into account, many tests for gene–environment interaction will be invalidated.

The common disease rare variant hypothesis assumes that disease etiology is caused collectively by multiple rare variants. To increase the power for testing interaction between rare variants and environment, in this chapter we detail canonical correlation analysis to develop group tests that record rare sequence variants at different genome positions and collectively test for interaction between multiple rare variants or (a gene) and environment.

As Liu pointed out, "the success of investigation of G×E interactions depends greatly on the selection of the optimal study design, the most accurate and precise assessment of genetic and environmental factors, and the most efficient statistical analysis" (Liu et al., 2004). Developing efficient analytic methods for evaluation of the gene–environment interactions is critical to the investigation of gene–environment interactions (Garcia-Closas and Lubin, 1999).

Odds ratio calculations, logistic regression analysis, data mining and multifactor dimensionality reduction (MDR) are some of the existing methods available to evaluate the gene–environment interactions (Winslow and Boguski, 2003; Yoon et al., 2003; Hahn et al., 2003, Luan et al., 2001; Gauderman, 2002; Goldstein et al., 2006, Goodman et al., 2007; Goodman and Dana Flanders, 2007; Chatterjee et al., 2006; Marchini et al., 2005; Chung et al., 2007; Ritchie et al., 2001; Bush et al., 2006). These methods have their merits, but also they have limitations.

As an alternative to these widely used methods for testing gene and environment interactions, we introduce a number of new gene–environment interaction measures and develop novel statistics that are based on these new gene–environment interaction measures. These new statistics are simple, less computationally intensive and easy to implement. We hope that these developments may open a new avenue for large-scale genome-wide gene–environment interaction analysis.

3.2 Measure of Interaction Between Gene and Binary Environment

3.2.1 Traditional Measure of Gene–Environment Interaction

Consider a binary genetic factor G and a binary environmental exposure E. The genetic factor G is coded as G = 1 (G = 0) if an individual carries risk increasing genotypes (or no risk genotypes). The environmental exposure is coded as E = 1, otherwise E is coded as 0. Let D be an indicator of disease. Two study designs: cohort study and case-control study are often used in investigating gene–environment interaction. In the cohort study, the measures of gene–environment interaction are usually defined by relative risk and in the case-control study they are often defined by odds ratio. There are two types of traditional measures of interaction between gene and environment: additive and multiplicative measures.

3.2.1.1 The Measure of Gene–Environment Interaction for the Cohort Study Design

We first introduce the measure of gene–environment interaction for the cohort study design. Define the disease risk for each of the four possible combinations of the genetic and environmental risk factor:

$$h_{11} = P(D=1|G=1,E=1), \qquad h_{12} = P(D=1|G=1,E=0)$$
$$h_{21} = P(D=1|G=0,E=1), \qquad h_{22} = P(D=1|G=0,E=0).$$

The relative risks are defined as

$$RR_{11} = \frac{h_{11}}{h_{22}}, \quad RR_{12} = \frac{h_{12}}{h_{22}}, \quad RR_{21} = \frac{h_{21}}{h_{22}}.$$

Additive and multiplicative measures of gene–environment interaction are, respectively, defined as

$$I_{add} = RR_{11} - RR_{12} - RR_{21} + 1 \quad \text{and} \quad I_{multip} = \frac{RR_{11}}{RR_{12}RR_{21}}.$$

In the absence of interaction, we have

$$RR_{11} - RR_{12} = RR_{21} - 1 \tag{1}$$

and

$$RR_{11} = RR_{12} {}^* RR_{21}. \tag{2}$$

Let

$$P_{11} = P(G = 1, E = 1), \quad P_{12} = P(G = 1, E = 0), \quad P_{21} = P(G = 0, E = 1),$$
$$P_{22} = P(G = 0, E = 0), \text{ and}$$
$$P^A_{11} = P(G = 1, E = 1|D = 1), \quad P^A_{12} = P(G = 1, E = 0|D = 1),$$
$$P^A_{21} = P(G = 0, E = 1|D = 1), \quad P^A_{22} = P(G = 0, E = 0|D = 1).$$

Then, from Equations (1) and (2), in the absence of interaction we can obtain that

$$\frac{P^A_{11}}{P_{11}} - \frac{P^A_{12}}{P_{12}} = \frac{P^A_{21}}{P_{21}} - \frac{P^A_{22}}{P_{22}} \tag{3}$$

and

$$\frac{P^A_{11}P^A_{22}}{P_{11}P_{22}} = \frac{P^A_{12}P^A_{21}}{P_{12}P_{21}}. \tag{4}$$

To gain into understanding measure of gene and environment interaction, we study several special cases.

Case 1: G is not the disease locus. If we assume that G is only a marker and will not cause disease, then we have

$$\frac{P^A_{11}}{P_{11}} = \frac{P(E = 1|D)P(G = 1|E = 1, D)}{P(E = 1)P(G = 1|E = 1)} = \frac{P(E = 1|D)P(G = 1|E = 1)}{P(E = 1)P(G = 1|E = 1)}$$
$$= \frac{P(E = 1|D)}{P(E = 1)}.$$

Similarly, we have

$$\frac{P^A_{12}}{P_{12}} = \frac{P(E = 0|D)}{P(E = 0)}, \quad \frac{P^A_{21}}{P_{21}} = \frac{P(E = 1|D)}{P(E = 1)}, \quad \frac{P^A_{22}}{P_{22}} = \frac{P(E = 0|D)}{P(E = 0)},$$

which implies that

$$\frac{P^A_{11}}{P_{11}} - \frac{P^A_{12}}{P_{12}} = \frac{P(E = 1|D)}{P(E = 1)} - \frac{P(E = 0|D)}{P(E = 0)} = \frac{P^A_{21}}{P_{21}} - \frac{P^A_{22}}{P_{22}},$$

and

$$\frac{P_{11}^A P_{22}^A}{P_{11}P_{22}} = \frac{P(E=1|D)P(E=0|D)}{P(E=1)P(E=0)} = \frac{P_{12}^A P_{21}^A}{P_{12}P_{21}}.$$

Thus, we obtain $I_{add} = 0$ and $I_{multip} = 1$. In other words, if the locus G is a marker, there is no interaction between the locus G and environment. Hence, both additive and multiplicative measures of gene–environment interaction correctly characterize the circumstance where the locus G is a marker. {Rewording is useful, what is a marker case?}

Case 2: Environmental exposure will not cause disease. If the environmental exposure will not cause disease, there will be no interaction between the gene and environment. We expect that the additive measure of gene and environment interaction should be equal to zero and the multiplicative measure of gene and environment interaction should be equal to 1. Indeed, by the same argument as that in case 1, we can show this.

The additive and multiplicative measures of gene–environment interaction have close relations with log-linear models. Consider the following log-linear model:

$$\log(P(D=1|G,E)) = \alpha + \beta_G G + \beta_E E + \beta_{GE} GE.$$

From this model it follows that

$$RR_{11} = e^{\beta_G+\beta_E+\beta_{GE}}, \quad RR_{12} = e^{\beta_G} \text{ and } RR_{21} = e^{\beta_E}.$$

The additive and multiplicative measures of gene–environment interaction are, respectively, given by

$$I_{add} = e^{\beta_G+\beta_E+\beta_{GE}} - e^{\beta_G} - e^{\beta_E} + 1 \quad \text{and} \quad I_{muliple} = e^{\beta_{GE}}.$$

The regression coefficient β_{GE} in the log-linear model is equal to logarithm of the multiplicative measure of gene–environment interaction.

The additive measure and multiplicative measures do not completely overlap. The question of which measure should be used to detect interaction has long been debated (Koopman, 1977; Ottman, 1996; Walter and Holford, 1978). What measure should be used to study interaction depends on the purpose of investigation (Ottman, 1996).

3.2.1.2 The Measure of Gene–Environment Interaction for the Case-Control Study Design

Next we study the measure of gene–environment interaction for the case-control study design. The gene–environment interaction for the case-control study design is usually measured by odds ratio. The genetic, environmental and interaction odds ratios are defined, respectively, by

$$OR_G = \frac{\frac{h_{12}}{1-h_{12}}}{\frac{h_{22}}{1-h_{22}}}, \quad OR_E = \frac{\frac{h_{21}}{1-h_{21}}}{\frac{h_{22}}{1-h_{22}}} \quad \text{and} \quad OR_{GE} = \frac{\frac{h_{11}}{1-h_{11}}}{\frac{h_{22}}{1-h_{22}}}.$$

Using odds ratios, we can define the additive and multiplicative measures of gene–environment interaction, respectively, as

$$I_{Oadd} = OR_{GE} - OR_G - OR_E + 1 \tag{5}$$

and

$$I_{Omultip} = \frac{OR_{GE}}{OR_G OR_E}. \tag{6}$$

Without gene–environment interaction, Equations (5) and (6) can be simplified as

$$OR_{GE} - OR_G - OR_E + 1 = 0 \text{ and } OR_{GE} = OR_G{}^* OR_E.$$

Let

$$P_{11}^N = P(G=1, E=1|D=0), \quad P_{12}^N = P(G=1, E=0|D=0),$$
$$P_{21}^N = P(G=0, E=1|D=0) \text{ and } P_{22}^N = P(G=0, E=0|D=0).$$

Similar to Equations (3) and (4), in the absence of interaction we have

$$\frac{P_{11}^A}{P_{11}^N} - \frac{P_{12}^A}{P_{12}^N} = \frac{P_{21}^A}{P_{21}^N} - \frac{P_{22}^A}{P_{22}^N} \tag{7}$$

and

$$\frac{P_{11}^A P_{22}^A}{P_{11}^N P_{22}^N} = \frac{P_{12}^A P_{21}^A}{P_{12}^N P_{21}^N}. \tag{8}$$

It is interesting to know that replacing population frequencies in Equations (3) and (4) by frequencies in controls will lead to Equations (7) and (8).

Consider the following logistic model:

$$P(D=1|G,E) = \frac{e^{\alpha+\beta_g G+\beta_e E+\beta_{ge} GE}}{1+e^{\alpha+\beta_g G+\beta_e E+\beta_{ge} GE}},$$

which gives the genetic, environmental and interaction odds ratios: $OR_G = e^{\beta_g}$, $OR_E = e^{\beta_e}$, and $OR_{GE} = e^{\beta_g+\beta_e+\beta_{ge}}$.

Using these expressions for the genetic, environmental and interaction odds ratios, we can obtain the following representation for the additive and multiplicative measures of gene–environment interaction:

$$I_{add} = e^{\beta_g+\beta_e+\beta_{ge}} - e^{\beta_g} - e^{\beta_e} + 1 \quad \text{and} \quad I_{multipl} = e^{\beta_{ge}}.$$

3.2.2 Disequilibrium Measure of Gene–Environment Interaction

Concept of linkage disequilibrium (LD) and measuring its value play an essential role in genetic studies of complex diseases (Sabatti and Risch, 2002). We can define LD as the measure for quantifying the magnitude of interaction between gene and environment, which allows us to borrow tools from LD studies, and is referred to as disequilibrium measure of interaction between gene and environment hereafter. Let D be an indicator of the disease status and P_D be the population prevalence of disease. Treating the environmental variable as a locus, the interaction between the gene and environment can be viewed as the interaction between two loci. Similar to the measure of LD, we can define a disequilibrium measure (covariance) between the gene and environment in the general population as follows: $\delta = P_{11}P_{22} - P_{12}P_{21}$. This mathematical form is precisely the same as the form of the measure of LD. The disequilibrium measure characterizes the dependence between the gene and environment. If two genetic and environmental variables are independent, the disequilibrium measure between the gene and environment will be equal to zero. To investigate whether the interaction between gene and environment create the disequilibrium between them, we derived the disequilibrium measure in the disease population under the general disease model:

$$\begin{aligned}\delta^A &= P_{11}^A P_{22}^A - P_{12}^A P_{21}^A \\ &= \frac{P_{11}P_{22}h_{11}h_{22} - P_{12}P_{21}h_{12}h_{21}}{P_D^2} \\ &= \frac{h_{11}h_{22}}{P_D^2}\delta + \frac{P_{12}P_{21}}{P_D^2}(h_{11}h_{22} - h_{12}h_{21}).\end{aligned}$$

The above equation motivates us to define the following measure of gene–environment interaction as

$$I_\delta = h_{11}h_{22} - h_{12}h_{21}. \tag{9}$$

If h_{ij} in Equation (9) is replaced by P_{ij} it becomes a measure of disequilibrium. Therefore, I_δ is referred to as the disequilibrium measure of gene–environment interaction. Surprisingly, we can show from Equations (4) and (12) that the disequilibrium measure I_δ is equal to zero if and only if the multiplicative measure of gene–environment interaction for the cohort study I_{multip} is equal to one. In other words, the absence of gene–environment interaction which is detected by the disequilibrium measure of gene–environment interaction can also be detected by multiplicative measure of gene–environment interaction.

With the aid of Equation (9), the measure of disequilibrium in the disease population can be expressed as

$$\delta^A = \frac{h_{11}h_{22}}{P_D^2}\delta + \frac{P_{12}P_{21}}{P_D^2}I_\delta. \tag{10}$$

Equation (10) shows that the disequilibrium between the gene and environment in the disease population comes from two parts. One part is from the disequilibrium between the gene and environment in the general population. Another is from the gene–environment interaction. Rewrite Equation (10) as

$$\delta^A - \frac{h_{11}h_{22}}{P_D^2}\delta = \frac{P_{12}P_{21}}{P_D^2}I_\delta,$$

which shows that the difference in the disequilibrium between disease population and general population is proportional to the disequilibrium measure of gene–environment interaction. This forms the basis for formal testing for the gene–environment interaction.

3.2.3 Information Measure of Gene–Environment Interaction

In studying information measure of gene–environment interaction, the locus G can be either coded as 0 and 1 as before or coded as 0, 1, and 2 indicating three genotypes. The environmental exposure is coded as before. Mutual information is to measure dependence between two random variables. The mutual information between gene and environment in the general population is defined as

$$I(G;E) = \sum_{i=0}^{2}\sum_{j=0}^{1} P(G=i,E=j)\log\frac{P(G=i,E=j)}{P(G=i)P(E=j)} \tag{11}$$

Information theory (Cover et al., 1991) shows that mutual information $I(G;E)$ is equal to zero if and only if

$$P(G=i,E=j) = P(G=i)P(E=j), \qquad (i=0,1,2; j=0,1)$$

i.e., gene and environment variables are independent.

The mutual information between gene and environment in the disease population is given by

$$I(G;E|D) = \sum_{i=0}^{2}\sum_{j=0}^{1} P(G=i,E=j|D=1)\log\frac{P(G=i,E=j|D=1)}{P(G=i|D=1)P(E=j|D=1)} \tag{12}$$

while can be reduced to

$$I(G;E|D) = \sum_{i=0}^{2}\sum_{j=0}^{1} P(G=i,E=j|D=1)\log\frac{P(G=i,E=j)}{P(G=i)P(E=j)} + \sum_{i=0}^{2}\sum_{j=0}^{1} P(G=i,E=j|D=1)\log\frac{P(D=1|G=i,E=j)/P_D}{\frac{P(D=1|G=i)}{P_D}\frac{P(D=1|E=j)}{P_D}} \quad (13)$$

where $P_D = P(D=1)$ is the prevalence of the disease.

Equation (13) shows that mutual information $I(G;E|D)$ has two components. The first term in Equation (13) is due to dependence between gene and environment in the general population. The second term in Equation (13) is due to interaction. Thus, we define information measure of interaction between gene and environment as

$$I_{GE} = \sum_{i=0}^{2}\sum_{j=0}^{1} P(G=i,E=j|D=1)\log\frac{P(D=1|G=i,E=j)/P_D}{\frac{P(D=1|G=i)}{P_D}\frac{P(D=1|E=j)}{P_D}} \quad (14)$$

which implies that $I_{GE} = 0$ if and only if

$$\frac{P(D=1|G=i,E=j)}{P_D} = \frac{P(D=1|G=i)}{P_D}\frac{P(D=1|E=j)}{P_D} \quad (i=0,1,2, j=0,1) \quad (15)$$

Information measure of interaction has two remarkable features. First, it is defined in terms of penetrance and hence related to the cause of the disease. Second, the interaction is measured by the interdependent operation of the gene and environment in causing disease. Absence of gene and environment interaction indicates that Equation (15) should hold. If G is coded as 0 or 1, then Equation (15) is equivalent to

$$h_{11}h_{22} = h_{12}h_{21} \quad \text{or} \quad \text{Equation (2) } RR_{11} = RR_{12}{}^{*}RR_{21}.$$

Equation (13) can be rewritten as

$$I(G;E|D) - \sum_{i=0}^{2}\sum_{j=0}^{1} P(G=i,E=j|D=1)\log\frac{P(G=i,E=j)}{P(G=i)P(E=j)} = I_{GE}. \quad (16)$$

The second term in the left side of Equation (16) is the mutual information between gene and environment in the general population if the probabilities $P(G=i,E=j|D)$ is replaced by $P(G=i,E=j)$. Equation (16) shows that the modified difference in mutual information between cases and general population is proportional to the information measure of gene–environment interaction.

If we assume that the gene and environment variables in the general population are independent, then

$$I(G;E|D) = I_{GE}$$

In this case, the mutual information between the gene and environment in the disease population is equal to the information measure of the interaction between gene and environment. This provides an easy way to calculate the information measure of gene–environment interaction.

To gain into understanding information measure of gene and environment interaction, we study several special cases.

Case 1: G is not the disease locus. If we assume that G is only a marker and will not cause disease, then we have

$$P(D=1|G=i,E=j) = P(D=1|E=j) \text{ and } P(D=1|G=i) = P_D$$

which implies that

$$\frac{P(D=1|G=i,E=j)/P_D}{\frac{P(D=1|G=i)}{P_D}\frac{P(D=1|E=j)}{P_D}} = 1$$

Thus, we obtain $I_{GE} = 0$. In other words, if the locus G is a marker, there is no interaction between the locus G and environment. The interaction measure I_{GE} between the marker and environment should be equal to zero. Hence, our information measure of gene–environment interaction correctly characterizes the circumstance where the locus G is a marker.

Case 2: Environmental exposure will not cause disease. If the environmental exposure will not cause disease, there will be no interaction between the gene and environment. We expect that the information measure of gene and environment interaction should be equal to zero. Indeed, by the same argument as that in case 1, we can show this.

3.3 Measure of Interaction Between Gene and Continuous Environment

Many environmental variables for example, age, income and gene expression are continuous variables. Generally, there is more information when a risk factor is represented by a continuous variable than a categorical variable. Dichotomization of continuous variable will lose information. Therefore, developing measures of interaction between gene and environment that can be applied to continuous environmental variables is indispensable in the studies of gene–environment interaction.

3.3.1 Multiplicative Measure of Interaction Between Gene and Continuous Environment

To extend multiplicative measure of gene–environment interaction for binary environment to continuous environment, we first introduce point-wise risk and relative risk. We take non-carrier of the susceptible genotype and average environment as the baseline. Denote the continuous environmental variable by e and its expectation by μ. Let the point-wise risk be defined as

$$h_{1e} = P(D = 1|G = 1, E = e), \quad h_{1\mu} = P(D = 1|G = 1, E = \mu)$$
$$h_{2e} = P(D = 1|G = 0, E = e), \quad h_{2\mu} = P(D = 1|G = 0, E = \mu).$$

Then, the point-wise relative risk can be defined as

$$RR_{1e} = \frac{h_{1e}}{h_{2\mu}}, \quad RR_{1\mu} = \frac{h_{1\mu}}{h_{2\mu}} \quad \text{and} \quad RR_{2e} = \frac{h_{2e}}{h_{2\mu}}. \tag{17}$$

Point-wise multiplicative measure of interaction between gene and continuous environment is then defined by

$$I_{PMGE} = \log \frac{RR_{1e}}{RR_{1\mu}RR_{2e}}. \tag{18}$$

If we assume that E is an environmental variable with normal density function of mean μ and variance σ^2 and that environmental variable E conditional on $G = i$ follows a normal density with mean μ_i and variance σ_i^2 and their corresponding densities in the disease population are normal density function with means μ_D, μ_{Di} and variances $\sigma_D^2, \sigma_{Di}^2$, then Equation (18) can be reduced to

$$I_{PMGE} = \log \frac{\mu_{D0}\mu_1}{\mu_{D1}\mu_0} + \frac{1}{2}\log \frac{\sigma_{D0}^2\sigma_1^2}{\sigma_{D1}^2\sigma_0^2} + \frac{(e-\mu_{D0})^2}{2\sigma_{D0}^2} + \frac{(e-\mu_0)^2}{2\sigma_0^2} - \frac{(e-\mu_{D1})^2}{2\sigma_{D1}^2} - \frac{(e-\mu_1)^2}{2\sigma_1^2} \tag{19}$$

We define expectation of point-wise multiplicative measure of gene–environment interaction I_{PMGE} as the multiplicative measure of interaction between gene and continuous environment:

$$I_{MGE} = E\left[\log \frac{RR_{1e}}{RR_{1\mu}RR_{2e}}\right]. \tag{20}$$

Under assumption of normal distribution of environmental variable, the multiplicative measure of interaction between gene and continuous environment is simplified to

$$I_{MGE} = \log \frac{\mu_{D0}\mu_1}{\mu_{D1}\mu_0} + \frac{1}{2}\log \frac{\sigma_{D0}^2\sigma_1^2}{\sigma_{D1}^2\sigma_0^2}. \tag{21}$$

In the absence of gene–environment interaction, the interaction measure I_{MGE} is equal to zero.

3.3.2 Disequilibrium Measure of Interaction Between Gene and Continuous Environment

Disequilibrium measure of interaction between a binary genetic factor and a continuous environmental factor can be defined as

$$I_\delta(e) = h_{1e}h_{2\mu} - h_{1\mu}h_{2e} \tag{22}$$

$I_\delta(e)$ is a function of the environmental factor. Let $P(G = 1, E = \mu)$, $P(G = 0, E = \mu)$, $P(G = 1, E = e)$ and $P(G = 0, E = e)$ be the joint probability density functions. The concept of disequilibrium measure between two random variables can be extended to measure dependence between a random variable and a random function. We first define a point-wise disequilibrium measure between the coded binary genotype and the continuous environment in general population as

$$\delta(e) = P(G = 1, E = e)P(G = 0, E = \mu) - P(G = 1, E = \mu)P(G = 0, E = e).$$

The point-wise disequilibrium measure in the disease population is then given by

$$\delta^A(e) = \frac{h_{1e}h_{2\mu}}{P_D^2}\delta(e) + \frac{P(G = 1, E = \mu)P(G = 0, E = e)}{P_D^2} I_\delta(e) \tag{23}$$

3.3.3 Mutual Information Measure of Interaction Between Gene and Continuous Environment

Mutual information between gene and a continuous environmental factor E is defined as $I(G;E) = \sum_{i=0}^{1} \int P(G = i, e) \log \frac{P(G=i,e)}{P(G=i)P(e)} de$, where $P(G = i, e)$ is the joint probability density function of $G = i$ and e, $P(e)$ is a density function of environmental variable and $P(G = i)$ is a probability mass function of the genotype. We define the mutual information measure of the interaction between the binary genetic factor and continuous environment as

$$I_{GCE} = \sum_{i=0}^{1} \int P(G = i, E = e|D = 1) \log \frac{P(D = 1|G = i, E = e)/P_D}{[P(D = 1|G = i)/P_D][P(D = 1|E = e)/P_D]} de, \tag{24}$$

The mutual information between the binary genetic factor and continuous environment in disease population is given by

$$I(G;E|D) = \sum_{i=0}^{1} \int P(G=i, E=e|D=1) \log \frac{P(G=i,E=e)}{P(G=i)P(E=e)} de + I_{GCE}. \quad (25)$$

Equation (25) shows that the mutual information in the disease population consists of two terms. The first term in the right side of equation is involved in mutual information between gene and environment in the general population and the second term is the mutual information measure of the interaction between the gene and the continuous environment.

Unlike mutual information between two discrete variables which is easy to calculate, the mutual information between the discrete variable and continuous variable requires calculation of integral that may involve intensive numerical computation. However, when environmental variable has a normal distribution with mean μ_D and variance σ_D^2 and conditional on the genotype $G = i$, it has normal distribution with mean μ_{Di} and variance σ_{Di}^2 in the disease population we can show that

$$I(G;E|D) = \frac{1}{2} \log \sigma_D^2 - \frac{1}{2} \left[P(G=0|D) \log \sigma_{D_0}^2 + P(G=1|D) \log \sigma_{D_1}^2 \right]$$

Similarly, for the general population if we assume that the environmental variable has a normal distribution with mean μ and variance σ^2 and it also has normal distributions with the conditional mean μ_i and variance σ_i^2, given the genotype $G = i$, we have

$$\begin{aligned}
&\sum_{i=0}^{1} \int P(G=i, E=e|D=1) \log \frac{P(G=i,E=e)}{P(G=i)P(E=e)} de \\
&= \tfrac{1}{2} \left[\log \sigma^2 - P(G=0|D) \log \sigma_0^2 - P(G=1|D) \log \sigma_1^2 \right] + \frac{\sigma_{D_1}^2 + (\mu_D - \mu)^2}{2\sigma^2} \\
&\quad - P(G=0|D) \frac{\sigma_{D_0}^2 + (\mu_{D_0} - \mu_0)^2}{2\sigma_0^2} - P(G=1|D) \frac{\sigma_{D_1}^2 + (\mu_{D_1} - \mu_1)^2}{2\sigma_1^2}.
\end{aligned}$$

Then, the mutual information measure of interaction between the binary genetic factor and continuous environmental variable with normal distributions is given by

$$\begin{aligned}
I_{GCE} = &\frac{1}{2} \log \frac{\sigma_D^2}{\sigma^2} - \frac{1}{2} \left[P(G=0|D) \log \frac{\sigma_{D_0}^2}{\sigma_0^2} + P(G=1|D) \log \frac{\sigma_{D_1}^2}{\sigma_1^2} \right] - \frac{\sigma_D^2 + (\mu_D - \mu)^2}{2\sigma^2} \\
&+ P(G=0|D) \frac{\sigma_{D_0}^2 + (\mu_{D_0} - \mu_0)^2}{2\sigma_0^2} + P(G=1|D) \frac{\sigma_{D_1}^2 + (\mu_{D_1} - \mu_1)^2}{2\sigma_1^2}.
\end{aligned} \quad (26)$$

3.4 Statistics for Testing Interaction Between Gene and Environment

In the previous section, we presented four types of measures of gene–environment interaction which provide the basis for developing statistics to formally test for gene–environment interaction. In this section we will study statistics for testing for gene–environment interaction based on the measure of gene–environment interaction. Some statistics are newly proposed.

3.4.1 Relative Risk and Odds-Ratio-Based Statistics for Testing Interaction Between Gene and Discrete Environment

Gene–environment interaction can be identified by formal tests. The test statistics can be developed parallel to the measure of gene–environment interaction. We first study test for gene–environment interaction in the cohort study design. The test statistics depend on the scale of the measurement of the gene–environment interaction.

Recall that the additive measure of gene–environment interaction is defined as

$$\begin{aligned} I_{add} &= RR_{11} - RR_{01} - RR_{10} + 1 \\ &= \frac{h_{11}}{h_{22}} - \frac{h_{12}}{h_{22}} - \frac{h_{21}}{h_{22}} + 1 \end{aligned}$$

Let n_1, n_2, n_3 and $n_4$be the number of individuals with both risk genotype and exposure, with risk genotype alone, with exposure alone and with neither the risk genotype nor the exposure, respectively. It can be shown that the variance of estimate of the additive interaction measure is given by (Lehmann, 1983)

$$\hat{V}_{Radd} = \frac{h_{11}(1-h_{11})}{n_1 h_{22}^2} + \frac{h_{12}(1-h_{12})}{n_2 h_{22}^2} + \frac{h_{21}(1-h_{21})}{n_3 h_{22}^2} + \frac{(1-h_{22})(h_{12}+h_{21}-h_{11})^2}{n_4 h_{22}^3}.$$

Define the statistic to test for gene–environment interaction for the additive scale of measurement as

$$T_{Radd} = \frac{I_{add}^2}{V_{Radd}}. \tag{27}$$

Then, under the null hypothesis of no gene–environment interaction, the statistic T_{Radd} is asymptotically distributed as a central $\chi^2_{(1)}$ distribution.

Similar to the additive measure of gene–environment interaction, we can develop statistics for testing gene–environment interaction based on the multiplicative measure of gene–environment interaction. The logarithm of the relative risk multiplicative measure of gene–environment interaction can be reduced to

$$\log(I_{Rmultip}) = \log \frac{RR_{11}}{RR_{12}RR_{21}}$$
$$= \log \frac{P^A_{11}P^A_{22}}{P^A_{12}P^A_{21}} - \log \frac{P_{11}P_{22}}{P_{12}P_{21}}$$

The variance of the estimate of the multiplicative measure of gene–environment interaction is given by

$$\hat{V}_{Rmultip} = \frac{1}{\frac{1}{n_A}\left(\frac{1}{P^A_{11}} + \frac{1}{P^A_{12}} + \frac{1}{P^A_{21}} + \frac{1}{P^A_{22}}\right) + \frac{1}{n_G}\left(\frac{1}{P_{11}} + \frac{1}{P_{12}} + \frac{1}{P_{21}} + \frac{1}{P_{22}}\right)},$$

where n_A and $n_G$are the number of sampled individuals in the disease population and general population, respectively.

The statistic for testing gene–environment interaction which is based on the multiplicative measure can be defined as

$$T_{Rmultip} = \frac{\left(\log \frac{P^A_{11}P^A_{22}}{P^A_{12}P^A_{21}} - \log \frac{P_{11}P_{22}}{P_{12}P_{21}}\right)^2}{\frac{1}{n_A}\left(\frac{1}{P^A_{11}} + \frac{1}{P^A_{12}} + \frac{1}{P^A_{21}} + \frac{1}{P^A_{22}}\right) + \frac{1}{n_G}\left(\frac{1}{P_{11}} + \frac{1}{P_{12}} + \frac{1}{P_{21}} + \frac{1}{P_{22}}\right)} \quad (28)$$

which is asymptotically distributed as a central $\chi^2_{(1)}$distribution under the null hypothesis of no gene–environment interaction.

To validate the null distribution of the test statistic $T_{Rmultip}$ we performed a series of simulation studies. MATLAB was used to generate the genotype and environment data of the individuals under the null hypothesis of no interaction between gene and environment. Individuals (n = 1,000,000) with $P(G = 1) = 0.8$, $\delta = P(G = 1, E = 1)P(G = 0, E = 0) - P(G = 1, E = 0)P(G = 0, E = 1) = 0.02$, $P(E = 1) = 0.2$, and preference of 0.01 in a cohort were generated. A total of 20,000 simulations were repeated. We plotted Fig. 3.1 showing the histograms of the test statistic $T_{Rmultip}$ for testing interaction between gene and environment, with sample size of 1,000. Figure 3.1 shows that the null distributions of the test statistics $T_{Rmultip}$ is similar to the theoretical $\chi^2_{(1)}$ distribution. Type I error rates were calculated by random sampling of 500–1,000 individuals from cases. In Table 3.1 we listed type I error rates for $T_{Rmultip}$, assuming $OR_g = 1$and $OR_e = 1$. Table 3.1 demonstrates that the estimated Type I error rates for the statistics $T_{Rmultip}$ to test the gene and environment interactions are not appreciably different from the nominal levels $\alpha = 0.05$, $\alpha = 0.01$ and $\alpha = 0.001$.

In case-control study design, we use odds ratio to measure gene–environment interaction. Similar to relative risk measure of gene–environment interaction in the cohort study design, there are also two odds ratio measures of gene–environment interaction in the case-control study design: additive and multiplicative measures.

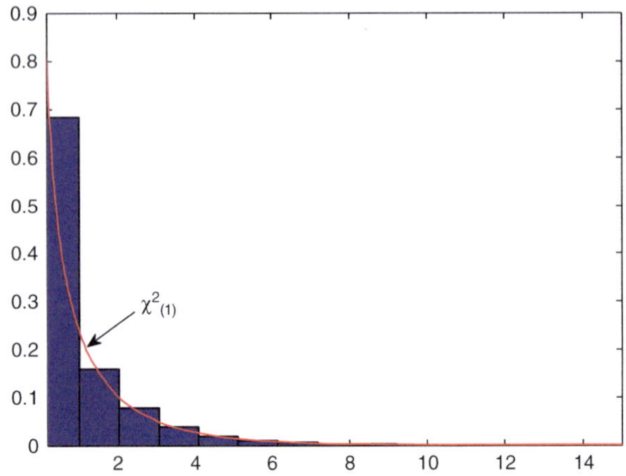

Fig. 3.1 Null distribution of the statistic $T_{Rmultip}$, sampling 1,000 cases from a cohort of 1,000,000 individual

Table 3.1 Type 1 error rates for the test statistic $T_{Rmultip}$ to test gene–environment interaction, assuming $OR_g = 1$ and $OR_e = 1$

	Nominal levels		
Sample sizes	α=0.05	α=0.01	α=0.001
500	0.0488	0.0088	0.0010
600	0.0514	0.0108	0.0009
700	0.0488	0.0097	0.0009
800	0.0515	0.0102	0.0007
900	0.0508	0.0110	0.0011
1,000	0.0492	0.0099	0.0009

The odds ratio additive measure of gene–environment interaction can be rewritten as

$$\begin{aligned} I_{Oadd} &= OR_{GE} - OR_G - OR_E + 1 \\ &= \frac{P_{11}^A P_{22}^N}{P_{22}^A P_{11}^N} - \frac{P_{12}^A P_{22}^N}{P_{22}^A P_{12}^N} - \frac{P_{21}^A P_{22}^N}{P_{22}^A P_{21}^N} + 1. \end{aligned}$$

The variance of I_{Oadd} is given by

$$\begin{aligned} V_{Oadd} = \frac{1}{n_A}\left(\frac{OR_{GE}^2}{P_{11}^A} + \frac{OR_G^2}{P_{12}^A} + \frac{OR_E^2}{P_{21}^A} + \frac{(OR_{GE} - OR_G - OR_E)^2}{P_{22}^A}\right) \\ + \frac{1}{n_G}\left(\frac{OR_{GE}^2}{P_{11}^N} + \frac{OR_G^2}{P_{12}^N} + \frac{OR_E^2}{P_{21}^N} + \frac{(OR_{GE} - OR_G - OR_E)^2}{P_{22}^N}\right) \end{aligned}$$

Therefore, for the additive measure, we define the statistic for testing gene–environment interaction as

$$T_{Oadd} = \frac{I^2_{Oadd}}{V_{Oadd}} \tag{29}$$

which is asymptotically distributed as a central $\chi^2_{(1)}$ distribution under the null hypothesis of no gene–environment interaction.

The logarithm of odds-ratio multiplicative measure of gene–environment interaction can be expressed as

$$\begin{aligned}\log(I_{Omultip}) &= \log\frac{OR_{GE}}{OR_G OR_E}\\ &= \log\frac{P^A_{11}P^A_{22}}{P^A_{12}P^A_{21}} - \log\frac{P^N_{11}P^N_{22}}{P^N_{12}P^N_{21}}.\end{aligned}$$

The statistics for testing gene–environment interaction which is based on the odds-ratio multiplicative measure is defined as (Mukherjee et al., 2008)

$$T_{Omultip} = \frac{\left(\log\frac{P^A_{11}P^A_{22}}{P^A_{12}P^A_{21}} - \log\frac{P^N_{11}P^N_{22}}{P^N_{12}P^N_{21}}\right)^2}{\frac{1}{n_A}\left(\frac{1}{P^A_{11}}+\frac{1}{P^A_{12}}+\frac{1}{P^A_{21}}+\frac{1}{P^A_{22}}\right)+\frac{1}{n_G}\left(\frac{1}{P^N_{11}}+\frac{1}{P^N_{12}}+\frac{1}{P^N_{21}}+\frac{1}{P^N_{22}}\right)}, \tag{30}$$

which is again asymptotically distributed as a central $\chi^2_{(1)}$ distribution under the null hypothesis of no gene–environment interaction. Difference between Equations (28) and (30) is that for cohort study design, cell frequencies P_{11}, P_{12}, P_{21} and P_{22}in Equation (28) are measured in the general population, but for the case-control study design, cell frequencies $P^N_{11}, P^N_{12}, P^N_{21}$ and P^N_{22} are measured in the controls.

To examine the null distribution of the test statistic $T_{Omultip}$ we performed a series of simulation studies. A total of 1,000,000 individuals as a general population with $P(G = 1) = 0.8$, $\delta = P(G = 1, E = 1)P(G = 0, E = 0) - P(G = 1, E = 0)P(G = 0, E = 1) = 0.02$, $P(E = 1) = 0.2$ were generated. A total of 20,000 simulations were repeated. We plotted Fig. 3.2 showing the histograms of the test statistic $T_{Omultip}$ for testing interaction between gene and environment, with 1,000 cases and 1,000 controls. Figure 3.2 shows that the null distributions of the test statistics $T_{Omultip}$ is similar to the theoretical $\chi^2_{(1)}$ distribution. Type I error rates were calculated by random sampling of 500–1,000 individuals as cases and controls from the general population. In Table 3.2 we listed type I error rates for $T_{Omultip}$, assuming $OR_g = 1$ and $OR_e = 1$. Table 3.2 demonstrates that the estimated Type I error rates for the statistic $T_{Omultip}$ to test the gene and environment interactions are not much different from the nominal levels $\alpha = 0.05$, $\alpha = 0.01$ and $\alpha = 0.001$.

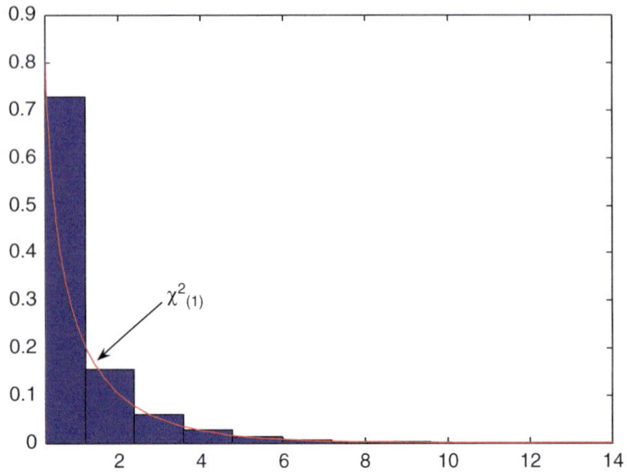

Fig. 3.2 Null distribution of the statistic $T_{Omultip}$, sampling 1,000 cases and controls from a general population with 1,000,000 individuals

Table 3.2 Type 1 error rates for the test statistic $T_{Rmultip}$ to test gene–environment interaction, assuming $OR_g = 1$ and $OR_e = 1$

	Nominal levels		
Sample sizes	α=0.05	α=0.01	α=0.001
500	0.0480	0.0097	0.0008
600	0.0493	0.0089	0.0011
700	0.0505	0.0089	0.0010
800	0.0498	0.0093	0.0010
900	0.0511	0.0097	0.0010
1,000	0.0515	0.0091	0.0012

If the gene and environment variable are independent in the general population or in the controls, the multiplicative interaction measure of gene–environment interaction can be estimated by the sample relative risk or odds-ratio between gene and environment among the cases alone and can be tested by (Piergorsch et al., 1994)

$$T_{multip} = \frac{\left(\log \frac{P^A_{11} P^A_{22}}{P^A_{12} P^A_{21}}\right)^2}{\frac{1}{n_A}\left(\frac{1}{P^A_{11}} + \frac{1}{P^A_{12}} + \frac{1}{P^A_{21}} + \frac{1}{P^A_{22}}\right)}. \tag{31}$$

The case-only design will increase the power of the test over case-control design by reduction of the variance associated with the estimation of relative risk or odds-ratio between gene and environment among the controls (Mukherjee et al., 2008).

3.4.2 Disequilibrium-Based Statistics for Testing Interaction Between Gene and Discrete Environment

In the previous section, we show that gene–environment interaction can create disequilibrium (dependence) between them. Intuitively, we can test gene–environment interaction by comparing the difference in the levels of the disequilibrium between gene-environment in the cases and general population. Precisely, the statistic for testing gene–environment interaction is defined as

$$T_{DIS} = \frac{\left(\delta_A - \frac{P_{11}^A P_{22}^A}{P_{11} P_{22}} \delta\right)^2}{V_A + \left(\frac{P_{11}^A P_{22}^A}{P_{11} P_{22}}\right)^2 V_N}, \tag{32}$$

where

$$V_A = \frac{P_G^A(1 - P_G^A)P_E^A(1 - P_E^A) + (1 - 2P_G^A)(1 - 2P_E^A)\delta_A - \delta_A^2}{n_A},$$

$$V_N = \frac{P_G(1 - P_G)P_E(1 - P_E) + (1 - 2P_G)(1 - 2P_E)\delta_N - \delta_N^2}{n_G},$$

$P_G^A = P(G = 1|D = 1), P_E^A = P(E = 1|D = 1), P_G = P(G = 1)$ and $P_E = P(E = 1)$. We can show that the statistic T_{DIS} is distributed as a central $\chi^2_{(1)}$ distribution under the null hypothesis of no gene–environment interaction. If we assume that the gene and environment variables in the general population are independent, then Equation (32) will be simplified to

$$T_{DIS} = \frac{\delta_A^2}{V_A}. \tag{33}$$

Equation (33) can be used to test for gene–environment interaction in case-only design.

To validate the null distribution of the test statistic T_{DIS} we performed a series of simulation studies. MATLAB was used to generate the genotype and environment data of the individuals under the null hypothesis of no interaction between gene and environment. A total of 1,000,000 individuals as a general population with $P(G = 1) = 0.8$, $\delta = P(G = 1, E = 1)P(G = 0, E = 0) - P(G = 1, E = 0)P(G = 0, E = 1) = 0.02$, $P(E = 1) = 0.2$ were generated. A total of 20,000 simulations were repeated. We plotted Fig. 3.3 showing the histograms of the test statistic T_{DIS} for testing interaction between gene and environment, with 1,000 cases and 1,000 individuals sampled from general population. Figure 3.3 shows that the null distributions of the test statistics T_{DIS} was similar to the theoretical $\chi^2_{(1)}$ distribution. Type I error rates were calculated by random

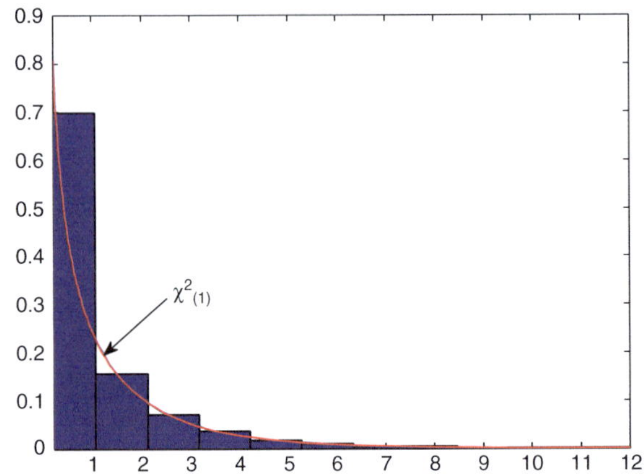

Fig. 3.3 Null distribution of the statistic T_{DIS}, sampling 1,000 cases and controls from a general population with 1,000,000 individuals

Table 3.3 Type 1 error rates for the test statistic T_{DIS} to test gene–environment interaction, assuming $OR_g = 1$ and $OR_e = 1$

	Nominal levels		
Sample sizes	α=0.05	α=0.01	α=0.001
500	0.0507	0.0102	0.0010
600	0.0511	0.0119	0.0008
700	0.0504	0.0103	0.0008
800	0.0515	0.0105	0.0010
900	0.0505	0.0108	0.0012
1,000	0.0504	0.0095	0.0009

sampling 500–1,000 individuals as cases and controls from the general population. Type I error rates for T_{DIS}, assuming $OR_g = 1$ and $OR_e = 1$, listed in Table 3.3 were similar to the nominal levels $\alpha = 0.05$, $\alpha = 0.01$ and $\alpha = 0.001$.

3.4.3 Information-Based Statistics for Testing Interaction Between Gene and Discrete Environment

Under the assumption that the gene and environment variables in the general population are independent, Wu et al. (2009) developed information-based statistics for testing gene–environment interaction. Let

$$f_{ij} = P(G = i, E = j) \log \frac{P(G = i, E = j)}{P(G = i)P(E = j)} \qquad (i = 0, 1, 2, j = 0, 1)$$

and $f_{D_{ij}} = P(G=i, E=j|D=1)\log \frac{P(G=i, E=j|D=1)}{P(G=i|D=1)P(E=j|D=1)}$

$(i=0,1,2, j=0,1)$. Let $f = \left[f_{11}, f_{12}, f_{21}, f_{22}, f_{31}, f_{32}\right]^T$

and $f_D = \left[f_{D_{11}}, f_{D_{12}}, f_{D_{21}}, f_{D_{22}}, f_{D_{31}}, f_{D_{32}}\right]^T$

$P_{ij} = P(G=i, E=j)$ and $P_{D_{ij}} = P(G=i, E=j|D=1)$

Define

$$P = [P_{00}, P_{01}, P_{10}, P_{11}, P_{20}, P_{21}]^T \text{ and } \quad P_D = \left[P_{D_{00}}, P_{D_{01}}, P_{D_{10}}, P_{D_{11}}, P_{D_{20}}, P_{D_{21}}\right]^T$$

The joint probabilities of the gene and environment variables in both the general population and disease population follow multinomial distributions with the following covariance matrices.

$$\Sigma = diag(P) - PP^T \quad \text{and} \quad \Sigma_D = diag(P_D) - P_D P_D^T.$$

Let the Jacobean matrices of f and f_D with respect to P and f_D be $B = \left(\frac{\partial f_D}{\partial P_D^T}\right)$ and $C = \left(\frac{\partial f}{\partial P^T}\right)$, respectively. It is easy to see that

$$\frac{\partial f_{ij}}{\partial P_{ij}} = \log \frac{P_{ij}}{P_{i.}P_{.j}} - \frac{P_{ij}}{P_{i.}} - \frac{P_{ij}}{P_{.j}} + 1, \underset{(l \neq j)}{\frac{\partial f_{ij}}{\partial P_{il}}} = -\frac{P_{ij}}{P_{i.}}, \underset{(k \neq i)}{\frac{\partial f_{ij}}{\partial P_{kj}}} = -\frac{P_{ij}}{P_{.j}}, \underset{(k \neq i, l \neq j)}{\frac{\partial f_{ij}}{\partial P_{kl}}} = 0$$

where $P_i = \sum_{j=0}^{1} P_{ij}$, and $P_j = \sum_{i=0}^{2} P_{ij}$. The partial derivatives of the function $f_{D_{ij}}$ with respect to $P_{D_{kl}}$ can be similarly defined. Let n_A be the number of sampled individuals in the cases and n_G be the number of sampled individuals in the controls. Define

$$\Lambda = \frac{B\Sigma_D B^T}{n_A} + \frac{C\Sigma C^T}{n_G}.$$

The statistic for testing the gene–environment interactions is then defined as

$$T_{MIS} = \left(\hat{f}_D - \hat{f}\right)^T \hat{\Lambda}^- \left(\hat{f}_D - \hat{f}\right) \tag{34}$$

where $\hat{f}, \hat{f}_D$, and $\hat{\Lambda}$ are the estimators of f, f_D, and Λ. $\hat{\Lambda}^-$ is a generalized inverse of the matrix $\hat{\Lambda}$

When the sample size is sufficiently large enough to ensure application of the large sample theory, the test statistic T_{MIS} is asymptotically distributed as a central $\chi^2_{(2)}$ distribution under the null hypothesis of the no gene–environment interactions, if we assume that the gene and environment variables in the general population are independent.

In many cases, the gene and environment variables may not be independent in general population. Therefore, in these cases, using the statistic T_{MIS} to test gene–environment interaction is inappropriate. We extend the information-based statistic for testing gene–environment interaction to a general case where the gene and environment variables can be dependent. Information measure of gene–environment interaction (Equation 16) can be rewritten as

$$I_{GE} = \sum_{i=0}^{2}\sum_{j=0}^{1} P_{Dij} \log \frac{P_{Dij}P_{i.}P_{.j}}{P_{Di.}P_{D.j}P_{ij}}. \tag{35}$$

To calculate the variance of the estimate of I_{GE}, we first calculate the partial derivatives of I_{GE}:

$$\frac{\partial I_{GE}}{\partial P_{Dij}} = \log \frac{P_{Dij}P_{i.}P_{.j}}{P_{Di.}P_{D.j}P_{ij}} - 1 \quad \text{and}$$

$$\frac{\partial I_{GE}}{\partial P_{ij}} = P_{Dij}\left(\frac{1}{P_{i.}} + \frac{1}{P_{.j}} - \frac{1}{P_{ij}}\right) + \frac{\sum\limits_{l \neq j} P_{Dil}}{P_{i.}} + \frac{\sum\limits_{k \neq i} P_{Dkj}}{P_{.j}}.$$

Then, using the delta method, we can obtain the approximate variance of I_{GE}:

$$V_{MI} = \frac{1}{n_A}\left\{\sum_{i=0}^{2}\sum_{j=0}^{1}\left(\frac{\partial I_{GE}}{\partial P_{Dij}}\right)^2 P_{Dij} - \left(\sum_{i=0}^{2}\sum_{j=0}^{1}\frac{\partial I_{GE}}{\partial P_{Dij}} P_{Dij}\right)^2\right\}$$
$$+\frac{1}{n_G}\left\{\sum_{i=0}^{2}\sum_{j=0}^{1}\left(\frac{\partial I_{GE}}{\partial P_{ij}}\right)^2 P_{ij} - \left(\sum_{i=0}^{2}\sum_{j=0}^{1}\frac{\partial I_{GE}}{\partial P_{ij}} P_{ij}\right)^2\right\}.$$

An information-based statistic for testing gene–environment interaction can then be defined as

$$T_{MI} = \frac{I_{GE}^2}{V_{MI}}, \tag{36}$$

which is asymptotically distributed as a central $\chi^2_{(1)}$ distribution under the null hypothesis of the no gene–environment interactions.

If we assume that the gene and environment variables in the general population are independent, then under the null hypothesis of no gene–environment interaction, the variance V_{MI} will become zero. In this case, the test statistic T_{MI} will become undefined. We either use statistic T_{MIS} defined in Equation (34) for testing gene–environment interaction or use the following statistic to test for gene–environment interaction:

$$T_{MII} = 2n_A \sum_{i=0}^{2} \sum_{j-0}^{1} P_{Dij} \log \frac{P_{Dij}}{P_{Di.}P_{D.j}} \quad (37)$$

which is asymptotically distributed as a central $\chi^2_{(1)}$ distribution (Brillinger, 2004). In practice, it is not convenient to test independence of gene and environment variables. Therefore, we need to develop statistics for testing gene–environment interaction which can be applied to both independent and dependent cases.

Let $x_{ij} = P_{Dij} \log \frac{P_{Dij}P_{i.}P_{.j}}{P_{Di.}P_{D.j}P_{ij}}$ and $X = [x_{00}, x_{01}, ..., x_{21}]^T$. Then, its partial derivatives with respect to P_{Dij} and P_{ij} are given by

$$\frac{\partial x_{ij}}{\partial P_{Dij}} = \log \frac{P_{Dij}P_{i.}P_{.j}}{P_{Di.}P_{D.j}P_{ij}} + P_{Dij}\left(\frac{1}{P_{Dij}} - \frac{1}{P_{Di.}} - \frac{1}{P_{D.j}}\right),$$

$$\underset{l \neq j}{\frac{\partial x_{ij}}{\partial P_{Dil}}} = -\frac{P_{Dij}}{P_{Di.}}, \underset{k \neq i}{\frac{\partial x_{ij}}{\partial P_{Dkj}}} = -\frac{P_{Dij}}{P_{D.j}}, \underset{k \neq i, l \neq j}{\frac{\partial x_{ij}}{\partial P_{Dkl}}} = 0,$$

$$\frac{\partial x_{ij}}{\partial P_{ij}} = P_{Dij}\left(\frac{1}{P_{i.}} + \frac{1}{P_{.j}} - \frac{1}{P_{ij}}\right), \underset{l \neq j}{\frac{\partial x_{ij}}{\partial P_{il}}} = \frac{P_{Dij}}{P_{i.}}, \underset{k \neq i}{\frac{\partial x_{ij}}{\partial P_{kj}}} = \frac{P_{Dij}}{P_{.j}} \text{ and}$$

$$\underset{k \neq i, l \neq j}{\frac{\partial x_{ij}}{\partial P_{kl}}} = 0.$$

Assume that the vectors P_{D} and P, the matrices Σ and Σ_D are defined as before. Let

$$B_I = \left(\frac{\partial X}{\partial P_D^T}\right) \quad \text{and} \quad C_I = \left(\frac{\partial X}{\partial P^T}\right).$$

Then, the covariance matrix of X is given by

$$\Lambda_I = \frac{B_I \Sigma_D B_I^T}{n_A} + \frac{C_I \Sigma C_I^T}{n_G}.$$

Define the statistic for testing gene–environment interaction as

$$T_{MIB} = \hat{X}^T \hat{\Lambda}_I^{-1} \hat{X}. \quad (38)$$

We can show that under null hypothesis of no gene–environment interaction, the statistic T_{MIB} is asymptotically distributed as a central $\chi^2_{(2)}$ distribution regardless of whether the gene and environment variables in the general population are independent or not. Therefore, statistic T_{MIB} can be used to test for gene–environment interaction in any cases.

3.4.4 Multiplicative Measure-Based Statistics for Testing Interaction Between Gene and Continuous Environment

Under the assumption of normal distribution of the continuous environment, the average multiplicative measure of gene–environment interaction is defined as

$$I_{MGE} = \log \frac{\mu_{D0}\mu_1}{\mu_{D1}\mu_0} + \frac{1}{2} \log \frac{\sigma_{D0}^2 \sigma_1^2}{\sigma_{D1}^2 \sigma_0^2}.$$

To develop statistic for testing interaction between discrete genotype and continuous environment, we first should study the distributions of the estimates of the means and variances of the environments in cases and general population. Let n_0, n_1, n_{D_0} and n_{D_1} be the number of individuals with the genotypes $G = 0$ and $G = 1$ in the general population and cases, respectively. Let $Y_n = \left[\hat{\mu}_0, \hat{\mu}_1, \hat{\mu}_{D_0}, \hat{\mu}_{D_1}, \hat{\sigma}_0^2, \hat{\sigma}_1^2, \hat{\sigma}_{D_0}^2, \hat{\sigma}_{D_1}\right]^T$. Then, from the standard asymptotical theory (Theorems 3.3.2 and 3.4.4 in Anderson, 1984), Y_n is asymptotically distributed as a normal distribution with the mean $\tau = \left[\mu_0, \mu_1, \mu_{D_0}, \mu_{D_1}, \sigma_0^2, \sigma_1^2, \sigma_{D_0}^2, \sigma_{D_1}\right]^T$ and covariance matrix $\Sigma = diag\left(\frac{\sigma_0^2}{n_0}, \frac{\sigma_1^2}{n_1}, \frac{\sigma_{D_0}^2}{n_{D_0}}, \frac{\sigma_{D_1}^2}{n_{D_1}}, \frac{2\sigma_0^4}{n_0-1}, \frac{2\sigma_1^4}{n_1-1}, \frac{2\sigma_{D_0}^2}{n_{D_0}-1}, \frac{2\sigma_{D_1}^2}{n_{D_1}-1}\right)$. Then, by the asymptotical theory of functions of asymptotically normal statistics (Lehmann, 1983), we can show that under the null hypothesis of no gene–environment interaction, the estimate of the multiplicative interaction measure of gene–environment interaction is distributed as a normal distribution with mean of zero and variance

$$V_{MGE} = \frac{\sigma_0^2}{n_0\mu_0^2} + \frac{\sigma_1^2}{n_1\mu_1^2} + \frac{\sigma_{D_0}^2}{n_{D_0}\mu_{D_0}^2} + \frac{\sigma_{D_1}^2}{n_{D_1}\mu_{D_1}^2} + \frac{1}{2(n_0-1)} + \frac{1}{2(n_1-1)} + \frac{1}{2(n_{D_0}-1)} + \frac{1}{2(n_{D_1}-1)}.$$

Therefore, we can define the following statistic for testing interaction between gene and continuous environment:

$$T_{GCE} = \frac{I_{MGE}^2}{V_{MGE}}. \tag{39}$$

Under the null hypothesis of no gene–environment interaction, the statistic T_{GCE} is asymptotically distributed as a central $\chi_{(1)}^2$ distribution.

3.4.5 Information Measure-Based Statistics for Testing Interaction Between Gene and Continuous Environment

Similar to Section 3.4.4, we can also use asymptotical theory of nonlinear transformation of given statistics to develop information measure-based statistic to test for interaction between gene and continuous variable. Let $n = n_0 + n_1$ and $n_D = n_{D_0} + n_{D_1}$. Other quantities are defined as before. Recall that the information measure of interaction between gene and continuous environment is defined as

$$\begin{aligned}
I_{GCE} &= \frac{1}{2}\log\frac{\sigma_D^2}{\sigma^2} - \frac{1}{2}\left[P(G=0|D)\log\frac{\sigma_{D_0}^2}{\sigma_0^2} + P(G=1|D)\log\frac{\sigma_{D_1}^2}{\sigma_1^2}\right] \\
&\quad - \frac{\sigma_D^2 + (\mu_D - \mu)^2}{2\sigma^2} + P(G=0|D)\frac{\sigma_{D_0}^2 + (\mu_{D_0} - \mu_0)^2}{2\sigma_0^2} \\
&\quad + P(G=1|D)\frac{\sigma_{D_1}^2 + (\mu_{D_1} - \mu_1)^2}{2\sigma_1^2}.
\end{aligned}$$

Then, the variance of the estimate of I_{GCE} is given by

$$\begin{aligned}
V_{GCE} &= \frac{P_{D_0}^2(\mu_{D_0} - \mu_0)^2}{n_0\sigma_0^2} + \frac{P_{D_1}^2(\mu_{D_1} - \mu_1)^2}{n_1\sigma_1^2} + \frac{P_{D_0}^2(\mu_{D_0} - \mu_D)^2\sigma_{D_0}^2}{n_{D_0}\sigma_0^4} \\
&\quad + \frac{P_{D_1}^2(\mu_{D_1} - \mu_1)^2\sigma_{D_1}^2}{n_{D_1}\sigma_1^4} + \frac{(\mu_D - \mu)^2}{n\sigma^2} + \frac{(\mu_D - \mu)^2\sigma_D^2}{n_D\sigma^4} \\
&\quad + \frac{P_{D_0}^2\sigma_0^4}{2n_0}\left[\frac{1}{\sigma_0^2} - \frac{\sigma_{D_0}^2 + (\mu_{D_0} - \mu_0)^2}{\sigma_0^4}\right] \\
&\quad + \frac{P_{D_1}^2\sigma_1^4}{n_1}\left[\frac{1}{\sigma_1^2} - \frac{\sigma_{D_1}^2 + (\mu_{D_1} - \mu_1)^2}{\sigma_1^4}\right] \\
&\quad + \frac{P_{D_0}^2\sigma_{D_0}^4}{2n_{D_0}}\left(\frac{1}{\sigma_0^2} - \frac{1}{\sigma_{D_0}^2}\right)^2 + \frac{P_{D_1}^2\sigma_{D_1}^4}{2n_{D_1}}\left(\frac{1}{\sigma_1^2} - \frac{1}{\sigma_{D_1}^2}\right)^2 \\
&\quad + \frac{\sigma^4}{2n}\left(\frac{1}{\sigma^2} - \frac{\sigma_D^2 + (\mu_D - \mu)^2}{\sigma^4}\right)^2 + \frac{\sigma_D^4}{2n_D}\left(\frac{1}{\sigma_D^2} - \frac{1}{\sigma^2}\right)^2.
\end{aligned}$$

After we calculate the variance of the estimate of I_{GCE} we can define the following information-based statistic to test for interaction between gene and continuous environment:

$$T_{MIGCE} = \frac{\hat{I}_{GCE}^2}{\hat{V}_{GCE}}, \tag{40}$$

which will asymptotically distributed as a central $\chi^2_{(1)}$ distribution under the null hypothesis of no gene–environment interaction.

3.5 Canonical Correlation for Testing Interaction Between a Gene (Multiple SNPs) and Environment

In the previous sections, the measure of interaction between gene and environment is defined as the interaction between an individual locus (or SNP) and environment. However, a gene consists of multiple loci. Some loci within the gene may have interactions with environment, and some may not. To accurately measure interaction between the gene and environment, we need to extend the concept of interaction between one locus and an environment to the interaction between multiple loci and an environment.

Assume that a gene has K loci: $G_1, ..., G_k$. Each locus G_j is coded as 1 or 0. Let $P_j = P(G_j = 1), P_E = P(E = 1), P_{j11} = P(E = 1, G_j = 1), P_{j21} = P(E = 0, G_j = 1), P_{j12} = P(E = 1, G_j = 0)$ and $P_{j22} = P(E = 0, G_j = 0)$. Define the linkage disequilibrium between two loci G_j and G_k:

$$\delta_{jk} = q_{jk} - P_j P_k,$$

where $q_{jk} = P(G_j = 1, G_k = 1)$. If we view the disequilibrium as a measure of dependence between two random variables, similar to linkage disequilibrium between two loci, we can define the disequilibrium between a locus G_j and an environment E as

$$\delta_{jGE} = P_{j11}P_{j22} - P_{j12}P_{j21}.$$

The corresponding quantities in the disease population are denoted by $P_j^A, P_E^A, P_{j11}^A, P_{j12}^A, P_{j21}^A, P_{j22}^A, q_{jk}^A, \delta_{jk}^A$ and δ_{jGE}^A. Define indicator variables:

$$Y_{ij} = \begin{cases} 1 & G_{ij} = 1 \\ 0 & G_{ij} = 0 \end{cases}$$

for the i-th individual cases and

$$X_{ij} = \begin{cases} 1 & G_{ij} = 1 \\ 0 & G_{ij} = 0 \end{cases}$$

for the i-th individual in general population. The variance and covariance of indicator variables are given by

$$\sigma_{jj} = \mathrm{cov}(Y_j, Y_j) = P_j^A\left(1 - P_j^A\right), \sigma_{jk} = \mathrm{cov}(Y_j, Y_k) = q_{jk}^A - P_j^A P_k^A = \delta_{jk}^A$$

Let E^A and E be the environmental variable in cases and general population, respectively, $\overline{E}^A$ and $\overline{E}$ be their corresponding average, $\bar{Y}_j = \frac{1}{n_A}\sum_{i=1}^{n_A} Y_{ij}$ and $\bar{X}_j = \frac{1}{n_G}\sum_{i=1}^{n_G} X_{ij}$. Define

$$Z_j = \bar{Y}_j - \frac{P^A_{j11}P^A_{j22}}{P_{j11}P_{j22}}\bar{X}_j$$

and

$$E^* = n_A\overline{E}^A + n_G\overline{E}.$$

Let $Z = [Z_1, Z_2, ..., Z_k]^T$. Their variance and covariance are given by

$$\sigma_{z_iz_i} = \frac{1}{n_A}P^A_j\left(1 - P^A_j\right) + \frac{1}{n_G}\left(\frac{P^A_{j11}P^A_{j22}}{P_{j11}P_{j22}}\right)^2 P_j(1 - P_j) \quad \text{and}$$

$$\sigma_{z_iz_j} = \frac{1}{n_A}\delta^A_{ij} + \frac{P^A_{i11}P^A_{i22}P^A_{j11}P^A_{j22}}{n_G P_{i11}P_{i22}P_{j11}P_{j22}}\delta_{ij}.$$

We can also calculate the variance of E^* and covariance of E^* and Z_j:

$$\Lambda_{EE} = \text{var}(E^*) = \frac{1}{n_A}P^A_E\left(1 - P^A_E\right) + \frac{1}{n_G}P_E\left(1 - P_E\right),$$

$$Cov(E^*, Z_j) = \delta^A_{jGE} - \frac{P^A_{j11}P^A_{j22}}{P_{j11}P_{j22}}\delta_{jGE}.$$

The covariance matrix of $[E^*, Z^T]^T$ is given by

$$\Lambda = \begin{bmatrix} \Lambda_{EE} & \Lambda_{EZ} \\ \Lambda_{ZE} & \Lambda_{ZZ} \end{bmatrix}, \qquad (41)$$

where the vectors $\Lambda_{EZ} = [\text{cov}(E^*Z_1), ..., \text{cov}(E^*, Z_k)]$, $\Lambda_{ZE} = \Lambda^T_{EZ}$ and $\Lambda_{ZZ} = (\sigma_{z_iz_j})_{k\times k}$.

Intuitively, interaction between a locus (SNP) and an environment indicates the strong dependence between SNP and environment. Since a gene consists of multiple loci, the interaction between a gene (multiple SNPs) and an environment implies the dependences between multiple SNPs and the environment. A powerful tool for studying the dependence between two sets of variables is canonical correlation analysis. Canonical correlation analysis investigates the correlation between a linear combination of the variables in one set and a linear combination of the variables in another set (Johnson and Wichern, 2002). The set of pairs of linear combinations that are orthogonal and have the largest correlations are referred to as canonical variables and their correlations are referred to as canonical correlations. The canonical correlations quantify the strength of association between the two set of variables. Canonical correlation analysis can be applied to investigation of interaction between the gene (multiple SNPs) and environment where we study correlation between a set of variables (SNPs) and an environmental variable (but not a set of variables).

We study the canonical correlations between the environment variable $E^*$and the group of SNPs represented by the vector Z. For convenience, we consider E^* and Z jointly and let $W = [E^*, Z^T]^T$. The covariance matrix of W is given by Equation (41). Motivated by canonical correlation between $E^*$and Z, we define the measure of interaction between the environment and K loci as

$$I_{GE}^{gene} = \frac{\Lambda_{EZ}\Lambda_{ZZ}^{-1}\Lambda_{ZE}}{\Lambda_{EE}}, \tag{42}$$

which is the square of the canonical correlation between E^* and Z. Let the ijth element of the matrix Λ_{ZZ}^{-1} be r_{ij}. Then, Equation (42) can be reduced to

$$\begin{aligned} I_{GE}^{gene} &= \frac{1}{\frac{1}{n_E}P_E^A\left(1-P_E^A\right)+\frac{1}{n_G}P_E(1-P_E)}\sum_{i=1}^{k}\sum_{j=1}^{k} r_{ij}\left(\delta_{iGE}^A - \frac{P_{i11}^A P_{i22}^A}{P_{i11}P_{i22}}\delta_{iGE}\right) \\ &\quad \left(\delta_{jGE}^A - \frac{P_{j11}^A P_{j22}^A}{P_{j11}P_{j22}}\delta_{jGE}\right) \\ &= \frac{1}{\frac{1}{n_E}P_E^A\left(1-P_E^A\right)+\frac{1}{n_G}P_E(1-P_E)}\sum_{i=1}^{k}\sum_{j=1}^{k}\frac{P_{i12}P_{i21}P_{j12}P_{j21}}{P_D^4} r_{ij} I_{EG_i} I_{EG_j} \end{aligned} \tag{43}$$

where P_D is the preference of the disease, I_{EG_i} and I_{EG_j} are the interaction between the environment and the i-th locus, j-th locus, respectively. Since Λ_{ZZ} is a positive definite matrix, from Equation (42) it is clear that the measure of interaction I_{GE}^{gene} is nonnegative, i.e. $I_{GE}^{gene} \geq 0$ and that $I_{GE}^{gene} = 0$ if and only if all the elements in the vector Λ_{EZ} are equal to zero. However, the elements in the vector Λ_{EZ} are given by

$$Cov(E^*, Z_j) = \delta_{jGE}^A - \frac{P_{j11}^A P_{j22}^A}{P_{j11}P_{j22}}\delta_{jGE} = \frac{P_{j12}P_{j21}}{P_D^2} I_{EG_j}.$$

Therefore, $I_{GE}^{gene} = 0$ if and only if all the measures of interaction between the locus $G_j(j = 1,..,k)$ and environment $I_{EG_j}, j = 1,...,k$ are equal to zero. In other words, The absence of interaction between the environment and gene (multiple SNPs) requires that there is no interaction between the environment and any SNP within the gene. To test for interaction between the environment and gene, we use a gene as the basic unit of analysis. Instead of testing for interaction between the environment and single SNP, we jointly test for interaction between the environment and all SNPs within the gene.

Thus, the null hypothesis of no gene–environment interaction is equivalent to the null hypothesis that $\Lambda_{EZ} = 0$. The likelihood ratio test of $H_0 : \Lambda_{EZ} = 0$ versus $H_a : \Lambda_{EZ} \neq 0$ is defined as

$$T_{GE}^{gene} = \log\left(\frac{|\hat{\Lambda}_{EE}||\hat{\Lambda}_{ZZ}|}{|\hat{\Lambda}|}\right) = -\log\left(1 - \hat{I}_{GE}^{gene}\right),$$

where $\hat{\Lambda}$, $\hat{\Lambda}_{EE}$, $\hat{\Lambda}_{ZZ}$ and $\hat{I}_{GE}^{gene}$ are the estimates of Λ, Λ_{EE}, Λ_{ZZ} and I_{GE}^{gene}.

Bartlett (Anderson, 1984) suggested to modify the above likelihood ratio statistic for testing the null hypothesis of $H_0 : \Lambda_{EZ} = 0$ as

$$T_{GE}^{gene} = \frac{k-2}{2}\log\left(1 - \hat{I}_{GE}^{gene}\right). \tag{44}$$

Therefore, we will use Bartlett's modification (44) to test for interaction between the gene (multiple SNPs) and environment. The statistic T_{GE}^{gene} is asymptotically distributed as a central $\chi^2_{(k)}$ distribution under the null hypothesis of no gene–environment interaction and a noncentral $\chi^2_{(k)}$ distribution under the alternative hypothesis of presence of gene–environment interaction. The noncentrality parameter is a function of the measure of gene–environment interaction. From Equation (44) it is clearly seen that $T_{GE}^{gene} = 0$ if and only if $I_{GE}^{gene} = 0$. If the prevalence of the disease is small, the statistic T_{GE}^{gene} can be applied to case-control study design.

3.6 Gene–Environment Interaction in Cancers

Cancer is the result of a series of somatic DNA alternations that are responsible for conversion of exogenous exposures into intermediate metabolites, affecting cell growth, DNA repair, cell cycle control, apoptosis, regulation and development of the immune system, angiogenesis, and influencing behaviors such as smoking, alcohol consumption and excess calorie intake (Brennan, 2002). For many years, genetic and environmental cancer risk factors have often been studied separately. However, genetic and environment exposure work together to cause cancers. In the absence of environmental exposure, the presence of genetic risk factors may not cause cancers. However, in the presence of exposure, genetic variants can modify the association of environmental exposure with cancer (Taioli, 2008). The environment can be taken as the context in which the genetic variants act (Giarelli and Jacobs, 2005). Research in the past several decades has concluded that large proportion of cancers may be caused by environmental exposure. Genetic variants often affect a person's response to environmental exposure, they are thus considered as effect modifiers.

Interaction between tobacco smoke and genetic factors is a typical example of gene–environment interaction in cancers. More than 3,000 chemicals have been isolated from tobacco leaves and more than 4,000 reaction products are generated when tobacco is burned (Taioli, 2008). It is also found that approximately 60 known carcinogens are present in tobacco smoke. Many constituents of tobacco are entered into the body via the airways and then reach the tissues and organs. Tobacco smoking is not only an important risk factor of lung cancer, but also plays a crucial role in the development of nose, pancreas, bladder, kidney, stomach, liver, colon, oral cavity, oropharynx, hypopharynx, larynx, esophagus, cervix and myeloid leukemia cancers (Taioli, 2008). The interaction between tobacco smoke and the genetic variants involved in the pathway of tobacco metabolism and DNA repair such as GSTM1, GST1, CYP1A1 and NAT2 in number of cancer studies has been reported.

Thorgeirsson et al. (2008) conducted a genome-wide studies of lung cancer in which a set of 306,207 single-nucleotide polymorphisms (SNPs) were typed in 10,995 Icelandic smokers. Allele T of the SNP rs1051730 in the nicotinic acetylcholine receptor gene cluster on chromosome 15q24 was most strongly associated with smoking quantity. Two other studies (Hung et al., 2008, with 317,139 SNPs typed in 1,989 lung cancer cases and 2,625 controls from six central European countries, and Amos et al., 2008, with 315,450 tagging SNPs typed in 1,154 current and former (ever) smoking cases of European ancestry and 1,137 frequency-matched, ever-smoking controls from Houston, Texas) also detected the association of the nicotinic acetylcholine receptor gene cluster on chromosome 15q24 with lung cancer, but failed to detect interaction between the nicotinic acetylcholine receptor gene cluster and tobacco smoking.

Other examples of gene and environment interactions have been presented in the literature. Interaction between EXO1 genotypes and smoking habit is detected in oral cancer (Tsai et al., 2009). An interaction between TP53 intron 3 16-bp repeats and multiple X-ray exposures has been observed in lung cancer (Hall et al., 2009). Andrew et al. (2009) performed a population-based study of bladder cancer with XRCC3, ERCC2 genotype/haplotype and arsenic exposure data on 549 controls and 342 cases and found interaction between a variant allele of the double-strand break repair gene XRCC3 T241M and arsenic exposure (adjusted OR 2.8 (1.1–7.3)). A study with 471 gastric cancer patients and 471 age-and sex-matched control subjects was conducted and interaction between NAT2 genotype and environmental dietary carcinogens was detected (Zhang et al., 2009). Alcohol or tobacco use (both smoking and chewing) were also found to interact with variant genotypes of CYP2E1 in significantly enhancing head and neck squamous cell carcinoma (Ruwali et al., 2009). To test interaction between BRCA mutations and diet diversity in breast cancer (BC), a case-only study was carried out in 738 cases from a French-Canadian population. Unconditional logistic regression was used to reveal a significant interaction between BRCA mutations and vegetable and fruit diversity (COR = 0.27; 95%CI = 0.10–0.80; P = 0.03) (Ghadirian et al., 2009). To assess the interaction between Organochlorine exposure and immune gene variation in non-Hodgkin lymphoma, 61 polymorphisms were genotyped in 36 immune genes in 1,172 NHL cases and 982 controls from the National Cancer Institute-Surveillance, Epidemiology, and End Results (NCI-SEER) study. Three exposures with elevated risk in this study: PCB180 (plasma, dust measurements), the toxic equivalency quotient (an integrated functional measure of several organochlorines) in plasma, and alpha-chlordane (dust measurements, self-reported termiticide use) were investigated. Unconditional logistic regression was used to test interaction. The results showed that the NHL risk by organochlorine exposure may depend on particular variants in immune genes: IFNG, IL4, IL8, IL10 and IL16 (Colt et al., 2009). A molecular epidemiology of colorectal cancer study with 625 cases and 623 controls was performed to test for interaction between recreational physical activity and insulin-like growth factor (IGF-I). An association was reported with decreased risk among individuals with no physical activity (odds ratio, 0.76; 95% confidence interval, 0.52–0.98), whereas the same genotype was marginally associated with increased risk among individuals who reported physical activity (odds ratio, 1.38; 95% confidence interval, 0.98–1.94), which implied an interaction between physical activity and the growth hormone/IGF-I system. The interaction between physical activity and the growth hormone/IGF-I was replicated in second study with 777 cases, 1,016 controls (Khoury-Shakour et al., 2008). To test interaction of genetic polymorphisms in methylenetetrahydrofolate reductase (MTHFR) and cytochrome P4502E1 (CYP4502E1) and environmental risks: green vegetables and fresh fruits, alcohol drinking, and unsafe water (shallow well, or river) in esophageal cancer, a case-control study with 120 cases and 240 controls in a high incidence area of Xinjiang Uygur autonomous region, China was conducted. A conditional logistic regression model was used to assess interaction. MTHFR 677 gene polymorphism was correlated with consumption of green vegetables and fresh fruit, while CYP4502E1 C1/C1 was correlated with alcohol drinking and unsafe drinking water (Qin et al., 2008). A case-only analyses ($n = 577$) and case-unaffected sibling comparisons ($n = 307$ sibships) were used to test interaction between polymorphisms in the nucleotide excision repair (NER) (ERCC1 $3'$ untranslated region (UTR) G/T, XPD Asp312Asn and Lys751Gln, XPC intron 11 C/A, XPA $5'$ UTR C/T, XPF Arg415Gln and XPG Asp1104His) and mismatch repair (MLH1 Ile219Val and MSH2 Gly322Asp) pathways, and red meat and poultry intake in colorectal cancer. Interactions between intake of red meat heavily brown on the outside or inside and the XPD codon 751 Lys/Lys genotype (case-only interaction $P = 0.006$ and $P = 0.001$, respectively, for doneness outside or inside), or the XPD codon 312 Asp/Asp genotype (case-only interaction $P = 0.090$ and $P < 0.001$, respectively) were detected (Joshi et al., 2009).

3.7 Real Examples for Application of Different Measures of Gene and Environment Interactions

To illustrate how to test for gene–environment interactions, the odds ratio-based statistics, disequilibrium-based statistic and the mutual information-based statistics T_{GE} and T_{G_iE} were applied to three real data examples (Wu et al., 2009). Odds-ratio multiplicative model-based statistic and logistic regression are equivalent. Therefore, only logistic regression was listed in the results. The first example studied the interaction between the polymorphism of the gene excision repair cross-complementing group 2 (ERCC2) and smoking exposure in lung cancer (Zhou et al., 2002), where two ERCC2 polymorphisms Asp312Asn and Lys751Gln were typed in 1,092 Caucasian lung cancer patients and 1,240 spouse and friend controls collected at Massachusetts General Hospital. Both ERCC2 polymorphisms in the controls were in Hardy-Weinberg equilibrium. Smoking exposure was classified into four categories: non smoking, mild smoking, moderate smoking and heavy smoking. For simplicity of comparison, we performed only crude analysis. In other words, analysis was performed only for the raw data that were not adjusted for age and gender. Odds-ratio (additive), logistic regression or odds ratio (multiplicative), disequilibrium and the mutual information-based statistics were used to test interaction between the polymorphism of ERCC2 and smoking in lung cancer. The results were summarized in Table 3.4 where "Logistic" denoted logistic regression, "Odds (add)" denoted the odds ratio additive measure-based statistic defined in Equation (29) and "Disq" denoted disequilibrium-based statistic defined in Equation (32). In general, logistic regression, odds ratio and disequilibrium-based statistics will not be used to test interaction between a single genotype and environment, thus there was no p-value to test interaction between the single genotype and environment for logistic regression, odds ratio and disequilibrium-based statistics in Table 3.4. Two features emerge from Table 3.4. First, in general, the p-values of the global test statistic T_{GE} were smaller than that of the T_{G_iE} for testing interaction between the particular genotype (single genotype) and environment. Second, in most cases, the p-values of the mutual information-based global test statistic T_{GE} were smaller than that of other three statistics.

The second example is the interaction between the gene SULT1A1 and smoking/alcohol consumption for squamous cell carcinoma of the oesophagus (Dandara et al., 2006). The gene SULT1A1 catalyses sulfation that is related to the metabolism of a broad range of compounds such as phenolic xenobiotics, hydroxylated aromatic amines and drugs. The gene SULT1A1 is suspected to play a role in esophageal cancer. We applied mutual information-based statistics, logistic regression, odds ratio additive measure-based statistic and disequilibrium-based statistic to this dataset to test for gene–environment interactions. The data in Table 3.5 were from Dandara's Table 3.4 for the mixed ancestry South African group. The P-values of mutual information-based statistics and other three statistics were listed in Table 3.5. Using the mutual information-based statistics we detected the interaction between the gene SULT1A1 and smoking, or the combination of smoking and alcohol consumption in causing esophageal cancer in the mixed ancestry South African group. However, logistic regression analysis, odds ratio (additive model) and disequilibrium-based analysis failed to detect the interaction.

The third example is case-control study of interaction between smoking and HLA-DR SE (shared epitope) gene in the development of anticitrulline antibody-positive rheumatoid arthritis (RA) in the Swedish Epidemiological Investigation of Rheumatoid Arthritis (EIRA) study (Klareskog et al., 2006; Kallberg et al., 2007). The major environmental risk factor and genetic risk factor are smoking and HLA-DR shared epitope (SE), respectively. We analyzed data from Klareskog et al.

Table 3.4 Comparison of P-values for the mutual information-based statistics, Odds ratio-based statistics and disequilibrium-based statistic to the interaction between ERCC2 polymorphisms and smoking in lung cancer

	Smoking											
	Mild *P*-values				Moderate *P*-values				Heavy *P*-values			
	MI	Logistic	Odds (add)	Disq	MI	Logistic	Odds (add)	Disq	MI	Logistic	Odds (add)	Disq
Asp312Asn	0.003	0.015	0.408	0.116	5.7E-04	0.017	0.406	0.224	<E-10	0.001	0.043	0.001
Asp/Asp	0.068				0.345				5.1E-04			
Asp/Asn	0.112				0.246				0.474			
Asn/Asn	0.008				0.009				0.004			
Lys751Gln	0.054	0.161	0.300	0.256	1.2E-08	0.085	0.171	0.860	<E-10	0.006	0.023	0.002
Lys/Lys	0.020				0.087				9.50E-04			
Lys/Gln	0.639				0.388				0.242			
Gln/Gln	0.236				0.47				0.040			

Table 3.5 Comparison of *P*-values of the mutual information-based statistics, logistic regression (Odds ratio multiplicative model-based statistic), odds ratio (additive model) and disequilibrium based statistic for testing the interaction between the gene SULT1A1 and smoking (alcohol consumption) in the Mixed Ancestry South African group

					P-values			
SULT1A1 genotype	Patients		Controls		MI	Odds (add)	Disq	logistic
				Tobacco smoking				
	No	Yes	No	Yes	0.0194	0.2681	0.1040	0.2603
SULT1A1∗1/∗1	3	45	15	37	0.0536			
SULT1A1∗1/∗2	1	16	2	27	0.0096			
SULT1A1∗2/∗2	2	27	3	10	0.09152			
				Alcohol consumption				
	No	Yes	No	Yes	0.0863	0.4426	0.2390	0.3329
SULT1A1∗1/∗1	12	36	31	21	0.2443			
SULT1A1∗1/∗2	2	15	13	16	0.4105			
SULT1A1∗2/∗2	9	20	5	8	0.1648			
				Both smoking and alcohol consumption				
	No	Yes	No	Yes	0.0017	0.2218	0.0185	0.1105
SULT1A1∗1/∗1	2	35	15	21	0.0082			
SULT1A1∗1/∗2	1	15	2	16	0.0124			
SULT1A1∗2/∗2	2	20	2	7	0.4310			

(2006) which consisted of 827 RA patients and 1,216 controls and from Kallberg et al. (2007) which consisted of 1,883 RA patients and 1,589 controls. Clearly, the second study (Kallberg et al., 2007) is the extension of the first study (Klareskog et al., 2006). Mutual information-based, logistic regression, odds ratio (additive model)-based and disequilibrium-based statistics were applied to the dataset to test for interaction between the smoking and HLA-DR SE genes in the development of anticitrulline antibody-positive RA. The results are summarized in Table 3.6 and confirmed the recently described interaction between smoking and the HLA-DR SE in the development of RA (Linn-Rasker et al., 2006; Lundberg et al., 2005). We also see that as the sample size increased in the second dataset, the P-values became much smaller (from 0.0009 to $< 10^{-10}$). The results again showed that the P-values of the mutual information-based statistics are usually smaller than that of other three statistics and that the P-values of the global test statistic T_{GE} using all information at the locus are in general smaller than that of the test statistic T_{G_iE}. We also observe that in many cases the P-values of odds ratio (additive model) and disequilibrium-based statistics were smaller than that of logistic regression.

Table 3.6 Comparison of *P*-values of the mutual information-based statistics, logistic regression (Odds ratio multiplicative model-based statistic), odds ratio (additive model) and disequilibrium based statistic for testing the interaction between the smoking and HLA-DR SE genes in the development of anticitrulline antibody-positive RA

	Case		Control		*P*-values			
Sex, anti-CCP status and HLA-DR SE genes	Never smoked	Ever smoked	Never smoked	Ever smoked	MI	Odds (add)	Disq	Logistic
The data were from the paper (KLARESKOG et al. 2006)								
Male and Female								
Anti-CCP$^+$					9.3E-4	0.0006	0.0777	0.1362
No SE	20	58	87	184	0.0149			
Single SE	72	192	104	146	0.7090			
Double SE	36	126	31	31	0.0325			
Anti-CCP$^-$					0.2245	0.1583	0.1328	0.2055
No SE	65	84	87	184	0.2037			
Single SE	64	76	104	146	0.4170			
Double SE	18	18	31	31	0.4585			
Female								
Anti-CCP$^+$					0.2180	0.0112	0.5072	0.5202
No SE	18	41	74	115	0.4437			
Single SE	58	130	75	109	0.4989			
Double SE	30	89	25	25	0.0849			
Anti-CCP$^-$					0.3128	0.9722	0.9525	0.9561
No SE	50	62	74	115	0.4577			
Single SE	45	52	75	109	0.9805			
Double SE	15	11	25	25	0.8092			
Male								
Anti-CCP$^+$					6.7E-10	0.1780	0.0289	0.2853
No SE	2	17	13	69	2.6E-09			
Single SE	14	63	29	37	0.0574			
Double SE	6	37	6	6	0.2240			
Anti-CCP$^-$					0.0273			
No SE	15	24	13	69	0.0244	9.79E-04	5.06E-04	0.0199
Single SE	19	24	29	37	0.1519			
Double SE	3	7	6	6	0.1423			
Data were from the paper (KALLBERG et al. 2007)								
Anti-CCP$^+$					<E-10	4.54E-05	0.0312	0.0356
No SE	35	71	137	242	0.0240			
Single SE	105	270	138	198	0.6392			
Double SE	61	179	39	39	0.0455			
Anti-CCP$^-$					0.3844	0.3060	0.2560	0.2950
No SE	86	115	140	242	0.2795			
Single SE	87	123	138	198	0.3946			
Double SE	25	26	39	39	0.6170			

3.8 Conclusion

Genome-wide association studies (GWAS) that focused largely on the contribution of SNPs to diseases are the current major approach to dissecting complex genetic structure of the common diseases. In the past 2 years, these studies have identified more than 500 loci associated with common diseases. These results provide substantial information for understanding the mechanisms of the diseases. Although great progress in GWAS has been made, the significant SNP associations identified by GWAS account for only a few percent of the genetic variance. Complex disease are caused by genes, environment and their complex interactions. Identification of main genetic effects only might miss large proportion of genetic variants which interact with each other and with environments. Unraveling gene–gene and gene–environment interaction holds a key to the success of dissecting complex genetic structure of common diseases. To achieve this goal, several issues must be addressed.

The first issue is to define and measure interaction. Over the last three decades, epidemiologists have debated intensely about how to define and measure interaction in epidemiologic studies. The distinction between biological interaction and statistical interaction becomes an important issue. Biological interaction is often defined as interdependent operation of genetic and environmental factors that cause diseases. In other words, biological interaction means that joint presence of the genetic and environmental factors is the necessary condition for causing disease. Due to the complexity of disease development, it is difficult to directly observe biological interactions. Biological interactions are often indirectly inferred. The major challenge is to come up with a definition that is mathematically explicit and estimate the magnitude of the biological interaction as accurate as possible. In this chapter, we first review classical measures of gene–environment interaction for cohort and case-control designs. Then, we use the classical concept of conditional probability as a tool to define interaction. A key component to biological interaction is the dependence of developing disease with the presence of both genetic and environmental factors. Therefore, the conditional dependence of the genetic factor on the environmental factor in causing disease is a natural expression for biological interaction. This mathematical definition is an alternative to the definition of biological interaction as a departure from additivity. With this definition, interaction has a broader meaning and divergent statistical and computational tools available for measuring gene–environment interaction. In this chapter, we reviewed two recently proposed gene–environment interaction measures: disequilibrium and mutual information measures of gene–environment interaction for independent genetic and environmental factors in the general population, and extended them to the dependent cases of genetic and environmental variables in the general population.

The second issue is how to measure interaction between gene and continuous environmental exposure data. Widely used measures of interaction include relative risks or odds ratios which were originally defined for binary data. As a consequence, we often code genetic and environmental factors as binary variables for calculation of relative risks and odds ratios even if the genetic and environmental factors take multiple values or even continuous values. In this chapter, we extend relative risk, disequilibrium and mutual information measures of interaction between gene and binary environmental variable to measure interaction between gene and continuous environment. We proposed new concepts of point-wise interaction measure and average interaction measure. Under assumption of normal distribution of environment, we derive simple formula for calculation of average measures of interaction between gene and continuous environment.

The third issue is how to define measure of interaction between rare variants and environment. Next generation sequencing technologies will detect many rare variants. Rare variants have several inherent features that are largely different from the common genetic variants. First, rare variants are infrequent and irregularly spaced. Second, massive sequencing strategies result in the unbalanced sampling of parental alleles and produce large number of errors. The current measures of interaction between gene and environment are to quantify interaction between individual genetic variants and environment and are originally designed for common variants. These measures of gene–environment interaction are difficult to be applied to rare variants. Interaction between a single rare variant and environment may be small, but the overall measure of interaction between multiple rare variants and environment will be significant. In the presence of allelic heterogeneity, the power of current variant-by-variant tests for interaction between rare variants and environment will be too small. Therefore, instead of measuring interaction between individual rare variants and environment, we measure interaction between a group of rare variants and environment. We used canonical correlation analysis as a tool to develop a measure of interaction between a group of multiple variants and an environmental exposure and related statistic to test interaction between multiple rare variants and environment.

The forth issue is how to develop efficient statistics to detect gene–environment interactions. Despite current enthusiasm for investigation of interactions between the gene and environment, the essential issue of how to detect gene–environment interactions remains unresolved. Developing efficient analytical methods for evaluation of the gene–environment interactions is central to the investigation of gene–environment interactions. Logistic regression is predominantly used to test for gene–environment interactions in epidemiology. It depends on how to decompose the genetic effect. Most researchers use logistic regression to model odds as the additive combination of main effects of a single-locus and the environment, and a residual term. The residual term in the model is defined as a statistical interaction between the gene and environment. As a consequence, the major part of functional (or biological) gene–environment interactions may be included in the main effects. The remaining part of the functional gene–environment interactions which is treated as a residual term in the mathematical model is small. In this chapter, we presented several new statistics to detect gene–environment interactions. Preliminary results showed that these new statistics provide alternative to the classic statistics for testing gene–environment interaction.

The fifth issue is how to perform genome-wide gene–environment interaction analysis. Despite GWAS have become the current major approach to dissecting complex genetic structure of the common diseases, and the gene–gene and gene–environment interaction hold a key to uncovering the mechanism of complex diseases, few genome-wide gene–environment interaction analysis has been performed. Two major obstacles discourage genome-wide gene–environment interaction analysis. One is a lack of powerful statistics for testing interaction between gene and environment. Another one is P-value correction for multiple testing. If a million of SNPs are used for genome-wide gene–environment interaction analysis, the genome-wide P-values for declaring significant gene–environment interaction should be extremely small. In this chapter, instead of taking a single SNP as a basic unit for gene–environment interaction analysis, we take a whole gene containing a number of SNPs as a basic unit for gene–environment interaction analysis and develop statistic to jointly measure the interaction between the whole gene and environment. This approach has three important features. First, it uses all genetic information in the gene and hence may increase the magnitude of interaction. Second, it will reduce the number of tests for gene–environment interaction. Instead of testing million SNPs, we need only to test several tens of thousands of genes or regions. Third, it will dramatically reduce the computational time for genome-wide interaction analysis, which will make genome-wide interaction analysis practically feasible. We expect that the new paradigm for genome-wide interaction analysis will open a new avenue for interaction studies.

Gene–environment interactions are an important, but complex concept. There are a number of ways to define them. How the definition of gene–environment interactions in population level reflects their biochemical or physiological interaction is still a mystery. We hope that this review and introduction will provide further motivation to conduct theoretical research and large-scale data analysis in deciphering the genetic and physiological meaning of gene–environment interactions and to develop sophisticated statistical methods for testing gene–environment interactions. In the coming years, integration of gene–environment interactions into genome-wide association analysis will be a major task in genetic studies of complex diseases.

Acknowledgments M. Xiong are supported by grants from the National Institutes of Health NIAMS P01 AR052915-01A1 and NIAMS R01AR057120-01.

References

Altshuler D, Daly MJ, Lander ES (2008) Genetic mapping in human disease. Science. 322(5903):881–8.

Amos CI, Wu X, Broderick P, et al. (2008) Genome-wide association scan of tag SNPs identifies a susceptibility locus for lung cancer at 15q25.1. Nat Genet. 40:616–22.

Anderson TW (1984) An introduction to multivariate statistical analysis, 2nd Edition. John Wiley & Sons, New York.

Andrew AS, Mason RA, Kelsey KT, Schned AR, Marsit CJ, Nelson HH, Karagas MR (2009) DNA repair genotype interacts with arsenic exposure to increase bladder cancer risk. Toxicol Lett. 187(1):10–4.

Andrieu N, Goldstein AM (1998) Epidemiologic and genetic approaches in the study of gene–environment interaction: an overview of available methods. Epidemiol Rev. 20(2):137–47.

Ay N (2002) Locality of global stochastic interaction in directed acyclic networks. Neural Comput. 14:2959–80.

Brennan P (2002) Gene–environment interaction and aetiology of cancer: what does it mean and how can we measure it? Carcinogenesis. 3:381–7.

Brillinger DR (2004) Some data analyses using mutual information. Braz J Probab Stat. 18: 163–83.

Bush WS, Dudek SM, Ritchie MD (2006) Parallel multifactor dimensionality reduction: a tool for the large-scale analysis of gene–gene interactions. Bioinformatics. 22(17):2173–4.

Chaisson MJ, Brinza D, Pevzner PA (2009) De novo fragment assembly with short mate-paired reads: does the read length matter? Genome Res. 19(2):336–46.

Chatterjee N, Kalaylioglu Z, Moslehi R, Peters U, Wacholder S (2006) Powerful multilocus tests of genetic association in the presence of gene–gene and gene–environment interactions. Am J Hum Genet. 79(6):1002–100.

Cheverud JM, Routman EJ (1995) Epistasis and its contribution to genetic variance components. Genetics. 139:1455–61.

Chung Y, Lee SY, Elston RC, Park T (2007) Odds ratio based multifactor-dimensionality reduction method for detecting gene–gene interactions. Bioinformatics. 23(1):71–6.

Colt JS, Rothman N, Severson RK, Hartge P, Cerhan JR, Chatterjee N, Cozen W, Morton LM, De Roos AJ, Davis S, Chanock S, Wang SS (2009) Organochlorine exposure, immune gene variation, and risk of non-Hodgkin lymphoma. Blood. 113:1899–905.

Cordell HJ (2009) Detecting gene–gene interactions that underlie human diseases. Nat Rev Genet. 10:392–404.

Cover TM, Thomas JA (1991) Elements of information theory. John Wiley & Sons, New York.

Dandara C, Li DP, Walther G, Parker MI (2006) Gene–environment interaction: the role of SULT1A1 and CYP3A5 polymorphisms as risk modifiers for squamous cell carcinoma of the oesophagus. Carcinogenesis. 27:791–7.

Frazer KA, Murray SS, Schork NJ, Topol EJ (2009) Human genetic variation and its contribution to complex traits. Nat Rev Genet. 10(4):241–51.

Garcia-Closas M, Lubin JH (1999) Power and sample size calculations in case-control studies of gene–environment interactions: comments on different approaches. Am J Epidemiol. 149: 689–92.

Gauderman WJ (2002) Sample size requirements for matched case-control studies of gene–environment interaction. Stat Med. 21(1):35–50.

Ghadirian P, Narod S, Fafard E, Costa M, Robidoux A, Nkondjock A (2009). Breast cancer risk in relation to the joint effect of BRCA mutations and diet diversity. Breast Cancer Res Treat. 117:417–22.

Giarelli E, Jacobs LA (2005). Modifying cancer risk factors: the gene–environment interaction. Semin Oncol Nurs. 21:271–7.

Goldstein AM, Dondon MG, Andrieu N (2006) Unconditional analyses can increase efficiency in assessing gene–environment interaction of the case-combined-control design. Int J Epidemiol. 35(4):1067–73.

Goodman M, Dana Flanders W (2007) Study design options in evaluating gene–environment interactions: practical considerations for a planned case-control study of pediatric leukemia. Pediatr Blood Cancer. 48(4):375–9.

Hahn LW, Ritchie MD, Moore JH (2003) Multifactor dimensionality reduction software for detecting gene–gene and gene–environment interactions. Bioinformatics. 19:376–82.

Hall J, Marcel V, Bolin C, Fernet M, Tartier L, Vaslin L, Hainaut P (2009). The associations of sequence variants in DNA-repair and cell-cycle genes with cancer risk: genotype-phenotype correlations. Biochem Soc Trans. 37(Pt 3):527–33.

Hansen TF, Wagner GP (2001) Modeling genetic architecture a multilinear theory of gene interaction. Theor Popul Biol. 59:61–86.

Hindorff LA, Sethupathy P, Junkins HA, Ramos EM, Mehta JP, Collins FS, Manolio TA (2009). Potential etiologic and functional implications of genome-wide association loci for human diseases and traits. Proc Natl Acad Sci USA. 106(23):9362–7.

Hung RJ, McKay JD, Gaborieau V, Boffetta P, Hashibe M, Zaridze D, et al. (2008). A susceptibility locus for lung cancer maps to nicotinic acetylcholine receptor subunit genes on 15q25. Nature. 452:633–7.

Jakulin A (2005) Machine learning based on attribute interaction. Ph.D. Dissertation, University of Ljubljana, Sezana.

Johnson RA, Wichern DW (2002) Applied multivariate statistical analysis, 5th Edition. Prentice Hall, Upper Saddle River, NJ.

Johnson PL, Slatkin M (2007). Accounting for bias from sequencing error in population. Mol Biol Evol. 25:199–206.

Joshi AD, Corral R, Siegmund KD, Haile RW, Le Marchand L, Martínez ME, Ahnen DJ, Sandler RS, Lance P, Stern MC (2009). Red meat and poultry intake, polymorphisms in the nucleotide excision repair and mismatch repair pathways and colorectal cancer risk. Carcinogenesis. 30:472–9.

Kallberg H, Padyukov L, Plenge RM, Ronnelid J, Gregersen PK, et al. (2007) Gene–gene and gene–environment interactions involving HLA-DRB1, PTPN22, and smoking in two subsets of rheumatoid arthritis. Am J Hum Genet. 80:867–75.

Khoury MJ, Wacholder S (2009). Invited commentary: from genome-wide association studies to gene-environment-wide interaction studies-challenges and opportunities. Am J Epidemiol. 169:227–30.

Khoury-Shakour S, Gruber SB, Lejbkowicz F, Rennert HS, Raskin L, Pinchev M, Rennert G (2008). Recreational physical activity modifies the association between a common GH1 polymorphism and colorectal cancer risk. Cancer Epidemiol Biomarkers Prev. 17: 3314–18.

Klareskog L, Stolt P, Lundberg K, Kallberg H, Bengtsson C, et al. (2006) A new model for an etiology of rheumatoid arthritis: smoking may trigger HLA-DR (shared epitope)-restricted immune reactions to autoantigens modified by citrullination. Arthritis Rheum. 54:38–46.

Koopman JS (1977) Causal models and sources of interaction. Am J Epidemiol. 106:439–44.

Lehmann EL (1983) Theory of point estimation. John Wiley & Sons, New York, NY.

Liberman U, Puniyani A, Feldman MW (2007) On the evolution of epistasis II: a generalized Wright-Kimura framework. Theor Popul Biol. 71(2):230–8.

Linn-Rasker SP, Van der Helm-Van Mil AH, Van Gaalen FA, Kloppenburg M, De Vries RR, et al. (2006) Smoking is a risk factor for anti-CCP antibodies only in rheumatoid arthritis patients who carry HLA-DRB1 shared epitope alleles. Ann Rheum Dis. 65:366–71.

Liu X, Fallin MD, Kao WH (2004) Genetic dissection methods: designs used for tests of gene–environment interaction. Curr Opin Genet Dev. 14:241–5.

Luan JA, Wong MY, Day NE, Wareham NJ (2001) Sample size determination for studies of gene–environment interaction. Int J Epidemiol. 30(5):1035–40.

Lundberg K, Nijenhuis S, Vossenaar ER, Palmblad K, Van Venrooij WJ, et al. (2005) Citrullinated proteins have increased immunogenicity and arthritogenicity and their presence in arthritic joints correlates with disease severity. Arthritis Res Ther. 7:R458–67.

Manolio TA, Bailey-Wilson JE, Collins FS (2006) Genes, environment and the value of prospective cohort studies. Nat Rev Genet. 7(10):812–20.

Marchini J, Donnelly P, Cardon LR (2005) Genome-wide strategies for detecting multiple loci that influence complex diseases. Nat Genet. 37:413–17.

Mukherjee B, Ahn J, Gruber SB, Rennert G, Moreno V, Chatterjee N. (2008) Tests for gene environment interaction from case-control data: a novel study of type I error, power and designs. Genet Epidemiol. 32(7):615–26.

Murcary CE, lewinger JP, Gauderman WJ (2009) Gene–environment interaction in genome-wide association studies. Am J Epidemiol. 169:219–26.

Ottman R (1996) Theoretic epidemiology. Gene–environment interaction: definitions and study designs. Prev Med. 25:764–70.

Phillips PC (2008) Epistasis-the essential role of gene interactions in the structure and evolution of genetic systems. Nature Rev Genet. 9:855–67.

Piegorsch WW, Weinberg CR, Taylor JA (1994) Non-hierarchical logistic models and case only designs for assessing susceptibility in population-based case-control studies. Stat Med. 13(2):153–62.

Puniyani A, Liberman U, Feldman MW (2004) On the meaning of non-epistatic selection. Theor Popul Biol. 66:317–21.

Qin JM, Yang L, Chen B, Wang XM, Li F, Liao PH, He L (2008) Interaction of methylenetetrahydrofolate reductase C677T, cytochrome P4502E1 polymorphism and environment factors in esophageal cancer in Kazakh population. World J Gastroenterol. 14:6986–92.

Ritchie MD, Hahn LW, Roodi N, Bailey LR, Dupont WD, et al. (2001) Multifactor-dimensionality reduction reveals high-order interactions among estrogen-metabolism genes in sporadic breast cancer. Am J Hum Genet. 69:138–47.

Rothman KJ, Greenland S, Walker AM (1980) Concepts of interaction. Am J Epidemiol. 112(4):467–70.

Ruwali M, Khan AJ, Shah PP, Singh AP, Pant MC, Parmar D. (2009) Cytochrome P450 2E1 and head and neck cancer: interaction with genetic and environmental risk factors. Environ Mol Mutagen. 50:473–82.

Sabatti C, Risch N (2002) Homozygosity and linkage disequilibrium. Genetics. 160:1707–19.

Shendure J, Ji H (2008) Next-generation DNA sequencing. Nat Biotechnol. 26(10):1135–45.

Taioli E (2008). Gene–environment interaction in tobacco-related cancers. Carcinogenesis. 29:1467–74.

Thorgeirsson TE, Geller F, Sulem P, et al. (2008) A variant associated with nicotine dependence, lung cancer and peripheral arterial disease. Nature. 452:638–42.

Tsai MH, Tseng HC, Liu CS, Chang CL, Tsai CW, Tsou YA, Wang RF, Lin CC, Wang HC, Chiu CF, Bau DT (2009) Interaction of Exo1 genotypes and smoking habit in oral cancer in Taiwan. Oral Oncol. 45(9):e90–4.

Walter SD, Holford TR (1978) Additive, multiplicative, and other models for disease risks. Am J Epidemiol. 108:341–6.

Wang K (2008) Genetic association tests in the presence of epistasis or gene–environment interaction. Genet Epidemiol. 32:606–14.

Winslow RL, Boguski MS (2003) Genome informatics: current status and future prospects. Circ Res. 92:953–61.

Wu X, Jin L, Xiong M. (2009) Mutual information for testing gene–environment interaction. PLoS One. 4(2):e4578.

Yoon Y, Song J, Hong SH, Kim JQ (2003) Analysis of multiple single nucleotide polymorphisms of candidate genes related to coronary heart disease susceptibility by using support vector machines. Clin Chem Lab Med. 41:529–34.

Zhang YW, Eom SY, Kim YD, Song YJ, Yun HY, Park JS, Youn SJ, Kim BS, Kim H, Hein DW (2009) Effects of dietary factors and the NAT2 acetylator status on gastric cancer in Koreans. Int J Cancer. 125(1):139–45.

Zhou W, Liu G, Miller DP, Thurston SW, Xu LL, et al. (2002) Gene–environment interaction for the ERCC2 polymorphisms and cumulative cigarette smoking exposure in lung cancer. Cancer Res. 62(5):1377–81.

Chapter 4
Clustering Studies for Identifying the Role of Environmental Factors in Aetiology of Human Cancers

Richard J.Q. McNally

Abstract This chapter reviews studies that have analysed clustering of cancer. In general, clustering studies may be divided into two distinct categories: (i) studies that are based on post hoc reports of unusual case aggregations; and (ii) studies that are based on rigorous and systematic analyses of population-based data. For each type of analysis, the underlying methodology is briefly described and key findings are summarised and interpreted in relation to putative aetiological factors.

Keywords Methods · Limitations · Etiological interpretation · Clustering of cancer

4.1 Introduction

The study of disease clustering provides useful insights into aetiology. The presence of such clustering is usually interpreted as providing evidence for an environmental component to aetiology. A distinction must be made between studies of post hoc clusters and systematic investigation of population-based data. In general, there are three distinct types of systematic clustering study. These are studies of "space-time clustering", "spatial clustering" and "temporal clustering". Sometimes separate analyses are performed on the same data set, but the results are interpreted together.

A cluster is an aggregation of cases in terms of a specified disease grouping, time period and geographical location where the number of cases is statistically greater than would be expected when the natural occurrence of the disease and chance fluctuations are taken into account. It is important to make a clear distinction between post hoc and a priori clusters. Post hoc clusters rely on observations of past events,

R.J.Q. McNally (✉)
Institute of Health and Society, Newcastle University, Newcastle upon Tyne, UK
e-mail: richard.mcnally@ncl.ac.uk

D. Roy, M.T. Dorak (eds.), *Environmental Factors, Genes, and the Development of Human Cancers*, DOI 10.1007/978-1-4419-6752-7_4,

whilst a priori clusters are found as a result of systematic statistical analyses of population-based data (Arrundale et al., 1997).

It is also important to distinguish between systematic studies of "global" (i.e. overall) clustering and studies of individual clusters. Studies of global clustering are used to see if such patterning is a general feature of the disease distribution (thus providing general clues to aetiology). Conversely, studies of individual clusters (determined post hoc or a priori) often involve the examination of an association with a specific possible hazard (Arrundale et al., 1997).

There are many types of post hoc clusters. These include transient clusters, permanent clusters, familial clusters, household clusters, school clusters and occupational clusters. Sometimes reported clusters appear to contain a marked excess of cases. However, continued surveillance finds relatively few extra cases and the cluster apparently disappears. Such transient clusters can arise in familial, household, neighbourhood, school or occupational settings. Some cluster reports arise from monitoring a geographical area over a prolonged period of time. One example of such a prolonged cluster is the excess of childhood and adolescent leukaemia that has been reported in Seascale village, in the county of Cumbria, Northern England (Gardner et al., 1990; Draper et al., 1993; Dickinson and Parker, 1999). Sometimes cases of the same type of cancer occur in blood relatives, indicating that there may be a genetic component to aetiology. Examples includes Hodgkin lymphoma and in rare breast cancer and bowel cancer families (Hemminki et al., 2004; Hjalgrim et al., 2004; Chia, 2008). Household clusters occur when the same cancer is diagnosed either in spouse pairs or other genetically unrelated people living in the same residence. They may be diagnosed at similar points in time, or many years apart. Neighbourhood clusters are the commonest type of cluster reported and occur when a specific cancer occurs in a defined community (e.g. a small town or a village). Clusters in schools may reflect a neighbourhood cluster but may also include cases from a much wider geographical area (Arrundale et al., 1997; Heath, 2005).

Clusters of cancer not normally regarded as having an occupational association may occur at a particular industrial plant. For example, if the cluster has arisen at a factory where the majority of the workers were recruited soon after the plant had been constructed, this may be a "cohort" phenomenon due to an aging workforce (since many of the commoner cancer types are age-related). However, it would be much more difficult to explain an excess of a rare cancer in younger workers. Although this could be related to exposures at the plant, it could also be part of a neighbourhood cluster (Arrundale et al., 1997). An example of an occupational cluster investigation is a study of cancer incidence and mortality at a Scottish semiconductor manufacturing facility (McElvenny et al., 2003).

The aims of this chapter are: (i) to review recent studies of clustering of cancer and their etiological interpretation; (ii) to describe some of the methods that are used in clustering studies; and (iii) to indicate some of the limitations of clustering analyses. There is a vast literature and PubMed (http://www.ncbi.nlm.nih.gov/PubMed) has been used to obtain relevant key references. The main types of clustering study are discussed and interpreted. Due to limitations of space, it is not possible to be

of space, it is not possible to be fully comprehensive. There are a number of older reviews to which the reader is referred (Alexander and Boyle, 1996; Arrundale et al., 1997; Alexander, 1999; Little, 1999; McNally and Eden, 2004; Heath, 2005). Indeed, the present chapter updates and extends these previously published reviews. Much of the work on clustering has focussed on childhood cancers and this chapter uses many examples from that body of literature.

The chapter is structured into the following sections: post-hoc cluster investigations; systematic studies of global space-time clustering; systematic studies of global spatial clustering; systematic studies of global temporal clustering; systematic studies to identify individual clusters; and conclusions.

4.2 Post-hoc Cluster Investigations

Putative clustering of cases of cancers are often defined by ad hoc reports. For example, there are many anecdotal reports of clusters of cases of childhood cancer. One of the most dramatic reports concerned eight cases of childhood leukaemia that occurred in Niles, Illinois during a 4-year period in a population of only 20,000. This represented an observed excess of five times more cases than would be expected by chance alone. An investigation of this cluster suggested two plausible reasons for its occurrence. First of all, there were possible differences in the occurrence of common childhood illnesses (such as measles and chicken pox) between families of cases with leukaemia and other unaffected families. Secondly, the appearance of the cluster also coincided with a marked growth of population in the area (Heath and Hasterlik, 1963; Schwartz et al., 1963). Such an expansion in the inhabitants would be consistent with unusual population mixing. Excesses of childhood leukaemia have also been observed elsewhere where similar population expansions have occurred. These include excesses observed in new towns, areas populated by oil workers and areas populated by wartime evacuees (Kinlen et al., 1990, 1993; Kinlen and John, 1994).

Another recent notable cluster of childhood leukaemia was reported in Fallon, Nevada. Eleven cases of childhood leukaemia were diagnosed in 24,000 people residing in the county of Churchill. A statistical evaluation used data from the Surveillance, Epidemiology and End Results program (SEER). The analyses found that the age-standardised rate ratio (RR) in Churchill county was 12.0 (95% confidence interval (CI): 6.0–21.4, $P = 4.3 \times 10^{-9}$). Such a large cluster of childhood leukaemia would only be expected to occur in the USA by random fluctuation once every 22,000 years. Furthermore, the age-standardised RR for five cases diagnosed after the cluster was first reported was still markedly high (RR = 11.2; 95% CI: 3.6–26.3). Also, such excesses were not seen at other military airbases across the USA. Possible hypothesised causes that were considered included exposure to jet fuel and also an infectious agent carried by the military staff (Kinlen and Doll, 2004; Steinmaus et al., 2004).

In the UK, without doubt the most studied cluster has been the unusual excess of childhood leukaemia that has been observed in Seascale, in the county of Cumbria,

Northern England (Gardner et al., 1990; Draper et al., 1993; Dickinson and Parker, 1999). Extensive investigations of this cluster have been carried out. Overall, it has been concluded that the most plausible explanation is that the cluster has arisen due to unusual population mixing (see for example Little, 1999; COMARE, 2006).

The study of post hoc cluster reports must be carried out with extreme care. Otherwise, there is a danger of misinterpretation. To carry out a statistical analysis population-based cancer incidence data and corresponding population denominator data must be available at small-area level. Mapping can be used as a descriptive tool, but again great care must be taken to avoid making false associations.

All geographical analyses should be based on the computation of cancer rates. It is not enough to know the number of cases in the study area. It is necessary to compare the number of cases in the study area with the number of cases in a larger area (reference area) to determine if there are more cases in the study area than would be expected by chance alone. This is done by calculating the number of cases that would be expected to occur in the study area under the assumption that it has the same disease rates as the reference area. It is essential to choose a sufficiently broad age range and time span and not to be confined to the specific ages and dates of occurrence as the original case observation. A narrow definition could miss other relevant events or, conversely, could give a false overall picture. For example, four cases of a rare cancer occurring over 3 years might be unusual, but if no other cases occur during a further 20 years, this observation may well be a chance occurrence (Arrundale et al., 1997).

There are some possible problems with post hoc cluster investigations. These include: (i) the dangers of "data dredging"; (ii) the temptation to fit results to a pre-conceived pattern of events (known as "Texas sharpshooting"—the "Texas sharp-shooter" (Fig. 4.1) first fires his gun at a barn, then paints a target on the barn

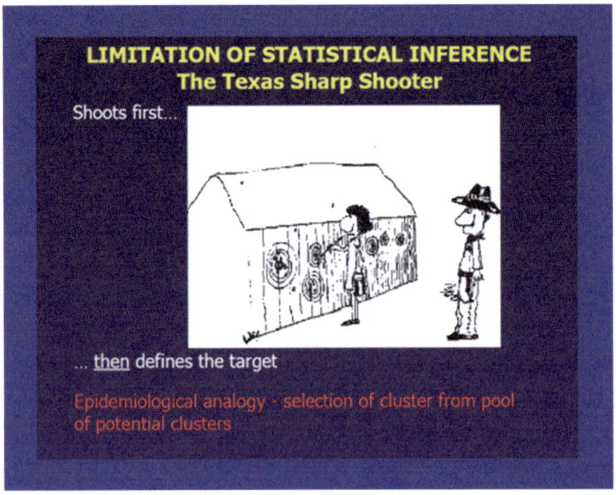

Fig. 4.1 The Texas sharp shooter

with a bulls-eye where most bullet holes have clustered and then shows this to his associates to demonstrate what a good marksman he is); (iii) the overuse of multiple comparisons; and (iv) errors in denominator data (Arrundale et al., 1997).

It is important that cases in the small area of interest should have the same definition as those from the larger area with which disease rates are being compared. Post hoc cluster reports should be interpreted with similar caution to the Texas sharpshooter's claims of good marksmanship. The local area in which the cluster is located has come to prominence simply because a number of cases were resident there. Disease rates will always fluctuate between different geographical locations. The "target" area should not have been drawn around the area only because of the high rates. There must be some other rationale or hypothesis underlying the definition of the target area boundary (Arrundale et al., 1997).

There are four possible outcomes to a post hoc cluster investigation: (i) observed number of cases less than expected; (ii) observed number of cases greater than expected, but not statistically significant; (iii) observed number of cases greater than expected and marginally significant; and (iv) observed number of cases greater than expected and statistically significant. Whilst outcome (iv) would certainly lead to further investigation, outcomes (i)–(iii) may lead to a curtailment of the study (although, in certain circumstances, surveillance may continue for public reassurance) (Arrundale et al., 1997).

In summary, post hoc cluster investigations are useful for determining whether particular local excesses can be explained as chance occurrences, or whether there may be a link with a putative environmental hazard. At the very least, such studies are a useful starting point to any more rigorous investigation. However, one review of eleven post hoc cluster reports determined that there was no causal factor that could explain a single cluster of childhood leukaemia (Alexander, 1999). Furthermore, Rothman (1990) has argued that studies of individual post hoc clusters are not very useful for testing general aetiological hypotheses.

Systematic studies of space-time, spatial or temporal clustering are advocated for determining whether clustering is a general feature related to the aetiology of a particular cancer type.

4.3 Systematic Studies of Global Space-Time Clustering

Studies of systematic "space-time clustering" require the availability of high quality population-based cancer data for a prolonged period of time. Analyses can provide global tests for statistically significant overall "space-time clustering". The time point may be taken as date of birth, date of diagnosis or another aetiologically relevant event. Similarly the spatial location may be address at birth or address at diagnosis (or other aetiologically relevant event).

Accurate geo-referenced spatial co-ordinates of addresses need to be obtained for analyses. These may be difficult or expensive to obtain at individual address level and can often only be obtained to a good approximation. Such accuracy is usually sufficient for determining the presence or absence of space-time clustering. In the UK, Ordnance Survey four-digit grid references (Easting and Northing) are available to geo-reference the centroid of every postcode to an accuracy of 0.1 km. In the whole of the UK, there are around 1.7 million postcodes that identify addresses for postal delivery. One postcode might identify fifteen to twenty houses, a smaller number of multiple occupancy residences, or a single commercial building (Bailey and Gatrell, 1995).

Global space-time clustering is observed when excess numbers of cases of a disease occur within highly localized geographical areas at limited time points and these excesses are not explained by general excesses in those areas or at those times. In other words, a disease that exhibits space-time clustering has an irregular occurrence of cases simultaneously both in space and time. Such an irregular distribution might arise from a number of scenarios. One possibility is a small number of locations with highly raised incidence over short, distinct, time periods. Another possibility is a large number of locations with moderately raised incidence at limited time periods. The statistical methods for analyses of space-time clustering adjust for constant excesses at specific locations, and also for short temporal peaks that are geographically widespread.

A finding of global space-time clustering is consistent with the involvement of a highly transient environmental exposure in aetiology. An example of such an agent would be a transmissible agent such as an infection. Indeed, a possible role for infections (both viruses and bacteria) has often been suggested to be relevant to the aetiology of a number of cancers. Furthermore, a causal link has been established between certain viruses and the subsequent development of leukaemia and osteosarcoma in animals (Penrose, 1970; Linenberger and Abkowitz, 1995; Nevins, 2005).

There is a body of evidence that indicates that some viruses are causally related to the aetiology of several human cancers (Evans and Mueller, 1990; Mueller, 1995). Recently a causal link has been made between infection with human papillomavirus (HPV) and subsequent occurrence of cervical cancer in a small number of infected women (Bosch and de Sanjose, 2007). It has also been established that a small number of adults infected with the retrovirus human T-cell lymphotropic virus type 1 (HTLV1) will develop Adult T-cell leukaemia/lymphoma (ATLL) (Kannagi et al., 2004). Epstein-Barr virus (EBV) has been identified in tumour tissue from cases of childhood Burkitt lymphoma (BL) in parts of sub-Saharan Africa, where BL is prevalent. Additionally, it has been shown that the spatial distribution of BL correlates with endemic malaria (Young and Rickinson, 2004).

If non-ubiquitous infections or non-endemic infections are involved in the aetiology of a cancer, then the case distribution may be predicted to show space-time clustering. It should be noted that this would only occur when the lag time from exposure to diagnosis (or birth) is short or at least relatively constant. The onset of cancer would happen as a rare consequence of infection and not from direct person-to-person infection.

A number of statistical methods have been developed to test for global space-time clustering (see Table 4.1). These include methods due to Pinkel and Nefzger

Table 4.1 Comparison of methods for analysing space-time clustering

Method	Critique
Pinkel and Nefzger (1959)	Combinatorial technique. Counts of cases in spatial and space-time units. Assumes uniform population density
Ederer et al. (1964)	Combinatorial technique. Counts of cases in spatial and space-time units. Does not assume uniform population density
Knox (1964)	Uses case time and co-ordinate data only, but only one set of critical values. Counts number of "close pairs." Repeated use of this test will result in multiple testing. Original test uses fixed distances to define "closeness in space", but modification uses variable nearest neighbour thresholds
Barton et al. (1965)	Uses case time and co-ordinate data only. Compares distances and times between case pairs. Extreme temporal or spatial values can distort the test statistic
Mantel (1967)	Uses case time and co-ordinate data only. Compares inverse distances and times between case pairs. Not good for detecting non-linear associations
Pike and Smith (1974)	Uses case and control data at a number of space and time strata. Calculates a test statistic based on matching of pairs of cases and controls
Diggle et al. (1995)	Uses case time and co-ordinate data only and range of critical values. Counts number of "close pairs". Overcomes multiple testing problems inherent with the Knox test. Original test uses fixed distances to define "closeness in space", but modification uses variable nearest neighbour thresholds
Jacquez (1996)	Uses case time and co-ordinate data only. Counts number of "close pairs." Repeated use of this test will result in multiple testing. Uses variable nearest neighbour thresholds. Most suitable for inhomogeneous populations
Melliker and Jacquez (2007)	Uses case and control co-ordinate data at a number of time points. Calculates a test statistic based on a nearest neighbour approach. Requires complete residential history data

(1959), Ederer et al. (1964), Knox (1964), Barton et al. (1965), Mantel (1967), Pike and Smith (1974) and Diggle et al. (1995). A recent method has enabled residential histories to be included in space-time clustering analyses (Meliker and Jacquez, 2007). However, complete residential history data are seldom available.

One of the most commonly used methods is due to Knox (1964). The Knox test considers a pair of cases to be in *close proximity* if they are both diagnosed (or born) at addresses that are both spatially close ($< s$ km apart, where, e.g., $s = 1$) and temporally close ($< t$ months apart, where, e.g., $t = 6$). The limits of *close proximity* are arbitrarily set by the investigator prior to the commencement of analyses. The number of pairs of cases that are in close proximity is obtained (denoted O). Also, the numbers of pairs of cases that are close in space (denoted D) and close in time (denoted T) are found. Under the null hypothesis, we assume that spatial and temporal proximity are independent. Then the expected value of O is denoted E and is equal to $D \times T/N$ (N is the total number of case pairs). We also assume (under the null hypothesis) that O follows a Poisson distribution, with mean E. If O is greater then E then there is evidence of possible space-time clustering. Statistical significance is then assessed. The strength of the clustering effect can be estimated by calculating $S = (O–E)/E$ (another related quantity is $R = (O–E)/\sqrt{E}$) (McNally et al., 2006a).

One of the main problems with the Knox (1964) and other similar tests is that the critical values of closeness in space (s) and time (t) are arbitrarily chosen. A more recent method due to Diggle et al. (1995) has overcome this problem (at least to some extent). The method of Diggle et al. uses a set of Knox-like calculations, in which the critical values are varied over a pre-specified set of values. For example, in a national study of childhood cancer from Great Britain, McNally et al. (2006a) used 225 Knox-like calculations with close points in space taken as $s = 0.5$, 1, 1.5,. . ., 7.5 km and close times taken as $t = 0.1$, 0.2,. . ., 1.5 years. The test statistic was formed by summing the values of R over all the 225 pre-specified pairs. Since the distribution of the K-function is not known, it was estimated by computer simulation, and hence statistical significance was assessed (see also COMARE, 2006).

Sometimes fixed geographical distances may not be appropriate to measure spatial proximity. This is especially true if the study region contains both urban and rural areas. A particular distance between two cases could have different interpretations in urban and rural areas. For example, the areas covered by school catchments would be markedly different. This problem was first recognised by Jacquez (1996), who developed a method to adjust for such variations in population density. In this method, for a particular "index" case, other cases that are adjacent are labelled as "nearest neighbours" (NNs). NNs are ranked by their proximity to the index case (1, 2, 3,. . .). All cases in a data set are treated as "index" cases and ranking is performed. An extension of this method has been applied to K-function analyses (see, for example, McNally et al., 2006a, 2009a; COMARE, 2006).

Further analyses can be done, including analyses by gender, level of population density and also cross-clustering between different diagnostic groups (see, for example, McNally et al., 2005, 2006a, 2009a; COMARE, 2006).

A number of studies from parts of Europe, Australia and the USA have found statistically significant space-time clustering amongst cases of childhood leukaemia, most notably cases of acute lymphoblastic leukaemia (ALL) occurring in the childhood peak at ages 1–4 years (Pinkel et al., 1963; Meighan and Knox, 1965; Mainwaring, 1966; Gunz and Spears, 1968; Klauber and Mustacchi, 1970; Zahalkova et al., 1970; Glass et al., 1971; Evatt et al., 1973; Larsen et al., 1973; Smith et al., 1976; Morris, 1990; Gilman and Knox, 1991, 1995; Alexander, 1992; Petridou et al., 1996; Alexander et al., 1998a; Gilman et al., 1999a; Birch et al., 2000; Gustafsson and Carstensen, 2000; McNally et al., 2002a, 2006a, 2009a; COMARE, 2006; Bellec et al., 2006). Other studies have not found evidence of space-time clustering (studies reviewed by Little, 1999).

Most of the studies that identified positive evidence of space-time clustering were based on place and date of diagnosis. However, three were based on place and date of birth (Gustafsson and Carstensen, 2000; McNally et al., 2002a, 2009a) and two were based on date of diagnosis and place of birth (Birch et al., 2000; McNally et al., 2009a).

The positive space-time clustering that has been found in a number of studies for childhood leukaemia in consistent with a role for infections in aetiology. Three recent hypotheses consider the role that infections may play (Greaves, 1988; Kinlen, 1988, 1995; Smith, 1997). Kinlen (1988, 1995) suggested that very high incidence of leukaemia would arise in previously isolated areas that had unusual population mixing. Greaves (1988) proposed that the final event that relates to onset of precursor B-cell acute lymphoblastic leukaemia (ALL) is related to delay in exposure to common infections in certain genetically susceptible children. Smith (1997) hypothesised that higher incidence rates of childhood leukaemia are related to exposure to an infection occurring in-utero.

The finding of space-time clustering, based on any combination of birth or diagnosis time and location, is consistent with Kinlen's hypothesis. However, the finding of space-time clustering based on place of birth and date of diagnosis, especially, is consistent with Greaves' hypothesis (and not Smith's hypothesis). Space-time clustering, based on time and place of diagnosis is also consistent with Greaves hypothesis (and not Smith's hypothesis). Conversely, space-time clustering, based on time and place of birth, is consistent with Smith's hypothesis (and not Greaves' hypothesis) (McNally and Eden, 2004).

A limited number of studies have identified statistically significant space-time clustering in childhood solid tumours, including Hodgkin lymphoma, non-Hodgkin lymphoma, central nervous system (CNS) tumours, soft tissue sarcomas, osteosarcoma and Wilms tumours (McNally, 2002b, 2003a, 2009a). Space-time clustering for both Hodgkin and non-Hodgkin lymphoma is consistent with the involvement of a directly transforming infectious agent. Infections that have been implicated include EBV, hepatitis C, human herpes virus 8 (HHV8), human immunodeficiency virus (HIV) and helicobacter pylori (Jarrett, 2006; Grulich and Vajdic, 2005; Engels, 2007). The finding of space-time clustering for CNS tumours also suggests an environmental, possibly infectious aetiology. Further support for infections is provided by evidence from other epidemiological studies (Linet et al., 1996; Fear et al., 2001; Dickinson et al., 2002; Shaw et al., 2006).

Space-time clustering of soft tissue sarcomas and osteosarcoma is suggestive of infectious involvement in aetiology. Additional support for an infectious aetiology for soft tissue sarcomas is provided by studies in adults that have found a causal association between HHV8 and Kaposi's sarcoma (with HIV also involved) (Viejo-Borbolla and Schulz, 2003). Osteosarcoma in hamsters has been shown to be induced by simian virus 40, but associations in humans are more tentative (Heinsohn et al., 2000; Jasani et al., 2001). There is little evidence linking Wilms tumour with infections. The space-time clustering (found amongst cases of Wilms tumour) may be due to other environmental factors (Little, 1999).

One study found cross-space-time clustering between cases of leukaemia and CNS tumour, suggesting a common environmental aetiology (McNally et al., 2005). Other studies have found no evidence of space-time clustering amongst certain childhood solid tumours (McNally et al., 2004, 2006a, 2009a; COMARE, 2006).

Studies of adolescents and adults have found evidence of space-time clustering amongst cases of Hodgkin lymphoma, CNS tumour and testicular cancer (Mangoud et al., 1985; Gilman et al., 1999b; Houben et al., 2005, 2006; McNally et al., 2006b). One study from the UK did not find space-time clustering amongst adult (including adolescent) cases of leukaemia (Gilman et al., 1999a). These findings were interpreted as supporting an infectious aetiology for Hodgkin lymphoma and possible infectious (or other environmental) aetiologies for CNS and testicular tumours.

There are some limitations to studies of space-time clustering. Kulldorf and Hjalmars (1999) have pointed out that small-area population shifts over short periods of time may induce artefactual space-time clustering. However, analysis at this level requires dynamic population data, which are not readily available in most countries. Also, population movements are implicitly linked with the aetiology of certain cancers (especially childhood leukaemia). Therefore, analyses that adjust for population shifts may actually over compensate. Furthermore, the distinctive space-time clustering is only apparent for a number of cancers (most notably childhood leukaemia) for which there are plausible aetiological explanations (for childhood leukaemia, see, for example, McNally and Eden, 2004).

4.4 Systematic Studies of Global Spatial Clustering

Studies of systematic “spatial clustering” require the availability of high quality population-based cancer data for a prolonged period of time. Analyses can provide global tests for statistically significant overall “spatial clustering”. The spatial location may be location at birth or (most often) location at diagnosis (or another aetiologically relevant event).

Studies of spatial clustering are dependent on the availability and accuracy of population (denominator) counts at small area level. These are usually stratified by age-group and sex and obtained from population censuses (which in the UK are carried out every 10 years). Any uncertainty in population data may result in either inflation or deflation of a possible clustering effect. Undercounting of a small area population may lead to an inflated estimate of a rate, whilst over-counting may lead to a deflated estimate of a rate.

Global spatial clustering is observed when excess numbers of cases of a disease occur within highly localized geographical areas for a prolonged period. Furthermore, these excesses are widespread and are not limited to one particular small area. In other words, a disease that exhibits spatial clustering has an irregular geographical occurrence of cases. Such an irregular distribution might arise from a number of scenarios. One possibility is a small number of locations with highly raised incidence. Another possibility is a large number of limited time periods with moderately raised incidence (McNally and Eden, 2004).

A finding of spatial clustering is consistent with an environmental component to aetiology. A number of environmental agents are likely to be geographically heterogeneous, including infections, ionizing radiation, electromagnetic fields, chemical exposures and contaminated drinking water.

A number of statistical methods have been developed to test for spatial clustering (see Table 4.2). These include methods due to Potthoff and Whittinghill (1966), Muirhead and Ball (1989) and Cuzick and Edwards (1990). A number of other methods are reviewed in Little (1999) and Alexander and Boyle (1996).

Recent studies from Europe, Hong Kong, Greece, the UK and New Zealand have found evidence of spatial clustering in childhood leukaemia (Draper, 1991; Knox and Gilman, 1992, 1996; Alexander et al., 1997, 1998b; Petridou et al., 1997; McNally et al., 2009b; COMARE, 2006). Another study, from New Zealand found limited evidence of clustering in 10–14 year olds (Dockerty et al., 1999). Other recent studies did not find general spatial clustering for childhood leukaemia (Hjalmars et al., 1996; McNally et al., 2003b; Bellec et al., 2006). Spatially clustering for childhood leukaemia is interpreted as providing support for an infectious component to aetiology. The persistent occurrence in a number of small areas is consistent with areas of high or unusual population mixing. Such situations have been predicted to lead to much higher incidence of childhood leukaemia (Kinlen, 1988, 1995).

There have been a limited number of studies that have examined childhood solid tumours. Recent studies from Great Britain found spatial clustering amongst cases of childhood soft tissue sarcoma and Wilms tumour (McNally et al., 2003c, 2009b). Clustering of soft tissue sarcoma may be associated with an infectious or other environmental aetiology. However, since there is little evidence linking Wilms tumour with infections, the clustering may be due to other environmental exposures, including hydrocarbons, lead, boron and pesticides (Little, 1999).

In older (non-childhood) cases of Hodgkin lymphoma, spatial clustering has been identified (Alexander et al., 1989) and this has been interpreted as providing support

Table 4.2 Comparison of methods for analysing spatial clustering

Method	Critique
Potthoff and Whittinghill (1966)	Uses case counts and population denominator data. Tests for departures from homogeneity. Requires accurate population denominator data
Muirhead and Ball (1989)	Modification of method of Potthoff and Whittinghill (1966)
Cuzick and Edwards (1990)	Use case data and control data from a population-based register. Test statistic based on whether nearest neighbours are cases or controls. Requires controls that reflect inhomogeneous population distribution
Besag and Newell (1991)	Uses case counts and population denominator data. Overall test statistic examines whether localized aggregations occur by chance or not. Requires very accurate population denominator data
Williams et al. (2001)	Further development of method of Besag and Newell (1991). Provides a test for an individual case being unusually close to its neighbours as well as a global test of clustering. Also requires very accurate population denominator data

for a transmissible aetiological agent. Higher prevalence (or transmission) of such a putative agent would be predicted to occur to a greater degree in certain small areas, such as those with greater levels of socio-economic deprivation.

4.5 Systematic Studies of Global Temporal Clustering

Global temporal clustering is observed when excess numbers of cases of a disease occur at very limited time periods over a wide geographical area. Furthermore, these excesses occur at a number of different time periods and are not limited to one particular point in time. Such temporal clustering might arise from a number of scenarios. One possibility is a small number of time points with highly raised incidence. Another possibility is a large number of limited time periods with moderately raised incidence.

Studies of temporal clustering are dependent on the availability and accuracy of (usually) annual population (denominator) counts. A finding of temporal clustering is consistent with an environmental component to aetiology. An example of such an environmental agent would be an infectious disease that exhibits an "epidemic" pattern of occurrence, such as influenza.

Studies of general temporal clustering are rarely reported in the literature. However, a special type of temporal clustering is seasonal variation which occurs when excesses are observed consistently at specific times of year. The presence of seasonal variation is indicative of an environmental aetiology. Putative agents would display a consistent, but seasonally heterogeneous patterning in their occurrence.

Statistical methods that have been developed to analyse seasonal variation include those due to Edwards (1961) and Walter and Elwood (1975).

A number of studies, from Iran, UK, Denmark, USA and Greece have found seasonal variation in the incidence of childhood leukaemia (reviewed in McNally and Eden, 2004). Seasonal variation was found with respect to date of birth, date of first symptom and date of diagnosis. Seasonal variation has also been found in Hodgkin lymphoma and CNS tumours (Westerbeek et al., 1998; McNally et al., 2002b). Seasonal variation in incidence is interpreted as supporting an environmental aetiology. Factors such as pesticides and infections are likely to exhibit this type of occurrence. The postulated mechanism for pesticides would be via seasonal consumption of fresh fruit and vegetable and for infections would be via regular seasonally occurring epidemics.

4.6 Systematic Studies to Identify Individual Clusters

Most of the literature has focussed on post hoc cluster investigations, or systematic investigations of global clustering. There have been far fewer systematic studies to identify individual (space-time, spatial or temporal) clusters.

Space-time and spatial clusters: Recent methodological developments have included techniques for systematically searching for individual space-time clusters (Kulldorff and Nagarwalla, 1995; Kulldorff, 1997; Kulldorff et al., 2005; Kulldorff, 2006). This approach is useful as a screening tool. Application to data has often led to negative findings and consequent public reassurance (Kulldorff et al., 1998; Bellec et al., 2006).

Temporal clusters: The identification of a temporal cluster of cancer may indicate a possible association with a carcinogen. Surveillance methods are used to identify such temporal excesses. These include both the sets and the cuscore techniques (Chen et al., 1997a).

One example of a systematic study is from Israel. Chen et al. (1997b) carried out a systematic investigation of cases of leukaemia registered during the period 1960–1990 in the city of Ashkelon. They found clustering both for acute lymphoblastic leukaemia and chronic myeloid leukaemia, and concluded that the findings were compatible with the involvement of a localised carcinogen, although other confounders could not be excluded.

4.7 Conclusions

In general clustering studies are useful for understanding the aetiology of different cancers. The finding of global clustering patterns suggests that widespread environmental factors are involved in aetiology. It is possible that chance may play a role in some of the studies. However, there has been consistency between different studies from different countries for certain cancer types. This is most notable for childhood leukaemia (McNally and Eden, 2004). In contrast, studies of individual clusters have a more limited role in providing general aetiological clues (Rothman, 1990; Neutra, 1990). However, such analyses may be useful for looking at specific putative risk factors. When findings are negative (as is commonly the situation for analyses of individual clusters), the studies provide public reassurance.

Acknowledgments Childhood cancer epidemiology at Newcastle University is supported by the North of England Children's Cancer Research Fund.

References

Alexander, F. E., Williams, J., McKinney, P. A., Ricketts, T. J., and Cartwright, R. A. 1989. A specialist leukaemia/lymphoma registry in the UK. Part 2: Clustering of Hodgkin's disease. Br. J. Cancer 60:948–952.

Alexander, F. E. 1992. Space-time clustering of childhood acute lymphoblastic leukaemia: indirect evidence for a transmissible agent. Br. J. Cancer 65:589–592.

Alexander, F. E., and Boyle, P., editors. 1996. Methods for investigating localized clustering of disease. Lyon: International Agency for Research on Cancer, Publ. no. 135.

Alexander, F. E., Chan, L. C., Lam, T. H., Yuen, P., Leung, N. K., Ha, S. Y., Yuen, H. L., Li, C. K., Li, C. K., Lau, Y. L., and Greaves, M. F. 1997. Clustering of childhood leukaemia in Hong Kong: association with the childhood peak and common acute lymphoblastic leukaemia and with population mixing. Br. J. Cancer 75:457–463.

Alexander, F. E., Boyle, P., Carli, P. M., Coebergh, J. W., Draper, G. J., Ekbom, A., Levi, F., McKinney, P. A., McWhirter, W., Magnani, C., Michaelis, J., Olsen, J. H., Peris-Bonet, R., Petridou, E., Pukkala, E., and Vatten, L. 1998a. Spatial temporal patterns in childhood leukaemia: further evidence for an infectious origin. EUROCLUS project. Br. J. Cancer 77:812–817.

Alexander, F. E., Boyle, P., Carli, P. M., Coebergh, J. W., Draper, G. J., Ekbom, A., Levi, F., McKinney, P. A., McWhirter, W., Michaelis, J. Peris-Bonet, R., Petridou, E., Pompe-Kirn, V., Plisko, I., Pukkala, E., Rahu, M., Storm, H., Terracini, B., Vatten, L., and Wray, N. 1998b. Spatial clustering of childhood leukaemia: summary results from the EUROCLUS project. Br. J. Cancer 77:818–824.

Alexander, F. E. 1999. Clusters and clustering of childhood cancer: a review. Eur. J. Epidemiol. 15:847–852.

Arrundale, J., Bain, M., Botting, B., Brewster, D., Cartwright, R., Chalmers, J., Coggon, D., Elliott, P., Jackson, I., McKinney, T., McNally, R., Miles, D. P., Quinn, M. J., Sharp, L., Staines, A., Stiller, C., and Wilkinson, P. 1997. Handbook and Guide to the Investigation of Clusters of Diseases. London: Leukaemia Research Fund.

Bailey, T. C., and Gatrell, A. 1995. Interactive Spatial Data Analysis. Harlow: Longman.

Barton, D. E., David, F. N., and Merrington, M. 1965. A criteria for testing contagion in time and space. Ann. Hum. Genet. 29:97–102.

Bellec, S., Hemon, D., Rudant, J., Goubin, A., and Clavel, J. 2006. Spatial and space-time clustering of childhood acute leukaemia in France from 1990 to 2000: a nationwide study. Br. J. Cancer 94:763–770.

Besag, J., and Newell, J. 1991. The detection of clusters in rare diseases. J. R. Stat. Soc. A 154: 143–155.

Birch, J. M., Alexander, F. E., Blair, V., Eden. O. B., Taylor, G. M., and McNally, R. J. 2000. Space-time clustering patterns in childhood leukaemia support a role for infection. Br. J. Cancer 82:1571–1576.

Bosch, F. X., and de Sanjose, S. 2007. The epidemiology of human papillomavirus infection and cervical cancer. Dis. Markers 23:213–227.

Chen, R., Connelly, R. R., and Mantel, N. 1997a. The efficiency of the sets and the cuscore techniques under biased baseline rates. Stat. Med. 16:1401–1411.

Chen, R., Iscovich, J., and Goldbourt, U. 1997b. Clustering of leukaemia cases in a city in Israel. Stat. Med. 16:1873–1887.

Chia, K. S. 2008. Gene–environment interactions in breast cancer. Novartis Found. Symp. 293:143–150.

Committee on Medical Aspects of Radiation in the Environment (COMARE). 2006. Eleventh report – the distribution of childhood leukaemia and other cancers in Great Britain 1969–1993. Chilton, Didcot, Oxfordshire: Health Protection Agency, Radiation Protection Division.

Cuzick, J., and Edwards, R. 1990. Spatial clustering for inhomogeneous populations (with discussion). J. R. Stat. Soc B 52:73–104.

Dickinson, H. O., and Parker, L. 1999. Quantifying the effect of population mixing on childhood leukaemia risk: the Seascale cluster. Br. J. Cancer 81:144–151.

Dickinson, H. O., Nyari, T. A., and Parker, L. 2002. Childhood solid tumours in relation to infections in the community in Cumbria during pregnancy and around the time of birth. Br. J. Cancer 87:746–750.

Diggle, P. J., Chetwynd, A. G., Haggkvist, R., and Morris, S. E. 1995. Second-order analysis of space-time clustering. Stat. Methods Med. Res. 4:124–136.

Dockerty, J. D., Sharples, K. J., and Borman, B. 1999. An assessment of spatial clustering of leukaemias and lymphomas among young people in New Zealand. J. Epidemiol. Comm. Health 53:154–158.

Draper, G. J., editor. 1991. The Geographical Epidemiology of Childhood Leukaemia and Non-Hodgkin Lymphomas in Great Britain, 1966–83. Studies on Medical and Population Subjects, no. 53. London: HMSO.

Draper, G. J., Stiller, C. A., Cartwright, R. A., Craft, A. W., and Vincent, T. J. 1993. Cancer in Cumbria and in the vicinity of the Sellafield nuclear installation, 1963–90. Br. Med. J. 306: 89–94.
Ederer, F., Myers, M. H., and Mantel, N. 1964. A statistical problem in space and time: do leukemia cases come in clusters? Biometrics 20:626–638.
Edwards, J. H. 1961. The recognition and estimation of cyclic trends. Ann. Hum. Genet. 25:83–86.
Engels, E. A. 2007. Infectious agents as causes of non-Hodgkin lymphoma. Cancer Epidemiol. Biomarkers Prev. 16:401–404.
Evans, A. S., and Mueller, N. E. 1990. Viruses and cancer. Causal associations. Ann. Epidemiol. 1:71–92.
Evatt, B. L., Chase, G. A., and Heath, C. W. 1973. Time-space clustering among cases of acute leukemia in two Georgia counties. Blood 41:265–272.
Fear, N. T., Roman, E., Ansell, P., and Bull, D. 2001. Malignant neoplasms of the brain during childhood: the role of prenatal and neonatal factors (United Kingdom). Cancer Causes Control 12:443–449.
Gardner, M. J., Snee, M. P., Hall, A. J., Powell, C. A., Downes, S., and Terrell, J. D. 1990. Results of case-control study of leukaemia and lymphoma among young people near Sellafield nuclear plant in West Cumbria. Br. Med. J. 300:423–429.
Gilman, E. A., and Knox, E. G. 1991. Temporal-spatial distribution of childhood leukaemias and non-Hodgkin's lymphoma in Great Britain. In: Draper, G. J., editor. The Geographical Epidemiology of Childhood Leukaemia and Non-Hodgkin Lymphomas in Great Britain, 1966–1983. Studies on Medical and Population Subjects no. 53. London: HMSO, 77–99.
Gilman, E. A., and Knox, E. G. 1995. Childhood cancers: space-time distribution in Britain. J. Epidemiol. Commun. Health 49:158–163.
Gilman, E. A., McNally, R. J., and Cartwright, R. A. 1999a. Space-time clustering of acute lymphoblastic leukaemia in parts of the UK (1984–1993). Eur. J. Cancer 35:91–96.
Gilman, E. A., McNally, R. J., and Cartwright, R. A. 1999b. Space-time clustering of Hodgkin's disease in parts of the UK, 1984–1993. Leuk. Lymphoma 36:85–100.
Glass, A. G., Mantel, N., Gunz, F. W., and Spears, G. F. 1971. Time-space clustering of childhood leukemia in New Zealand. J. Natl. Cancer Inst. 47:329–336.
Greaves, M. F. 1988. Speculations on the cause of childhood acute lymphoblastic leukemia. Leukemia 2:120–125.
Grulich, A. E., and Vajdic, C. M. 2005. The epidemiology of non-Hodgkin lymphoma. Pathology 37:409–419.
Gunz, F. W., and Spears, G. F. 1968. Distribution of acute leukaemia in time and space. Studies in New Zealand. Br. Med. J. 4:604–608.
Gustafsson, B., and Carstensen, J. 2000. Space-time clustering of childhood lymphatic leukaemias and non-Hodgkin's lymphomas in Sweden. Eur. J. Epidemiol. 16:1111–1116.
Heath, C. W., and Hasterlik, R. J. 1963. Leukemia among children in a suburban community. Am. J. Med. 34:796–812.
Heath, C. W. 2005. Community clusters of childhood leukemia and lymphoma: evidence of infection? Am. J. Epidemiol. 162:817–822.
Heinsohn, S., Scholz, R. B., Weber, B., Wittenstein, B., Werner, M., Delling, G., Kempf-Bielack, B., Setlak, P., Bielack, S., and Kabisch, H. 2000. SV40 sequences in human osteosarcoma of German origin. Anticancer Res. 20:4539–4545.
Hemminki, K., Rawal, R., Chen, B., and Bermejo, J. L. 2004. Genetic epidemiology of cancer: from families to heritable genes. Int. J. Cancer 111:944–950.
Hjalgrim, H., Rasmussen, S., Rostgaard, K., Nielsen, N. M., Koch-Henriksen, N., Munksgaard, L., Storm, H. H., and Melbye, M. 2004. Familial clustering of Hodgkin lymphoma and multiple sclerosis. J. Natl. Cancer Inst. 96:780–784.
Hjalmars, U., Kulldorff, M., Gustafsson, G., and Nagarwalla, N. 1996. Childhood leukaemia in Sweden: using GIS and a spatial scan statistic for cluster detection. Stat. Med. 15:707–715.

Houben, M. P., Coebergh, J. W., Birch, J. M., Tijssen, C. C., van Duijn, C. M., and McNally, R. J. 2005. Space-time clustering patterns of gliomas in The Netherlands suggest an infectious aetiology. Eur. J. Cancer 41:2917–2923.

Houben, M. P., Coebergh, J. W., Birch, J. M., Tijssen, C. C., van Duijn, C. M., and McNally, R. J. 2006. Space-time clustering of glioma cannot be attributed to specific histological subgroups. Eur. J. Epidemiol. 21:197–201.

Jacquez, G. M. 1996. A *k* nearest neighbour test for space-time interaction. Stat. Med. 15: 1935–1949.

Jarrett R. F. 2006. Viruses and lymphoma/leukaemia. J. Pathol. 208:176–186.

Jasani, B., Cristaudo, A., Emri, S. A., Gazdar, A. F., Gibbs, A., Krynska, B., Miller, C., Mutti, L., Radu, C., Tognon, M., and Procopio, A. 2001. Association of SV40 with human tumours. Semin. Cancer Biol. 11:49–61.

Kannagi, M., Ohashi, T., Harashima, N., Hanabuchi, S., and Hasegawa, A. 2004. Immunological risks of adult T-cell leukemia at primary HTLV-I infection. Trends Microbiol. 12:346–352.

Kinlen, L. 1988. Evidence for an infective cause of childhood leukaemia: comparison of a Scottish new town with nuclear reprocessing sites in Britain. Lancet 2:1323–1327.

Kinlen, L. J., Clarke, K., and Hudson, C. 1990. Evidence from population mixing in British new towns 1946–85 of an infective basis for childhood leukaemia. Lancet 336:577–582.

Kinlen, L. J., O'Brien, F., Clarke, K., Balkwill, A., and Matthews, F. 1993. Rural population mixing and childhood leukaemia: effects of the North Sea oil industry in Scotland, including the area near Dounreay nuclear site. Br. Med. J. 306:743–748.

Kinlen, L. J., and John, S. M. 1994. Wartime evacuation and mortality from childhood leukaemia in England and Wales in 1945–49. Br. Med. J. 309:1197–1202.

Kinlen, L. J. 1995. Epidemiological evidence for an infective basis in childhood leukaemia. Br. J. Cancer 71:1–5.

Kinlen, L., and Doll, R. 2004. Population mixing and childhood leukaemia: Fallon and other US clusters. Br. J. Cancer 91:1–3.

Klauber, M. R., and Mustacchi, P. 1970. Space-time clustering of childhood leukemia in San Francisco. Cancer Res. 30:1969–1973.

Knox, E. G. 1964. The detection of space-time interactions. Appl. Stat. 13:25–29.

Knox, E. G., and Gilman, E. 1992. Leukaemia clusters in Great Britain. 2. Geographical concentrations. J. Epidemiol. Community Health 46:573–576.

Knox, E. G., and Gilman, E. A. 1996. Spatial clustering of childhood cancers in Great Britain. J. Epidemiol. Community Health 50:313–319.

Kulldorff, M., and Nagarwalla, N. 1995. Spatial disease clusters: detection and inference. Stat. Med. 14:799–810.

Kulldorff, M. 1997. A spatial scan statistic. Commun. Stat. – Theory Meth. 26:1481–1496.

Kulldorff, M., Athas, W. F., Feurer, E. J., Miller, B. A., and Key, C. R. 1998. Evaluating cluster alarms: a space-time scan statistic and brain cancer in Los Alamos, New Mexico. Am. J. Public Health 88:1377–1380.

Kulldorff, M., and Hjalmars, U. 1999. The Knox method and other tests for space-time interaction. Biometrics 55:544–552.

Kulldorff, M., Heffernan, R., Hartman, J., Assuncao, R., and Mostashari, F. 2005. A space-time permutation scan statistic for disease outbreak detection. PLoS Med. 2:e59.

Kulldorff, M., Information Management Services, Inc. 2006. SaTScanTM v7.0: Software for the spatial and space-time scan statistics. http://www.satscan.org/

Larsen, R. J., Holmes, C. L., and Heath, C. W. 1973. A statistical test for measuring unimodal clustering: a description of the test and of its application to case of acute leukemia in metropolitan Atlanta, Georgia. Biometrics 29:301–309.

Linenberger, M. L., and Abkowitz, J. L. 1995. Haematological disorders associated with feline retrovirus infections. Baillieres Clin. Haematol. 8:73–112.

Linet, M. S., Gridley, G., Cnattingius, S., Nicholson, H. S., Martinsson, U., Glimelius, B., Adami, H. O., and Zack, M. 1996. Maternal and perinatal risk factors for childhood brain tumors (Sweden). Cancer Causes Control 7:437–448.

Little, J. 1999. Epidemiology of Childhood Cancer. Lyon: International Agency for Research on Cancer, Publ. no. 149.
Mainwaring, D. 1966. Epidemiology of acute leukaemia of childhood in the Liverpool area. Br. J. Prev. Soc. Med. 20:189–194.
Mangoud, A., Hillier, V. F., Leck, I., and Thomas, R. W. 1985. Space-time interaction in Hodgkin's disease in Greater Manchester. J. Epidemiol. Community Health 39:58–62.
Mantel, N. 1967. The detection of disease clustering and a generalized regression approach. Cancer Res. 27:209–220.
McElvenny, D. M., Darnton, A. J., Hodgson, J. T., Clarke, S. D., Elliott, R. C., and Osman, J. 2003. Investigation of cancer incidence and mortality at a Scottish semiconductor manufacturing facility. Occup. Med. (Lond). 53:419–430.
McNally, R. J., Alexander, F. E., and Birch, J. M. 2002a. Space-time clustering analyses of childhood acute lymphoblastic leukaemia by immunophenotype. Br. J. Cancer 87: 513–515.
McNally, R. J., Cairns, D. P., Eden, O. B., Alexander, F. E., Taylor, G. M., Kelsey, A. M., and Birch, J. M. 2002b. An infectious aetiology for childhood brain tumours? Evidence from space-time clustering and seasonality analyses. Br. J. Cancer 86:1070–1077.
McNally, R. J., Kelsey, A. M., Eden, O. B., Alexander, F. E., Cairns, D. P., and Birch, J. M. 2003a. Space-time clustering patterns in childhood solid tumours other than central nervous system tumours. Int. J. Cancer 103:253–258.
McNally, R. J., Alston, R. D., Cairns, D. P., Eden, O. B., and Birch, J. M. 2003b. Geographical and ecological analyses of childhood acute leukaemias and lymphomas in North-West England. Br. J. Haematol. 123:60–65.
McNally, R. J., Alston, R. D., Cairns, D. P., Eden, O. B., Kelsey, A. M., and Birch, J. M. 2003c. Geographical and ecological analyses of childhood Wilms' tumours and soft-tissue sarcomas in North West England. Eur. J. Cancer 39:1586–1593.
McNally, R. J., and Eden, T. O. 2004. An infectious aetiology for childhood acute leukaemia: a review of the evidence. Br. J. Haematol. 127:243–263.
McNally, R. J., Alexander, F. E., Eden, O. B., and Birch, J. M. 2004. Little or no space-time clustering found amongst cases of childhood lymphoma in North West England. Eur. J. Cancer 40:585–589.
McNally, R. J., Eden, T. O., Alexander, F.E., Kelsey, A. M., and Birch, J. M. 2005. Is there a common aetiology for certain childhood malignancies? Results of cross-space-time clustering analyses. Eur. J. Cancer 41:2911–2916.
McNally, R. J., Alexander, F. E., and Bithell, J. F. 2006a. Space-time clustering of childhood cancer in Great Britain: a national study, 1969–1993. Int. J. Cancer 118:2840–2846.
McNally, R. J., Pearce, M. S., and Parker, L. 2006b. Space-time clustering analyses of testicular cancer amongst 15–24-year-olds in Northern England. Eur. J. Epidemiol. 21:139–144.
McNally, R. J., Bithell, J. F., Vincent, T. J., and Murphy, M. F. 2009a. Space-time clustering of childhood cancer around the residence at birth. Int. J. Cancer 124:449–455.
McNally, R. J., Alexander, F. E., Vincent, T. J., and Murphy, M. F. 2009b. Spatial clustering of childhood cancer in Great Britain during the period 1969–1993. Int. J. Cancer 124:932–936.
Meighan, S. S., and Knox, G. 1965. Leukaemia in childhood: epidemiology in Oregon. Cancer 18:811–814.
Meliker, J. R., and Jacquez, G. M. 2007. Space-time clustering of case-control data with residential histories: insights into empirical induction periods, age-specific susceptibility, and calendar year-specific effects. Stoch. Environ. Res. Risk Assess. 21:625–634.
Morris, V. 1990. Space-time interactions in childhood cancers. J. Epidemiol. Community Health 44:55–58.
Mueller, N. 1995. Overview: viral agents and cancer. Environ. Health Perspect. 103(Suppl 8): 259–261.
Muirhead, C. R., and Ball, A. M. 1989. Contribution to the discussion at the Royal Statistical Society meeting on cancer near nuclear establishments. J. R. Stat. Soc A 152:376.

Neutra, R. R. 1990. Counterpoint from a cluster buster. Am. J. Epidemiol. 132:1–8.
Nevins, J. R. 2005. Cell transformation by viruses. In: Knipe, D. M., Howley, P. M., Griffin, D. E., Lamb, R. A., Martin, M. A., Roizman, B., and Straus, S., editors. Fields Virology. Philadelphia, PA: Lippincott Williams and Wilkins.
Penrose, M. 1970. Cat leukaemia. Br. Med. J. 1:755.
Petridou, E., Revinthi, K., Alexander, F. E., Haidas, S., Koliouskas, D., Kosmidis, H., Piperopoulou, F., Tzortzatou, F., and Trichopoulos, D. 1996. Space-time clustering of childhood leukaemia in Greece: evidence supporting a viral aetiology. Br. J. Cancer 73:1278–1283.
Petridou, E., Alexander, F. E., Trichopoulos, D., Revinthi, K., Dessypris, N., Wray, N., Haidas, S., Koliouskas, D., Kosmidis, H., Piperopoulou, F., and Tzortzatou, F. 1997. Aggregation of childhood leukemia in geographic areas of Greece. Cancer Causes Control 8:239–245.
Pinkel, D., and Nefzger, D. 1959. Some epidemiological features of childhood leukemia in the Buffalo, NY area. Cancer 12:351–358.
Pinkel, D., Dowd, J. E., and Bross, I. D. 1963. Some epidemiological features of malignant solid tumors of children in the Buffalo, NY area. Cancer 16:28–33.
Pike, M. C., and Smith, P. G. 1974. Case-control approach to examine diseases for evidence of contagion, including disease with long latent periods. Biometrics 30:263–279.
Potthoff, R. F., and Whittinghill, M. 1966. Testing for homogeneity: II. The Poisson distribution. Biometrika 53:183–190.
Rothman, K. J. 1990. A sobering start for the cluster busters' conference. Am. J. Epidemiol. 132(Suppl 1):S6–S13.
Schwartz, S. O., Greenspan, I., and Brown, E. R. 1963. Leukemic clusters in Niles, ILL. Immunologic data on families of leukemic patients and others. JAMA 186;106–108.
Shaw, A. K., Li, P., and Infante-Rivard, C. 2006. Early infection and risk of childhood brain tumors (Canada). Cancer Causes Control 17:1267–1274.
Smith, P. G., Pike, M. C., Till, M. M., and Hardisty, R. M. 1976. Epidemiology of childhood leukaemia in Greater London: a search for evidence of transmission assuming a possibly long latent period. Br. J. Cancer 33:1–8.
Smith, M. 1997. Considerations on a possible viral etiology for B-precursor acute lymphoblastic leukemia of childhood. J. Immunother. 20:89–100.
Steinmaus, C., Lu, M., Todd, R. L., and Smith, A. H. 2004. Probability estimates for the unique childhood leukemia cluster in Fallon, Nevada, and risks near other US military aviation facilities. Environ. Health Perspect. 112:766–771.
Viejo-Borbolla, A., and Schulz, T. F. 2003. Kaposi's sarcoma-associated herpesvirus (KSHV/HHV8): key aspects of epidemiology and pathogenesis. AIDS Rev. 5:222–229.
Walter, S. D., and Elwood, J. M. 1975. A test for seasonality of events with a variable population at risk. Br. J. Prevent. Soc. Med. 29:18–21.
Westerbeek, R. M., Blair, V., Eden, O. B., Kelsey, A. M., Stevens, R. F., Will, A. M., Taylor, G. M., and Birch, J. M. 1998. Seasonal variations in the onset of childhood leukaemia and lymphoma. Br. J. Cancer 78:119–124.
Williams, J. R., Alexander, F. E., Cartwright, R. A., and McNally, R. J. 2001. Methods for eliciting aetiological clues from geographically clustered cases of disease, with application to leukaemia-lymphoma data. J. R. Stat. Soc. A 164:49–60.
Young, L. S., and Rickinson, A. B. 2004. Epstein-Barr virus: 40 years on. Nat. Rev. Cancer 4: 757–768.
Zahalkova, M., Bilek, O., Kubikova, A., and Belusa, M. 1970. The incidence of leukaemias in children and their clustering in space and time in South Moravian Province, Czechoslovakia. Blut 21:180–185.

Chapter 5
Discovering Gene–Gene and Gene–Environment Causal Interactions Using Bioinformatics Approaches

Changwon Yoo

Abstract The exponential growth of molecular biology data led to an intense focus on the study of interactions among DNA, RNA, protein biosynthesis, and environment. Using advanced genomics revolution tools, large datasets generated by the gene expression profiling experiments and next generation sequences technologies enable us to link molecular states and environmental effects to physiological states through the reverse engineering of gene–gene and gene–environment interaction networks that sense DNA and environmental perturbations. This will ultimately let us understand variations in physiological states associated with disease. In this chapter we review different mathematical and statistical bioinformatics approaches to discover and model gene–gene and gene–environment causal interactions. We also present new additional modeling methods in probabilistic networks to incorporate various interventions to perturb the system.

Keywords Gene–gene and gene–environment interactions · Bioinformatics · Causal discovery · Causal modeling · Causal bayesian networks

The genome sequences of a number of different organisms have been characterized recently. For example, an international effort to sequence the entire genome of the yeast *Saccharomyces cerevisiae* was completed in April 1996. The first complete DNA sequence of a plant, *Arabidopsis thaliana*, was finished in December 1999. In June 2000, the Human Genome Project and representatives of the biotechnology company Celera announced the completion of a working draft reference of the DNA sequence of the human genome.

Gene expression profiling and next generation DNA and RNA sequencing are related technologies that have opened a new era for systems biology studies. They allow a quick and easy way to measure the level of cDNA or mRNA and sequences from different genes among different cells. Large datasets generated by

---

C. Yoo (✉)
Department of Epidemiology and Biostatistics, Robert Stempel School of Public Health, Florida International University, Miami, FL 33199-0001, USA
e-mail: cyoo@fiu.edu

D. Roy, M.T. Dorak (eds.), *Environmental Factors, Genes, and the Development of Human Cancers*, DOI 10.1007/978-1-4419-6752-7_5,

the gene expression profiling experiments and next generation sequences technologies provide good opportunities to learn gene–gene and gene–environment causal interactions, and compilation of the causal knowledge will help us associate more genotypes with phenotypes.

Good experimental design generally permits meaningful analyses of experimental results. But most current gene expression computational tools concentrate only on issues related to the analysis of gene expression data. They do not help with the experimental design of gene expression profiling experiments.

In this chapter we will review bioinformatics approaches in modeling the gene–gene and gene–environment causal interactions of systems biology studies. Many gene–gene causal interactions models have been introduced recently. However, not many bioinformatics approaches are available in modeling gene-environment causal interactions. Thus, in Section 5.4 we introduce a promising probabilistic causal model, i.e., causal Bayesian networks, and discuss how to represent gene-environment causal interactions using the probabilistic causal model. Note that Section 5.4 is dense with mathematical formulas. If you are not comfortable with mathematical formulas, you may skip Section 5.4 without losing the entire idea of this chapter. We conclude this chapter with promising research directions of gene–gene and gene–environment causal interactions models using bioinformatics approaches.

5.1 Introduction

The field of bioinformatics has been rapidly growing in recent years especially since the completion of human genome project (The Genome International Sequencing Consortium, 2001). Bioinformatics is the study of representing and analyzing biological systems from different types of information from molecular level measurements (genome sequence, gene expression, protein structure, etc.) and also from patient, ecological, and population data.

In bioinformatics, the ultimate goal of studies in discovering gene–gene and gene–environment interactions is to discover *causal* relationship among genes and environmental factors. Many bioinformatics approaches will use a causal probabilistic model to discover interactions among hundreds and thousands of genes and environmental factors. In the causal probabilistic model, we typically model genes and environmental factors as variables or random variables. Some examples of the causal probabilistic models are shown in Fig. 5.1.

Figure 5.1a shows a Bayesian network that represents hypothetical interaction among genes and transcription factors (denoted as Gene1, Gene2, TF1, TF2, and TF3). Nodes represent random variables and arcs represent interaction among the random variables. Bayesian networks will be described in further detail in Section 5.3.3. Figure 5.1b shows the same gene network that is presented in EcoCyc (Karp et al., 1999). EcoCyc is a bioinformatics pathway database that describes the genome and the biochemical machinery of *E. coli*. As opposed to Bayesian

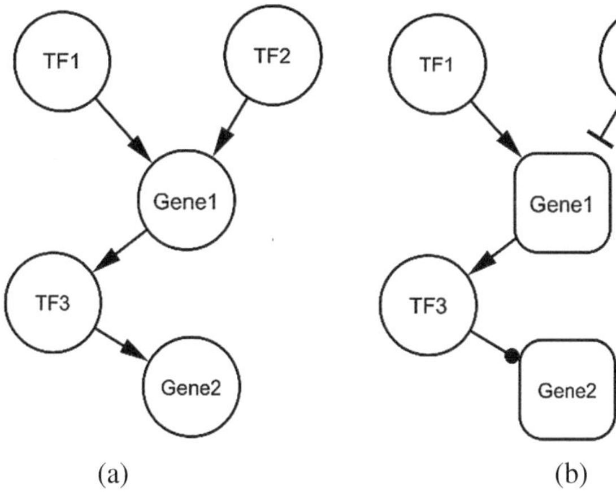

Fig. 5.1 Examples of causal probabilistic models

networks, EcoCyc uses different representations for genes (as rectangles), and for some arcs (blunt arrow indicates repression; a brown circle-ended arrow indicates that the factor can activate or repress, depending on circumstances). Although Bayesian networks and EcoCyc use different representations, they can represent the same underlying causal relationships.

Causal modeling and discovery are fundamental pursuits of science. Causal relationship discovery among genes and their surrounding environment is promising more than ever, since recent sequencing and high throughput gene expression measurement technologies have enabled us to observe the sequence of the genome and the activities of thousands of genes at a time (Brown and Botstein, 1999; Lipshutz et al., 1999; Margulies et al., 2005). Novel causal discoveries that are enabled by sequencing and high throughput technologies are likely to have a large impact on science. For better causal discovery, not only is the causal analysis method and data important, but good experimental design is also crucial. Recent systems biology research approaches (Schadt, 2009) benefit from a causal analysis method that incorporates a recommendation of experimental design for causal discovery (Tong and Koller, 2001; Yoo and Cooper, 2004) and knowledge discovery from published scientific papers (Schuemie et al., 2007; Steele et al., 2009).

Most research on causal discovery using causal networks has been based on using passive observational data (Cooper and Herskovits, 1992; Heckerman, 1995; Spirtes et al., 2000). There are limitations in learning causal relationships from observational data only. For example, if the generating process contains a latent factor (confounder) that influences two variables, it can be difficult, if not impossible, to learn the causal relationships between those two variables from observational data alone.

To uncover such causal relationships, a scientist generally needs to design a study that involves manipulating a variable (or variables) and then observing the changes (if any) in other variables of interest. For example, if a biologist is interested in the causal relationship between gene A and gene B, he or she may knock out gene A, observe the expression level of gene B, and compare that level with the expression level of gene B when gene A was not knocked out ("wild-type"). In this simple study, in one group that acts as a control, the biologist observed both gene A and gene B, in the other group, the biologist manipulated gene A and observed gene B. The biologist could also knock out gene B, observe the expression level of gene A, and compare it with the control group. Limited time and funds restrict the number of variables that can be manipulated and the number of *experimental repeats*[1] that can be collected for the control and experimental groups. For example, a molecular biologist who is interested in discovering the causal pathway of the genes involved in galactose metabolism first has to select the genes he or she is interested in understanding at a causal level. These genes are usually selected based on previously published results or by the molecular biologist's personal interest. Many aspects are considered in order to decide the number of experimental repeats to obtain for each variable in the study design. Having more experimental repeats will typically tighten the statistical confidence intervals in the data analysis. Considering available time, budget, and other constraints, the biologist will make a decision about the number of *cases*[2] to obtain, that is, the number of experimental repeats to perform for each type of experiment.

This process, also known as a systems biology cycle (Kitano, 2002), is shown in Fig. 5.3. In Fig. 5.3, the gene–gene and gene-environment models uses large scale and high dimensional data, e.g., microarray expression data, in light of the user's prior beliefs about causal relationships among the models under study. These models recommend the best possible experiments to the experimenter. The experimenter then chooses the next experiment to perform, which may or may not be the one suggested by the models. When the experiment results are available, they can be submitted to the models for a new round of analysis.

Developing causal analysis methods is a key focus of several fields. In statistics, jointly with medicine, issues related to randomized clinical trials (RCTs) are studied, including methods for finding an optimal number of cases using stopping rules (Spiegelhalter et al., 1994; Berry and Stangl, 1996; Friedman et al., 1996). In molecular biology, developing techniques that generate efficient experimental designs for high throughput methods, such as cDNA microarrays, is widely used (Karp et al., 1999; Kerr and Churchill, 2001; Smith and Kruglyak, 2008). In artificial intelligence, techniques using graphical models have been used to model experimentation and have been applied to suggest the next experiment for causal discovery (Karp et al., 1999; Ideker et al., 2000; Tong and Koller, 2001).

All these prior approaches have made significant contributions to efficient causal study design (see Section 5.2 for details), but they are not sensitive to issues of limited resources and experimenter preferences. Theoretically, modeling gene–gene

[1] Measurements of different microarray chips under same experimental condition.

[2] Refers to a vector of gene expression levels extracted from a single microarray chip. Generally, it refers to a record in a database.

and gene–environment causal interactions is, to put it in a simplistic term, nothing but adding more modeled variables into the mathematical model. As we will see in this chapter that many bioinformatics approaches that are applied to model gene–gene (Yoo et al., 2002; Jones et al., 2008; Yoo and Blitz, 2008) or gene-environment (Hahn et al., 2003; Smith and Kruglyak, 2008) causal interactions. As we gather more and more data, we will see more bioinformatics approaches that will be applied to gene–gene *and* gene–environment causal interactions.

We will first review bioinformatics models that have been developed for gene–gene causal interactions and then we use one of the bioinformatics models, causal Bayesian networks, to show how gene-environment causal interactions can be modeled.

5.2 Background

This section introduces background for gene–gene and gene–environment causal modeling in bioinformatics systems biology analyses. Many different fields concentrate on study design for causal discovery. Traditionally, in statistics and medicine, research on causal discovery is actively pursued in research on controlled trials. In computer science, causal discovery is also an active research topic, especially in the machine learning community. In biology, recent microarray technologies have fueled a field known as *systems biology*, which seeks to discover causal relationships among a large number of genes and other cellular constituents. In this section, we will introduce background of causal modeling in systems biology analysis, concentrating especially on the fields just mentioned.

5.2.1 Medicine and Statistics

The randomized clinical trial (RCT) is a well-known method for deciding the effect of a new clinical treatment, such as a drug. Although the clinical trial (CT) dates back to the eighteenth century (Lilienfield, 1982), the concept of randomization was first introduced by Fisher (1925).

For a long time, statistics and medicine worked jointly on issues related to the RCT, such as choosing how to randomize, selecting a treatment, finding an efficient sample size, and specifying a length of time for the experiment (Friedman et al., 1996). Chaloner and Verdinelli (1995) give a good review of the Bayesian approach to experimental design. Their review is based on the decision theoretic approach to experimental design (Lindley, 1972), which states the problem as follows:

> An experimental design e should be chosen from some set E and data y should be observed from a sample space Y. Based on y, a decision d will be chosen from some set D. The decision is in two parts: first the selection of e and then the choice of a decision d. For any design e, the expected utility of the best decision is given by

$$U(e) = \int_Y \max_{d \in D} \int_\Theta U(d, \theta, y, e) \cdot p(\theta | y, e) \cdot (y | e)\, d\theta\, dy$$

where θ are unknown parameters from the parameter space Θ. Then the Bayesian solution to the experimental design problem is provided by the design e^* that maximizes the above equation namely:

$$U(e^*) = \max_{e \in E} \int_Y \max_{d \in D} \int_\Theta U(d, \theta, y, e) \cdot p(\theta | y, e) \cdot p(y | e)\, d\theta\, dy$$

Bayesian calculation of the sample size for the CT was studied by Achcar (1984) using a Weibull distribution. Brooks (1987) used the expected gain in information from a two-group experiment with Weibull lifetimes. Sylvester (1988) studied the sample size for a phase II CT using a Bayesian approach when the outputs follow a Bernoulli distribution. Spiegelhalter et al. (1994) showed a Bayesian approach to RCTs that include modeling the experimenter's priors. To provide an efficient stopping rule of the RCT, Berry and Stangl (1996) modeled all possible outcomes of two therapies and calculated the expected value of the outcomes. They used these expected values to recommend which therapy the experimenter should choose next.

Although issues related to the experimental designs of CTs are closely related to the experimental designs of gene expression studies, there is a major difference between the two. The design of the CT concentrates more on high-level causal relationships. For example, a typical CT is designed to learn whether a drug has a significant effect on treating a disease. The main interest in the CT design is not the pathophysiological causal pathways by which the patient's body reacts to the drug. Thus, the intervention in the CT is whether to give (usually randomly) a patient the drug or placebo. In experimental designs of gene expression studies the causes and effects can involve detailed networks of relationships among the genes. The experimental combinatorics are huge, because—for example—every possible multi-gene knock-out of a set of genes is a possible experimental intervention. Also in the CT design, a patient model incorporates compliance, noncompliance, and switchover (Lakatos, 1988; Dupont and Plummer, 1990) whereas in the design of a gene expression study, those issues are not relevant.

5.2.2 *Molecular Biology*

Microarray techniques opened a new era of studies in molecular biology. Before these techniques existed, there were labor-intensive methods like Northern blot analyses to measure a single gene's expression patterns in cells. Current microarray techniques can measure the expression level of about 10,000 genes at a time. A successful sequencing of the entire genome of yeast *Saccharomyces cerevisiae* in April 1996 initiated many gene expression experimental studies in yeast (Spellman et al.,

1998; Ideker et al., 2001; Smith and Kruglyak, 2008). These studies, as well as many other studies that are related to them, fit under a new approach in biology that is called *systems biology*. Systems biology seeks in part to model large networks of cellular function, including the causal pathways that capture how genes regulate each other. A recent review of system biology is provided by Ideker et al. (2001) and Kitano (2002).

The more that experimental studies of gene expression are performed, the greater is the benefit of having standardized components of experimental design are needed. A standard representation of gene experimental design was suggested and a Web-based experimentation search tool was implemented in (Heiman and Walter, 2000). A standard representation of genes of different species has been proposed (The Gene Ontology Consortium, 2000). Several metabolic causal pathway representations have also been suggested using a hybrid method that combines Boolean ON OFF switches and continuous input–output functions (McAdams and Shapiro, 1995; Yuh et al., 1998). Metabolic causal pathway representation has been implemented into computer systems (KEGG; MIPS; Karp et al., 1999). Kerr and Churchill (2001) talked about a different way to pair the targets in the cDNA microarray experimental design. They argued that more variance can be modeled using a "balanced design" than with the widely used "reference design" in microarray studies. They used analysis of variance (ANOVA) to model microarray experiments with multiple categorical factors such as microarray chip effect, dye effect, and experimental condition effect (Kerr and Churchill, 2001).

The gene expression experimental study cycle consists of three large steps: first, form a hypothesis; second, model and perform experiments; and third, update the hypothesis. It is likely that gene pathways from published articles (Blaschke et al., 2001; Stephens et al., 2001) will help the first step of the experimental study. Developing a system that recommends how to design and analyze experimentation will help the second and third steps of the cycle. Having a standard representation of a gene pathway will also help the overall experimental study cycle. Unfortunately there is as yet no accepted standard representation of gene pathways, although as suggested above, such standards are quickly evolving.

5.2.3 Artificial Intelligence

We design experimental studies in either a clinical trial or a gene pathway study to learn the causal relationships among the modeled variables. In artificial intelligence (AI) research there have been two main approaches to inferring causal relationships using directed acyclic graphs as a representation of causation. One approach involves searching the data for patterns of conditional independence and dependence that reveal some information about the underlying causal structure (Pearl, 2000; Spirtes et al., 2000). The other approach uses a Bayesian method to calculate the posterior probability of some causal model hypothesis given data and prior belief about causation (Cooper and Herskovits, 1992; Heckerman, 1995; Heckerman et al., 1999).

To review related work on modeling gene–gene and gene–environment causal interactions, we will first review the different models that have been used to represent the underlying gene–gene causal interactions (genetic pathway) itself. Next we will review related work on modeling gene–environment causal interactions using genetic pathway models.

5.3 Gene–Gene Causal Interaction Model

Before describing gene–gene causal interaction (genetic pathway) models, we first place them in the context of gene clustering methods, which have been very popular the last few years. Indeed most of the early work on gene expression data analyses used clustering methods. Gene expression levels that were measured by cDNA microarray in the yeast cell-division cycle were analyzed for the first time using a cluster analysis (Spellman et al., 1998). A cluster analysis typically searches for groups of genes that show similar expression pattern among different experimental conditions. Other analyses followed using similar cluster analyses applied to microarray data (Michaels et al., 1998; Golub et al., 1999; Herwig et al., 1999).

Clinical studies also used cluster analysis on microarray data (Alizadeh et al., 2000; Getz et al., 2000). For example, Alizadeh et al. (2000) used cluster analysis to find different types of diffuse large B-cell lymphoma (DLBCL) among DLBCL patients by comparing the clusters of similarly expressed genes and whether or not they responded to the current therapy. Recently many microarray clinical studies have been published (see section on *Human Genome Variation: Linking Genotypes to Clinical Phenotypes* in Pacific Symposium on Biocomputing 2001). Along with classification or cluster analyses, gene pathway (network) analyses were performed on the gene expression data. Analyses to construct pathways among the genes yield more information than do cluster or classification analyses. Cluster and classification analyses do not necessarily provide causal information, which is at the heart of gene pathway discovery. On the other hand, knowledge of causal pathways can be used to produce a causal clustering of the genes.

In the following subsections, we will review gene–gene causal interaction (genetic pathway or network) models. Tsang (1999) and Dutilh (1999) give a short review of genetic networks. A more thorough review based on biological context was published by Smolen et al. (2000), who suggested that current microarray techniques are limited in delineating intracellular signaling pathways. Smolen et al. (2000) argues that since microarray technology is measuring an average expression level of a gene among millions of cells, there is little we can learn about gene-regulation pathways information from the data. A review of genetic networks that is focused more on modeling methods (see Section 5.2.3) is given by de Jong (2002).

Wessels et al. (2001) conducted a limited comparison study of selected continuous genetic network models (Arkin et al., 1997; Chen et al., 1999; Weaver et al.,

1999). Again, using three different published models, they generated 165 datasets and tested them on selected continuous genetic network models. They concluded that the Arkin et al. (1997) model performs relatively better than other models, and that the linear model performed well in complex models.

5.3.1 Boolean Networks

Boolean networks were first introduced by Somogyi and Sniegoski (1996). A structure search algorithm in Boolean networks called REVEAL (REVerse Engineering ALgorithm) was introduced by Liang et al. (1998).

REVEAL uses mutual information among nodes in search of a structure. Liang et al. (1998) defined entropy of a gene X_i as $H(X_i) = -p_0 \log p_0 - p_1 \log p_1$, where p_0 and p_1 are the maximum likelihood of 0s and 1s (as an expression level of the gene X_i) from data respectively. Also defined is $H(X_i, X_j) = -\sum_{k,l \in \{0,1\}} p_{kl} \log p_{kl}$, where p_{kl} represents the maximum likelihood estimate from the data of the joint expression level of X_i as k and X_j as l. Finally, mutual information is defined as follows:

$$M(X_i, X_j) = H(X_j) - H(X_j|X_i) = H(X_i) - H(X_i|X_j)$$

where $H(X_i \mid X_j) = H(X_i, X_j) - H(X_j)$ and $H(X_j \mid X_i) = H(X_i, X_j) - H(X_i)$. Using mutual information their search algorithm has three stages: (1) search for all pairs X_i and X_{j1} and check whether $M(X_i, X_{j1}) = H(X_i)$. Whenever the condition is satisfied, a Boolean function is assigned between X_i and X_{j1}, i.e., X_{j1} determines X_i; (2) if there is any X_i with no function assignment, then test whether $M(X_i, X_{j1}, X_{j2}) = H(X_i)$ for all X_{j1}, X_{j2}; (3) repeat the second stage by adding additional X_j to the previous condition. In the worst case, the search algorithm will check the condition $M(X_i, X_{j1}, X_{j2}, \ldots, X_{jn-1}) = H(X_i)$, where n is the number of modeled genes. Akutsu et al. (1999) gave a mathematical proof of the observation of Liang et al. (1998) that a small number of state transition (INPUT/OUTPUT) pairs are sufficient in order to infer the original Boolean network. More systems that use Boolean networks were introduced with some added functions (Karp et al., 1999; Samsonova and Serov, 1999; Ideker et al., 2000).

With its simple representation, Boolean networks were easily implemented as genetic networks. However, since Boolean networks do not explicitly model uncertainty, they cannot model the stochastic behavior of a biological system. Also note that Boolean networks do not use any arrows for the arcs among gene–gene and gene–environment interactions. Thus, there is no sense of causality in the model. In Fig. 5.2, we show an example of a Boolean network that represents the hypothetical gene–gene interaction that was previously introduced in Fig. 5.1.

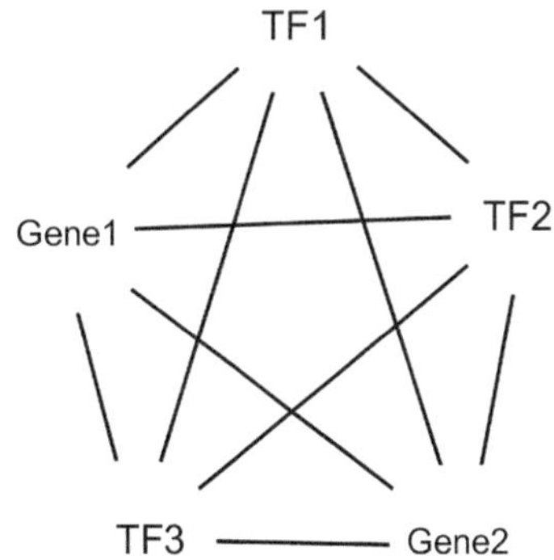

Fig. 5.2 An example of a Boolean network

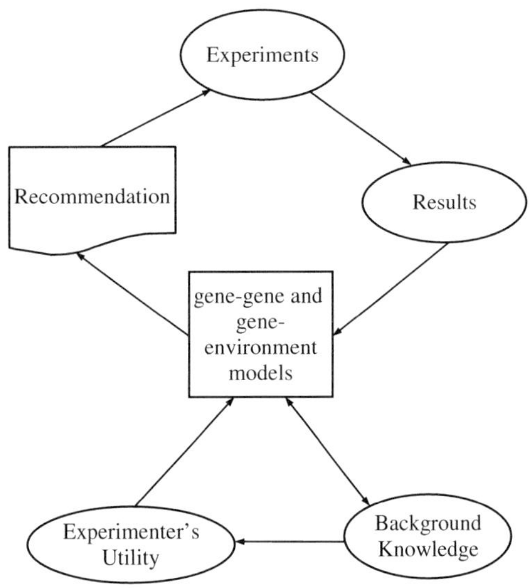

Fig. 5.3 Systems biology analysis cycle in bioinformatics

5.3.2 Continuous Models

In mathematics, using differential equations to model a biological system has a long history (Goodwin, 1965; Griffith, 1968; Griffith, 1968). Chen et al. (1999) modeled a dynamic system of genes using differential equations. They modeled a simplified dynamic system of gene regulation (with feedback on transcription) as shown in Fig. 5.4.

In Fig. 5.4, C and L are transcription and translation constant ($n \times n$ matrices) respectively, V and U are degradation rates ($n \times n$ matrices), and n represents the number of genes.

Figure 5.4 can be modeled as a nonlinear dynamic system as follows:

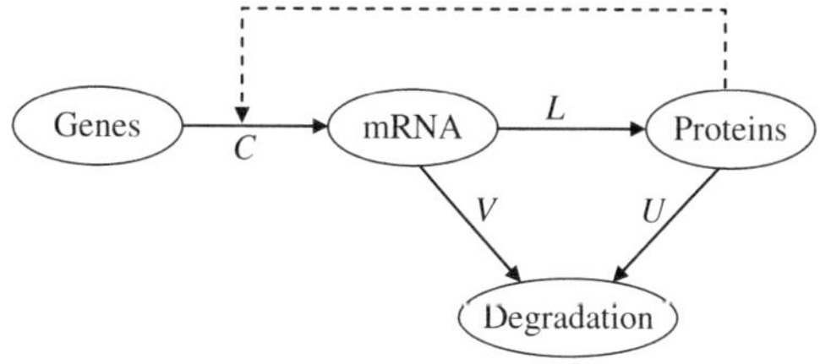

Fig. 5.4 A simplified dynamic system of gene regulation

$$\frac{d\boldsymbol{r}}{dt} = f(\boldsymbol{p}) - V\boldsymbol{r} \qquad \frac{d\boldsymbol{p}}{dt} = L\boldsymbol{r} - U\boldsymbol{p}$$

where $\boldsymbol{r}$ and $\boldsymbol{p}$ are the mRNA and protein concentration (n-dimensional vector) respectively and f is a transcription function. Chen et al. (1999) assumed $f(\boldsymbol{p})$ to be a linear function of $\boldsymbol{p}$ and constructed the model from a set of temporal samples of mRNA and protein. They argue that this approach can model most of gene regulation in a genome from a relatively small set of accurate temporal gene-expression data. Several other models of differential equations were used to describe the genetic pathway (Snoussi and Thomas, 1993; Mestl et al., 1996; Plahte et al., 1998).

Weaver et al. (1999) used a simple weighted model, which assumes that the net regulatory effect of gene j on gene i at some state t is simply the expression level of gene j times its regulatory influence (modeled as a weight) on gene i. Similar to Weaver et al. (1999), D'haeseleer et al. (1999) used a linear weighted model to analyze the time series gene expression data from a rat cervical spinal cord and hippocampus. Reis et al. (2001) looked at the dynamics to search for causal relationships among genes with a cluster analysis, where dynamics refers to the rate of change of genetic expression over time.

Differential equations can model biological dynamics more specifically than Boolean networks, but the computational cost of the differential equation model is high, and often many of the parameters needed in the differential equation model are not available. Since most of the dynamics of the actual genetic pathways appear to be non-linear, a linear model seems to work on only limited dynamics of the genetic pathway.

5.3.3 Bayesian Networks

The Bayesian network (BN) model, also known as a probabilistic causal network, has been widely used to learn predictive models from data. The BN overcomes the shortcomings of the simple Bayesian method, first explored extensively in the early 1960s, that assumed conditional independence of the evidence given an hypothesis. BNs can model causality based on expert's knowledge, data or both. It is also used in many medical related domains because of its ability to perform inference in the forward direction, backward direction, or any combination (Citro et al., 1997; Chevrolat et al., 1998; Lucas et al., 2000). One practical limitation of BNs is that inference within them is NP-hard (Cooper, 1987), which is a frequent limitation of powerful reasoning methodologies; in response, researchers have developed approximate inference methods to apply to complex BN inference tasks.

A causal Bayesian network (or *causal network* for short) is a Bayesian network in which each arc is interpreted as a direct causal influence between a parent node (variable) and a child node, relative to the other nodes in the network (Pearl, 1988). Figure 5.5 illustrates the structure of a hypothetical causal Bayesian network structure containing five nodes that represent genes. The probabilities associated with this causal network structure are not shown.

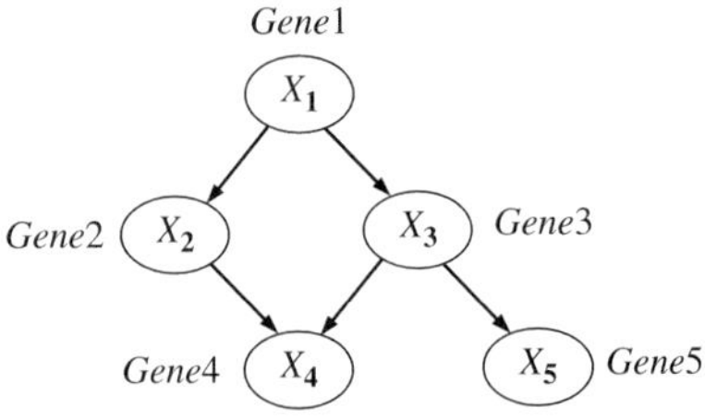

Fig. 5.5 A causal Bayesian network that represents a hypothetical gene-regulation pathway

The causal network structure in Fig. 5.5 indicates, for example, that the *Gene*1 can regulate (causally influence) the expression level of the *Gene*3, which in turn can regulate the expression level of the *Gene*5. The causal Markov condition gives the conditional independence relationships specified by a causal Bayesian network:

> A variable is independent of its non-descendants (i.e., non-effects) given its parents (i.e., its direct causes).

The causal Markov condition permits the joint distribution of the n variables in a causal Bayesian network to be factored as follows (Pearl, 1988):

$$P(x_1, x_2, ..., x_n|K) = \prod_{i=1}^{n} P(x_i|\pi_i, K) \quad (1)$$

where x_i denotes a state of variable X_i, π_i denotes a joint state of the parents of X_i, and K denotes background knowledge. Bayesian networks have been used in analyzing gene expression data from microarray experiments in order to model gene regulated pathways (Friedman et al., 2000; Hartemink et al., 2001).

Murphy and Mian (1999) showed that the Boolean network model (Somogyi and Sniegoski, 1996), the linear model (D'haeseleer et al., 1999), and the nonlinear weighted model (Weaver et al., 1999) are all special cases of dynamic Bayesian networks (DBN). A DBN incorporates time in Bayesian networks (which is then usually called a temporal Bayesian network). Yeast cell-cycle-regulated gene expression data (Spellman et al., 1998) was first analyzed using Bayesian networks by Friedman et al. (2000). Hartemink et al. (2001) used Bayesian networks with annotated arcs to represent promotion and inhibition reactions. Spirtes et al. (2001) discuss issues of sample size, measurement error and averaging effects on gene expression studies using causal Bayesian networks.

5.3.4 Mixture Models and Other Models

McAdams and Shapiro (1995) modeled the *E. coli* λ phage lysis-lysogeny genetic switch using a mixture of Boolean switches and continuous input-output relations. Yuh et al. (1998) modeled gene *endo16* in the sea urchin embryo with a similar hybrid model. Matsuno et al. (2000) used a Petri net that models continuous variables and analyzes the genetic switch mechanism of λ phage. Goss and Peccoud (1999) used stochastic Petri nets to model the stabilizing effect of the protein ROM on the genetic network regulating ColE1 plasmid replication.

There are many different kinds of statistical classification methods. A method commonly used for statistical classification is *k*-Nearest Neighbor (kNN), which classifies a new case by calculating the minimum distance (according to some metric) between the new case and a set of training cases. kNN has been used in areas such as the classification of radiology reports and the modeling of the immune system. Variations of kNN have more recently been used in classifying and clustering genes from large gene expression datasets (Michaels et al., 1998; Spellman et al., 1998; Golub et al., 1999; Herwig et al., 1999).

Petri nets is a formal graphical language appropriate for modeling systems with concurrency. Petri nets are based on a general theory for discrete parallel systems. Petri nets were used in guidelines for patient care flow (Quaglini et al., 2001). It has also been used in modeling mechanisms in a cell (Boucher et al., 1998; Goss and Peccoud, 1999; Matsuno et al., 2000).

Genetic programming uses the three basic mechanisms that drive natural evolution—*reproduction*, *mutation*, and *selection*—in its search for a model that best fits the training data. Evolutionary methods allow a program to evolve, giving it great freedom to search through a large space of possible models. Koza et al. (2001) has used genetic programming to learn gene networks from simulated data that was generated by a computer model of the cell, called E-cell (Tomita et al., 1999).

5.4 Gene-Environment Causal Interaction Models

Many developments have been made in gene–gene causal interaction models. These models are usually referred as gene networks, gene pathways, or gnomonic networks, however, molecular networks may be used to refer more general networks (Schadt, 2009). Many studies investigated relationships between polymorphism and environmental factors to study gene-environment causal interactions in humans, e.g., heart disease (Talmud, 2007), depression (Caspi et al., 2003), and cancer (Ulrich et al., 1999). However, we are still limited in collecting and analyzing molecular data for gene-environment causal interactions in human. Recent high throughput sequencing technologies enable us to identify large number of DNA sequence variations in population. The first and second phases of the International Haplotype Map, including, millions of single nucleotide polymorphisms (SNPs) were recently completed (The International Haplotype Map Consortium, 2005; Sabeti et al., 2007). Advance in high throughput sequencing technologies are already identifying rare DNA variations in different cancer types (Jones et al., 2008; Parsons et al., 2008).

Since it is difficult to learn molecular mechanisms of gene–environment interactions in human, there are limited bioinformatics approaches in modeling gene–environment interactions in human. However, transcript level of gene–environment causal interactions in other organisms such as yeast (Landrya et al., 2005; Smith and Kruglyak, 2008) and worms (Li et al., 2006) have been reported. Bayesian networks have been widely used and accepted in modeling molecular networks (Pe'er et al., 2001; Yoo et al., 2002; Yoo and Blitz, 2008; Zhu et al., 2008) We will introduce *causal* Bayesian networks and show how *causal* Bayesian networks can be use to model both gene–gene and gene–environment causal interactions. This section describes causal Bayesian networks.

5.4.1 Modeling Experiments in Bayesian Networks

In this section we will first explain Bayesian network models in general, and then describe how experimental manipulations can be modeled in causal Bayesian networks.

5.4.1.1 A General Bayesian Analysis

This section derives the posterior probability that variable[3] X causes variable Y given database D on measured variables V. Let H denote an additional set of latent (hidden) variables. Use $V+$ to designate the union of V and H. Let S denote an arbitrary causal Bayesian network structure containing all of the variables in $V+$. Let K denote any background knowledge that may influence our beliefs about the causal relationships among the variables in $V+$. Such background knowledge could come from scientific laws, common sense, expert opinion, or accumulated personal experience, as well as other sources. As we will see later in this section, K can also include knowledge of which cases (also known as records, instances, or samples) in D are experimental and which are observational. We can derive the posterior probability that X causes Y as:

$$P(X \rightarrow Y|D, K) = \sum_{S:\{X \rightarrow Y\} \text{ is in } S} P(S|D, K) \tag{2}$$

where the sum is taken over all causal network structures that (1) contain just the nodes in $V+$, and (2) contain an arc from X to Y.[4] Based on the properties

[3]We use the terms *variable* and *node* are used interchangeably in this section.

[4]In Equation (2) and subsequent equations in this section, the substructure $X \rightarrow Y$ can be replaced by any other substructure containing a subset of the variables in $V+$. For simplicity of exposition, however, we focus in this section on a pairwise causal relationship of the form $X \rightarrow Y$.

of probabilities, the term within the sum in Equation (2) may be rewritten as follows:

$$P(S|D,K) = \frac{P(S,D|K)}{P(D|K)} = \frac{P(S,D|K)}{\sum_S P(S,D|K)} \tag{3}$$

Since the probability $P(D \mid K)$ is a constant relative to the entire set of causal structures being considered, Equation (3) shows that the posterior probability of causal structure S is proportional to $P(S, D \mid K)$, which we can view as a *score* of S in the context of D. In this section, we use $P(S \mid D, K)$ and $P(S, D \mid K)$ interchangeably to refer the structure score. The probability terms on the right side of Equation (3) may be expanded as follows:

$$P(S,D|K) = P(S|K)P(D|S,K) = P(S|K)\int P(D|S,\theta_S,K)P(\theta_S|S,K)\,d\theta_S \tag{4}$$

where (1) $P(S \mid K)$ is a prior belief that network structure S correctly captures the qualitative causal relationships among the variables in $V+$; (2) θ_S are the probabilities (parameters) that relate the nodes in S quantitatively to their respective direct causes (represented as parents); (3) $P(D \mid S, \theta_S, K)$ is the likelihood of data D being produced, given that the causal process generating the data is a causal Bayesian network given by S and θ_S; and (4) $P(\theta_S \mid S, K)$ is the expression of a prior belief about the probability distributions that serve to model the underlying causal process. The integral in Equation (4) integrates out the parameters θ_S in a causal Bayesian network with structure S to derive $P(D \mid S, K)$, which is called the *marginal likelihood*. Combining Equations (2), (3), and (4), we obtain Equation (5):

$$P(X \to Y|D,K) = \frac{\sum_{S:\{X\to Y\}\text{ is in }S} P(S|K)\int P(D|S,\theta_S,K)P(\theta_S|S,K)\,d\theta_S}{\sum_S P(S|K)\int P(D|S,\theta_S,K)P(\theta_S|S,K)\,d\theta_S} \tag{5}$$

The only assumption made in this equation is that causal relationships are represented using causal Bayesian networks.

The full Bayesian approach to causal discovery expressed by Equation (5) considers—at least in principle—all causal Bayesian networks that are a priori possible. Thus, for example, the sums in Equation (5) are over all possible causal Bayesian network structures on $V+$, and the integrals are over all possible parameters for each possible causal structure. The result of such a global analysis of causality is that the derived posterior probabilities summarize a comprehensive, normative belief about the causal relationships among a set of variables.

5.4.2 Gene–Environment Causal Interaction Models Through Modeling Manipulation

In this section, first, we consider the situation in which manipulation of a variable may not be deterministic. A classic example from medicine is when a patient who has volunteered to participate in a study is randomized to receive a certain medication, but he or she decides not to take it. Let M_{X_i} be a variable that represents the value k (from 1 to r_i) to which the experimenter wishes to manipulate X_i. Let $M_{X_i} = 0$ denote that the experimenter does not wish to manipulate X_i, but merely wants to observe its value. Augment the model variables V in Section 5.4.1.1 to include M_{X_i}. Finally, carry out the analysis in Section 5.4.1.1 assuming only observational data. The causal network hypotheses used in that analysis will include probabilities that specify prior beliefs about the causal influence of M_{X_i} on X_i. Those prior beliefs (on structure and parameters) will be updated by data on stated experimental intentions and observed variable value outcomes. For the special case of deterministic manipulation, we have that (1) with probability 1, variable M_{X_i} is a parent of X_i; and (2) $P(X_i = x_i|M_{X_i} = k, \pi'_i) = 1$, where π'_i are the parents of X_i other than M_{X_i}. Note that M_{X_i} can also represent allele variation (natural variation, single nucleotide polymorphism) (Benfey and Mitchell-Olds, 2008).

For example, Fig. 5.6 shows a causal network structure which has an additional variable M_{X_2} relative to the network structure in Fig. 5.5. In Fig. 5.6, variable X_2 (*Gene*2) is modeled as being manipulated in some experiments by the researcher, such as the researcher knocking out (deleting) the *Gene*2.

Fig. 5.6 A causal Bayesian network structure that represents the manipulation of the *Gene*2

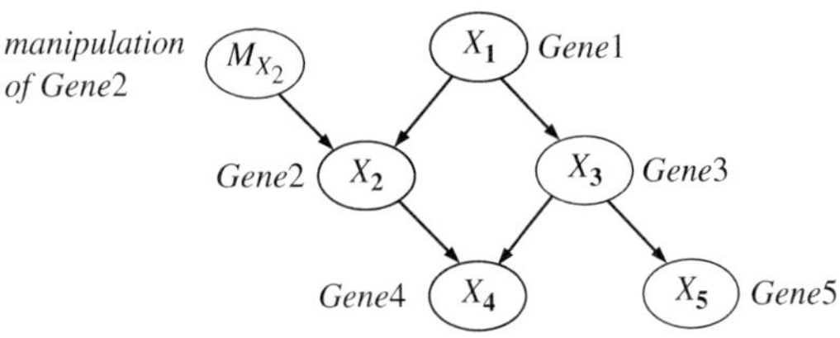

Now consider the situation in which the effects of the manipulation are either unknown or not well understood. These types of manipulations are most common in studies to learn gene-environment causal interactions. For example, Fig. 5.7 shows a causal network structure which has an additional variable M_E and E, which represent a manipulation (M_E) of an environmental condition (E) where its effects are unknown or not well understood. In Fig. 5.7, all genes are modeled as being manipulated by E because we do not know what genes are actually being affected by E. Some examples of such experiments are a study exposing genes to different chemicals, a study between smoker and non-smokers and difference in their gene expression patterns, and an RCT study of a new drug's molecular effects.

The advantage of representing manipulations (interventions) explicitly, as is done in Fig. 5.6, is that all variables in the causal Bayesian network model become

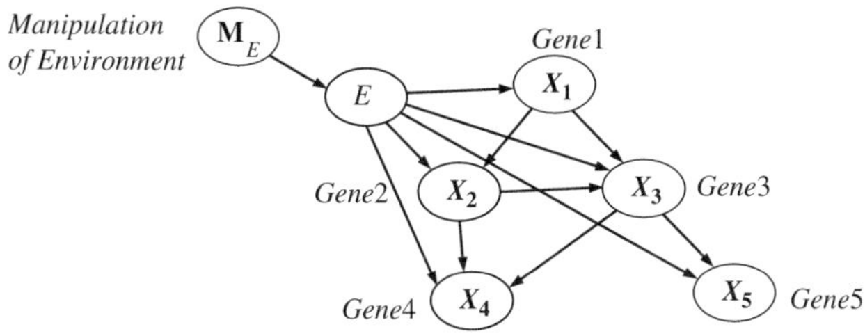

Fig. 5.7 A causal Bayesian network structure that represents the manipulation of an environmental condition *E*

observational. That is, by explicitly representing the act of manipulating a variable, we make that process an observational one, because we are simply observing it. Therefore, we can apply previously developed methods for evaluating Bayesian networks with observational data alone (see the next section).

5.4.2.1 Evaluating Causal Bayesian Networks

In this section, we show how causal Bayesian network models are evaluated (scored) assuming some conditions.[5] Under these assumptions, a causal Bayesian network *B* has a marginal likelihood that is given by the following equation (Cooper and Herskovits, 1992; Heckerman et al., 1995):

$$P(D|S,K) = \prod_{i=1}^{n}\prod_{j=1}^{q_i}\frac{\Gamma(\alpha_{ij})}{\Gamma(\alpha_{ij}+N_{ij})}\prod_{k=1}^{r_i}\frac{\Gamma(\alpha_{ijk}+N_{ijk})}{\Gamma(\alpha_{ijk})} \tag{6}$$

where r_i is the number of states that X_i can have, q_i denotes the number of joint states that the parents of X_i can have, N_{ijk} is the number of cases[6] in *D* in which node X_i is *passively observed* to have state *k* when its parents have states as given by *j*, Γ is the gamma function, α_{ijk} and α_{ij} express parameters of Dirichlet prior distributions, and $N_{ij} = \sum_{k=1}^{ri} N_{ijk}$. We use the BDe metric (Heckerman et al., 1995) with $\alpha_{ijk} = \frac{1}{r_i q_i}$, which is a commonly applied, non-informative parameter prior for the BDe metric.

[5]They are (1) discrete variables (2) Dirichlet prior parameter distributions (3) multinomial likelihood functions (4) parameter independence, and (5) parameter modularity, and (6) no missing data For assumptions (4) and (5), please refer Cooper and Herskovits (1992), Heckerman et al. (1995) for further information. However, in short, assumption (4) states: given network structure *S*, if $p(S|K)$>0 then (1) $p(\theta_S|S,K) = \prod_{i=1}^{n} p(\theta_i|S,K)$ (2) for *i*=1,. . .,*n*: $p(\theta_i|S,K) = \prod_{j=1}^{n} p(\theta_{ij}|S,K)$, where θ_{ijk} denote the multinomial parameter corresponding to $p(x_i{=}\,k|\pi_i{=}\,j, K)$ and $\theta_{ij}{=} \cup_k \theta_{ijk}$ and $\theta_j{=} \cup_j \theta_{ij}$. Assumption (5) states: given two network structures *S* and S' such that $p(S|K)$>0 and $p(S'|K)$>0, if x_i has the same parents in *S* and S', then for *j*=1,. . ., *n*: $p(\theta_{ij}|S, K) = p(\theta_{ij}|\, S', K)$.

[6]In this section, the term *case(s)* is used to represent the measurement(s) that was (were) taken under a specified experimental condition.

The *score for causal Bayesian network B* is $P(D \mid S, K)\, P(S \mid K)$, where $P(S \mid K)$ is the prior probability of causal network structure S in light of background knowledge K.

If the manipulation of a variable is deterministic, that is, we are able to set the variable to a desired value with probability 1, then it allow us to simplify the handling of interventions even beyond the straightforward analysis given in the previous section. In particular, in order to incorporate experimental data when manipulations are deterministic, we simply evaluate Equation (6) by not adding those cases to N_{ijk} where X_i is manipulated (Cooper and Yoo, 1999).

It also follows from the results in Cooper and Herskovits (1992) and Heckerman et al. (1995) that when X_i is observed, we estimate its conditional distribution as follows:

$$P(X_i = k|\pi_i = j, D, S, K) = \frac{\alpha_{ijk} + N_{ijk}}{\alpha_{ij} + N_{ij}} \tag{7}$$

Thus, parameter estimates are simply smoothed versions of frequencies, where the smoothing is due to the Bayesian parameter priors.

5.5 Conclusion and Future Direction

With an exponential growth of biological data, it is not surprising to foresee causal models, which represent gene–gene and gene–environment interactions, having to integrate a deluge of large scale, high-dimensional molecular and physiological data. We also need to recognize that the biological data is coming from many different sources, e.g., whole genome transcription measurements, next generation DNA and RNA sequencing technologies, genome wide single nucleotide polymorphism genotyping technologies, cDNA, mRNA, and protein expression measurements.

We have shown in this chapter that bioinformatics approaches such as causal probabilistic networks (e.g., causal Bayesian networks) will provide an elegant tool to integrate these large scale biological data from different sources. Note that since Bayesian analyses incorporate prior knowledge into the model, the Bayesian model easily benefits from many research projects in statistics, artificial intelligence, machine learning, and natural language processing for knowledge discovery from published scientific articles (Schuemie et al., 2007; Steele et al., 2009).

With these causal probabilistic networks, we will be able to run *dry experiments*[7] and make wise predictions about the future. Dry experiments and predictions are bases for the recommendations that are given in systems biology analysis cycle (Fig. 5.3). The recommendations can be any useful information that will be helpful for experimenter to perform new rounds of *wet experiments*, e.g., novel plausible gene–gene causal interactions.

---

[7] Contrast to the laboratory based *wet experiments*, dry experiments refer to simulations conducted based on computational models.

Fisher (1971) noted that the statistical analysis procedure and experiment design are merely two different aspects of the same whole. In molecular biology in particular, Karp (1990) created systems in bacterial gene regulation that could describe the initial conditions of an experiment, generate a hypothesis, and refine it. Future bioinformatics approaches in gene–gene and gene–environment causal interactions will need to incorporate larger heterogeneous datasets and even data from different disciplines, such as public health and medicine. We have shown that advance in bioinformatics modeling approaches will lead us to manage our knowledge in gene–gene and gene–environment causal interactions effectively. To do so, we should use systems biology approach (that is shown in Fig. 5.3), which is a systematical way to discover and update such knowledge.

In conclusion, experimental design recommendations and knowledge discovery from published scientific papers are two major promising areas for discovering gene–gene and gene–environmental causal interactions using bioinformatics approaches. Here we wrap up this chapter with reviews of experiment design recommendation models in bioinformatics:

Yoo and Cooper (2004) introduced a system called GEEVE (causal discovery in Gene Expression data using Expected Value of Experimentation), which implements expected value of experimentation in discovering gene–gene causal interactions using gene expression data. GEEVE provides the following assistance, which is intended to help biologists in their quest to discover gene-regulation pathways:

- Recommending which experiments to perform (with a focus on "knock-out" experiments) using an expected value of experimentation (EVE) method.
- Recommending the number of measurements (observational and experimental) to include in the experimental design, again using an EVE method.
- Providing a Bayesian analysis that combines prior knowledge with the results of recent microarray experimental results to derive posterior probabilities of gene regulation relationships.

In recommending which experiments to perform (and how many times to repeat them) the EVE approach considers the biologist's preferences for which genes to focus the discovery process. Also, since exact EVE calculations are exponential in time, GEEVE incorporates approximation methods. GEEVE is able to combine data from knock-out experiments with data from wild-type experiments to suggest additional experiments to perform and then to analyze the results of those microarray experimental results. It models the possibility that unmeasured (latent) variables may be responsible for some of the statistical associations among the expression levels of the genes under study (Yoo and Cooper, 2004).

An extension of supervised learning, *active learning* was applied to learning causal Bayesian networks in scientific discovery (Tong and Koller, 2001). Tong and Koller used edge entropy loss functions and a myopic search in order to recommend the next best experiment to perform. Their main assumptions are: (1) discrete variables only; (2) no missing data; and (3) no modeling of latent (hidden) variables.

They modeled all variables in their experiments as a query variable Q and the particular instantiation for Q as a query $\mathbf{q}$. A query represents the variables that can be experimentally manipulated. The result of the query is called the response and it is a randomly sampled instance $\mathbf{x}$ from the distribution of all non-query variables. They modeled manipulation and selection using the manipulation representation that was introduced in the previous section and was introduced by Cooper and Yoo (1999).

Ideker et al. (2000) used binary networks to model the perturbation on a gene network and used entropy loss function to recommend the next best perturbation to perform, where perturbation on a gene means forcing the gene to take a fixed value. They implemented two methods to infer a genetic network built from a gene expression dataset. To implement the genetic network, they used a deterministic Boolean model. This model is a simplified version of Bayesian networks (see Section 5.3.3) where all variables are binary and all conditional distribution tables are simply truth tables.

Similar Boolean networks were used to model the experiments involving the gene networks, and the set-covering method was used to recommend the next best experiment for more than one experimental repeat (Karp et al., 1999). Karp et al., used a Boolean circuit model of a biological pathway (Akutsu et al., 1999) to model experimentation. As an example of a Boolean circuit model, the following diagram represents three classes of genes: (1) class 1 represents the genes that are expressed when drug d is present and protein p is absent; (2) class 2 represents the genes that are expressed when drug d is absent and protein p is present; and (3) class 3 represents the genes that are expressed when drug d and protein p are both present.

References

Achcar, J. A. (1984). "Use of Bayesian analysis to design of clinical trials with one treatment." Communications in Statistics, Theory, and Methods **13**: 1693–1707.

Akutsu, T., S. Miyano, et al. (1999). Identification of genetic networks from a small number of gene expression patterns under the Boolean network model. Pacific Symposium on Biocomputing, Maui, Hawaii.

Alizadeh, A. A., M. B. Eisen, et al. (2000). "Distinct types of diffuse large B-cell lymphoma identified by gene expression profiling." Nature **403**(6769): 503–511.

Arkin, A., P. Shen, et al. (1997). "A test case of correlation metric construction of a reaction pathway from measurements." Science **277**: 1275–1279.

Benfey, P. N. and T. Mitchell-Olds (2008). "From genotype to phenotype: systems biology meets natural variation." Science **320**: 495–497.

Berry, D. A. and D. K. Stangl (1996). Bayesian methods in health-related research. Bayesian Biostatistics D. A. Berry and D. K. Stangl. New York, Marcel Dekker: 3–66.

Blaschke, C., J. C. Oliveros, et al. (2001). "Mining functional information associated with expression arrays." Functional and Integrative Genomics **4**: 256–268.

Boucher, A., A. Doisy, et al. (1998). "A society of goal-oriented agents for the analysis of living cells." Artificial Intelligence in Medicine **14**(1–2): 183–199.

Brooks, R. J. (1987). "On the design of comparative lifetime studies." Communications in Statistics Theory and Methods **16**: 1221–1240.

Brown, P. O. and D. Botstein (1999). "Exploring the new world of the genome with DNA microarrays." Nature Genetics **21**(supplement): 33–37.
Caspi, A., K. Sugden, et al. (2003). "Influence of life stress on depression: moderation by a polymorphism in the 5-HTT gene." Science **301**(5631): 386–389.
Chaloner, K. and I. Verdinelli (1995). "Bayesian experimental design: a review." Statistical Science **10**: 273–304.
Chen, T., V. Filkov, et al. (1999). Identifying gene regulatory networks from experimental data. ACM-SIGAT, Proceedings of the Third Annual International Conference on Computational Molecular Biology (RECOMB99), Lyon, France.
Chen, T., H. L. He, et al. (1999). Modeling gene expression with differential equations. Pacific Symposium on Biocomputing, Maui, Hawaii.
Chevrolat, J., J. Golmard, et al. (1998). "Modelling behavioral syndromes using Bayesian networks." Artificial Intelligence in Medicine **14**(3): 259–277.
Citro, G., G. Banks, et al. (1997). "INKBLOT: A neurological diagnostic decision support system integrating causal and anatomical knowledge." Artificial Intelligence in Medicine **10**: 257–267.
Cooper, G. F. (1987). Probabilistic inference using belief networks is NP-hard, Stanford University, Stanford, CA.
Cooper, G. F. and E. Herskovits (1992). "A Bayesian method for the induction of probabilistic networks from data." Machine Learning **9**: 309–347.
Cooper, G. F. and C. Yoo (1999). Causal discovery from a mixture of experimental and observational data. Proceedings of the Conference on Uncertainty in Artificial Intelligence, San Fransisco, CA, Morgan Kaufmann.
D'haeseleer, P., X. Wen, et al. (1999). Linear modeling of mRNA expression levels during CNS development and injury. Pacific Symposium on Biocomputing, Maui, Hawaii.
de Jong, H. (2002). "Modeling and simulation of genetic regulatory systems: a literature review." Journal of Computational Biology **9**(1): 67–103.
Dupont, W. D. and W. D. Plummer (1990). "Power and sample size calculations: a review and computer program." Controlled Clinical Trials **11**: 116–128.
Dutilh, B. (1999). Gene Networks from Microarray Data. Unpublished manuscript, Literature thesis, Utrecht University.
Fisher, R. A. (1925). Statistical Methods for Research Workers. London, Oliver and Boyd.
Fisher, R. A. (1971). The Design of Experiments. New York, Hafner Publishing Company.
Friedman, L. M., C. D. Furberg, et al. (1996). Chapter 7, sample size. Fundamentals of Clinical Trials, 3rd Edition. St. Louis, MO, Mosby-Year Book: 94–129.
Friedman, N., M. Linial, et al. (2000). "Using Bayesian networks to analyze expression data." Journal of Computational Biology **7**: 601–620.
Getz, G., E. Levine, et al. (2000). "Coupled two-way clustering analysis of gene microarray data". Proceedings of the National Academy of Sciences **97**(22): 12079–12084.
Golub, T. R., D. K. Slonim, et al. (1999). "Molecular classification of cancer: class discovery and class prediction by gene expression monitoring." Science **286**: 531–537.
Goodwin, B. C. (1965). "Oscillatory behavior of enzymatic control processes." Advances in Enzyme Regulation **3**: 425–439.
Goss, P. J. E. and J. Peccoud (1999). Analysis of the stabilizing effect of ROM on the genetic network controlling ColE1 plasmid replication. Pacific Symposium on Biocomputing, Maui, Hawaii.
Griffith, J. S. (1968). "Mathematics of cellular control processes I. Negative feedback to one gene." Journal of Theoretical Biology **20**: 202–208.
Griffith, J. S. (1968). "Mathematics of cellular control processes II. Positive feedback to one gene." Journal of Theoretical Biology **20**: 209–216.
Hahn, L. W., M. D. Ritchie, et al. (2003). "Multifactor dimensionality reduction software for detecting gene–gene and gene–environment interactions." Bioinformatics **19**(3): 376–382.

Hartemink, A. J., D. K. Gifford, et al. (2001). Using graphical models and genomic expression data to statistically validate models of genetic regulatory networks. Pacific Symposium on Biocomputing, Maui, Hawaii.

Heckerman, D. (1995). A Bayesian approach to learning causal networks. Proceedings of the Conference on Uncertainty in Artificial Intelligence, San Francisco, CA, Morgan Kaufmann.

Heckerman, D., D. Geiger, et al. (1995). "Learning Bayesian networks: the combination of knowledge and statistical data." Machine Learning **20**: 197–243.

Heckerman, D., C. Meek, et al. (1999). A Bayesian approach to causal discovery. Computation, Causation, and Discovery. C. Glymour and G. F. Cooper. Menlo Park, CA, AAAI Press: 141–165.

Heiman, M. G. and P. Walter (2000). "Prm1p, a pheromone-regulated multispanning membrane protein, facilitates plasma membrane fusion during yeast mating." Journal of Cell Biology **151**: 719–730.

Herwig, R., A. J. Poustka, et al. (1999). "Large-scale clustering of cDNA-fingerprinting data." Genome Research **9**: 1093–1105.

Ideker, T., T. Galitski, et al. (2001). "A new approach to decoding life: system biology." Annual Review of Genomics and Human Genetics **2**: 343–372.

Ideker, T., V. Thorsson, et al. (2000). Discovery of regulatory interactions through perturbation: inference and experimental design. Pacific Symposium Biocompution, Maui, Hawaii.

Ideker, T., V. Thorsson, et al. (2001). "Integrated genomic and proteomic analysis of a systematically perturbed metabolic network." Science **292**: 929–934.

Jones, S., X. Zhan, et al. (2008). "Core signaling pathways in human pancreatic cancers revealed by global genomic analyses". Science **321**(5897): 1801–1806.

Karp, P. D. (1990). Hypothesis formation as design. Computational Models of Discovery and Theory Formation. J. Shrager and P. Langley. San Mateo, CA, Morgan Kaufman: 276–317.

Karp, P. D., M. Krummenacker, et al. (1999). "Integrated pathway/genome database and their role in drug discovery". Trends in Biotechnology **17**(7): 275–281.

Karp, R. M., R. Stoughton, et al. (1999). Algorithms for choosing differential gene expression experiments. Annual Conference on Research in Computational Biology, Lyon, France.

KEGG (Kyoto Encyclopedia of Genes and Genomes). Available at: http://www.genome.ad.jp/kegg/

Kerr, M. K. and G. A. Churchill (2001). "Experimental design for gene expression microarrays." Biostatistics **2**: 183–201.

Kitano, H. (2002). "Systems biology: a brief overview." Science **295**: 1662–1664.

Koza, J., W. Mydlowec, et al. (2001). Reverse engineering of metabolic pathways from observed data using genetic programming. Pacific Symposium on Biocomputing, Maui, Hawaii.

Lakatos, E. (1988). "Sample sizes based on the log-rank statistic in complex clinical trials." Biometrics **44**: 229–242.

Landrya, C. R., J. Ohb, et al. (2005). "Genome-wide scan reveals that genetic variation for transcriptional plasticity in yeast is biased towards multi-copy and dispensable genes". Gene **366**(2): 343–351.

Li, Y., Alvarez, O. A., Gutteling, E. W., et al. (2006). "Mapping determinants of gene expression plasticity by genetical genomics in C. elegans." PLoS Genetics **2**(12): e222.

Liang, S., S. Fuhrman, et al. (1998). REVEAL, A general reverse engineering algorithm for inference of genetic network architectures. Pacific Symposium on Biocomputing, Maui, Hawaii.

Lilienfield, A. M. (1982). "Ceteris paribusthe evolution of the clinical trial." Bulletin of the History of Medicine **56**: 1–18.

Lindley, D. V. (1972). Bayesian Statistics, a Review. Philadelphia, PA, SIAM.

Lipshutz, R. J., S. P. A. Fodor, et al. (1999). "High density synthetic oligonucleotide arrays." Nature Genetics **21**(supplement): 20–24.

Lucas, P. J. F., de Bruijn, N. C., et al. (2000). "A probabilistic and decision-theoretic approach to the management of infectious disease at the ICU." Artificial Intelligence in Medicine **19**(3): 251–279.

Margulies, M., M. Egholm, et al. (2005). "Genome sequencing in microfabricated high-density picolitre reactors." Nature **437**: 376–380.

Matsuno, H., A. Doi, et al. (2000). Hybrid Petri net representation of gene regulatory network. Pacific Symposium on Biocomputing, Maui, Hawaii.

McAdams, H. and L. Shapiro (1995). "Circuit simulation of genetic networks". Science **269**(4): 650–656.

Mestl, T., C. Lemay, et al. (1996). "Chaos in high-dimensional neural and gene networks." Physica D **98**: 33–52.

Michaels, G. S., D. B. Carr, et al. (1998). Cluster analysis and data visualization of large-scale gene expression data. Pacific Symposium on Biocomputing, Maui, Hawaii.

MIPS (Munich Information Center for Protein Sequences). Yeast pathway. Available at: http://mips.gsf.de/proj/yeast/CYGD/db/pathway_index.html

Murphy, K. and S. Mian (1999). Modelling gene expression data using dynamic Bayesian networks. Technical report, Department of Computer Science, University of California, Berkeley.

Parsons, D. W., S. Jones, et al. (2008). "An integrated genomic analysis of human glioblastoma multiforme". Science **26**(5897): 1807–1812.

Pe'er, D., A. Regev, et al. (2001). Inferring subnetworks from perturbed expression profiles. Proceedings in 9th International Conference on Intelligent Systems for Molecular Biology (ISMB), Copenhagen, Denmark.

Pearl, J. (1988). Probabilistic Reasoning in Intelligent Systems. San Mateo, CA, Morgan Kaufmann.

Pearl, J. (2000). Causality: Models, Reasoning, and Inference. Cambridge, UK, Cambridge University Press.

Plahte, E., T. Mestl, et al. (1998). "A methodological basis for description and analysis of systems with complex switch-like interactions." Journal of Mathematical Biology **36**: 321–348.

Quaglini, S., M. Stefanelli, et al. (2001). "Flexible guideline-based patient careflow systems". Artificial Intelligence in Medicine **22**(1): 65–80.

Reis, B. Y., A. S. Butte, et al. (2001). "Extracting knowledge from dynamics in gene expression." Journal of Biomedical Informatics **1**(1): 1–13.

Sabeti, P. C., P. Varilly, et al. (2007). "Genome-wide detection and characterization of positive selection in human populations." Nature **449**: 913–919.

Samsonova, M. G. and V. N. Serov (1999). NetWork: an interactive interface to the tools for analysis of genetic network structure and dynamics. Pacific Symposium on Biocomputing, Maui, Hawaii.

Schadt, E. E. (2009). "Molecular networks as sensors and drivers of common human diseases." Nature **461**: 218–223.

Schuemie, M., C. Chichester, et al. (2007). "Assignment of protein function and discovery of novel nucleolar proteins based on automatic analysis of MEDLINE." Proteomics **7**: 921–931.

Smith, E. N. and L. Kruglyak (2008). "Gene–environment interaction in yeast gene expression". PLoS Biology **6**(4): 810–824.

Smolen, P., D. A. Baxter, et al. (2000). "Modeling transciptional control in gene networks – methods, recent results and future directions." Bulletin of Mathematical Biology **62**: 247–292.

Snoussi, E. H. and R. Thomas (1993). "Logical identification of all steady states: the concept of feedback loop characteristic states." Bulletin of Mathematical Biology **55**: 973–991.

Somogyi, R. and C. Sniegoski (1996). "Modeling the complexity of genetic networks: understanding multigenetic and pleiotropic regulation." Complexity **1**(6): 45–63.

Spellman, P. T., G. Sherlock, et al. (1998). "Comprehensive identification of cell cycle-regulated genes of the yeast saccharomyces cerevisiae by microarray hybridization." Molecular Biology of the Cell **9**: 3273–3297.

Spiegelhalter, D. J., L. S. Freedman, et al. (1994). "Bayesian approach to randomized trials." Journal of the Royal Statistical Society **157**(Part 3): 357–416.

Spirtes, P., C. Glymour, et al. (2000). Causation, Prediction, and Search. Cambridge, MA, MIT Press.

Spirtes, P., C. Glymour, et al. (2001). Constructing Bayesian network models of gene expression networks from microarray data. The Proceedings of the Atlantic Symposium on Computational Biology, Genome Information Systems and Technology (to appear).

Steele, E., A. Tucker, et al. (2009). "Literature-based priors for gene regulatory networks." Bioinformatics **25**(14): 1768–1774.

Stephens, M., M. Palakal, et al. (2001). Detecting gene relations from MEDLINE abstracts. Pacific Symposium on Biocomputing, Maui, Hawaii.

Sylvester, R. J. (1988). "A Bayesian approach to the design of phase II clinical trials." Biometrics **44**: 823–836.

Talmud, P. (2007). "Gene–environment interaction and its impact on coronary heart disease risk". Nutrition, Metabolism, and Cardiovascular Diseases **17**(2): 148–152.

The Gene Ontology Consortium (2000). "Gene ontology: tool for the unification of biology." Nature Genetics **25**: 25–29.

The Genome International Sequencing Consortium (2001). "Initial sequencing and analysis of the human genome." Nature **409**: 860–921.

The International Haplotype Map Consortium (2005). "A haplotype map of the human genome." Nature **437**: 1299–1320.

Tomita, M., K. Hashimoto, et al. (1999). "E-CELL: software environment for whole cell simulation." Bioinformatics **15**(1): 72–84.

Tong, S. and D. Koller (2001). Active learning for structure in Bayesian networks. International Joint Conference on Artificial Intelligence, Seattle, WA.

Tsang, J. (1999). Gene expression, DNA arrays, and genetic network. Unpublished manuscript, Bioinformatics Laboratory, University of Waterloo.

Ulrich, C. M., E. Kampman, et al. (1999). "Colorectal adenomas and the C677T MTHFR polymorphism: evidence for gene–environment interaction?" Cancer Epidemiology, Biomarkers & Prevention **8**(669): 659–668.

Weaver, D. C., C. T. Workman, et al. (1999). Modeling regulatory networks with weight matrices. Pacific Symposium on Biocomputing, Maui, Hawaii, 123.

Wessels, L. F. A., E. P. V. Someren, et al. (2001). A comparison of genetic network models. Pacific Symposium on Biocomputing, Maui, Hawaii.

Yoo, C. and E. Blitz (2008). "Local causal discovery algorithm using causal Bayesian networks." Annals of the New York Academy of Science **1158**: 93–101.

Yoo, C. and G. Cooper (2004). "An evaluation of a system that recommends microarray experiments to perform to discover gene-regulation pathways." Journal of Artificial Intelligence in Medicine **31**: 169–182.

Yoo, C., V. Thorsson, et al. (2002). Discovery of a gene-regulation pathway from a mixture of experimental and observational DNA microarray data. Pacific Symposium on Biocomputing, Maui, Hawaii, World Scientific.

Yuh, C., H. Bolouri, et al. (1998). "Genomic Cis-regulatory logic: experimental and computational analysis of a sea urchin gene." Science **279**: 1896–1902.

Zhu, J., B. Zhang, et al. (2008). "Integrating large-scale functional genomic data to dissect the complexity of yeast regulatory networks." Nature Genetics **40**(7): 854–861.

Chapter 6
Gene Environment Interactions and Vascular Lesions

Quentin Felty

Abstract Despite the extensive research in the field of tumor angiogenesis, the complex interaction of genes with environmental factors is not yet understood in terms of development and aggressiveness of vascular lesions in different human tumor types. Environmental risk factors such as tobacco smoke, alcohol, xenobiotics, arsenic, and air pollutants are the exposures studied most frequently for interactions with genetic polymorphisms in cancer. To date, results from the literature show no direct studies of angiogenic gene environment interactions. However, it is important to study angiogenic gene environment interactions because of the influence that vascular lesions have on the invasiveness of cancer. In this chapter, we review the literature to determine the possible role of angiogenic gene environment interactions in vascular lesion formation. We have focused our efforts using mainly estrogenic compounds as the model to describe the role of gene environment interactions in the pathogenesis of vascular lesions.

Keywords Environmental estrogens · Oxidative stress · Genetic susceptibility · Angiogenesis

6.1 Introduction

In pathological circumstances, such as breast cancer, solid human tumors cannot continue growing without an adequate network of blood vessels from normal tissue to supply oxygen and nutrients and to remove waste products. Continued growth of a malignant tumor beyond a certain size is dependent on the tumor's ability to attract and develop a network of blood vessels that serve to provide nutrients to the expanding mass of cells. Despite the extensive research in the field of angiogenesis

---

Q. Felty (✉)
Department of Environmental and Occupational Health, FIU Stempel School of Public Health, Florida International University, Miami, FL 33199, USA
e-mail: feltyq@fiu.edu

D. Roy, M.T. Dorak (eds.), *Environmental Factors, Genes, and the Development of Human Cancers*, DOI 10.1007/978-1-4419-6752-7_6,

still many of the genetic risk factors for vascular disease have not been identified, and the complex interaction of genes with other genes and genes with environmental factors is not yet understood in terms of development and aggressiveness of vascular lesions in different human tumor types.

The vascular system is an important target of estrogenic compounds much like the reproductive tissues, brain, liver, and bone through genomic and nongenomic pathways (Chambliss et al., 2002). Estrogen receptor alpha (ERα) has been shown in human coronary arteries and endothelial cells (Kim-Schulze et al., 1996); while ERβ has been observed in primary human cardiomyocytes (Yang et al., 2004). Under normal conditions estrogens exert important regulatory functions on different components of the vascular wall, including the endothelium, smooth muscle cells, vascular stromal cells and different leukocyte species (Stork et al., 2004). However, use of synthetic estrogens can produce thromboembolic disorders. An increased incidence of deep vein thrombosis and pulmonary embolism has been reported in young women who use oral contraceptives (OC) (Ramos et al., 1996). Intracranial venous thrombosis and secondary increases in the risk of stroke have also been noted. In experimental animal studies, estrogen has been shown to promote stroke in hypertensive rats (Stier et al., 2003), produce severe degenerative atherosclerotic effects on coronary arteries (Toda et al., 1981), and increase susceptibility to early atherosclerosis in male mice via the ERα (Villablanca et al., 2004). In this chapter, we have focused our efforts using mainly estrogenic compounds as the model to describe the role of gene environment interactions in the pathogenesis of vascular lesions.

6.2 Angiogenic Lesion Development

Angiogenesis, or blood vessel growth, is a critical element of tumor progression that may involve growth factors, oxygen, nutrients, and metabolic wastes. Hypoxia within tumors induces the expression of angiogenic factors, which prompt an influx of vessels from surrounding tissues. Neovascularization also facilitates the spread of cancer cells to other tissues; which contributes to the metastatic potential and tumor vascularity. A specific example of vascular lesion formation mimicking in vivo conditions is described below. Although the matrigel culture is a frequently used method for detection of vascular formation in vitro, Donovan et al. (2001) have demonstrated that vessel formation on matrigel is not specific for endothelial cells. Moreover, they reported that the morphology of vessels when endothelial cells are co-cultured with fibroblasts is more representative of vascular formation in vivo. HUVECs were seeded on top of a confluent layer of fibroblasts and treated with 17β-estradiol, PCB153, and PCB77, or the vehicle control (DMSO). Co-cultures immunostained for endothelial marker CD31 showed a well developed vascular network in the PCB treatment groups compared to 17β-estradiol and control. A representative illustration is shown below.

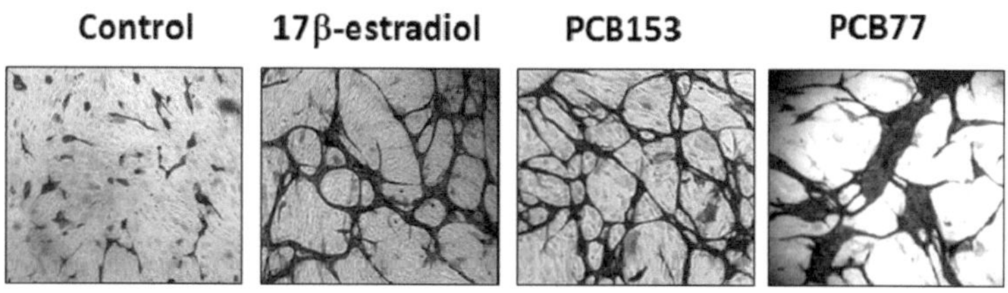

6.3 Environment and Vascular Lesions

There is a growing body of evidence establishing exposure to environmental agents as a risk factor for vascular lesions. Angiogenic genes underexpressed or overexpressed in relevant tissues after exposure to environmental pollutants in humans or animals may be potential candidates for studies of gene–environment interaction. Some examples of environmental factors that are currently attracting interest with respect to contribution to vascular lesion development are included in Table 6.1.

Table 6.1 Influence of the environment on angiogenic genes

Environment	Angiogenic gene	Response
Arsenic	↑ VEGF, NOS3, bFGF	↑ Endothelial cell proliferation and tube formation ↑ VEGF secretion and NO production (Kao et al., 2003)
Arsenic + ethanol	↑ VEGF, IGF1	Co-exposure ↑ Endothelial cell tube formation (Klei and Barchowsky, 2008)
Cigarette smoke	↑ VEGF, MCP1	Second hand smoke ↑ tumor vessel density in xenograft model (Zhu et al., 2003)
	↑ PIGF	Cigarette smoke extract ↑ secretion of placental growth factor (Mehendale et al., 2007)
Estrogen therapy	↑ VEGF	↑ Angiogenesis under hypoxic and normoxic conditions (Nematbakhsh et al., 2008)
	↑ SDF1	Promoted myocardial angiogenesis (Chen et al., 2008)
Ethanol	↑ VEGF	↑ Tumor microvessel density ↑ Tumor growth (Tan et al., 2007)
Human cytomegalovirus	↑ Various growth factors (i.e. TGFB, VEGF)	↑ Endothelial cell tube formation (Dumortier et al., 2008)
Hypoxia	↑ VEGF	Inhalational hypoxia ↑ VEGF protein expression in rat myocardium (Sasaki et al., 2000) Chronic systemic hypoxia ↑ angiogenesis of adult rat retina (Shortt et al., 2004)
Nicotine	↑ VEGF	↑ Tumor vessel density in xenograft model (Wong et al., 2007)
Polychlorinated biphenyl 104	↑ VEGF	↑ Endothelial hyperpermeability (Eum et al., 2004)

Table 6.1 (continued)

Environment	Angiogenic gene	Response
Roxarsone (3-nitro-4-hydroxy benzene arsonic acid)	↑ HGF	↑ Endothelial cell tube formation greater than inorganic As^{III} (Basu et al., 2008)
A poultry feed additive		↑ NOS3 activity
Soluble manganese [Mn(II)]	↑ VEGF, VEGFR1, HIF1A subunits	Subchronic inhalation ↑ angiogenic gene expression in mouse lung (Bredow et al., 2007)
Xenoestrogens (i.e. BPA, OP, dieldrin, phthalates)	↑ VEGF	Potential for ↑ breast tumor angiogenesis (Buteau-Lozano et al., 2008)

6.4 Redox Signaling and Vascular Lesions

Chronic systemic inflammation is not confined to a particular tissue, but involves the lining of blood vessels. This inflammatory process is often associated with free radical damage and oxidative stress. Several studies have demonstrated that PCBs can induce oxidative stress and inflammatory effects in human vascular endothelial cells (Hennig et al., 2002a; Ramadass et al., 2003; Lim et al., 2007; Arzuaga et al., 2007; Hennig et al., 2002b). In the animal model, mice exposed orally to estrogenic PCB 153 and PCB 77 were shown to have increased inflammatory responses (Tavolari et al., 2006; Sipka et al., 2008). Considering clinical studies that have also shown estrogen to increase inflammation which has been implicated in vascular lesion formation (Stork et al., 2004; Roy and Cai, 2002), we postulate that PCB-induced redox signaling is a critical process in the pathology of vascular lesions. It is generally believed that the primary target of estrogens in the cardiovascular system is endothelial nitric oxide synthase (eNOS). Estrogen is known to mediate the production of nitric oxide (NO) and similarly PCBs have been shown to increase eNOS phosphorylation and NO production in human vascular endothelial cells (Lim et al., 2007). Even though estrogen-induced NO contributes to its beneficial cardiovascular effects, when eNOS becomes "uncoupled" in the absence of the NOS cofactor tetrahydrobiopterin (BH_4), then eNOS produces the free radical $O_2{\bullet}^-$ rather than NO (Channon, 2004). Estrogen exposure has been demonstrated to increase $O_2{\bullet}^-$ production rather than the beneficial NO in NOS uncoupled cells (White et al., 2005). A recent study has implicated eNOS uncoupling in vascular disease pathogenesis. In transgenic mice with endothelial-targeted NOS overexpression, atherosclerotic plaque formation increased in the ApoE knockout model (Ozaki et al., 2002). Although NOS overexpression modestly increased NO production, there was a much larger increase in endothelial $O_2{\bullet}^-$ release. These features were reduced by BH_4, directly implicating BH_4-mediated eNOS regulation in vascular disease pathogenesis. As a woman ages there is a decline in cofactors for maintaining NOS in the coupled (i.e. NO producing) state. Interestingly, the conclusions of the WHI were based on older postmenopausal women (mean age 63.3). Since aging is associated with the depletion of NOS cofactors such as BH_4, it is biologically plausible that NOS activity becomes increasingly uncoupled as women age thereby increasing their predisposition to oxidative stress when exposed to estrogenic compounds. This point may form the basis of an explanation as to why the WHI observed mainly harmful effects of estrogen in postmenopausal women: simply stated estrogen stimulated oxidative stress. Since PCBs are widespread and persistent environmental contaminants known to induce oxidative stress in human vascular endothelial cells (Hennig et al., 2002b; Ramadass et al., 2003; Lim et al., 2007); research defining the mechanism of how estrogenic PCBs may promote vascular lesions is highly relevant to public health.

Vascular lesions have been proposed to occur as a result of the monoclonal expansion of a mutated vascular cell (Benditt and Benditt, 1973) and are characterized by abnormal cell proliferation that can lead to vascular blockage, myocardial infarction, and stroke (Boehm and Nabel, 2003). Evidence in support of this concept comes from PCR based studies of dissected tissue from an atherosclerotic lesion that showed vascular cells present in lesions were monoclonal in origin (Schwartz and Murry, 1998). The origin of a monoclonal population of cells may be explained by previously reported oxidative DNA damage and subsequent genetic alterations including mutations produced by estrogens (Roy et al., 1991; Roy and Abul-Hajj, 1997; Roy and Liehr, 1999). Regardless of monoclonal cell origin, vascular lesions undergo a cell proliferation stage that is associated with the progression of cancer. Growing evidence indicates that chronic and acute overproduction of ROS such as superoxide anion ($O_2{\bullet}^-$) and even reactive nitrogen species are integral in the development of cancer. We have shown that estrogen-induced ROS act as signal transducing messengers that mediate the growth of vascular endothelial cells (Felty, 2006; Felty and Porther, 2008). Vascular endothelial cells are important biological signal transducers that respond to a variety of input from the circulation including estrogenic chemicals. Blood vasculature formation, a process linked to the proliferation of endothelial cells, is virtually absent in adult organisms; however, physiological exceptions are found in wound healing and in the female reproductive tract during the menstrual cycle and pregnancy (Hyder and Stancel, 1999; Pare et al., 2002). Our preliminary findings suggest that PCB-induced redox signaling is involved in vessel formation and this process is mediated by redox sensitive molecules Pyk2 and Id3. The concentration of PCBs used in our study is well within the reported range of PCB 153 [0.60–1.63 ng/ml] found in human serum and highlights the potential damaging consequences of PCBs to the vascular system (Charlier et al., 2004). Since the dysfunction of blood vasculature formation is associated with the development of vascular disease (Folkman, 1995), estrogenic PCBs that we and others have shown to mediate endothelial cell vessel formation should be considered potentially harmful to the human vascular system (Tavolari et al., 2006).

High concentrations [10 μM] of 17β-estradiol (E2) have been shown to act as antioxidants in vitro (Behl et al., 1997). In contrast, we have demonstrated that physiological concentrations of E2 (100 pg/ml–1 ng/ml) which do not act as antioxidants actually induce the formation of reactive oxygen species (ROS) (Felty, 2006; Felty et al., 2005a, b). Evidence in support of the role of ROS signaling endothelial cell proliferation comes from our studies showing that antioxidants block E2-induced DNA synthesis and endothelial vessel formation (Felty, 2006; Felty and Porther, 2008). Similarly, we have shown that overexpression of the antioxidant enzymes MnSOD and catalase or co-treatment with chemical antioxidants significantly inhibit PCB-induced vessel formation. The conventional paradigm of estrogen action is based on binding to its receptors, ERα/β, which initiates transcription by binding to estrogen response elements of genes involved in cell growth. Discrepancies between the binding affinity of various estrogens to the ER and their growth potency both in vitro and in vivo have been reported (DuMond et al., 2001; Bocchinfuso et al., 1999). Furthermore, we have shown that antioxidants N-acetylcysteine and ebselen, which are not ER antagonist, prevented both PCB- and E2-induced DNA synthesis and vessel formation. This suggests that this signaling mechanism does not solely rely on ER genomic signaling, but rather an oxidative stress sensitive signaling pathway.

Epidemiologic studies have demonstrated a strong correlation between levels of arsenic in the drinking water and increased incidence of peripheral vascular disease (Tseng et al., 1997). Since environmentally relevant concentrations of arsenic have been shown to induce oxidant formation that increased DNA synthesis and endothelial cell proliferation (Barchowsky et al., 1999), PCB-induced oxidants may also participate in this process. Arsenic has been shown to activate the focal adhesion kinase Pyk2 as well as increased the expression of angiogenic genes and vascular formation in human endothelial cells (Klei and Barchowsky, 2008). G protein coupled receptors (GPCRs) have been implicated in the pathogenesis of vascular cell proliferation, leading to the development of vascular lesions (Schieffer et al., 1997). Pyk2 plays an important role in coupling GPCRs and growth factor receptors to classic MAPK pathway activation in a number of cell types. Several lines of evidence demonstrate that stimulation of GPCRs leads to the formation of protein complexes. For instance, activation of the G protein-coupled m1 muscarinic acetylcholine receptor has been shown to form a Pyk2/c-Src/Grb2 protein complex (Felsch et al., 1998). Interestingly, many of these complexes are composed of oxidant sensitive proteins such as Pyk2 (Cheng et al., 2002), c-src (Pu et al., 1996), Vav1, and Grb2 (Huang et al., 1996). In patients undergoing coronary artery bypass graft surgery, GPR30 expression was shown in both arteries and veins (Haas et al., 2007). GPR30 expression has also been shown in human umbilical vein endothelial cells and may play an important role in the regulation of endothelial function (Takada et al., 1997). Since GPR30 has been shown to signal estrogen-induced cell proliferation and DNA synthesis (Kanda and Watanabe, 2004), it is biologically plausible that GPR30 could play a role in estrogen-induced vascular lesion formation. Pyk2 has also been shown to associate with the cytoskeletal protein Vav1 upon GPCR activation (Okabe et al., 2005). Vav proteins participate in the reorganization of the actin cytoskeleton which is critical to processes such as cell division, growth, and adhesion. Overexpression of wild-type Vav1 has been shown to cause uncontrolled proliferation of cells (Hornstein et al., 2004). More recently, tyrosine phosphorylation of Pyk2 has been shown to activate Vav1 (Zhao and Bokoch, 2005). From these studies, it is apparent that many environmental contaminants exhibit their adverse vascular lesions via redox signaling (see Fig. 6.1).

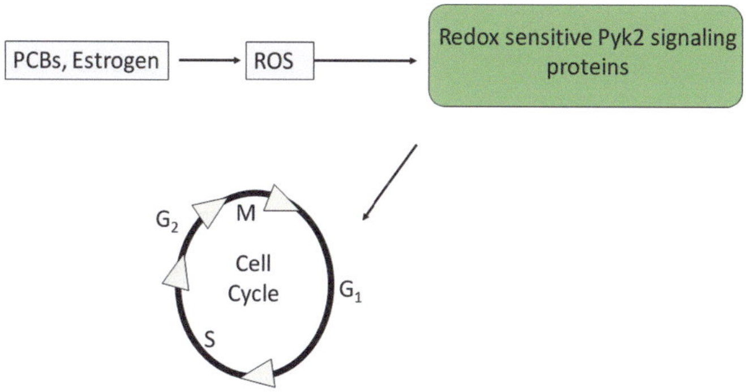

Fig. 6.1 Potential redox signaling pathway involved in environmental estrogen associated vascular lesion development

6.5 Angiogenic Genes

Solid human tumors cannot continue growing (generally 1–2 mm in diameter) without an adequate network of blood to supply oxygen and to remove waste products. In response to the environment, endothelial cells branch off from nearby blood vessels to form a network of "new" vessels that supply oxygen and nutrients to the growing tumor, a process termed "angiogenesis." Genes that play a role in angiogenesis include growth factors and receptors, adhesion molecules, proteases, cytokines, chemokines and transcription factors. Table 6.1 reports a list of these angiogenic genes.

6.6 Genetic Susceptibility to Vascular Lesions

Currently, our review of the literature did not find any gene–environment interaction studies on vascular lesions. However, since metastatic or invasiveness of cancer depends on tumor angiogenesis than it can be inferred that polymorphisms in angiogenic genes may increase susceptibility to vascular lesions. Therefore, we searched the literature for gene variant studies on cancer. Table 6.2 reports a list of the main proposed associations between common genetic variations in angiogenic genes and the risk for cancer.

Table 6.2 Angiogenic gene polymorphisms associated with cancer

Gene name	Genotypic variant	Cancer risk
VEGF	VEGF-1498 CC	OR = 2.01; 95% CI = 1.08–3.76 Increased breast cancer risk (Schneider et al., 2008)
	VEGF-2578 AA	OR = 1.99; 95% CI = 1.06–3.74 Increased breast cancer risk
NOS3	NOS3-894 TT	OR = 2.18; 95% CI = 0.99–4.81 Women who took iron-containing multivitamin supplements showed an increased breast cancer risk (Hong et al., 2007)
	NOS3-786 TT NOS3-894 GG	Greater likelihood of invasive and metastatic breast cancer (Schneider et al., 2008)
TNF-β	TNFB-intron 1 GG	OR = 5.33; 95% CI = 2.33–12.19 Increased breast cancer risk (Park et al., 2002)
HIF-1α	HIF1A-1772 CT/TT	OR = 3.84; 95% CI = 1.65–8.93 Increased cervical cancer risk OR = 7.41; 95% CI = 2.33–23.59 Increased risk for endometrial cancer (Konac et al., 2007)
EGF	EGF-61 GG	OR = 4.9; 95% CI = 2.3–10.2 Increased risk for malignant melanoma (Shahbazi et al., 2002)
Endostatin (COL18A1 is the formal name)	Endostatin-4349 GA	OR = 2.4; 95% CI = 1.4–4.16 Increased prostate cancer risk (Iughetti et al., 2001)
MMP-1	MMP1-1607 2G/2G	OR = 2.21; 95% CI = 1.17–4.16 Increased risk for colorectal cancer (Ghilardi et al., 2001) OR = 1.76; 95% CI = 1.29–2.39 Increased lung cancer risk (Zhu et al., 2001)
IL-10	IL10-1082AG	OR = 3.05; 95% CI = 1.84–5.05 Increased risk for oral cancer (Vairaktaris et al., 2008)

6.7 Gene–Environment Interactions and Vascular Lesion Development

Only about 5% of all cancers can be attributed to genetic susceptibility, and therefore environmental insults play a significant role in cancer. Thus, both genetic and environmental factors also influence tumor angiogenesis that facilitates the spread of cancer cells to other tissues. Gene–environment interaction implies that, in combination, the impact of the genotype and the environmental factor is more than the additive effects of each factor alone. The importance of gene–environment interaction is that, only when a genetically susceptible individual enters into a high-risk environment, will the effect be so great that premature disease will develop. Furthermore, few studies have shown the environment linked to abnormal changes in epigenetic pathways involved in angiogenesis. Epigenetics refers to three interrelated mechanisms: DNA methylation, post-translational modifications, and RNA-based mechanisms. The effect of the environment on the epigenome offers a new perspective on transcriptional control of angiogencic genes in vascular endothelial cells. There is recent evidence of how the environment impacts the epigenome in humans. For instance, a study showed altered DNA methylation in gas station workers and traffic police officers who were exposed to benzene; and these alterations were similar to aberrant epigenetic patterns found in malignant cells (Bollati et al., 2007). More recently, a study showed that particulate matter (PM) exposure in steel furnace workers caused a decrease in DNA methylation of the iNOS promoter (Tarantini et al., 2009). Interestingly, animals exposed to PM have shown an increase in iNOS expression (Carmeliet et al., 1998) and iNOS overexpression has been shown to correlate with tumor angiogenesis (Cullis et al., 2006). Thus, further studies are warranted to determine the role of such alterations in mediating the effects of particles on human vascular lesion development. We have summarized in Table 6.3 examples of environmental factors that are related to changes in epigenetic pathways involved in angiogenesis.

Table 6.3 Influence of the environment on epigenetic pathways involved in angiogenesis

Environment	Epigenetic alteration	Response
Oxidative stress	FoxO1 (deacetylation)	↑ Angiogenesis (Potente et al., 2007; Laurent et al., 2008)
Hypoxia	HIF-1α (deacetylation)	↑ VEGF (Carmeliet et al., 1998) ↑ Tumor angiogenesis
Particulate matter (PM)	iNOS (demethylation)	↓ Methylation of iNOS gene promoter in workers (Tarantini et al., 2009, Environ Health Perspect) ↑ iNOS seen in animals exposed to PM (Folkmann et al., 2007)

6.8 Summary

It has long been accepted that environmental chemicals can cause cancer through changes in the genome. Angiogenic gene–environment interactions are important to study because of their potential to increase the metastatic potential or invasiveness of cancer via vascular lesion formation. The lack of firm findings of interaction between angiogenic genes and environmental factors is not surprising, given the early stage of the field. How these genetic variants interact with one another and with environmental risk factors to form vascular lesions should be the subject of future research studies.

References

Arzuaga X, Reiterer G, Majkova Z, Kilgore MW, Toborek M, Hennig B 2007 PPARalpha ligands reduce PCB-induced endothelial activation: possible interactions in inflammation and atherosclerosis. Cardiovasc Toxicol 7:264–272

Barchowsky A, Roussel RR, Klei LR, James PE, Ganju N, Smith KR, Dudek EJ 1999 Low levels of arsenic trioxide stimulate proliferative signals in primary vascular cells without activating stress effector pathways. Toxicol Appl Pharmacol 159:65–75

Basu P, Ghosh RN, Grove LE, Klei L, Barchowsky A 2008 Angiogenic potential of 3-nitro-4-hydroxy benzene arsonic Acid (roxarsone). Environ Health Perspect 116:520–523

Behl C, Skutella T, Lezoualc'h F, Post A, Widmann M, Newton CJ, Holsboer F 1997 Neuroprotection against oxidative stress by estrogens: structure-activity relationship. Mol Pharmacol 51:535–541

Benditt EP, Benditt JM 1973 Evidence for a monoclonal origin of human atherosclerotic plaques. Proc Natl Acad Sci USA 70:1753–1756

Bocchinfuso WP, Hively WP, Couse JF, Varmus HE, Korach KS 1999 A mouse mammary tumor virus-Wnt-1 transgene induces mammary gland hyperplasia and tumorigenesis in mice lacking estrogen receptor-alpha. Cancer Res 59:1869–1876

Boehm M, Nabel EG 2003 The cell cycle and cardiovascular diseases. Prog Cell Cycle Res 5: 19–30

Bollati V, Baccarelli A, Hou L, Bonzini M, Fustinoni S, Cavallo D, Byun HM, Jiang J, Marinelli B, Pesatori AC, Bertazzi PA, Yang AS 2007 Changes in DNA methylation patterns in subjects exposed to low-dose benzene. Cancer Res 67:876–880

Bredow S, Falgout MM, March TH, Yingling CM, Malkoski SP, Aden J, Bedrick EJ, Lewis JL, Divine KK 2007 Subchronic inhalation of soluble manganese induces expression of hypoxia-associated angiogenic genes in adult mouse lungs. Toxicol Appl Pharmacol 221:148–157

Buteau-Lozano H, Velasco G, Cristofari M, Balaguer P, Perrot-Applanat M 2008 Xenoestrogens modulate vascular endothelial growth factor secretion in breast cancer cells through an estrogen receptor-dependent mechanism. J Endocrinol 196:399–412

Carmeliet P, Dor Y, Herbert JM, Fukumura D, Brusselmans K, Dewerchin M, Neeman M, Bono F, Abramovitch R, Maxwell P, Koch CJ, Ratcliffe P, Moons L, Jain RK, Collen D, Keshert E 1998 Role of HIF-1alpha in hypoxia-mediated apoptosis, cell proliferation and tumour angiogenesis. Nature 394:485–490

Chambliss KL, Yuhanna IS, Anderson RG, Mendelsohn ME, Shaul PW 2002 ERbeta has nongenomic action in caveolae. Mol Endocrinol 16:938–946

Channon KM 2004 Tetrahydrobiopterin: regulator of endothelial nitric oxide synthase in vascular disease. Trends Cardiovasc Med 14:323–327

Charlier CJ, Albert AI, Zhang L, Dubois NG, Plomteux GJ 2004 Polychlorinated biphenyls contamination in women with breast cancer. Clin Chim Acta 347:177–181

Chen Y, Jin X, Zeng Z, Liu W, Wang B, Wang H 2008 Estrogen-replacement therapy promotes angiogenesis after acute myocardial infarction by enhancing SDF-1 and estrogen receptor expression. Microvasc Res 77(2):71–77

Cheng JJ, Chao YJ, Wang DL 2002 Cyclic strain activates redox-sensitive proline-rich tyrosine kinase 2 (PYK2) in endothelial cells. J Biol Chem 277:48152–48157

Cullis ER, Kalber TL, Ashton SE, Cartwright JE, Griffiths JR, Ryan AJ, Robinson SP 2006 Tumour overexpression of inducible nitric oxide synthase (iNOS) increases angiogenesis and may modulate the anti-tumour effects of the vascular disrupting agent ZD6126. Microvasc Res 71:76–84

Donovan D, Brown NJ, Bishop ET, Lewis CE 2001 Comparison of three in vitro human 'angiogenesis' assays with capillaries formed in vivo. Angiogenesis 4:113–121

DuMond JW, Jr, Singh KP, Roy D 2001 Regulation of the growth of mouse Leydig cells by the inactive stereoisomer, 17alpha-estradiol: lack of correlation between the elevated expression of ERalpha and difference in sensitivity to estradiol isomers. Oncol Rep 8:899–902

Dumortier J, Streblow DN, Moses AV, Jacobs JM, Kreklywich CN, Camp D, Smith RD, Orloff SL, Nelson JA 2008 Human cytomegalovirus secretome contains factors that induce angiogenesis and wound healing. J Virol 82:6524–6535

Eum SY, Lee YW, Hennig B, Toborek M 2004 VEGF regulates PCB 104-mediated stimulation of permeability and transmigration of breast cancer cells in human microvascular endothelial cells. Exp Cell Res 296:231–244

Felsch JS, Cachero TG, Peralta EG 1998 Activation of protein tyrosine kinase PYK2 by the m1 muscarinic acetylcholine receptor. Proc Natl Acad Sci USA 95:5051–5056

Felty Q 2006 Estrogen-induced DNA synthesis in vascular endothelial cells is mediated by ROS signaling. BMC Cardiovasc Disord 6:16

Felty Q, Porther N 2008 Estrogen-induced redox sensitive Id3 signaling controls the growth of vascular cells. Atherosclerosis 198:12–21

Felty Q, Singh KP, Roy D 2005a Estrogen-induced G(1)/S transition of G(0)-arrested estrogen-dependent breast cancer cells is regulated by mitochondrial oxidant signaling. Oncogene 24:4883–4893

Felty Q, Xiong WC, Sun D, Sarkar S, Singh KP, Parkash J, Roy D 2005b Estrogen-induced mitochondrial reactive oxygen species as signal-transducing messengers. Biochemistry 44: 6900–6909

Folkman J 1995 Angiogenesis in cancer, vascular, rheumatoid and other disease. Nat Med 1: 27–31

Folkmann JK, Risom L, Hansen CS, Loft S, Moller P 2007 Oxidatively damaged DNA and inflammation in the liver of dyslipidemic $ApoE^{-/-}$ mice exposed to diesel exhaust particles. Toxicology 237:134–144

Ghilardi G, Biondi ML, Mangoni J, Leviti S, DeMonti M, Guagnellini E, Scorza R 2001 Matrix metalloproteinase-1 promoter polymorphism 1G/2G is correlated with colorectal cancer invasiveness. Clin Cancer Res 7:2344–2346

Haas E, Meyer MR, Schurr U, Bhattacharya I, Minotti R, Nguyen HH, Heigl A, Lachat M, Genoni M, Barton M 2007 Differential effects of 17beta-estradiol on function and expression of estrogen receptor alpha, estrogen receptor beta, and GPR30 in arteries and veins of patients with atherosclerosis. Hypertension 49:1358–1363

Hennig B, Hammock BD, Slim R, Toborek M, Saraswathi V, Robertson LW 2002a PCB-induced oxidative stress in endothelial cells: modulation by nutrients. Int J Hyg Environ Health 205: 95–102

Hennig B, Meerarani P, Slim R, Toborek M, Daugherty A, Silverstone AE, Robertson LW 2002b Proinflammatory properties of coplanar PCBs: in vitro and in vivo evidence. Toxicol Appl Pharmacol 181:174–183

Hong CC, Ambrosone CB, Ahn J, Choi JY, McCullough ML, Stevens VL, Rodriguez C, Thun MJ, Calle EE 2007 Genetic variability in iron-related oxidative stress pathways (Nrf2, NQ01, NOS3, and HO-1), iron intake, and risk of postmenopausal breast cancer. Cancer Epidemiol Biomarkers Prev 16:1784–1794

Hornstein I, Alcover A, Katzav S 2004 Vav proteins, masters of the world of cytoskeleton organization. Cell Signal 16:1–11

Huang RP, Wu JX, Fan Y, Adamson ED 1996 UV activates growth factor receptors via reactive oxygen intermediates. J Cell Biol 133:211–220

Hyder SM, Stancel GM 1999 Regulation of angiogenic growth factors in the female reproductive tract by estrogens and progestins. Mol Endocrinol 13:806–811

Iughetti P, Suzuki O, Godoi PH, Alves VA, Sertie AL, Zorick T, Soares F, Camargo A, Moreira ES, di LC, Moreira-Filho CA, Simpson A, Oliva G, Passos-Bueno MR 2001 A polymorphism in endostatin, an angiogenesis inhibitor, predisposes for the development of prostatic adenocarcinoma. Cancer Res 61:7375–7378

Kanda N, Watanabe S 2004 17beta-estradiol stimulates the growth of human keratinocytes by inducing cyclin d2 expression. J Invest Dermatol 123:319–328

Kao YH, Yu CL, Chang LW, Yu HS 2003 Low concentrations of arsenic induce vascular endothelial growth factor and nitric oxide release and stimulate angiogenesis in vitro. Chem Res Toxicol 16:460–468

Kim-Schulze S, McGowan KA, Hubchak SC, Cid MC, Martin MB, Kleinman HK, Greene GL, Schnaper HW 1996 Expression of an estrogen receptor by human coronary artery and umbilical vein endothelial cells. Circulation 94:1402–1407

Klei LR, Barchowsky A 2008 Positive signaling interactions between arsenic and ethanol for angiogenic gene induction in human microvascular endothelial cells. Toxicol Sci 102:319–327

Konac E, Onen HI, Metindir J, Alp E, Biri AA, Ekmekci A 2007 An investigation of relationships between hypoxia-inducible factor-1 alpha gene polymorphisms and ovarian, cervical and endometrial cancers. Cancer Detect Prev 31:102–109

Laurent G, Solari F, Mateescu B, Karaca M, Castel J, Bourachot B, Magnan C, Billaud M, Mechta-Grigoriou F 2008 Oxidative stress contributes to aging by enhancing pancreatic angiogenesis and insulin signaling. Cell Metab 7:113–124

Lim EJ, Smart EJ, Toborek M, Hennig B 2007 The role of caveolin-1 in PCB77-induced eNOS phosphorylation in human-derived endothelial cells. Am J Physiol Heart Circ Physiol 293:H3340–H3347

Mehendale R, Hibbard J, Fazleabas A, Leach R 2007 Placental angiogenesis markers sFlt-1 and PlGF: response to cigarette smoke. Am J Obstet Gynecol 197:363–365

Nematbakhsh M, Ghadesi M, Hosseinbalam M, Khazaei M, Gharagozlo M, Dashti G, Rajabi P, Rafieian S 2008 Oestrogen promotes coronary angiogenesis even under normoxic conditions. Basic Clin Pharmacol Toxicol 103:273–277

Okabe S, Fukuda S, Kim YJ, Niki M, Pelus LM, Ohyashiki K, Pandolfi PP, Broxmeyer HE 2005 Stromal cell-derived factor-1alpha/CXCL12-induced chemotaxis of T cells involves activation of the RasGAP-associated docking protein p62Dok-1. Blood 105:474–480

Ozaki M, Kawashima S, Yamashita T, Hirase T, Namiki M, Inoue N, Hirata K, Yasui H, Sakurai H, Yoshida Y, Masada M, Yokoyama M 2002 Overexpression of endothelial nitric oxide synthase accelerates atherosclerotic lesion formation in apoE-deficient mice. J Clin Invest 110:331–340

Pare G, Krust A, Karas RH, Dupont S, Aronovitz M, Chambon P, Mendelsohn ME 2002 Estrogen receptor-alpha mediates the protective effects of estrogen against vascular injury. Circ Res 90:1087–1092

Park KS, Mok JW, Ko HE, Tokunaga K, Lee MH 2002 Polymorphisms of tumour necrosis factors A and B in breast cancer. Eur J Immunogenet 29:7–10

Potente M, Ghaeni L, Baldessari D, Mostoslavsky R, Rossig L, Dequiedt F, Haendeler J, Mione M, Dejana E, Alt FW, Zeiher AM, Dimmeler S 2007 SIRT1 controls endothelial angiogenic functions during vascular growth. Genes Dev 21:2644–2658

Pu M, Akhand AA, Kato M, Hamaguchi M, Koike T, Iwata H, Sabe H, Suzuki H, Nakashima I 1996 Evidence of a novel redox-linked activation mechanism for the Src kinase which is independent of tyrosine 527-mediated regulation. Oncogene 13:2615–2622

Ramadass P, Meerarani P, Toborek M, Robertson LW, Hennig B 2003 Dietary flavonoids modulate PCB-induced oxidative stress, CYP1A1 induction, and AhR-DNA binding activity in vascular endothelial cells. Toxicol Sci 76:212–219

Ramos KS, Chacon E, Acosta D Jr 1996 Toxic responses of the heart and vascular systems. In: Klaassen CD, ed. Casarett & Doull's Toxicology: The Basic Science of Poisons, 5th ed. New York: McGraw-Hill; 487–527

Roy D, Abul-Hajj YJ 1997 Estrogen-nucleic acid adducts: guanine is major site for interaction between 3,4-estrone quinone and COIII gene. Carcinogenesis 18:1247–1249

Roy D, Cai Q 2002 Estrogen, immunoactivation, gene damage, and development of breast, endometrial, ovarian, prostate, and testicular cancers. Recent Res Devel Steroid Biochem Mol Biol 3:1–32

Roy D, Floyd RA, Liehr JG 1991 Elevated 8-hydroxydeoxyguanosine levels in DNA of diethylstilbestrol-treated Syrian hamsters: covalent DNA damage by free radicals generated by redox cycling of diethylstilbestrol. Cancer Res 51:3882–3885

Roy D, Liehr JG 1999 Estrogen, DNA damage and mutations. Mutat Res 424:107–115

Sasaki H, Ray PS, Zhu L, Galang N, Maulik N 2000 Oxidative stress due to hypoxia/reoxygenation induces angiogenic factor VEGF in adult rat myocardium: possible role of NFkappaB. Toxicology 155:27–35

Schieffer B, Drexler H, Ling BN, Marrero MB 1997 G protein-coupled receptors control vascular smooth muscle cell proliferation via pp60c-src and p21ras. Am J Physiol 272:C2019–C2030

Schneider BP, Radovich M, Sledge GW, Robarge JD, Li L, Storniolo AM, Lemler S, Nguyen AT, Hancock BA, Stout M, Skaar T, Flockhart DA 2008 Association of polymorphisms of angiogenesis genes with breast cancer. Breast Cancer Res Treat 111:157–163

Schwartz SM, Murry CE 1998 Proliferation and the monoclonal origins of atherosclerotic lesions. Annu Rev Med 49:437–460

Shahbazi M, Pravica V, Nasreen N, Fakhoury H, Fryer AA, Strange RC, Hutchinson PE, Osborne JE, Lear JT, Smith AG, Hutchinson IV 2002 Association between functional polymorphism in EGF gene and malignant melanoma. Lancet 359:397–401

Shortt AJ, Howell K, O'Brien C, McLoughlin P 2004 Chronic systemic hypoxia causes intra-retinal angiogenesis. J Anat 205:349–356

Sipka S, Eum SY, Son KW, Xu S, Gavalas VG, Hennig B, Toborek M 2008 Oral administration of PCBs induces proinflammatory and prometastatic responses. Environ Toxicol Pharmacol 25:251–259

Stier CT Jr, Chander PN, Rosenfeld L, Powers CA 2003 Estrogen promotes microvascular pathology in female stroke-prone spontaneously hypertensive rats. Am J Physiol Endocrinol Metab 285:E232–E239

Stork S, van der Schouw YT, Grobbee DE, Bots ML 2004 Estrogen, inflammation and cardiovascular risk in women: a critical appraisal. Trends Endocrinol Metab 15:66–72

Takada Y, Kato C, Kondo S, Korenaga R, Ando J 1997 Cloning of cDNAs encoding G protein-coupled receptor expressed in human endothelial cells exposed to fluid shear stress. Biochem Biophys Res Commun 240:737–741

Tan W, Bailey AP, Shparago M, Busby B, Covington J, Johnson JW, Young E, Gu JW 2007 Chronic alcohol consumption stimulates VEGF expression, tumor angiogenesis and progression of melanoma in mice. Cancer Biol Ther 6:1211–1217

Tarantini L, Bonzini M, Apostoli P, Pegoraro V, Bollati V, Marinelli B, Cantone L, Rizzo G, Hou L, Schwartz J, Bertazzi PA, Baccarelli A 2009 Effects of particulate matter on genomic DNA methylation content and iNOS promoter methylation. Environ Health Perspect 117:217–222

Tavolari S, Bucci L, Tomasi V, Guarnieri T 2006 Selected polychlorobiphenyls congeners bind to estrogen receptor alpha in human umbilical vascular endothelial (HUVE) cells modulating angiogenesis. Toxicology 218:67–74

Toda T, Leszczynski D, Kummerow F 1981 Vasculotoxic effects of dietary testosterone, estradiol, and cholesterol on chick artery. J Pathol 134:219–231

Tseng CH, Chong CK, Chen CJ, Tai TY 1997 Lipid profile and peripheral vascular disease in arseniasis-hyperendemic villages in Taiwan. Angiology 48:321–335

Vairaktaris E, Yapijakis C, Serefoglou Z, Derka S, Vassiliou S, Nkenke E, Vylliotis A, Spyridonidou S, Neukam FW, Schlegel KA, Patsouris E 2008 The interleukin-10 (-1082A/G) polymorphism is strongly associated with increased risk for oral squamous cell carcinoma. Anticancer Res 28:309–314

Villablanca A, Lubahn D, Shelby L, Lloyd K, Barthold S 2004 Susceptibility to early atherosclerosis in male mice is mediated by estrogen receptor alpha. Arterioscler Thromb Vasc Biol 24:1055–1061

White RE, Han G, Dimitropoulou C, Zhu S, Miyake K, Fulton D, Dave S, Barman SA 2005 Estrogen-induced contraction of coronary arteries is mediated by superoxide generated in vascular smooth muscle. Am J Physiol Heart Circ Physiol 289:H1468–H1475

Wong HP, Yu L, Lam EK, Tai EK, Wu WK, Cho CH 2007 Nicotine promotes colon tumor growth and angiogenesis through beta-adrenergic activation. Toxicol Sci 97:279–287

Yang SH, Liu R, Perez EJ, Wen Y, Stevens SM Jr, Valencia T, Brun-Zinkernagel AM, Prokai L, Will Y, Dykens J, Koulen P, Simpkins JW 2004 Mitochondrial localization of estrogen receptor beta. Proc Natl Acad Sci USA 101:4130–4135

Zhao T, Bokoch GM 2005 Critical role of proline-rich tyrosine kinase 2 in reversion of the adhesion-mediated suppression of reactive oxygen species generation by human neutrophils. J Immunol 174:8049–8055

Zhu BQ, Heeschen C, Sievers RE, Karliner JS, Parmley WW, Glantz SA, Cooke JP 2003 Second hand smoke stimulates tumor angiogenesis and growth. Cancer Cell 4:191–196

Zhu Y, Spitz MR, Lei L, Mills GB, Wu X 2001 A single nucleotide polymorphism in the matrix metalloproteinase-1 promoter enhances lung cancer susceptibility. Cancer Res 61:7825–7829

Chapter 7
Epigenetic Changes in Cancer: Role of Environment

Zdenko Herceg and Paolo Boffetta

Abstract It is now recognized that epigenetic heredity is important for understanding the causes of complex diseases such as cancer. Recent discoveries provided strong evidence arguing that epigenetic mechanisms play key roles in virtually all stages of cancer development and progression. A number of critical processes found in cancer cells, such as silencing of tumour suppressor genes, activation of oncogenes, aberrant cell cycle, and defects in DNA repair, can be a consequence of not only genetic but also epigenetic changes. Various environmental agents that are either known or suspected risk factors for human cancer may promote tumorigenesis by eliciting epigenetic changes. Better understanding of the contribution of aberrant epigenetic mechanisms induced by environment may prove critical in the development of novel strategies for cancer prevention.

Keywords Environmental epigenetics · Epigenetic changes · Environment · DNA methylation · Histone modifications · Cancer

7.1 Introduction

The term "epigenetics" refers to all changes that are heritable and stable over many rounds of cell divisions without altering the nucleotide sequence (genetic code) within the DNA molecule (Bird, 2007). Although most of these features are considered dynamic over the course of development of multicellular organisms, some epigenetic features show transgenerational inheritance arguing that they can be inherited not only from one cellular generation to the next, but also transmitted through the germ line. The term "epigenetic" was introduced by Conrad Waddington in 1942 to describe "the interactions of genes with their environment that bring

---

Z. Herceg (✉)
Epigenetics Group, International Agency for Research on Cancer (IARC), F-69008 Lyon, France
e-mail: herceg@iarc.fr

D. Roy, M.T. Dorak (eds.), *Environmental Factors, Genes, and the Development of Human Cancers*, DOI 10.1007/978-1-4419-6752-7_7,

the phenotype into being" (Holliday, 2006). Currently, "epigenetics" also refers to the study of cellular mechanisms that control somatically heritable gene expression states without changing the underlying DNA sequence. Epigenetic variations between individuals were detected and in some cases these epigenetic variants were found to be inherited by the offspring: this represents a biological inheritance that is not DNA-based and that adds a layer of complexity to the field of epigenetics (Rakyan and Beck, 2006).

The outbred nature of human populations makes it difficult to identify phenotypes that are truly due to epigenetic variants and not genetic or environmental influences. However, monozygotic twins that are genetically identical and generally brought up in similar environments may show a difference in limited number of phenotypic traits. A number of groups have studied twins that are discordant for the phenotype of interest. These studies found epigenetic differences between monozygotic twins suffering from Beckwith-Wiedemann syndrome (Weksberg et al., 2002), caudal duplications (Oates et al., 2006) or schizophrenia (Petronis et al., 2003). The alleles that are genetically similar (or identical) but differ in their epigenetic properties are termed "epialleles". The existence of epialleles in human populations was also demonstrated by a pilot study for the Human Epigenome Project (Rakyan et al., 2004).

Along normal mammalian development, genome-wide epigenetic profiles are reprogrammed during gametogenesis, and then again following fertilization of the egg. Thus the epialleles are usually lost and are not passed on to the next generation. However, occasionally, epialleles can escape reprogramming both during gametogenesis in the parent and during early embryogenesis, and then persist in the somatic cells of an individual (Rakyan and Whitelaw, 2003; Rakyan et al., 2003). As epigenetic inheritance is less stable than DNA-based inheritance, it results in a non-Mendelian type of inheritance.

DNA methylation, histone modifications and RNA-mediated gene silencing are three major types of epigenetic inheritance, however epigenetics also encompasses a wide variety of events including paramutation, bookmarking, imprinting, X-chromosome inactivation, reprogramming, transvection, infection agents like prions, and maternal conditioning. In this chapter, we will focus on DNA methylation and histone modifications and how they can be modified by environmental factors in the course of cancer development.

DNA methylation is the best understood epigenetic modification and represents the addition of a methyl group to the 5-carbon (C^5) position of cytosine bases that are located 5′ to a guanosine base in a CpG dinucleotide (Bird, 2002). This covalent modification of the DNA molecule is carried out by a number of DNA methyltransferase enzymes (DNMTs). Methylation of DNA is important in development and plays multiple roles in cellular processes, including regulation of gene expression and the defence against parasitic DNA sequences such as viruses (Jones and Baylin, 2002). Importantly, aberrant levels and patterns of DNA methylation may lead to unscheduled gene silencing and thus compromise cellular regulatory processes such as DNA repair and cell cycle control.

Histone modifications encompass a number of post-translational markings of specialized proteins (histones) that form DNA-protein structure (chromatin). Histone modifications include acetylation, phosphorylation, ubuiquitination, methylation, and poly(ADP) ribosylation of conserved lysine residues on the amino-terminal portions ("tails") of histones (Jenuwein and Allis, 2001; Strahl and Allis, 2000; Turner, 2002). The different histone modifications appear to act in a combinatorial and consistent fashion in regulation of several cellular processes. This led to the concept known as the "histone code" (Jenuwein and Allis, 2001; Strahl and Allis, 2000; Turner, 2002), which postulates that different histone modifications generate a code that is read by cellular machineries. Thus histone code may extend and modulate genetic (DNA) code in dictating functional outcomes (Jenuwein and Allis, 2001; Kurdistani and Grunstein, 2003; Loizou et al., 2006; Strahl and Allis, 2000).

A number of recent studies suggested that distinct epigenetic mechanisms do not act in an isolated fashion, rather they are intimately linked and reinforce each other in the maintaining functional and morphologic identity of the cell over many generations (Fig. 7.1) (Bird and Wolffe, 1999; Cameron et al., 1999; Fuks et al., 2000; Johnson et al., 2002; Lehnertz et al., 2003; Nan et al., 1998; Shukla et al., 2008; Soppe et al., 2002; Strahl and Allis, 2000). However, disruption of epigenetic mechanisms and aberrant epigenetic patterns (both DNA methylation and histone modifications) are associated with several human diseases, most notably cancer. The work on the role of epigenetic mechanisms in the regulation of cellular processes and cancer development has been recently reviewed (Belinsky, 2004; Bird, 2002; Cairns, 2001; Callinan and Feinberg, 2006; Egger et al., 2004; Esteller, 2005; Feinberg and Tycko, 2004; Jenuwein and Allis, 2001; Jones and Baylin, 2002; Loizou et al., 2006; Murr et al., 2007; Nan et al., 1998; Rowley, 1998; Wolffe, 2001; Yang, 2004). Here, we will focus on recent developments establishing a link between epigenetic changes induced by environmental factors and human cancer and discuss its implication for cancer therapy and prevention.

7.2 Epigenetic Changes Play an Important Role in the Development of Cancer

Cancer epigenetics is now recognised as an important field of cancer research and a flurry or recent reports and conceptual advances are likely to make this field to flourish in coming years. The importance of cancer epigenetics has also been recognised by funding agencies and at the end of 2007 this resulted in a launch of a comprehensive programme on cancer epigenetics as a part of new NIH Roadmap Initiative (nihroadmap.nih.gov/epigenomics/index.asp). It is now widely accepted that epigenetic events are universally present in human cancer and that they appear to be mechanistically implicated in virtually every step of tumour development and progression (Feinberg et al., 2006; Feinberg and Tycko, 2004; Jones and Baylin, 2002).

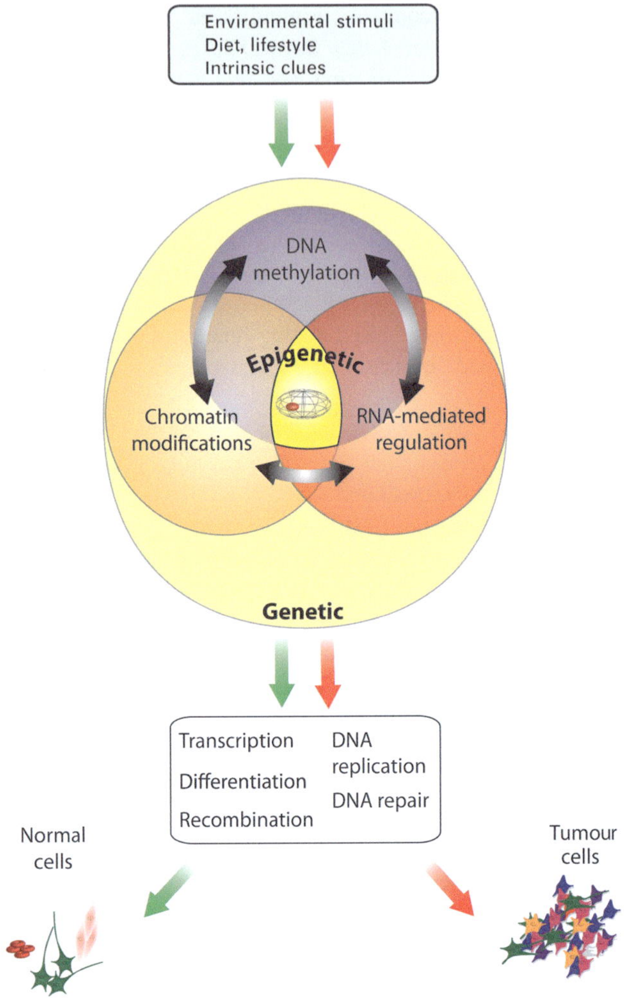

Fig. 7.1 Different epigenetic mechanisms regulate critical cellular processes directly or indirectly and play critical roles in cellular responses to environmental and endogenous stimuli. There is an intimate and self-reinforcing cross-talk between different types of epigenetic mechanisms. This is proposed to constitute the "epigenetic code" that extends and modulates genetic (DNA) code in response to endogenous and environmental cues. Epigenetic mechanisms are important to maintain gene expression profiles and chromatin structure in heritable manner over many cell generations and therefore they may dictate cellular outcomes by regulating cellular processes such as gene transcription, proliferation, and DNA repair. *Green* and *red arrows* indicate physiological and adverse exposure/response, respectively

Furthermore, aberrant epigenetic states are implicated in several developmental syndromes (Egger et al., 2004; Feinberg and Tycko, 2004; Jiang et al., 2004), and other human disease such as cardiovascular disorders and type-2 diabetes (Maier and Olek, 2002; McKinsey and Olson, 2004).

An important aspect of cancer epigenetics concerns its application in the clinic (Belinsky, 2004; Egger et al., 2004; Laird, 2003). One of distinguishing features between epigenetic and genetic alterations is that the epigenetic changes are in principle reversible, as they do not implicate irreversible modifications in DNA sequence. This means that aberrant states of DNA methylation and/or histone modifications may represent an attractive targets for the epigenetic therapy aiming to re-activate epigenetically silenced tumour suppressor genes or DNA repair genes (Egger et al., 2004; Esteller, 2005). A number of drugs capable of altering aberrant DNA methylation and histone modifications are currently in clinical trials (Egger et al., 2004). DNA demethylating agents (such as 5-azacytidine and zebularine) and HDAC inhibitors (such as Valporic acid and suberoylanilide hydroxamic acid, SAHA) are examples of epigenetic drugs that are able to reactivate the expression of epigenetically silenced genes. In addition, the intrinsic reversibility of epigenetic alterations may also be exploited in the development of novel strategies for cancer prevention.

7.3 DNA Methylation Changes in Cancer

DNA methylation, the covalent addition of a methyl group to the cytosine base in DNA, is an epigenetic event that is believed to affect cell functions and behaviour by altering gene expression. In somatic cells, methylated cytosine accounts for approximately 1% of total nucleotides; thus it affects ~75% of all CpG dinucleotides in the human genome (Ehrlich et al., 1982). Analysis of DNA methylation patterns in eukaryotes revealed the presence of so-called CpG islands, typically 0.5–4 kb long GC-rich regions containing high relative densities of CpG sites, positioned in the promoters of many genes. It is estimated that the human genome contains ~29,000 CpG islands and that around 60% of total human genes are associated with CpG islands (Bird, 2002). Previous studies have demonstrated that DNA hypermethylation is associated with gene silencing, and that genes with high levels of methylcytosine in their promoter region are usually transcriptionally silent. DNA methylation is essential during embryonic development, and in somatic cells, patterns of DNA methylation are generally passed faithfully to daughter cells. However, aberrant DNA methylation has been associated with a large number of human malignancies, other non-neoplastic diseases and aging (Feinberg and Tycko, 2004; Jones and Baylin, 2002; Richardson, 2003).

Aberrant DNA methylation is found in two distinct forms: hypermethylation and hypomethylation (Fig. 7.2). DNA hypermethylation is most studied epigenetic change to date and is found in all types of cancer. Hypermethylation typically occurs at CpG islands and is associated with gene inactivation (Fig. 7.3). A number of tumour suppressor genes and other cancer-related genes, including retinoblastoma (*RB*), p16 (*CDKN2A*), VHL, MLH1, E-cadherin, RASSF1A, CDH1, LKB1, GSTP1 and MGMT, have been found to be silenced by promoter hypermethylation (Feinberg and Tycko, 2004; Jones and Baylin, 2002). The list of genes altered by

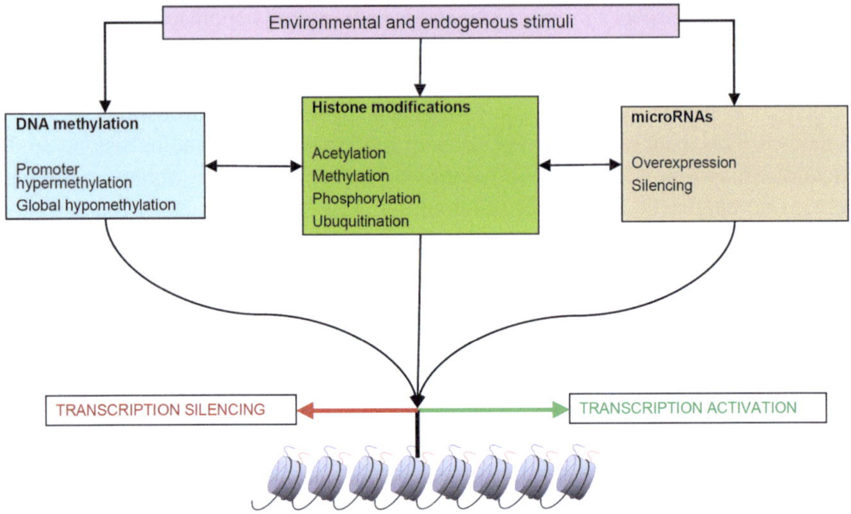

Fig. 7.2 Epigenetic mechanisms that regulate gene activation and silencing in response to environmental stimuli and endogenous cues

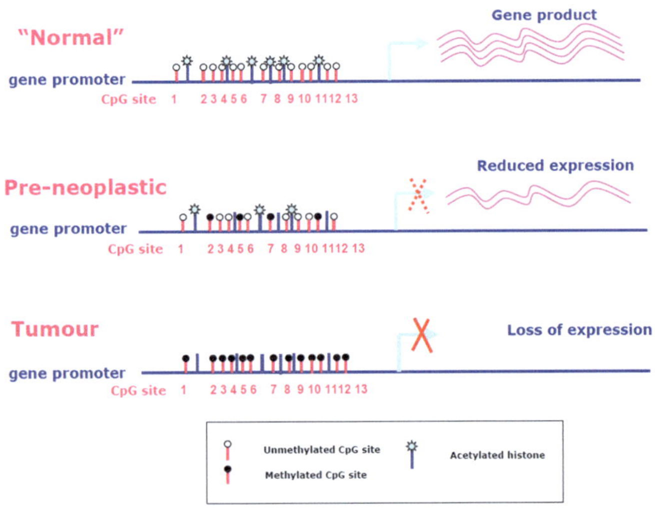

Fig. 7.3 Silencing of tumour suppressors by epigenetic deregulation is gradual and reversable process. In normal tissues, the promoter region of the active genes are typically unmethylated and histones at local chromatin are acetylated. During tumour development, concomitant and gradual deacetylation of histones and increased methylation of cytosines in CpG island is associated with progressive silencing of the gene expression

epigenetic mechanisms is rapidly expanding (over 600 genes have been reported to be modified by epigenetic mechanisms to date) and with the Human Epigenome Project (HEP) in preparation (Jones and Martienssen, 2005), a more comprehensive repertoire of aberrant human epigenome will be available.

Although the loss of DNA methylation was the first epigenetic alteration identified in cancer (Feinberg and Vogelstein, 1983), global hypomethylation has been overlooked in favor of gene promoter-associated hypermethylation. However, recent studies have shown that global hypomethylation is found in virtually all human cancers (Adorjan et al., 2002; Cho et al., 2003; Feinberg and Tycko, 2004; Sato et al., 2003). Although the precise mechanism by which the global loss of DNA methylation contributes to the neoplastic process is unknown, it is believed that it may act through induction of chromosomal instability and activation of cellular proto-oncogenes (Feinberg and Tycko, 2004; Qu et al., 1999; Sato et al., 2003).

7.4 Role of Histone Modifications in Cancer

In addition to aberrant DNA methylation, recent discoveries have revealed that deregulation of histone modifications and chromatin remodelling is also implicated in cancer (Fig. 7.2). Different modifications at several amino acids at different histone tails are possible, and there is interdependence between them. For example, acetylation, methylation and ubiquitination occur at lysines, whereas phosphorylation can occur on serine or threonine residues. The importance of histone modifications is demonstrated by the fact that mechanisms involving these modifications are essential during development and that their deregulation can lead to human malignancies (Cairns, 2001; Feinberg et al., 2006; Lund and van Lohuizen, 2004; Roberts and Orkin, 2004; Wolffe, 2001; Yang, 2004). Histone proteins have thus emerged as key carriers of epigenetic information, constituting a fundamental and critical regulatory system that extends beyond the genetic information.

Interest in histone modifications has further grown over the last few years with the discovery and characterization of a large number of histone-modifying molecules and protein complexes. Different chromatin-modifying complexes act in physiological contexts to modulate DNA accessibility to the transcriptional and DNA repair machineries (Herceg and Wang, 2005; Jazayeri et al., 2004; Loizou et al., 2006; Murr et al., 2006; Peterson and Cote, 2004). Alterations in these chromatin-based processes could lead to mutations in oncogenes, tumor suppressor genes or DNA repair genes resulting in genomic instability, oncogenic transformation and the development of cancer. The histone-modifying complexes include histone acetyltransferases (HATs), enzymes responsible for acetylation of the tails of core histones (Carrozza et al., 2003; Herceg and Wang, 2005), and histone methyltransferases (HMTases), a group of enzymes that add methyl epitope on several histone residues and are responsible for diverse functions including gene-silencing and generation of heterochromatin (Jenuwein and Allis, 2001).

Importantly, aberrant activity of histone modifying factors may promote cancer development by misregulating chromatin structure and activity, an example of which is frequently found in human leukaemia (Cairns, 2001; Rowley, 1998; Wolffe, 2001; Yang, 2004). Aberrant epigenetic regulation of key cellular processes, most notably gene transcription and DNA repair, is likely to be involved in oncogenesis. However, despite the fact that progress in determining different forms of epigenetic information in chromatin has been remarkably rapid, the way histone modifications are disrupted in cancer remains largely unknown.

7.5 Epigenetic Changes Induced by Environmental Factors in Human Cancer

An important role of environmental factors in the development of a wide variety of cancers is well supported by both epidemiological and laboratory-based studies (Peto, 2001). Environmental factors known to play important roles in the aetiology of human cancer include chemical carcinogens (for example, occupational carcinogen), dietary toxins (aflatoxin B1), and physical carcinogens (UV and ionizing radiation), whereas tobacco smoking, alcohol and fat consumption, and excess exposure to sunlight are lifestyle factors known to contribute to human malignancies (Doll and Peto, 1981; Mathers, 2004; Peto, 2001). Epigenetic mechanisms are believed to play a critical role in response to both endogenous stimuli and exogenous (environmental) factors. These mechanisms are thus physiological tools used by cells to establish and maintain gene expression patterns that are appropriate for specific environmental cues (Feil, 2006; Herceg, 2007; Jaenisch and Bird, 2003). Studies on plants as model systems provided important information on the role of epigenetic mechanism in response to environmental stresses (Gendall et al., 2001; Sheldon et al., 2000). It is believed that epigenetic mechanisms in animals also play key roles in the adaptation and response to environmental exposures. In many instances, however, clear-cut causal relationship between epigenetic states and environmental factors proved to be difficult to establish. This stems from the fact that environmental factors are likely to induce subtle changes. These changes may often be cumulative and thus quantitative manifestation of phenotypic traits occurs after repetitive exposure over a long period of time. For these reasons, epidemiology proved to be incapable of identifying complex environmental factors and dietary regimes that induce or promote tumour development by inducing epigenetic changes. This stems in part from the lack of epidemiological and laboratory-based studies that addressed the role of epigenetic changes induced by environment and nutrition with sufficient statistical power and sound technology (Herceg, 2007). Finally, the difficulty in identifying specific environmental factors that trigger epigenetic alterations is further complicated by the fact that the prevalence of different epigenetic mechanisms is likely to vary among different types of cancer, depending on the tissue-specific genes and gene networks affected and specific environmental exposures.

Recent studies implicated epigenetic changes induced by environment in virtually all types of human cancer. A number of physical and chemical carcinogens and infectious (viral and bacterial) agents in the environment are believed to promote neoplastic process through disruption of epigenetically maintained patterns of gene expression. These agents are also known as epigenetic carcinogens (epimutagens) (Feinberg and Tycko, 2004; Herceg, 2007; Jablonka, 2004; Sutherland and Costa, 2003). The effects of epimutagens on epigenetic states have been demonstrated either experimentally using different animal and cellular models or inferred from epidemiological studies (Herceg, 2007). Environmental epimutagens include tobacco smoke (Belinsky et al., 1998, 2002; Pulling et al., 2004), arsenic (Okoji et al., 2002; Sutherland and Costa, 2003), cadmium (Takiguchi et al., 2003), nickel (Conway and Costa, 1989; Klein et al., 1991; Sutherland and Costa, 2003), ionizing and UV radiation (Belinsky et al., 2004; Mittal et al., 2003; van Doorn et al., 2005). Different infectious agents such as HBV. HCV, and HPV viruses and bacteria *Helicobacter pylori (H. pylori)* may be considered as infectious epimutagens as they are shown to deregulate proliferation, cell division and gene expression pattern of the host cell via an epigenetic strategy (de Capoa et al., 2003; Herceg, 2007; Li and Minarovits, 2003). Among dietary factors, alcohol and fat consumption may act as epimutagens (Heijmans et al., 2003; Herceg, 2007; James et al., 2002; Poirier, 2002; Pufulete et al., 2003).

It should be noted that many epimutagens may promote tumour development through the induction of both epigenetic changes (aberrant DNA methylation and histone modifications) and genetic alterations (mutations). However, individual genetic polymorphism and epigenetic make-up ("epigenetic polymorphism") may also play pivotal roles in cellular response to environmental stress and thus may represent a part of individual predisposition to the development of cancer. Therefore, individual cancer susceptibility is likely to depend not only on genetic but also epigenetic make-up that dictates an individual's response and adaptation response. These responses involve the action of diverse cellular machineries such as those involved in DNA repair, carcinogen detoxification, cell cycle control, and cell death. The technological advances in epigenomics (high throughput and genome-wide profiling) will soon allow identification of entire epigenomes (genome-wide patterns of DNA methylation and histone modifications). This may provide critical information for testing the notion that differences in individual susceptibility may also be attributed to epigenetic make-up.

Environmental epimutagens can be broadly divided into two groups: (1) epimutagens that induce changes, either directly or indirectly, in genomic DNA, and (2) epimutagens that do not induce DNA changes but disrupt cellular processes pertinent to tumorigenesis such as carcinogen detoxification, gene transcription, DNA repair, DNA damage response, cell cycle and cell division control, and apoptosis. Among the epimutagens that induce DNA changes are those that disrupt DNA methylation patterns. This may indirectly alter cellular processes but also trigger other changes in DNA sequence (mutation and chromosomal aberrations). For example, the transcriptional inactivation by hypermethylation of promoters of a particular set of genes involved in DNA repair (MLH1, MGMT and BRCA1) and carcinogen detoxification (GSTP1) can cause genetic changes leading to cancer (Esteller et al., 2001c, 2000d; Herman et al., 1998; Jacinto and Esteller, 2007; Jones and Baylin, 2002; Kane et al., 1997). Another mechanism by which epigenetic changes may trigger genetic events involve preferential binding of environmental carcinogens to epigenetically modified DNA (presence of methyl group at CpG sites). This is exemplified by benzo(a)pyrene diol epoxide (BPDE) (Chen et al., 1998), a tobacco smoke carcinogen that seems to preferentially bind methyl-cytosine, leading to the formation of DNA adducts and G to T mutations (Denissenko et al., 1996; Yoon et al., 2001b). These studies represent examples of the most remarkable recent developments linking epigenetic deregulation and induction of genetic changes in human maliganacies. This resulted in a growing awareness that aberrant epigenetic states may predispose to genetic events during tumour development and progression. Therefore, epigenetic and genetic changes may work together to deregulate key cellular genes and pathways and destabilize the genome, leading to neoplastic process.

The epimutagens from the second group include those agents that alter the pattern of histone modifications and expression of microRNAs. These agents may act in a transient manner to deregulate "histone code" or microRNA expression profiles leading to abnormal function of cellular regulatory processes such as gene transcription, replication, DNA repair and cell death. Epimutagens from this group may target specific histone modifications (histone acetylation or methylation) or enzymes responsible for histone modifications including histone acetyltyransferases (HATs), histone deacetylases (HDACs), and histone methyltransferase (HMTs). Interestingly, emerging evidence suggest that HATs and HDACs are involved in the process of DNA repair and cell cycle control (Downs et al., 2004; Jazayeri et al., 2004; Li et al., 2004; Loizou et al., 2006; Murr et al., 2006, 2007; Peterson and Cote, 2004; Tamburini and Tyler, 2005), and that HAT activity is frequently deregulated in human neoplasms (Cairns, 2001; Lund and van Lohuizen, 2004; Yang, 2004). Therefore, it is likely that even moderate and transient inhibition of HAT and HDAC enzymes induced by environmental stress may impair critical cellular processes, resulting in abnormal cell growth and proliferation.

Epimutagens from the second group may also target methyl-C binding proteins (MBDs), a group of specialized proteins that bind to methylated CpG sites (Bird, 2002; Jaenisch and Bird, 2003; Lund and van Lohuizen, 2004). These include MBD1, MBD2, MBD3, MeCP2, and KAISO, and some members of this family seem to be a part of the cross-talk between different epigenetic mechanisms. For example, MeCP2 is shown to bind and recruit HDAC activity to chromatin (Jones et al., 1998; Nan et al., 1998), consistent with the notion that different epigenetic mechanisms are intimately linked and reinforce each other in stably maintaining the patterns of gene expression. Therefore, epimutagens in the environment that alter MBD protein stability and function may compromise the establishment and maintenance of the patterns of permissive or repressive chromatin states, essential for the propagation of cell identity and proliferation properties. This area of research is in its infancy, however better understanding of the epigenetic mechanism by which environmental epimutagens promotes tumour development will be important for better understanding of tumorigenesis and the design of new strategies for cancer therapy and prevention.

7.6 Examples of Environmental Epimutagens

Here, the term "environment" is used in its broadest sense, that is to refer to the sum of all external factors, both biotic (living) and abiotic (nonliving), to which an organism is exposed. Thus, diet and lifestyle are considered as integral parts of the environment. There is a growing list of agents in the environment that are shown or suspected to exhibit epimutagenic properties. These epimutagens may affect normal patterns of DNA methylation and/or histone modifications, however underlying mechanisms remain poorly understood. It should be noted that many of these agents are also known to induce genetic events, although it is possible that these events may turn out to be, at least in some instances, a consequence of primary epigenetic change.

Tobacco smoke A strong association between tobacco smoking and human cancer, most notably lung cancer, is know since the pioneering epidemiological studies by Doll and other investigators (Doll and Hill, 1950, 1952; Wynder and Graham, 1950). More recent experimental studies from different laboratories provided evidence that a number of different substances in tobacco smoke induce a variety of genetic changes that contribute to cancer development (Hainaut and Pfeifer, 2001; Pfeifer et al., 2002; Wistuba et al., 2002). More recently, an association between tobacco smoke and epigenetic events in human cancer has also been documented (Herceg, 2007), although the identity of tobacco epimutagens and the molecular mechanism by which these agents disrupt epigenetic states resulting in unscheduled gene silencing/activation remain unknown. Although laboratory-based studies on lung carcinogenesis induced by tobacco smoke have been largely focused on polycyclic aromatic hydrocarbons (PAHs), mostly benzo[a]pyrene (BP), considered the most carcinogenic (Rubin, 2001), it should be noted that tobacco smoke is a complex aerosol and carcinogenic effects for more than 44 substances in tobacco smoke have been demonstrated either in humans or laboratory animals (IARC-Monograph, 1986) Moreover, recent studies have suggested that among 4,800 identified compounds in tobacco smoke, as many as 69 may be carcinogens (Hoffmann et al., 2001).

Generally, the mechanisms by which epimutagens contributes to carcinogenesis may involve an enhanced binding of carcinogens, increased mutability of epigenetically modified DNA or histones, and silencing of tumour suppressors and DNA repair genes. Therefore, one plausible epigenetic mechanism by which the PAHs from tobacco smoke promotes tumorigenesis may involve preferential binding of PAH compounds to methylated cytosine (Jones and Baylin, 2002), a phenomenon already demonstrated for BPDE, a carcinogen found in tobacco smoke (Chen et al., 1998; Yoon et al., 2001b). Furthermore, aberrant silencing of several cancer-associated genes in lung cancer has been associated with tobacco smoking. The genes that are frequently silenced by hypermethylation in lung cancers include p16 (CDKN2A) and MGMT (Belinsky, 2004). The p16 gene is shown to be frequently mutated in lung cancer of smokers (Osada and Takahashi, 2002), therefore tobacco smoke exemplifies an agent that promote carcinogenesis by targeting one regulatory pathways through both genetic and epigenetic mechanisms. Although largely unexplored, it is also possible that epimutagens in tobacco smoke disrupt the pattern of histone modifications (histone code) leading to epigenetic silencing of cancer-associated genes.

While epigenetic changes seems to be frequently present in tobacco-associated lung cancer, it was not clear whether these changes are causally involved in the development of cancer or rather appear as a secondary event associated with tumour development (Belinsky, 2004; Laird, 2003; Palmisano et al., 2000). However, several studies demonstrated that DNA methylation changes could be detected in bodily fluids, such as sputum of lung cancer patients several years prior to clinical diagnosis (Belinsky, 2004; Laird, 2003; Palmisano et al., 2000). This argues that epigenetic changes often precede and are causes of neoplastic process. Therefore, almost universal presence and early occurrence are features that renders DNA methylation as powerful biomarker for early diagnosis and risk assessment.

It should be noted that tobacco causes cancer of many organs other than lung and given the complex composition of tobacco smoke the mechanisms are likely to vary in different organs. PAHs are belived to be important for lung and other organs in direct contact with smoke (larynx, oral cavity), aromatic amins target bladder, whereas nitrosamines seems to be important for oesophagus and pancreas (and probably lung). Therefore, epigenetic modifications induced by tobacco smoke in different organs may reflect the preferential organ and pathway targeted by distinct tobacco component.

Nickel: Occupational nickel exposure causes cancer of the nose and sinuses, as well as lung cancer (IARC-Monograph, 1990). In contrast to tobacco smoke, nickel, a potent cancer-promoting agent in both humans and animals (1990), appears to exert its carcinogenic effect through disrupting histone modifications states (Sutherland and Costa, 2003). For example, studies in yeast showed that nickel can induce gene silencing by altering patterns of histone acetylation (Broday et al., 1999). Interestingly, nickel seems to target acetyl mark at specific residues of histone "tail" (lysine 12 and 16 of histone H4) (Broday et al., 2000). Another study suggested that non-lysine residues of the same histone tail (histidine-18) may be preferential binding site for nickel, and that nickel molecules bound to histidine-18 impair accessibility of neighbouring lysines to HAT complexes, resulting in local hypoacetylation and consequently gene silencing (Zoroddu et al., 2000). Studies in cultured cells showed that the exposure to nickel may damage histone proteins such as truncation, deamidation, and oxidation of histone variants including histone H2B and histone H2A (Bal et al., 2000; Karaczyn et al., 2003, 2005). Loss of acetylation of H2A, H2B, H3 and H4, abnormally high levels of dimethyl-K9 at histone H3 as well as increased ubiquitination of H2A and H2B have also been observed in cells exposed to nickel compounds (Ke et al., 2006). Together, these observations suggest that environmental epimutagens can trigger a wide range of epigenetic alterations that can silence critical regulatory genes, leading to cancer development.

Arsenic: Arsenic is an important human carcinogen. Workers exposed to different arsenic salts have shown an excess risk of skin and lung cancer (Hayes, 1997). However, the most important source of exposure is via contaminated drinking water, resulting in an increased risk of several cancers, including lung, skin, bladder, liver, and kidney (IARC-Monograph, 2004). Arsenic may be considered epimutagen as it possesses the capacity to alter epigenetic states (Sutherland and Costa, 2003). Chronic exposure to arsenic induces transformed phenotype in cultured cells (Zhao et al., 1997), a property attributed to the capacity of arsenic to deplete cellular pools of S-adenosylmethionine (SAM), a metabolite needed for both the metabolism of arsenic and physiological DNA methylation (Zhao et al., 1997). This hypothesis predicts that chronic exposure to arsenic leads to the depletion of cellular pools of SAM resulting in so-called global DNA hypomethylation, a phenomenon proposed to activate cellular proto-oncogenes and parasitic DNA sequences (Feinberg and Tycko, 2004; Walsh et al., 1998).

Viruses and bacteria: A number of infectious agents are causally involved in the development of human cancer (Table 7.1). Different viruses and bacteria can be considered as environmental epimutagens as they are shown to be able to promote carcinogenesis through deregulation of epigenetic information. Among these agents human hepatitis virus (HBV), human papillomavirus (HPV), Epstein-Barr virus (EBV), and *Helicobacter pylori* have been reported to be associated with epigenetic changes in cancer. These infectious agents appear to adopt epigenetic strategy to either deregulate cellular regulatory mechanisms for their own benefit

Table 7.1 Infectious agents causally associated with human cancer, from IARC 1994a (Monographs Vol. 59), 1994b (Vol. 61), 1996 (Vol. 67), 1997 (Vol. 70) and 2007 (Vol. 90)

	Target organs	IARC Mono-graphs Vol.
Viruses:		
Hepatitis B virus	Liver	59
Hepatitis C virus	Liver	59
Human papilloma virus type 16	Cervix, vulva, vagina, penis, anus, oral cavity, oropharynx	90
Human papillomavirus types 18, 31, 33, 35, 39, 45, 51, 52, 56, 58, 59, 66	Cervix	90
Human immunodeficiency virus 1	Kaposi sarcoma, non-Hodgkin lymphoma	67
Human T-cell lymphotrophic virus I	Adult T-cell leukemia/lymphoma	67
Epstein-Barr virus	Burkitt lymphoma, Hodgkin disease, nasopharynx	70
Bacteria:		
Helicobacter pylori	Stomach	61
Parasites:		
Schistosoma haematobium	Bladder	61
Opistorchis viverrini	Liver	61
Clonorchis sinensis	Liver	61

or to protect themselves from cellular defence systems (de Capoa et al., 2003; Li and Minarovits, 2003; Maekita et al., 2006; Van Tine et al., 2004). It should be noted that epigenetic mechanism is a part of arsenal of tools used by cells to defend itself against foreign DNA sequences. This often include a prompt de novo hypermethylation of integrated viral genomes with the aim to silence and neutralise the activity of potentialy harmful viral gene products. For example, it has been shown that methylation of integrated HPV-associated cervical cancer or cell lines inhibits the transcription of the most viral genes (Van Tine et al., 2004). However, the level of DNA methylation correlates with HPV pathogenesis, suggesting that methylation of HPV DNA is implicated in the development and progression of cervical cancer (Kalantari et al., 2004; Van Tine et al., 2004; Wiley et al., 2005). Therefore, by using DNA methylation as a defense mechanism the cell may inflict adverse effects on itself. This can be explained by the fact that epigenetic silencing may spread from integrated viral genome to neighbouring host sequences, although alternative epigenetic mechanisms may contribute to the deregulation of cellular processes.

EBV virus, when integrated into host genome, may also be subject to host cell-dependent epigenetic modifications including DNA methylation, binding of regulatory proteins and histone modifications, and different EBV latency types are associated with distinct viral epigenotypes (Li and Minarovits, 2003). Associations between EBV and HBV infection and promoter hypermethylation of several genes were commonly found in different cancer types including gastric and nasopharyngeal cancer (Zazula et al., 2006; Zhou et al., 2005).

HBV virus can be considered as a potent epimutagen as its integration is often associated with epigenetic changes (Herceg, 2007). HBV virus is one of major risk factors for hepatocellular carcinoma (HCC). Although other risk factors such as chronic alcoholism, tobacco smoking, and aflatoxins are believed to be also important risk factors. Most HCC patients exhibit chronic hepatitis or cirrhosis caused by persistent infection with HBV. HBV infection is endemic in all areas with high incidence of HCC implying its primary role in the development of the disease (Custer et al., 2004; Ganem and Prince, 2004; Poynard et al., 2003). It is estimated that HBV carriers have about 20-fold higher risk of developing HCC than non carriers and that HBV accounts for about 53% of HCC cases worldwide (Parkin et al., 2001). The molecular mechanisms by which HBV virus induce tumour remains poorly understood (Block et al., 2003; Ganem and Prince, 2004; Wright, 2006). HBV, a member of a virus family called *Hepadnaviridae*, is a small circular DNA virus of about 3.2 kb, partially double-stranded because it has a complete strand and a partially synthesized strand. Unlike other oncogenic viruses HBV does not contain classical oncogenes and cannot immortalize hepatocytes in vitro. Since epigenetic mechanisms are believed to be important in protection against viral genomes (Herceg, 2007; Jaenisch and Bird, 2003), it is possible that aberrant epigenetic changes associated with integration of viral genomes may trigger events that promote tumorigenesis. Previous studies have shown that HBV integration may lead to epigenetic modifications (DNA hypermethylation) at the level of both viral and host genomes (Herceg, 2007). These epigenetic changes that persist in HBV infected hepatocytes may act indirectly by creating conditions that increase the chance of generating hepatocyte populations containing critical combinations of structurally and functionally aberrant genes. Therefore, it is possible that HBV virus may apply an epigenetic strategy to alter cellular growth and proliferation through both silencing of cellular genes and inhibition of host surveillance systems such DNA repair and checkpoint control (de Capoa et al., 2003; Li and Minarovits, 2003). Previous studies have shown partial methylation of HBV genome in cancer cells (Bowyer et al., 1987), consistent with the idea that methylation can play a role in viral repression, however, the precise patterns of DNA methylation in viral genome, surrounding host sequences and their significance to HCC carcinogenesis remain mysterious. Nevertheless, associations between HBV infection and promoter hypermethylation of cancer-associated genes were frequently found in hepatocellular carcinoma (Jicai et al., 2006), and can be exploited as a potential biomarker for diagnostic and prognostic purposes.

DNA methylation in certain virus-associated cancers (eg. cervical cancers associated with HPV infection) does not appear to be specific for viral DNA, but rather occurs as a frequent event throughout the host genome (Feng et al., 2005; Zhang et al., 2005), suggesting that viral proteins may also induce long-range epigenetic changes, likely through binding to promoter regions of host genes and by recruiting epigenetic modifiers. For example, viral proteins may interact with methyl-CpG-binding proteins and thus recruit histone deacetylase that will silence the gene promoter by deacetylating local histones. Future studies are needed to provide critical information for better understanding of epigenetic events associated with viral infection and viral genome integration.

Helicobacter pylori is a bacterium that lives in the stomach and duodenum and has a unique way of adapting in the harsh environment of the stomach. This agent has been recently linked to epigenetic changes (DNA methylation) in gastric cancer (Maekita et al., 2006). *H. pylori* infection may induce DNA hypermethylation in promoters of several genes in gastric mucosa, which appears to reflect gastric cancer risk. Although the mechanism underlying *H. pylori*-induced changes in DNA methylation is unknown, it is proposed that H. pylori infection may enhance cancer incidence after initiation with mutagens such as N-methyl-N-nitrosourea (Sugiyama et al., 1998). Given that *H. pylori* infection in turn induces chronic inflammation and cell proliferation (Szaleczky et al., 2000), it is possible that these events induced by bacterial infection trigger de novo hypermethylation (Issa et al., 2001; Szaleczky et al., 2000; Velicescu et al., 2002). Alternatively, transcriptional suppression of host genes through different mechanisms associated with inflammation process may "attract" DNA methylation machinery to the inactive gene promoters (De Smet et al., 2004; Song et al., 2002b), a phenomenon proposed to lock irrevocably silent state of the gene activity (Bird, 2002).

Aflatoxin: Aflatoxin B1 (AFB1) is an environmental carcinogen naturally occurring as a result of contamination of food by some species of the fungus *Aspergillus*. Several recent studies suggested that AFB1 can promote tumour development by deregulation of epigenetic mechanisms. For example, AFB1 exposure has been associated with abnormal status of DNA methylation in several cancer-associated genes such as RASSF1A (Zhang et al., 2002), MGMT (Zhang et al., 2003) and p16

(Zhang et al., 2006) in hepatocellular carcinoma. However, the mechanism by which AFB1 deregulates the pattern of DNA methylation in target tissue (liver) remains unknown.

Epimutagenic effects of nutrition: Although it is widely accepted that nutrition is very important in human cancer, the knowledge of specific dietary factors (other than alcohol and aflatoxin) remain fragmentary (IARC-Monograph, 2003). A diet rich in fresh fruits and vegetables is generally considered to entail a decrease in cancer risk, however the evidence from epidemiological studies is not fully consistent. The effect of other dietary components (such as fat and fibre) are unclear. Therefore, with several exceptions, the relationship between dietary factors and abnormal epigenetic states is poorly understood, likely owing to the chemical and physical complexity of the diet. However, there are studies that implicate specific dietary components in the regulation of epigenetic heredity (Herceg, 2007). For example, it was shown that methionine, an essential amino acid, may play a critical role in the process of DNA methylation (Waterland, 2006). Methionine serves as methyl donor for methylation reactions, therefore abnormal levels of methionine in the diet may compromise the establishment and maintenance of DNA methylation patterns, and consequently normal patterns of gene expression.

Cytosine methylation is carried out by DNMT enzymes that converts S-adenosylmethionine (SAM) to S-adenosylhomocysteine (SAH). For this reason, it is believed that an optimal supply of SAM or removal of SAH may be important for the physiological establishment and maintenance of genome-wide patterns of methylated cytosines in CpG sites. DNA methylation marks are erased to some extend during early embryonic development (soon after fertilisation) and then re-established in a tissue-specific manner (Reik et al., 2001). This dramatic and dynamic process may thus be highly sensitive to the supply of methionine (mainly through intake of fresh vegetables) and other dietary components essential for normal function of DNMT enzymes. One can imagine that methionine deficiency in the mother's diet may result in a deregulation of CpG island methylation leading to an aberrant establishment of DNA methylation patterns that may persist to the adulthood. This notion is supported by studies in mice demonstrating that dietary methyl supplementation during early embryonic development may increase CpG island methylation at specific genes resulting in lasting changes in gene expression (Waterland and Jirtle, 2003). However, methionine levels are also likely to be important in childhood and adulthood. For example, the treatment of adult men with hyperhomocysteinemia, with high doses of folate increases methylation levels at specific genes and restore normal expression (Ingrosso et al., 2003), suggesting that folate treatment may be a potent therapeutic or preventive agent in certain human conditions.

Alcohol: Alcohol drinking has long been known to cause cancers of different organs including upper aero-digestive tract, liver, colorectum and female breast (IARC-Monograph, 1988). As in the case of other multi-organ carcinogens, distinct mechanisms are likely to be responsible for alcohol-induced cancers in different organs (Boffetta and Hashibe, 2006). Alcohol consumption has been suspected to contribute to cancer development through epigenetic mechanisms. Two large epidemiological studies showed that colorectal cancer patients with high alcohol intake exhibited a higher frequency of promoter hypermethylation of a number of cancer-associated genes such as p16, p15, MGMT, RASSF1A, hMLH1, and APC-1A (Giovannucci et al., 1995; van Engeland et al., 2003). Chronic alcoholism is believed to be one of major etiological factors in the development of liver cancer. Carcinogenic effect of alcohol is likely to be associated with liver damage and consequent cirrhosis, the pathological change considered as precancerous lesion (Farber, 1996). In contrast, the mechanism by which alcohol promote the development of head and neck cancer is unclear, although studies on head and neck squamous cell carcinoma demonstrated that tumour tissue from alcoholics exhibited a higher prevalence of aberrant DNA methylation of cancer associated genes, including MGMT gene and the genes involved in the regulation of the WNT signalling pathway (Marsit et al., 2006; Puri et al., 2005).

Alcohol consumption may have direct and indirect carcinogenic effect in different tissues. Indirect effects of alcohol on tumorigenesis may be exerted through the induction of nutritional deficiency and compromising the organism's tumour defence. For example, alcohol consumption may abrogate the protective role of folate (Giovannucci et al., 1995; van Engeland et al., 2003). In addition, alcohol may act as a potent cocarcinogen, and exhibits strong synergistic effects with other carcinogens including HBV virus and aflatoxin. One important mechanism by which alcohol exerts its carcinogenic effect may involve acetaldehyde, the main metabolite of alcohol. Acetaldehyde is known to induce DNA damage and lesions in liver parenchyma which may result in cirrhosis and consequently liver tumour. Alcohol may alter epigenetic patterns through deregulation of SAM equilibrium. SAM is a metabolite regenerated from demethylated SAM via the methionine cycle that involves folate. Alcohol consumption may deregulate the cycle of SAM regeneration resulting in SAM depletion and consequent disruption of DNA methylation process.

Furthermore, epigenetic silencing of the class I alcohol dehydrogenases (ADHs), the genes encoding dehydrogenase enzymes that serve to break down alcohol which could otherwise be toxic by facilitating the interconversion between alcohols and aldehydes or ketones. For example, the class I ADH genes were found to be repressed in human hepatoma cell lines, but could be reactivated after the treatment with HDAC inhibitor or DNA demethylating agent (Dannenberg et al., 2006). Therefore, disrupted patterns of DNA methylation or histone modifications associated with alcohol-metabolizing genes compromise organism's detoxifying capacity making different organs particularly vulnerable to tissue damage and tumorigenesis. Finally, alcohol may also alter metabolism of different dietary compounds including vitamins. Together, these studies indicate that alcohol and its metabolites may promote tumorigenesis through multiple epigenetic mechanisms, however further studies are needed to elucidate precise molecular mechanisms and to identify gene targets in specific types of human cancer.

Epimutagensis and transgenerational epigenetic inheritance: The transmission of phenotypic variations that do not depend on nucleotide sequence (genetic code) from one generation to the next is known as epigenetic inheritance (Jablonka, 2004). It has long been thought that the patterns of epigenetic modifications (DNA methylation and histone modifications) are entirely cleared between generations and that only genetic code (DNA molecule) is transmitted with high fidelity to the next generation of organisms, at least in mammals. Studies demonstrated that this is only partially true, and that the passage through the germ line does not completely erase epigenetic marks, including DNA methylation (Campbell and Perkins, 1988; Morgan et al., 1999). The most flagrant example for this phenomenon is genomic imprinting, the conditioning of parental genomes during gametogenesis ensuring that a specific locus is exclusively expressed from either maternal or paternal genome in the offspring (John and Surani, 2000; Oakey and Beechey, 2002; Surani et al., 1984). Imprinting is a normal mechanisms of gene expression regulation and is mediated by epigenetic modifications, most notably DNA methylation. However, an unscheduled and incomplete erasure of epigenetic marks between generations may also occur. In this way, abnormal epigenetic "imprint" caused by parental exposure to epimutagens may be transmitted to the offspring resulting in a pathological phenotype. This unusual mechanism of inheritance from one generation to the next is known as transgenerational epigenetic inheritance. Although several epidemiological and experimental studies suggested the existence of transgenerational impact of both maternal nutrition and paternal exposure, the evidence supporting this notion is rather limited. Recent epidemiological studies suggested that effects of environmental exposures in humans may be transmitted trangenerationally to more than one generation (Pembrey et al., 2006). These studies suggested that transgenerational effects of dietary exposure of grandparents may be male-line specific (Kaati et al., 2002; Pembrey et al., 2006). This was exemplified by the correlation between father's mid-childhood smoking and body mass index (BMI) in his child at young age. In mice, it has been shown that DNA methylation patterns at specific gene locus associated with characteristic phenotype can be transmitted from one generation of mice to the next both through maternal and paternal lines (Rakyan and Whitelaw, 2003). Moreover, a study in the fruit fly (*Drosphila melanogaster*) demonstrated that altered epigenetic states induced by specific stimuli could be transmitted to subsequent generations through altered chromatin states (Sollars et al., 2003). Thus, it appears that human germline is capable of "remembering" epigenetic imprint of environmental exposure and passing it to next generation(s), although further studies are needed to substantiate these observations.

7.7 Susceptibility to Epigenetic Changes and Cancer

Cancer is a complex disease arising through multi-step genetic and epigenetic changes that alter multiple cellular regulatory pathways. Traditionally, differences in cancer incidence in populations have been attributed to variation in the exposure to environmental stimuli. For example, variation in susceptibility to diseases in identical twins and inbred strains of laboratory mice have been explained by distinct environmental impact. However, evidence is accumulating to suggest that epigenetic patterns (including DNA methylation and histone modifications) may be responsible for differential susceptibility to diseases, most notably cancer. A flurry of screening studies identified many genes (tumour suppressors and other cancer-associated genes) that are epigenetically silenced in human cancer (Table 7.2). Recent studies also suggested that there are many genes that may be prone to altered expression through epigenetic disruption in response to different environmental stresses, although the identity of environmental factors and the critical windows of vulnerability to environmentally induced epigenetic alterations are largely unknown. Gaining better insights into these phenomena would be critical for better understanding of cancer aetiology and efficient interventions in cancer control.

Table 7.2 A list of genes frequently silenced by promoter hypermethylation in human cancer

Gene	Tumour type	References
14-3-3 Sigma	Breast, stomach	Ferguson et al. (2000), Iwata et al. (2000), Suzuki et al. (2000), Umbricht et al. (2001)
AR (androgen receptor)	Prostate, colon, cell lines	Jarrard et al. (1998), Kinoshita et al. (2000), Sasaki et al. (2002)
APC	Colon, stomach, esophagus, breast	Jin et al. (2001), Muller et al. (2003), Virmani et al. (2001), Xu et al. (2004)
BRCA1	Breast, ovaries	Baldwin et al. (2000), Catteau et al. (1999), Dobrovic and Simpfendorfer (1997), Esteller et al. (2000c), Magdinier et al. (1998), Rice et al. (1998, 2000)
CDH1	Breast, stomach, leukaemia	Corn et al. (2001), Esteller et al. (2001a, c), Grady et al. (2000), Machado et al. (2001), Wheeler et al. (2001), Widschwendter et al. (2004)
CDH13	Lung, breast, lymphoma	Hibi et al. (2004), Ogama et al. (2004), Sakai et al. (2004), Widschwendter et al. (2004)
CDX2	Gastric cancer (in relation with diet)	Guo et al. (2007), Yuasa et al. (2005)
CHFR	Liver	Sakai et al. (2005)
COX2	Colon, colon, breast and prostate cell lines	Chan et al. (2003a), Toyota et al. (2000)
CRBP1	Stomach, colon, lymphoma, prostate, kidney	Jeronimo et al. (2004)
cystatin M	Breast	Ai et al. (2006a), Schagdarsurengin et al. (2007)
DAPK	Bladder	Tada et al. (2002)
DKK1	Colon	Aguilera et al. (2006)
ER	Breast	Falette et al. (1990), Issa et al. (1996a, 1994), Issa et al. (1996b), Lapidus et al. (1996), Li et al. (2000), Piva et al. (1990)
FAT	Colon	Paz et al. (2003)
GATA-4	Colon, stomach, lung, cell lines	Guo et al. (2004)
GATA-5	Colon, stomach, lung, cell lines	Guo et al. (2004)
Gadd45	Breast, pituitary gland	Bahar et al. (2004), Wang et al. (2005)

Table 7.2 (continued)

Gene	Tumour type	References
gelsolin	Breast	Mielnicki et al. (1999)
GSTP1	Breast, prostate, kidney, bladder, liver, stomach	Chan et al. (2002), Esteller et al. (1998a), Jhaveri and Morrow (1998), Kang et al. (2003), Lee et al. (1994), Millar et al. (1999), Morris et al. (2003), Song et al. (2002a), Tchou et al. (2000), Zhong et al. (2002)
HIC1	Multiple tumours	Fujii et al. (1998), Issa et al. (1997)
HOXA9	Neuroblastoma	Alaminos et al. (2004)
ID4	Stomach, leukaemia	Chan et al. (2003b), Hagiwara et al. (2007), Umetani et al. (2005)
IGFBP3	Lung, skin	Fraga et al. (2004)
LKB1	Lung, breast, colon	Esteller et al. (2000a, 2001a), Sato et al. (2001), Trojan et al. (2000)
MAGEA1	Colon, liver	Kim et al. (2006), Qiu et al. (2006), Xu et al. (2004)
MINT1	Colon	Xu et al. (2004)
MLH1	Colon, stomach, endometrium	Brucher et al. (2006), Cunningham et al. (1998), Esteller et al. (1998b), Fleisher et al. (1999), Kane et al. (1997), Leung et al. (1999), Nan et al. (2005), Toyota et al. (1999)
MGMT	Lymphoma, glioma, colon, lung, breast, oligodendrogliomas	Esteller et al. (2002, 2000b), Mollemann et al. (2005)
NORE1A	Lung	Hesson et al. (2003), Irimia et al. (2004)
P14 (ARF)	Colon, kidney, stomach	Baur et al. (1999), Calmon et al. (2007), Esteller et al. (2000e), Iida et al. (2000), Sato et al. (2002)
P15 (INK4B)	Leukemia	Baur et al. (1999), Herman et al. (1996), Uchida et al. (1998)
P16 (INK4A, CDKN2A)	Multiple tumors	Baur et al. (1999), Calmon et al. (2007), Esteller et al. (2001b, 2000e), Gonzalez-Zulueta et al. (1995), Jin et al. (2000), Kim et al. (2001), Lee et al. (2002), van der Velden et al. (2001)
P73	Lymphoma	Corn et al. (1999)
PR (progesterone receptor)	Breast	Lapidus et al. (1996)
RARbeta2	Head and neck, lung, colon	Esteller et al. (2001a), Sirchia et al. (2002), Virmani et al. (2000)
RASSF1A	Multiple types	Agathanggelou et al. (2001), Astuti et al. (2001), Burbee et al. (2001), Byun et al. (2001), Dammann et al. (2000), (2001a, b), Hogg et al. (2002), Lee et al. (2001), Liu et al. (2002), Lo et al. (2001), Lusher et al. (2002), Morrissey et al. (2001), Muller et al. (2003), Wagner et al. (2002), Yoon et al. (2001a)

Table 7.2 (continued)

Gene	Tumour type	References
Rb	Retinoblastoma	Greger et al. (1994, 1989), Ohtani-Fujita et al. (1993), Sakai et al. (1991)
RIZ1	Liver, breast, stomach	Chang et al. (2003), Du et al. (2001), Nomoto et al. (2007), Oshimo et al. (2004), Tokumaru et al. (2003)
SFRP1	Bladder, lung, colon	Fukui et al. (2005), Suzuki et al. (2002)
SOCS1	Liver, pancreas, stomach, mieloma, Barrett's adenocarcinoma	Fukushima et al. (2003), Galm et al. (2003), Oshimo et al. (2004), Tischoff et al. (2007), Yoshikawa et al. (2001), Zardo et al. (2002)
SOCS3	Lung, liver, ovaries, breast, head and neck, Barrett's adenocarcinoma	He et al. (2003), Niwa et al. (2005), Sutherland et al. (2004), Tischoff et al. (2007), Weber et al. (2005)
SRBC	Breast, lung	Xu et al. (2001), Zochbauer-Muller et al. (2005)
SYK	Breast, stomach	Wang et al. (2004), Yuan et al. (2001)
VHL	Kidney	Herman et al. (1994)
TIMP3	Breast, colon	Brueckl et al. (2005), Lui et al. (2005)
TMS1	Breast, lung	Conway et al. (2000), Virmani et al. (2003)
TSHR	Thyroid	Xing et al. (2003)
WIF1	Lung, colon, stomach, breast, leukemia	Ai et al. (2006b), Chim et al. (2006), Mazieres et al. (2004), Taniguchi et al. (2005)
WRN	Colon, stomach, sarcoma	Agrelo et al. (2006)

Many studies in experimental animals indicated that the exposure to environmental factors during early development may promote the development of disease through alterations in epigenetic states (Jirtle and Skinner, 2007). Different epigenetic mechanisms are believed to be important for organism's adaptation to environmental stress and differences in epigenetic patterns are likely to represent the bases for differential susceptibility to diseases. Studies in mice provided evidence for the existence of gene loci that are susceptible to prenatal and postnatal environmental exposures. These loci are known as metastable epialleles and are believed to be responsible for differential phenotypes in post-natal period and adult age. Various environmental exposures including chemical and physical agents and dietary and lifestyle factors are likely to modify epigenetic states of epialleles and consequently alter susceptibility to diseases, such as cancer. Environmentally-induced epigenetic changes may involve DNA methylation, histone modifications, and microRNAs all of which can produce phenotypic changes through altered expression of specific genes and pathways. Epigenetic deregulation of gene expression may intervene at the level of gene promoter (CpG island hypermethylation, histone deacetylation), regulatory regions of imprinted genes, and transposable elements (sequences adjacent to genes with metastable epialleles), as well as post-transcriptionally (RNA interference). Different gene loci may be affected through different epigenetic mechanisms although it is possible that a single gene may be the subject to epigenetic deregulation through multiple mechanisms.

Environment and metastable epialleles: Studies of inheritance in different model systems identified several loci that are, despite identical genetic sequence, responsible for variable and reversible phenotype due to differential epigenetic modifications. These metastable epialleles have been identified in plants and laboratory animals although it is likely that they exist in all species of animal kingdom including humans. One of the best characterized epiallele is the *Avy* (viable yellow agouti) locus in mice. Agouti yellow allele arise spontaneously through epigenetic deregulation of the retrotransposon particle inserted in the gene locus. The expression of the aguti locus is modified by DNA methylation status of the transposable element in its promoter. While transposons are typically methylated and thus silenced, DNA methylation levels of certain transposable elements are not stable and may vary in a stochastic manner. Therefore, epigenetic variability at transponons may affect the transcriptional activity of the adjacent gene (*Avy* locus) providing an example that the variability in epigenetic states may result in phenotypic variability among genetically identical mice. This allele has been used as a sensitive indicator of diet-induced changes in epigenetic information and proved to be very useful in studying the role of environment (Duhl et al., 1994; Jirtle and Skinner, 2007; Waterland and Jirtle, 2003). In particular, the agouti epiallele has been exploited to investigate the influence of maternal diet during pregnancy on the phenotype. For example, it has been shown that supplementation of diet of pregnant females with high doses of methyl donors (folic acid, choline and vitamin B12) may shift the phenotype (coat colour distribution) of their offspring (Cooney et al., 2002; Waterland and Jirtle, 2003). Detailed studies have confirmed that this methyl-donor-induced shift in coat-colour is a direct consequence of DNA methylation changes at IAP transponson in the regulatory region of the *Avy* locus. These observations argue that changes in the nutritional composition of mother during pregnancy may result in subtle shift in the epigenetic states and consequently induce phenotypic changes in the offspring.

The existence of other epialleles has also been reported. These include the *AxinFu* (axin fused) (Vasicek et al., 1997) and *CabpIAP* (CDK5 activator binding protein–intra-cisternal A particle (IAP)) locus (Druker et al., 2004). It is likely that there are many other metastable epialleles in mammalian genomes, however the phenotypic readout of such loci may be less discernable. This is consistent with the notion that changes of epigenetic states in multiple genomic loci may be susceptible to changes in response to environmental factors (Jirtle and Skinner, 2007). Therefore, future studies are likely to substantiate the notion that the existence of epialleles susceptible to environmental modulation is a general feature of human genome. Better insights into the regulation of epialleles by the environmental stimuli may prove critical for our understanding of the aetiology of human diseases including cancer.

Another epigenetic target that may be responsible for variable phenotype in response to environmental exposure is imprinted genes. Imprinted genes represent a fraction of autosomal genes that are expressed preferentially from either maternal or paternal allele.

Although around 80 genes have so far been found imprinted in humans and mice, it is estimated that there may be as many as 600 genes susceptible to imprinting (Luedi et al., 2005). Imprinted genes are randomly distributed throughout the genome, but rather are found in clusters (imprinted domains). An example of a genomic region containing a high density of imprinted genes is in chromosome 7, however functional significance of this phenomenon is unknown (http://www.mgu.har.mrc.ac.uk/research/imprinting). Imprinted genes have been shown to play critical roles in developmental and different cellular processes and are regulated through epigenetic modifications (DNA methylation and histone marking). Deregulation of imprinting (loss of imprinting, LOI) results in unscheduled biallelic expression of the imprinted genes and typically abnormal dosage of gene product. The importance of imprinting is highlighted by the fact that deregulation of this process is associated with several developmental and cancer-prone syndromes. These include Angelman syndrome (AS), Prader–Willi syndrome (PWS), and Beckwith–Wiedemann syndrome (BWS) (Feinberg et al., 2006; Feinberg and Tycko, 2004). In addition, it has been suggested that some human behavioural disorders including autism may be caused by deregulation of genomic imprinting during brain development (Badcock and Crespi, 2006). One of the best-studied example of genomic imprinting and its deregulation in human diseases is the IGF2/H19 locus. The H19 gene, which encodes a nontranslated RNA, is monoallelically expressed as the paternal allele is normally silenced by promoter hypermethylation. Since H19 gene lies at 100 kb downstream from the IGF2 gene, the maternal specific expression of H19 induces silencing of IGF2 in cis, resulting in monoallelic expression of IGF2 from opposite (paternal) copy. Because the reciprocal expression of these two genes is a tightly regulated mechanism, unscheduled methylation of both alleles of the H19 promoter results in abnormal hyperexpression of the IGF2 gene. The importance of IGF2/H19 locus imprinting has been highlighted by the study showing that its deregulation is strongly associated with Wilms tumours in children and overgrowth syndromes such as the Beckwith-Wiedemann syndrome (Feinberg and Tycko, 2004). LOI occurs at much higher frequency compared to genetic mutations in human malignancies (King et al., 1994), arguing that deregulation of genomic imprinting may play more important role in human malignancies than previously thought.

Because imprinting is a heritable (although non-Mendelian) form of gene regulation, it is obvious that the expression of imprinted genes in the offspring may be influenced by the parental environment. Furthermore, it is important to bear in mind that loss of imprinting may also occur in somatic cells during adult life. Considering that one allele of imprinted genes is typically silenced, imprinted loci may be particularly vulnerable to epigenetic alterations induced by the environmental factors. Certain developmental phases that involve major epigenetic reconfiguration, such as the early gametogenesis and genome-wide demethylation and remethylation after fertilization, represent highly sensitive windows for environmentally-induced deregulation of imprinted genes. It is thus likely that imprinted loci may be candidate susceptibility genes for environmentally induced diseases such as cancer, although further studies are needed to establish the identity of these loci and their biological effects.

7.8 Concluding Remarks and Perspectives

It is now widely recognized that deregulated epigenetic mechanisms are involved in virtually every step of cancer development and progression and that cancer is as much a disease of abnormal epigenetics as it is a disease of genetic mutations. Recent studies provided important information on the mechanisms by which epigenetic inheritance mediates critical regulatory processes and how epigenetic patterns are disrupted in human malignancies. However, we may have revealed only "the tip of the iceberg" of epigenetic disruption induced by environmental factors (epimutagens) in human cancers. Numerous physical and chemical carcinogens and infectious agents in the environment are believed to promote neoplastic process through disruption of epigenetically maintained patterns of gene expression. The list of environmental epimutagens is likely to grow rapidly with the completion of large-scale molecular epidemiology studies aiming to identify new cancer risk factors in the environment.

The effects of epimutagens on epigenetic states have been demonstrated either experimentally using different animal and cellular models or inferred from epidemiological studies. Epimutagens appear to be capable of deregulating a number of critical processes found in cancer cells, such as silencing of tumour suppressor genes, activation of oncogenes, aberrant cell cycle control, defects in DNA repair and detoxification of carcinogens (Fig. 7.4). However, further studies are needed to elucidate molecular mechanisms by which epimutagens impair the establishment and maintenance of normal patterns of epigenetic modifications, and associated abnormal events leading to cancer development. A number of studies demonstrated that epigenetic events frequently co-exist with genetic changes. Importantly, epigenetic changes may occur early in tumour development and may trigger a spectrum of genetic alterations such as mutations and chromosomal aberrations. There are different pathways by which disruption of epigenetic states (DNA methylation, histone modifications, and microRNAs) either individually or in combination may trigger genetic changes. These include unscheduled silencing of tumour suppressor genes, DNA repair genes and carcinogene detoxifying genes, abrogation of DNA repair, inactivation of cell cycle checkpoints and apoptosis impairment. Therefore, it is of great interest to identify what are the primary and what are secondary genetic and epigenetic events induced by specific environmental exposures. This will be important for a better mechanistic understanding of the process of tumorigenesis but also for the development of novel strategies for cancer prevention.

Two important features that distinguish epigenetic changes from genetic alterations are gradual appearance and reversibility of epigenetic events. In other words,

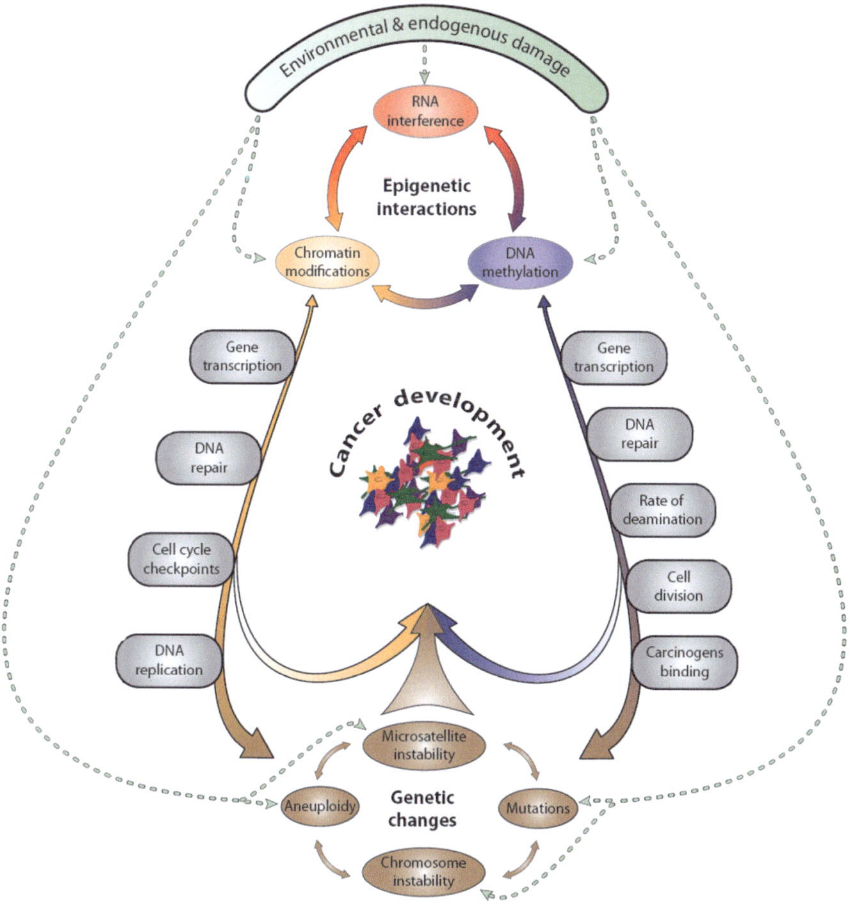

Fig. 7.4 Cellular processes disrupted by epigenetic and genetic changes in response to the environmental and endogenous factors. Epigenetic changes induced by a variety of environmental stimuli or endogenous cues may deregulate, directly or indirectly (through of genetic alterations), a spectrum of critical regulatory processes including DNA repair, cell cycle checkpoints, carcinogen detoxification, gene transcription, and cell death. Disrupted epigenetic mechanisms (DNA methylation, chromatin modifications, and RNA mediated gene silencing) may induce alone or in combination with secondary ("passenger") genetic alterations the deregulation of different cellular processes that contribute to cancer development and malignant phenotype. The disruption of one or multiple of critical cellular processes promotes different steps in the development and progression of cancer

epigenetic changes are in turn reversible as they do not implicate changes in DNA sequence. These features make epigenetic alterations an attractive target for therapeutic intervention and for preventive strategies. For example, aberrant patterns of DNA methylation, histone acetylation and methylation can be targeted by epigenetic drugs aiming to re-activate epigenetically silenced genes (Egger et al., 2004;

Esteller, 2005). Re-expression of such silenced genes can lead to suppression of tumour growth or sensitisation to anticancer therapies. Many drugs capable of targeting changes in DNA methylation and histone modifications are currently in clinical trials (Egger et al., 2004). Two drugs, 5-azacytidine (Vidaza), and decitabine (Dacogen), are the first epigenetic compounds approved by the Food and Drug Administration (FDA) for second-line treatment of myelodysplastic syndrome and leukemias. Current efforts in clinics will likely to result in the emergence of many other drugs capable of efficient targeting epigenetic changes in other caner types.

Despite the fact that epigenetic changes induced by environmental factors are likely to be important mechanisms of cancer development, epigenetic epidemiology is in its infancy, and little is known of the precise contribution of epigenetic changes to cancer burden. A list of genes and gene networks that are targets of epigenetic alterations are likely to grow with the development of powerful screening approaches and the Human Genome Project (HGP) in preparation (Jones and Martienssen, 2005). While studies have so far been focused largely on DNA methylation, likely due to the availability of sensitive and quantitative techniques for detection of methyl-cytosine, disruption of histone modifications (histone code) in human cancer remains largely unexplored. Given their critical role in cellular regulatory process, it seems inevitable that changes in normal patterns of histone modifications are induced by environmental factors that contribute to human cancer development. However, a formal proof of such a relationship remains to be established.

Recent advances in epigenomics and emergence of powerful technologies for detection of epigenetic changes in high throughput and genome-wide settings (Callinan and Feinberg, 2006; Esteller, 2007; van Steensel and Henikoff, 2003) will further advance our capacity to evaluate the contribution of epigenetic changes induced by the environmental epimutagens to human cancer. These powerful tools will be applied to large population-based and case-control studies which offer some of the most exciting opportunities to study the contribution of epigenetic events to specific human cancers. Application of epigenetic markers to epidemiological studies requires careful considerations in the design of such studies. Specifically, random and systematic errors should be avoided. Control of random error takes place through the enrolment of a sufficiently large series of patients and controls. Sample size should be estimated based on power calculations which depend on the background rate of the marker (e.g. among controls) and the expected strength of the association (e.g. difference in the marker frequencies between cases—or exposed—and controls). In general few, large-scale investigations are preferable to a larger number of small, under-powered studies. Systematic error (bias) might arise because of the observational nature of epidemiology. Sources of errors in the measurement of the biomarkers (e.g., inter-batch variability) can be controlled, e.g., by implementing quality control procedures, and non-differential misclassification from measurement error can be controlled by blind allocation of samples with respect to exposure and disease status. A potentially more important, and after not appreciated, source of bias is selection of study subjects. Lack of comparability of cases and controls can originated from biased selection of either group (e.g. selection of cases based on severity of disease, or selection of hospital-based controls with diseases potentially linked to the exposure or the marker). These considerations are not different from those relevant to other types of epidemiological studies, and the adoption of stringent criteria for the design, conduct and analysis of studies in which epigenetic markers are applied should reduce opportunity for bias.

Together, spectacular advances in cancer genomics and epigenomics combined with epidemiological population-based studies will provide unique opportunity to address critical issues in environmental cancer epigenetics. Therefore, in the near future, we are likely to obtain long-awaited answers on the contribution of environmental factors to specific human cancers and critical information for the development of novel and efficient strategies for cancer prevention, one of major public health challenges in coming decades.

Acknowledgment We apologize to colleagues whose relevant publications were not cited due to space limitation. Our work is supported by the National Institutes of Health/National Cancer Institute (NIH/NCI), United States; Association for International Cancer Research (AICR), United Kingdom; Institut National du Cancer (Epigenetic profiling Network, EpiPro), France; L'Association pour la Recherche sur le Cancer (ARC), France; la Ligue Nationale (Française) Contre le Cancer, France; the European Network of Excellence Environmental Cancer Risk, Nutrition and Individual Susceptibility (ECNIS), the Swiss Bridge Award, and the European Molecular Biology Organisation (EMBO).

References

Adorjan, P., Distler, J., Lipscher, E., Model, F., Muller, J., Pelet, C., Braun, A., Florl, A.R., Gutig, D., Grabs, G., Howe, A., Kursar, M., Lesche, R., Leu, E., Lewin, A., Maier, S., Muller, V., Otto, T., Scholz, C., Schulz, W.A., Seifert, H.H., Schwope, I., Ziebarth, H., Berlin, K., Piepenbrock, C. and Olek, A. (2002) Tumour class prediction and discovery by microarray-based DNA methylation analysis. *Nucleic Acids Res*, **30**, e21.

Agathanggelou, A., Honorio, S., Macartney, D.P., Martinez, A., Dallol, A., Rader, J., Fullwood, P., Chauhan, A., Walker, R., Shaw, J.A., Hosoe, S., Lerman, M.I., Minna, J.D., Maher, E.R. and Latif, F. (2001) Methylation associated inactivation of RASSF1A from region 3p21.3 in lung, breast and ovarian tumours. *Oncogene*, **20**, 1509–1518.

Agrelo, R., Cheng, W.H., Setien, F., Ropero, S., Espada, J., Fraga, M.F., Herranz, M., Paz, M.F., Sanchez-Cespedes, M., Artiga, M.J., Guerrero, D., Castells, A., von Kobbe, C., Bohr, V.A. and Esteller, M. (2006) Epigenetic inactivation of the premature aging Werner syndrome gene in human cancer. *Proc Natl Acad Sci USA*, **103**, 8822–8827.

Aguilera, O., Fraga, M.F., Ballestar, E., Paz, M.F., Herranz, M., Espada, J., Garcia, J.M., Munoz, A., Esteller, M. and Gonzalez-Sancho, J.M. (2006) Epigenetic inactivation of the Wnt antagonist DICKKOPF-1 (DKK-1) gene in human colorectal cancer. *Oncogene*, **25**, 4116–4121.

Ai, L., Kim, W.J., Kim, T.Y., Fields, C.R., Massoll, N.A., Robertson, K.D. and Brown, K.D. (2006a) Epigenetic silencing of the tumor suppressor cystatin M occurs during breast cancer progression. *Cancer Res*, **66**, 7899–7909.

Ai, L., Tao, Q., Zhong, S., Fields, C.R., Kim, W.J., Lee, M.W., Cui, Y., Brown, K.D. and Robertson, K.D. (2006b) Inactivation of Wnt inhibitory factor-1 (WIF1) expression by epigenetic silencing is a common event in breast cancer. *Carcinogenesis*, **27**, 1341–1348.

Alaminos, M., Davalos, V., Cheung, N.K., Gerald, W.L. and Esteller, M. (2004) Clustering of gene hypermethylation associated with clinical risk groups in neuroblastoma. *J Natl Cancer Inst*, **96**, 1208–1219.

Astuti, D., Agathanggelou, A., Honorio, S., Dallol, A., Martinsson, T., Kogner, P., Cummins, C., Neumann, H.P., Voutilainen, R., Dahia, P., Eng, C., Maher, E.R. and Latif, F. (2001) RASSF1A promoter region CpG island hypermethylation in phaeochromocytomas and neuroblastoma tumours. *Oncogene*, **20**, 7573–7577.

Badcock, C. and Crespi, B. (2006) Imbalanced genomic imprinting in brain development: an evolutionary basis for the aetiology of autism. *J Evol Biol*, **19**, 1007–1032.

Bahar, A., Bicknell, J.E., Simpson, D.J., Clayton, R.N. and Farrell, W.E. (2004) Loss of expression of the growth inhibitory gene GADD45gamma, in human pituitary adenomas, is associated with CpG island methylation. *Oncogene*, **23**, 936–944.

Bal, W., Liang, R., Lukszo, J., Lee, S.H., Dizdaroglu, M. and Kasprzak, K.S. (2000) Ni(II) specifically cleaves the C-terminal tail of the major variant of histone H2A and forms an oxidative damage-mediating complex with the cleaved-off octapeptide. *Chem Res Toxicol*, **13**, 616–624.

Baldwin, R.L., Nemeth, E., Tran, H., Shvartsman, H., Cass, I., Narod, S. and Karlan, B.Y. (2000) BRCA1 promoter region hypermethylation in ovarian carcinoma: a population-based study. *Cancer Res*, **60**, 5329–5333.

Baur, A.S., Shaw, P., Burri, N., Delacretaz, F., Bosman, F.T. and Chaubert, P. (1999) Frequent methylation silencing of p15(INK4b) (MTS2) and p16(INK4a) (MTS1) in B-cell and T-cell lymphomas. *Blood*, **94**, 1773–1781.

Belinsky, S.A. (2004) Gene-promoter hypermethylation as a biomarker in lung cancer. *Nat Rev Cancer*, **4**, 707–717.

Belinsky, S.A., Klinge, D.M., Liechty, K.C., March, T.H., Kang, T., Gilliland, F.D., Sotnic, N., Adamova, G., Rusinova, G. and Telnov, V. (2004) Plutonium targets the p16 gene for inactivation by promoter hypermethylation in human lung adenocarcinoma. *Carcinogenesis*, **25**, 1063–1067.

Belinsky, S.A., Nikula, K.J., Palmisano, W.A., Michels, R., Saccomanno, G., Gabrielson, E., Baylin, S.B. and Herman, J.G. (1998) Aberrant methylation of p16(INK4a) is an early event in lung cancer and a potential biomarker for early diagnosis. *Proc Natl Acad Sci USA*, **95**, 11891–11896.

Belinsky, S.A., Palmisano, W.A., Gilliland, F.D., Crooks, L.A., Divine, K.K., Winters, S.A., Grimes, M.J., Harms, H.J., Tellez, C.S., Smith, T.M., Moots, P.P., Lechner, J.F., Stidley, C.A. and Crowell, R.E. (2002) Aberrant promoter methylation in bronchial epithelium and sputum from current and former smokers. *Cancer Res*, **62**, 2370–2377.

Bird, A. (2002) DNA methylation patterns and epigenetic memory. *Genes Dev*, **16**, 6–21.

Bird, A. (2007) Perceptions of epigenetics. *Nature*, **447**, 396–398.

Bird, A.P. and Wolffe, A.P. (1999) Methylation-induced repression – belts, braces, and chromatin. *Cell*, **99**, 451–454.

Block, T.M., Mehta, A.S., Fimmel, C.J. and Jordan, R. (2003) Molecular viral oncology of hepatocellular carcinoma. *Oncogene*, **22**, 5093–5107.

Boffetta, P. and Hashibe, M. (2006) Alcohol and cancer. *Lancet Oncol*, **7**, 149–156.

Bowyer, S.M., Dusheiko, G.M., Schoub, B.D. and Kew, M.C. (1987) Expression of the hepatitis B virus genome in chronic hepatitis B carriers and patients with hepatocellular carcinoma. *Proc Natl Acad Sci USA*, **84**, 847–850.

Broday, L., Cai, J. and Costa, M. (1999) Nickel enhances telomeric silencing in Saccharomyces cerevisiae. *Mutat Res*, **440**, 121–130.

Broday, L., Peng, W., Kuo, M.H., Salnikow, K., Zoroddu, M. and Costa, M. (2000) Nickel compounds are novel inhibitors of histone H4 acetylation. *Cancer Res*, **60**, 238–241.

Brucher, B.L., Geddert, H., Langner, C., Hofler, H., Fink, U., Siewert, J.R. and Sarbia, M. (2006) Hypermethylation of hMLH1, HPP1, p14(ARF), p16(INK4A) and APC in primary adenocarcinomas of the small bowel. *Int J Cancer*, **119**, 1298–1302.

Brueckl, W.M., Grombach, J., Wein, A., Ruckert, S., Porzner, M., Dietmaier, W., Rummele, P., Croner, R.S., Boxberger, F., Kirchner, T., Hohenberger, W., Hahn, E.G. and Jung, A. (2005) Alterations in the tissue inhibitor of metalloproteinase-3 (TIMP-3) are found frequently in human colorectal tumours displaying either microsatellite stability (MSS) or instability (MSI). *Cancer Lett*, **223**, 137–142.

Burbee, D.G., Forgacs, E., Zochbauer-Muller, S., Shivakumar, L., Fong, K., Gao, B., Randle, D., Kondo, M., Virmani, A., Bader, S., Sekido, Y., Latif, F., Milchgrub, S., Toyooka, S., Gazdar, A.F., Lerman, M.I., Zabarovsky, E., White, M. and Minna, J.D. (2001) Epigenetic inactivation of RASSF1A in lung and breast cancers and malignant phenotype suppression. *J Natl Cancer Inst*, **93**, 691–699.

Byun, D.S., Lee, M.G., Chae, K.S., Ryu, B.G. and Chi, S.G. (2001) Frequent epigenetic inactivation of RASSF1A by aberrant promoter hypermethylation in human gastric adenocarcinoma. *Cancer Res*, **61**, 7034–7038.

Cairns, B.R. (2001) Emerging roles for chromatin remodeling in cancer biology. *Trends Cell Biol*, **11**, S15–21.

Callinan, P.A. and Feinberg, A.P. (2006) The emerging science of epigenomics. *Hum Mol Genet*, **15 Spec No 1**, R95–101.

Calmon, M.F., Colombo, J., Carvalho, F., Souza, F.P., Filho, J.F., Fukuyama, E.E., Camargo, A.A., Caballero, O.L., Tajara, E.H., Cordeiro, J.A. and Rahal, P. (2007) Methylation profile of genes CDKN2A (p14 and p16), DAPK1, CDH1, and ADAM23 in head and neck cancer. *Cancer Genet Cytogenet*, **173**, 31–37.

Cameron, E.E., Bachman, K.E., Myohanen, S., Herman, J.G. and Baylin, S.B. (1999) Synergy of demethylation and histone deacetylase inhibition in the re-expression of genes silenced in cancer. *Nat Genet*, **21**, 103–107.

Campbell, J.H. and Perkins, P. (1988) Transgenerational effects of drug and hormonal treatments in mammals: a review of observations and ideas. *Prog Brain Res*, **73**, 535–553.

Carrozza, M.J., Utley, R.T., Workman, J.L. and Cote, J. (2003) The diverse functions of histone acetyltransferase complexes. *Trends Genet*, **19**, 321–329.

Catteau, A., Harris, W.H., Xu, C.F. and Solomon, E. (1999) Methylation of the BRCA1 promoter region in sporadic breast and ovarian cancer: correlation with disease characteristics. *Oncogene*, **18**, 1957–1965.

Chan, M.W., Chan, L.W., Tang, N.L., Tong, J.H., Lo, K.W., Lee, T.L., Cheung, H.Y., Wong, W.S., Chan, P.S., Lai, F.M. and To, K.F. (2002) Hypermethylation of multiple genes in tumor tissues and voided urine in urinary bladder cancer patients. *Clin Cancer Res*, **8**, 464–470.

Chan, A.O., Kim, S.G., Bedeir, A., Issa, J.P., Hamilton, S.R. and Rashid, A. (2003a) CpG island methylation in carcinoid and pancreatic endocrine tumors. *Oncogene*, **22**, 924–934.

Chan, A.S., Tsui, W.Y., Chen, X., Chu, K.M., Chan, T.L., Chan, A.S., Li, R., So, S., Yuen, S.T. and Leung, S.Y. (2003b) Downregulation of ID4 by promoter hypermethylation in gastric adenocarcinoma. *Oncogene*, **22**, 6946–6953.

Chang, H.W., Chan, A., Kwong, D.L., Wei, W.I., Sham, J.S. and Yuen, A.P. (2003) Detection of hypermethylated RIZ1 gene in primary tumor, mouth, and throat rinsing fluid, nasopharyngeal swab, and peripheral blood of nasopharyngeal carcinoma patient. *Clin Cancer Res*, **9**, 1033–1038.

Chen, J.X., Zheng, Y., West, M. and Tang, M.S. (1998) Carcinogens preferentially bind at methylated CpG in the p53 mutational hot spots. *Cancer Res*, **58**, 2070–2075.

Chim, C.S., Chan, W.W., Pang, A. and Kwong, Y.L. (2006) Preferential methylation of Wnt inhibitory factor-1 in acute promyelocytic leukemia: an independent poor prognostic factor. *Leukemia*, **20**, 907–909.

Cho, B., Lee, H., Jeong, S., Bang, Y.J., Lee, H.J., Hwang, K.S., Kim, H.Y., Lee, Y.S., Kang, G.H. and Jeoung, D.I. (2003) Promoter hypomethylation of a novel cancer/testis antigen gene CAGE is correlated with its aberrant expression and is seen in premalignant stage of gastric carcinoma. *Biochem Biophys Res Commun*, **307**, 52–63.

Conway, K. and Costa, M. (1989) Nonrandom chromosomal alterations in nickel-transformed Chinese hamster embryo cells. *Cancer Res*, **49**, 6032–6038.

Conway, K.E., McConnell, B.B., Bowring, C.E., Donald, C.D., Warren, S.T. and Vertino, P.M. (2000) TMS1, a novel proapoptotic caspase recruitment domain protein, is a target of methylation-induced gene silencing in human breast cancers. *Cancer Res*, **60**, 6236–6242.

Cooney, C.A., Dave, A.A. and Wolff, G.L. (2002) Maternal methyl supplements in mice affect epigenetic variation and DNA methylation of offspring. *J Nutr*, **132**, 2393S–2400S.

Corn, P.G., Heath, E.I., Heitmiller, R., Fogt, F., Forastiere, A.A., Herman, J.G. and Wu, T.T. (2001) Frequent hypermethylation of the 5′ CpG island of E-cadherin in esophageal adenocarcinoma. *Clin Cancer Res*, **7**, 2765–2769.

Corn, P.G., Kuerbitz, S.J., van Noesel, M.M., Esteller, M., Compitello, N., Baylin, S.B. and Herman, J.G. (1999) Transcriptional silencing of the p73 gene in acute lymphoblastic leukemia and Burkitt's lymphoma is associated with 5′ CpG island methylation. *Cancer Res*, **59**, 3352–3356.

Cunningham, J.M., Christensen, E.R., Tester, D.J., Kim, C.Y., Roche, P.C., Burgart, L.J. and Thibodeau, S.N. (1998) Hypermethylation of the hMLH1 promoter in colon cancer with microsatellite instability. *Cancer Res*, **58**, 3455–3460.

Custer, B., Sullivan, S.D., Hazlet, T.K., Iloeje, U., Veenstra, D.L. and Kowdley, K.V. (2004) Global epidemiology of hepatitis B virus. *J Clin Gastroenterol*, **38**, S158–168.

Dammann, R., Li, C., Yoon, J.H., Chin, P.L., Bates, S. and Pfeifer, G.P. (2000) Epigenetic inactivation of a RAS association domain family protein from the lung tumour suppressor locus 3p21.3. *Nat Genet*, **25**, 315–319.

Dammann, R., Takahashi, T. and Pfeifer, G.P. (2001a) The CpG island of the novel tumor suppressor gene RASSF1A is intensely methylated in primary small cell lung carcinomas. *Oncogene*, **20**, 3563–3567.

Dammann, R., Yang, G. and Pfeifer, G.P. (2001b) Hypermethylation of the cpG island of Ras association domain family 1A (RASSF1A), a putative tumor suppressor gene from the 3p21.3 locus, occurs in a large percentage of human breast cancers. *Cancer Res*, **61**, 3105–3109.

Dannenberg, L.O., Chen, H.J., Tian, H. and Edenberg, H.J. (2006) Differential regulation of the alcohol dehydrogenase 1B (ADH1B) and ADH1C genes by DNA methylation and histone deacetylation. *Alcohol Clin Exp Res*, **30**, 928–937.

de Capoa, A., Musolino, A., Della Rosa, S., Caiafa, P., Mariani, L., Del Nonno, F., Vocaturo, A., Donnorso, R.P., Niveleau, A. and Grappelli, C. (2003) DNA demethylation is directly related to tumour progression: evidence in normal, pre-malignant and malignant cells from uterine cervix samples. *Oncol Rep*, **10**, 545–549.

De Smet, C., Loriot, A. and Boon, T. (2004) Promoter-dependent mechanism leading to selective hypomethylation within the 5′ region of gene MAGE-A1 in tumor cells. *Mol Cell Biol*, **24**, 4781–4790.

Denissenko, M.F., Pao, A., Tang, M. and Pfeifer, G.P. (1996) Preferential formation of benzo[a]pyrene adducts at lung cancer mutational hotspots in P53. *Science*, **274**, 430–432.

Dobrovic, A. and Simpfendorfer, D. (1997) Methylation of the BRCA1 gene in sporadic breast cancer. *Cancer Res*, **57**, 3347–3350.

Doll, R. and Hill, A.B. (1950) Smoking and carcinoma of the lung; preliminary report. *Br Med J*, **2**, 739–748.

Doll, R. and Hill, A.B. (1952) A study of the aetiology of carcinoma of the lung. *Br Med J*, **2**, 1271–1286.

Doll, R. and Peto, R. (1981) The causes of cancer: quantitative estimates of avoidable risks of cancer in the United States today. *J Natl Cancer Inst*, **66**, 1191–1308.

Downs, J.A., Allard, S., Jobin-Robitaille, O., Javaheri, A., Auger, A., Bouchard, N., Kron, S.J., Jackson, S.P. and Cote, J. (2004) Binding of chromatin-modifying activities to phosphorylated histone H2A at DNA damage sites. *Mol Cell*, **16**, 979–990.

Druker, R., Bruxner, T.J., Lehrbach, N.J. and Whitelaw, E. (2004) Complex patterns of transcription at the insertion site of a retrotransposon in the mouse. *Nucleic Acids Res*, **32**, 5800–5808.

Du, Y., Carling, T., Fang, W., Piao, Z., Sheu, J.C. and Huang, S. (2001) Hypermethylation in human cancers of the RIZ1 tumor suppressor gene, a member of a histone/protein methyltransferase superfamily. *Cancer Res*, **61**, 8094–8099.

Duhl, D.M., Stevens, M.E., Vrieling, H., Saxon, P.J., Miller, M.W., Epstein, C.J. and Barsh, G.S. (1994) Pleiotropic effects of the mouse lethal yellow (Ay) mutation explained by deletion of a maternally expressed gene and the simultaneous production of agouti fusion RNAs. *Development*, **120**, 1695–1708.

Egger, G., Liang, G., Aparicio, A. and Jones, P.A. (2004) Epigenetics in human disease and prospects for epigenetic therapy. *Nature*, **429**, 457–463.

Ehrlich, M., Gama-Sosa, M.A., Huang, L.H., Midgett, R.M., Kuo, K.C., McCune, R.A. and Gehrke, C. (1982) Amount and distribution of 5-methylcytosine in human DNA from different types of tissues of cells. *Nucleic Acids Res*, **10**, 2709–2721.

Esteller, M. (2005) DNA methylation and cancer therapy: new developments and expectations. *Curr Opin Oncol*, **17**, 55–60.

Esteller, M. (2007) Cancer epigenomics: DNA methylomes and histone-modification maps. *Nat Rev Genet*, **8**, 286–298.

Esteller, M., Avizienyte, E., Corn, P.G., Lothe, R.A., Baylin, S.B., Aaltonen, L.A. and Herman, J.G. (2000a) Epigenetic inactivation of LKB1 in primary tumors associated with the Peutz-Jeghers syndrome. *Oncogene*, **19**, 164–168.

Esteller, M., Corn, P.G., Urena, J.M., Gabrielson, E., Baylin, S.B. and Herman, J.G. (1998a) Inactivation of glutathione S-transferase P1 gene by promoter hypermethylation in human neoplasia. *Cancer Res*, **58**, 4515–4518.

Esteller, M., Fraga, M.F., Guo, M., Garcia-Foncillas, J., Hedenfalk, I., Godwin, A.K., Trojan, J., Vaurs-Barriere, C., Bignon, Y.J., Ramus, S., Benitez, J., Caldes, T., Akiyama, Y., Yuasa, Y., Launonen, V., Canal, M.J., Rodriguez, R., Capella, G., Peinado, M.A., Borg, A., Aaltonen, L.A., Ponder, B.A., Baylin, S.B. and Herman, J.G. (2001a) DNA methylation patterns in hereditary human cancers mimic sporadic tumorigenesis. *Hum Mol Genet*, **10**, 3001–3007.

Esteller, M., Gaidano, G., Goodman, S.N., Zagonel, V., Capello, D., Botto, B., Rossi, D., Gloghini, A., Vitolo, U., Carbone, A., Baylin, S.B. and Herman, J.G. (2002) Hypermethylation of the DNA repair gene O(6)-methylguanine DNA methyltransferase and survival of patients with diffuse large B-cell lymphoma. *J Natl Cancer Inst*, **94**, 26–32.

Esteller, M., Garcia-Foncillas, J., Andion, E., Goodman, S.N., Hidalgo, O.F., Vanaclocha, V., Baylin, S.B. and Herman, J.G. (2000b) Inactivation of the DNA-repair gene MGMT and the clinical response of gliomas to alkylating agents. *N Engl J Med*, **343**, 1350–1354.

Esteller, M., Gonzalez, S., Risques, R.A., Marcuello, E., Mangues, R., Germa, J.R., Herman, J.G., Capella, G. and Peinado, M.A. (2001b) K-ras and p16 aberrations confer poor prognosis in human colorectal cancer. *J Clin Oncol*, **19**, 299–304.

Esteller, M., Levine, R., Baylin, S.B., Ellenson, L.H. and Herman, J.G. (1998b) MLH1 promoter hypermethylation is associated with the microsatellite instability phenotype in sporadic endometrial carcinomas. *Oncogene*, **17**, 2413–2417.

Esteller, M., Risques, R.A., Toyota, M., Capella, G., Moreno, V., Peinado, M.A., Baylin, S.B. and Herman, J.G. (2001c) Promoter hypermethylation of the DNA repair gene O(6)-methylguanine-DNA methyltransferase is associated with the presence of G:C to A:T transition mutations in p53 in human colorectal tumorigenesis. *Cancer Res*, **61**, 4689–4692.

Esteller, M., Silva, J.M., Dominguez, G., Bonilla, F., Matias-Guiu, X., Lerma, E., Bussaglia, E., Prat, J., Harkes, I.C., Repasky, E.A., Gabrielson, E., Schutte, M., Baylin, S.B. and Herman, J.G. (2000c) Promoter hypermethylation and BRCA1 inactivation in sporadic breast and ovarian tumors. *J Natl Cancer Inst*, **92**, 564–569.

Esteller, M., Sparks, A., Toyota, M., Sanchez-Cespedes, M., Capella, G., Peinado, M.A., Gonzalez, S., Tarafa, G., Sidransky, D., Meltzer, S.J., Baylin, S.B. and Herman, J.G. (2000d) Analysis of adenomatous polyposis coli promoter hypermethylation in human cancer. *Cancer Res*, **60**, 4366–4371.

Esteller, M., Tortola, S., Toyota, M., Capella, G., Peinado, M.A., Baylin, S.B. and Herman, J.G. (2000e) Hypermethylation-associated inactivation of p14(ARF) is independent of p16(INK4a) methylation and p53 mutational status. *Cancer Res*, **60**, 129–133.

Falette, N.S., Fuqua, S.A., Chamness, G.C., Cheah, M.S., Greene, G.L. and McGuire, W.L. (1990) Estrogen receptor gene methylation in human breast tumors. *Cancer Res*, **50**, 3974–3978.

Farber, E. (1996) Alcohol and other chemicals in the development of hepatocellular carcinoma. *Clin Lab Med*, **16**, 377–394.

Feil, R. (2006) Environmental and nutritional effects on the epigenetic regulation of genes. *Mutat Res*, **600**, 46–57.

Feinberg, A.P., Ohlsson, R. and Henikoff, S. (2006) The epigenetic progenitor origin of human cancer. *Nat Rev Genet*, **7**, 21–33.

Feinberg, A.P. and Tycko, B. (2004) The history of cancer epigenetics. *Nat Rev Cancer*, **4**, 143–153.

Feinberg, A.P. and Vogelstein, B. (1983) Hypomethylation distinguishes genes of some human cancers from their normal counterparts. *Nature*, **301**, 89–92.

Feng, Q., Balasubramanian, A., Hawes, S.E., Toure, P., Sow, P.S., Dem, A., Dembele, B., Critchlow, C.W., Xi, L., Lu, H., McIntosh, M.W., Young, A.M. and Kiviat, N.B. (2005) Detection of hypermethylated genes in women with and without cervical neoplasia. *J Natl Cancer Inst*, **97**, 273–282.

Ferguson, A.T., Evron, E., Umbricht, C.B., Pandita, T.K., Chan, T.A., Hermeking, H., Marks, J.R., Lambers, A.R., Futreal, P.A., Stampfer, M.R. and Sukumar, S. (2000) High frequency of hypermethylation at the 14-3-3 sigma locus leads to gene silencing in breast cancer. *Proc Natl Acad Sci USA*, **97**, 6049–6054.

Fleisher, A.S., Esteller, M., Wang, S., Tamura, G., Suzuki, H., Yin, J., Zou, T.T., Abraham, J.M., Kong, D., Smolinski, K.N., Shi, Y.Q., Rhyu, M.G., Powell, S.M., James, S.P., Wilson, K.T., Herman, J.G. and Meltzer, S.J. (1999) Hypermethylation of the hMLH1 gene promoter in human gastric cancers with microsatellite instability. *Cancer Res*, **59**, 1090–1095.

Fraga, M.F., Herranz, M., Espada, J., Ballestar, E., Paz, M.F., Ropero, S., Erkek, E., Bozdogan, O., Peinado, H., Niveleau, A., Mao, J.H., Balmain, A., Cano, A. and Esteller, M. (2004) A mouse skin multistage carcinogenesis model reflects the aberrant DNA methylation patterns of human tumors. *Cancer Res*, **64**, 5527–5534.

Fujii, H., Biel, M.A., Zhou, W., Weitzman, S.A., Baylin, S.B. and Gabrielson, E. (1998) Methylation of the HIC-1 candidate tumor suppressor gene in human breast cancer. *Oncogene*, **16**, 2159–2164.

Fuks, F., Burgers, W.A., Brehm, A., Hughes-Davies, L. and Kouzarides, T. (2000) DNA methyltransferase Dnmt1 associates with histone deacetylase activity. *Nat Genet*, **24**, 88–91.

Fukui, T., Kondo, M., Ito, G., Maeda, O., Sato, N., Yoshioka, H., Yokoi, K., Ueda, Y., Shimokata, K. and Sekido, Y. (2005) Transcriptional silencing of secreted frizzled related protein 1 (SFRP 1) by promoter hypermethylation in non-small-cell lung cancer. *Oncogene*, **24**, 6323–6327.

Fukushima, N., Sato, N., Sahin, F., Su, G.H., Hruban, R.H. and Goggins, M. (2003) Aberrant methylation of suppressor of cytokine signalling-1 (SOCS-1) gene in pancreatic ductal neoplasms. *Br J Cancer*, **89**, 338–343.

Galm, O., Yoshikawa, H., Esteller, M., Osieka, R. and Herman, J.G. (2003) SOCS-1, a negative regulator of cytokine signaling, is frequently silenced by methylation in multiple myeloma. *Blood*, **101**, 2784–2788.

Ganem, D. and Prince, A.M. (2004) Hepatitis B virus infection – natural history and clinical consequences. *N Engl J Med*, **350**, 1118–1129.

Gendall, A.R., Levy, Y.Y., Wilson, A. and Dean, C. (2001) The VERNALIZATION 2 gene mediates the epigenetic regulation of vernalization in Arabidopsis. *Cell*, **107**, 525–535.

Giovannucci, E., Rimm, E.B., Ascherio, A., Stampfer, M.J., Colditz, G.A. and Willett, W.C. (1995) Alcohol, low-methionine–low-folate diets, and risk of colon cancer in men. *J Natl Cancer Inst*, **87**, 265–273.

Gonzalez-Zulueta, M., Bender, C.M., Yang, A.S., Nguyen, T., Beart, R.W., Van Tornout, J.M. and Jones, P.A. (1995) Methylation of the 5′ CpG island of the p16/CDKN2 tumor suppressor gene in normal and transformed human tissues correlates with gene silencing. *Cancer Res*, **55**, 4531–4535.

Grady, W.M., Willis, J., Guilford, P.J., Dunbier, A.K., Toro, T.T., Lynch, H., Wiesner, G., Ferguson, K., Eng, C., Park, J.G., Kim, S.J. and Markowitz, S. (2000) Methylation of the CDH1 promoter as the second genetic hit in hereditary diffuse gastric cancer. *Nat Genet*, **26**, 16–17.

Greger, V., Debus, N., Lohmann, D., Hopping, W., Passarge, E. and Horsthemke, B. (1994) Frequency and parental origin of hypermethylated RB1 alleles in retinoblastoma. *Hum Genet*, **94**, 491–496.

Greger, V., Passarge, E., Hopping, W., Messmer, E. and Horsthemke, B. (1989) Epigenetic changes may contribute to the formation and spontaneous regression of retinoblastoma. *Hum Genet*, **83**, 155–158.

Guo, M., House, M.G., Hooker, C., Han, Y., Heath, E., Gabrielson, E., Yang, S.C., Baylin, S.B., Herman, J.G. and Brock, M.V. (2004) Promoter hypermethylation of resected bronchial margins: a field defect of changes? *Clin Cancer Res*, **10**, 5131–5136.

Guo, M., House, M.G., Suzuki, H., Ye, Y., Brock, M.V., Lu, F., Liu, Z., Rustgi, A.K. and Herman, J.G. (2007) Epigenetic silencing of CDX2 is a feature of squamous esophageal cancer. *Int J Cancer*, **121**, 1219–1226.

Hagiwara, K., Nagai, H., Li, Y., Ohashi, H., Hotta, T. and Saito, H. (2007) Frequent DNA methylation but not mutation of the ID4 gene in malignant lymphoma. *J Clin Exp Hematop*, **47**, 15–18.

Hainaut, P. and Pfeifer, G.P. (2001) Patterns of p53 G–>T transversions in lung cancers reflect the primary mutagenic signature of DNA-damage by tobacco smoke. *Carcinogenesis*, **22**, 367–374.

Hayes, R.B. (1997) The carcinogenicity of metals in humans. *Cancer Causes Control*, **8**, 371–385.

He, B., You, L., Uematsu, K., Zang, K., Xu, Z., Lee, A.Y., Costello, J.F., McCormick, F. and Jablons, D.M. (2003) SOCS-3 is frequently silenced by hypermethylation and suppresses cell growth in human lung cancer. *Proc Natl Acad Sci USA*, **100**, 14133–14138.

Heijmans, B.T., Boer, J.M., Suchiman, H.E., Cornelisse, C.J., Westendorp, R.G., Kromhout, D., Feskens, E.J. and Slagboom, P.E. (2003) A common variant of the methylenetetrahydrofolate reductase gene (1p36) is associated with an increased risk of cancer. *Cancer Res*, **63**, 1249–1253.

Herceg, Z. (2007) Epigenetics and cancer: towards an evaluation of the impact of environmental and dietary factors. *Mutagenesis*, **22**, 91–103.

Herceg, Z. and Wang, Z.Q. (2005) Rendez-vous at mitosis: TRRAPed in the chromatin. *Cell Cycle*, **4**, 383–387.

Herman, J.G., Jen, J., Merlo, A. and Baylin, S.B. (1996) Hypermethylation-associated inactivation indicates a tumor suppressor role for p15INK4B. *Cancer Res*, **56**, 722–727.

Herman, J.G., Latif, F., Weng, Y., Lerman, M.I., Zbar, B., Liu, S., Samid, D., Duan, D.S., Gnarra, J.R., Linehan, W.M., et al. (1994) Silencing of the VHL tumor-suppressor gene by DNA methylation in renal carcinoma. *Proc Natl Acad Sci USA*, **91**, 9700–9704.

Herman, J.G., Umar, A., Polyak, K., Graff, J.R., Ahuja, N., Issa, J.P., Markowitz, S., Willson, J.K., Hamilton, S.R., Kinzler, K.W., Kane, M.F., Kolodner, R.D., Vogelstein, B., Kunkel, T.A. and Baylin, S.B. (1998) Incidence and functional consequences of hMLH1 promoter hypermethylation in colorectal carcinoma. *Proc Natl Acad Sci USA*, **95**, 6870–6875.

Hesson, L., Dallol, A., Minna, J.D., Maher, E.R. and Latif, F. (2003) NORE1A, a homologue of RASSF1A tumour suppressor gene is inactivated in human cancers. *Oncogene*, **22**, 947–954.

Hibi, K., Kodera, Y., Ito, K., Akiyama, S. and Nakao, A. (2004) Methylation pattern of CDH13 gene in digestive tract cancers. *Br J Cancer*, **91**, 1139–1142.

Hoffmann, D., Hoffmann, I. and El-Bayoumy, K. (2001) The less harmful cigarette: a controversial issue. a tribute to Ernst L. Wynder. *Chem Res Toxicol*, **14**, 767–790.

Hogg, R.P., Honorio, S., Martinez, A., Agathanggelou, A., Dallol, A., Fullwood, P., Weichselbaum, R., Kuo, M.J., Maher, E.R. and Latif, F. (2002) Frequent 3p allele loss and epigenetic inactivation of the RASSF1A tumour suppressor gene from region 3p21.3 in head and neck squamous cell carcinoma. *Eur J Cancer*, **38**, 1585–1592.

Holliday, R. (2006) Epigenetics: a historical overview. *Epigenetics*, **1**, 76–80.

IARC-Monograph. (1986) IARC Monographs programme on the evaluation of the carcinogenic risk of chemicals to humans. Preamble. *IARC Monogr Eval Carcinog Risk Chem Hum*, **39**, 13–32.

IARC-Monograph (1988) IARC Monographs on the evaluation of carcinogenic risks to humans, alcohol drinking. *IARC Monogr Eval Carcinog Risks Hum*, **44**, 1–416.

IARC-Monograph. (1994a) Hepatitis Viruses. *IARC Monogr Eval Carcinog Risk Chem Hum*, **59**, 45–257.

IARC-Monograph. (1994b) Schistosomes, Liver Flakes and Helicobacter pylori. *IARC Monogr Eval Carcinog Risk Chem Hum*, **61**, 45–241.

IARC-Monograph. (1996) Human Immunodeficiency Viruses and Human T-Cell Lymphotropic Viruses. *IARC Monogr Eval Carcinog Risk Chem Hum*, **67**, 31–395.

IARC-Monograph. (1997) Epstein-Barr Virus and Kaposi's Sarcoma Herpesvirus/Human Herpesvirus 8. *IARC Monogr Eval Carcinog Risk Chem Hum*, **70**, 33–495.

IARC-Monograph (2003) World Cancer Report, Eds Bernard W. Stewart and Paul Kleihues. *IARC Monogr Eval Carcinog Risks Hum*, **1**, 33–38.

IARC-Monograph (2004) Arsenic in drinking water. *IARC Monogr Eval Carcinog Risks Hum*, **84**, 41–477.

IARC-Monograph. (2007) Human papillomaviruses. IARC Monographs programme on the evaluation of the carcinogenic risk of chemicals to humans. Preamble. *IARC Monogr Eval Carcinog Risk Chem Hum*, **90**, 47–634.

IARC-Monograph (1990) Chromium, nickel and welding. *IARC Monogr Eval Carcinog Risks Hum*, **49**, 1–648.

Iida, S., Akiyama, Y., Nakajima, T., Ichikawa, W., Nihei, Z., Sugihara, K. and Yuasa, Y. (2000) Alterations and hypermethylation of the p14(ARF) gene in gastric cancer. *Int J Cancer*, **87**, 654–658.

Ingrosso, D., Cimmino, A., Perna, A.F., Masella, L., De Santo, N.G., De Bonis, M.L., Vacca, M., D'Esposito, M., D'Urso, M., Galletti, P. and Zappia, V. (2003) Folate treatment and unbalanced methylation and changes of allelic expression induced by hyperhomocysteinaemia in patients with uraemia. *Lancet*, **361**, 1693–1699.

Irimia, M., Fraga, M.F., Sanchez-Cespedes, M. and Esteller, M. (2004) CpG island promoter hypermethylation of the Ras-effector gene NORE1A occurs in the context of a wild-type K-ras in lung cancer. *Oncogene*, **23**, 8695–8699.

Issa, J.P., Ahuja, N., Toyota, M., Bronner, M.P. and Brentnall, T.A. (2001) Accelerated age-related CpG island methylation in ulcerative colitis. *Cancer Res*, **61**, 3573–3577.

Issa, J.P., Baylin, S.B. and Belinsky, S.A. (1996a) Methylation of the estrogen receptor CpG island in lung tumors is related to the specific type of carcinogen exposure. *Cancer Res*, **56**, 3655–3658.

Issa, J.P., Ottaviano, Y.L., Celano, P., Hamilton, S.R., Davidson, N.E. and Baylin, S.B. (1994) Methylation of the oestrogen receptor CpG island links ageing and neoplasia in human colon. *Nat Genet*, **7**, 536–540.

Issa, J.P., Zehnbauer, B.A., Civin, C.I., Collector, M.I., Sharkis, S.J., Davidson, N.E., Kaufmann, S.H. and Baylin, S.B. (1996b) The estrogen receptor CpG island is methylated in most hematopoietic neoplasms. *Cancer Res*, **56**, 973–977.

Issa, J.P., Zehnbauer, B.A., Kaufmann, S.H., Biel, M.A. and Baylin, S.B. (1997) HIC1 hypermethylation is a late event in hematopoietic neoplasms. *Cancer Res*, **57**, 1678–1681.

Iwata, N., Yamamoto, H., Sasaki, S., Itoh, F., Suzuki, H., Kikuchi, T., Kaneto, H., Iku, S., Ozeki, I., Karino, Y., Satoh, T., Toyota, J., Satoh, M., Endo, T. and Imai, K. (2000) Frequent hypermethylation of CpG islands and loss of expression of the 14-3-3 sigma gene in human hepatocellular carcinoma. *Oncogene*, **19**, 5298–5302.

Jablonka, E. (2004) Epigenetic epidemiology. *Int J Epidemiol*, **33**, 929–935.

Jacinto, F.V. and Esteller, M. (2007) Mutator pathways unleashed by epigenetic silencing in human cancer. *Mutagenesis*, **22**, 247–253.

Jaenisch, R. and Bird, A. (2003) Epigenetic regulation of gene expression: how the genome integrates intrinsic and environmental signals. *Nat Genet*, **33 Suppl**, 245–254.

James, S.J., Melnyk, S., Pogribna, M., Pogribny, I.P. and Caudill, M.A. (2002) Elevation in S-adenosylhomocysteine and DNA hypomethylation: potential epigenetic mechanism for homocysteine-related pathology. *J Nutr*, **132**, 2361S–2366S.

Jarrard, D.F., Kinoshita, H., Shi, Y., Sandefur, C., Hoff, D., Meisner, L.F., Chang, C., Herman, J.G., Isaacs, W.B. and Nassif, N. (1998) Methylation of the androgen receptor promoter CpG island is associated with loss of androgen receptor expression in prostate cancer cells. *Cancer Res*, **58**, 5310–5314.

Jazayeri, A., McAinsh, A.D. and Jackson, S.P. (2004) Saccharomyces cerevisiae Sin3p facilitates DNA double-strand break repair. *Proc Natl Acad Sci USA*, **101**, 1644–1649.

Jenuwein, T. and Allis, C.D. (2001) Translating the histone code. *Science*, **293**, 1074–1080.

Jeronimo, C., Henrique, R., Oliveira, J., Lobo, F., Pais, I., Teixeira, M.R. and Lopes, C. (2004) Aberrant cellular retinol binding protein 1 (CRBP1) gene expression and promoter methylation in prostate cancer. *J Clin Pathol*, **57**, 872–876.

Jhaveri, M.S. and Morrow, C.S. (1998) Methylation-mediated regulation of the glutathione S-transferase P1 gene in human breast cancer cells. *Gene*, **210**, 1–7.

Jiang, Y.H., Bressler, J. and Beaudet, A.L. (2004) Epigenetics and human disease. *Annu Rev Genomics Hum Genet*, **5**, 479–510.

Jicai, Z., Zongtao, Y., Jun, L., Haiping, L., Jianmin, W. and Lihua, H. (2006) Persistent infection of hepatitis B virus is involved in high rate of p16 methylation in hepatocellular carcinoma. *Mol Carcinog*, **45**, 530–536.

Jin, M., Piao, Z., Kim, N.G., Park, C., Shin, E.C., Park, J.H., Jung, H.J., Kim, C.G. and Kim, H. (2000) p16 is a major inactivation target in hepatocellular carcinoma. *Cancer*, **89**, 60–68.

Jin, Z., Tamura, G., Tsuchiya, T., Sakata, K., Kashiwaba, M., Osakabe, M. and Motoyama, T. (2001) Adenomatous polyposis coli (APC) gene promoter hypermethylation in primary breast cancers. *Br J Cancer*, **85**, 69–73.

Jirtle, R.L. and Skinner, M.K. (2007) Environmental epigenomics and disease susceptibility. *Nat Rev Genet*, **8**, 253–262.

John, R.M. and Surani, M.A. (2000) Genomic imprinting, mammalian evolution, and the mystery of egg-laying mammals. *Cell*, **101**, 585–588.

Johnson, L., Cao, X. and Jacobsen, S. (2002) Interplay between two epigenetic marks. DNA methylation and histone H3 lysine 9 methylation. *Curr Biol*, **12**, 1360–1367.

Jones, P.A. and Baylin, S.B. (2002) The fundamental role of epigenetic events in cancer. *Nat Rev Genet*, **3**, 415–428.

Jones, P.A. and Martienssen, R. (2005) A blueprint for a Human Epigenome Project: the AACR Human Epigenome Workshop. *Cancer Res*, **65**, 11241–11246.

Jones, P.L., Veenstra, G.J., Wade, P.A., Vermaak, D., Kass, S.U., Landsberger, N., Strouboulis, J. and Wolffe, A.P. (1998) Methylated DNA and MeCP2 recruit histone deacetylase to repress transcription. *Nat Genet*, **19**, 187–191.

Kaati, G., Bygren, L.O. and Edvinsson, S. (2002) Cardiovascular and diabetes mortality determined by nutrition during parents' and grandparents' slow growth period. *Eur J Hum Genet*, **10**, 682–688.

Kalantari, M., Calleja-Macias, I.E., Tewari, D., Hagmar, B., Lie, K., Barrera-Saldana, H.A., Wiley, D.J. and Bernard, H.U. (2004) Conserved methylation patterns of human papillomavirus type 16 DNA in asymptomatic infection and cervical neoplasia. *J Virol*, **78**, 12762–12772.

Kane, M.F., Loda, M., Gaida, G.M., Lipman, J., Mishra, R., Goldman, H., Jessup, J.M. and Kolodner, R. (1997) Methylation of the hMLH1 promoter correlates with lack of expression of hMLH1 in sporadic colon tumors and mismatch repair-defective human tumor cell lines. *Cancer Res*, **57**, 808–811.

Kang, G.H., Lee, S., Kim, J.S. and Jung, H.Y. (2003) Profile of aberrant CpG island methylation along the multistep pathway of gastric carcinogenesis. *Lab Invest*, **83**, 635–641.

Karaczyn, A.A., Bal, W., North, S.L., Bare, R.M., Hoang, V.M., Fisher, R.J. and Kasprzak, K.S. (2003) The octapeptidic end of the C-terminal tail of histone H2A is cleaved off in cells exposed to carcinogenic nickel(II). *Chem Res Toxicol*, **16**, 1555–1559.

Karaczyn, A.A., Golebiowski, F. and Kasprzak, K.S. (2005) Truncation, deamidation, and oxidation of histone H2B in cells cultured with nickel(II). *Chem Res Toxicol*, **18**, 1934–1942.

Ke, Q., Davidson, T., Chen, H., Kluz, T. and Costa, M. (2006) Alterations of histone modifications and transgene silencing by nickel chloride. *Carcinogenesis*, **27**, 1481–1488.

Kim, K.H., Choi, J.S., Kim, I.J., Ku, J.L. and Park, J.G. (2006) Promoter hypomethylation and reactivation of MAGE-A1 and MAGE-A3 genes in colorectal cancer cell lines and cancer tissues. *World J Gastroenterol*, **12**, 5651–5657.

Kim, D.H., Nelson, H.H., Wiencke, J.K., Zheng, S., Christiani, D.C., Wain, J.C., Mark, E.J. and Kelsey, K.T. (2001) p16(INK4a) and histology-specific methylation of CpG islands by exposure to tobacco smoke in non-small cell lung cancer. *Cancer Res*, **61**, 3419–3424.

King, C.M., Gillespie, E.S., McKenna, P.G. and Barnett, Y.A. (1994) An investigation of mutation as a function of age in humans. *Mutat Res*, **316**, 79–90.

Kinoshita, H., Shi, Y., Sandefur, C., Meisner, L.F., Chang, C., Choon, A., Reznikoff, C.R., Bova, G.S., Friedl, A. and Jarrard, D.F. (2000) Methylation of the androgen receptor minimal promoter silences transcription in human prostate cancer. *Cancer Res*, **60**, 3623–3630.

Klein, C.B., Conway, K., Wang, X.W., Bhamra, R.K., Lin, X.H., Cohen, M.D., Annab, L., Barrett, J.C. and Costa, M. (1991) Senescence of nickel-transformed cells by an X chromosome: possible epigenetic control. *Science*, **251**, 796–799.

Kurdistani, S.K. and Grunstein, M. (2003) Histone acetylation and deacetylation in yeast. *Nat Rev Mol Cell Biol*, **4**, 276–284.

Laird, P.W. (2003) The power and the promise of DNA methylation markers. *Nat Rev Cancer*, **3**, 253–266.

Lapidus, R.G., Ferguson, A.T., Ottaviano, Y.L., Parl, F.F., Smith, H.S., Weitzman, S.A., Baylin, S.B., Issa, J.P. and Davidson, N.E. (1996) Methylation of estrogen and progesterone receptor gene 5′ CpG islands correlates with lack of estrogen and progesterone receptor gene expression in breast tumors. *Clin Cancer Res*, **2**, 805–810.

Lee, M.G., Kim, H.Y., Byun, D.S., Lee, S.J., Lee, C.H., Kim, J.I., Chang, S.G. and Chi, S.G. (2001) Frequent epigenetic inactivation of RASSF1A in human bladder carcinoma. *Cancer Res*, **61**, 6688–6692.

Lee, S., Kim, W.H., Jung, H.Y., Yang, M.H. and Kang, G.H. (2002) Aberrant CpG island methylation of multiple genes in intrahepatic cholangiocarcinoma. *Am J Pathol*, **161**, 1015–1022.

Lee, W.H., Morton, R.A., Epstein, J.I., Brooks, J.D., Campbell, P.A., Bova, G.S., Hsieh, W.S., Isaacs, W.B. and Nelson, W.G. (1994) Cytidine methylation of regulatory sequences near the pi-class glutathione S-transferase gene accompanies human prostatic carcinogenesis. *Proc Natl Acad Sci USA*, **91**, 11733–11737.

Lehnertz, B., Ueda, Y., Derijck, A.A., Braunschweig, U., Perez-Burgos, L., Kubicek, S., Chen, T., Li, E., Jenuwein, T. and Peters, A.H. (2003) Suv39h-mediated histone H3 lysine 9 methylation directs DNA methylation to major satellite repeats at pericentric heterochromatin. *Curr Biol*, **13**, 1192–1200.

Leung, S.Y., Yuen, S.T., Chung, L.P., Chu, K.M., Chan, A.S. and Ho, J.C. (1999) hMLH1 promoter methylation and lack of hMLH1 expression in sporadic gastric carcinomas with high-frequency microsatellite instability. *Cancer Res*, **59**, 159–164.

Li, L.C., Chui, R., Nakajima, K., Oh, B.R., Au, H.C. and Dahiya, R. (2000) Frequent methylation of estrogen receptor in prostate cancer: correlation with tumor progression. *Cancer Res*, **60**, 702–706.
Li, H., Cuenin, C., Murr, R., Wang, Z.Q. and Herceg, Z. (2004) HAT cofactor Trrap regulates the mitotic checkpoint by modulation of Mad1 and Mad2 expression. *Embo J*, **23**, 4824–4834.
Li, H. and Minarovits, J. (2003) Host cell-dependent expression of latent Epstein-Barr virus genomes: regulation by DNA methylation. *Adv Cancer Res*, **89**, 133–156.
Liu, L., Yoon, J.H., Dammann, R. and Pfeifer, G.P. (2002) Frequent hypermethylation of the RASSF1A gene in prostate cancer. *Oncogene*, **21**, 6835–6840.
Lo, K.W., Kwong, J., Hui, A.B., Chan, S.Y., To, K.F., Chan, A.S., Chow, L.S., Teo, P.M., Johnson, P.J. and Huang, D.P. (2001) High frequency of promoter hypermethylation of RASSF1A in nasopharyngeal carcinoma. *Cancer Res*, **61**, 3877–3881.
Loizou, J.I., Murr, R., Finkbeiner, M.G., Sawan, C., Wang, Z.Q. and Herceg, Z. (2006) Epigenetic information in chromatin: the code of entry for DNA repair. *Cell Cycle*, **5**, 696–701.
Luedi, P.P., Hartemink, A.J. and Jirtle, R.L. (2005) Genome-wide prediction of imprinted murine genes. *Genome Res*, **15**, 875–884.
Lui, E.L., Loo, W.T., Zhu, L., Cheung, M.N. and Chow, L.W. (2005) DNA hypermethylation of TIMP3 gene in invasive breast ductal carcinoma. *Biomed Pharmacother*, **59 Suppl 2**, S363–365.
Lund, A.H. and van Lohuizen, M. (2004) Epigenetics and cancer. *Genes Dev*, **18**, 2315–2335.
Lusher, M.E., Lindsey, J.C., Latif, F., Pearson, A.D., Ellison, D.W. and Clifford, S.C. (2002) Biallelic epigenetic inactivation of the RASSF1A tumor suppressor gene in medulloblastoma development. *Cancer Res*, **62**, 5906–5911.
Machado, J.C., Oliveira, C., Carvalho, R., Soares, P., Berx, G., Caldas, C., Seruca, R., Carneiro, F. and Sobrinho-Simoes, M. (2001) E-cadherin gene (CDH1) promoter methylation as the second hit in sporadic diffuse gastric carcinoma. *Oncogene*, **20**, 1525–1528.
Maekita, T., Nakazawa, K., Mihara, M., Nakajima, T., Yanaoka, K., Iguchi, M., Arii, K., Kaneda, A., Tsukamoto, T., Tatematsu, M., Tamura, G., Saito, D., Sugimura, T., Ichinose, M. and Ushijima, T. (2006) High levels of aberrant DNA methylation in Helicobacter pylori-infected gastric mucosae and its possible association with gastric cancer risk. *Clin Cancer Res*, **12**, 989–995.
Magdinier, F., Ribieras, S., Lenoir, G.M., Frappart, L. and Dante, R. (1998) Down-regulation of BRCA1 in human sporadic breast cancer; analysis of DNA methylation patterns of the putative promoter region. *Oncogene*, **17**, 3169–3176.
Maier, S. and Olek, A. (2002) Diabetes: a candidate disease for efficient DNA methylation profiling. *J Nutr*, **132**, 2440S–2443S.
Marsit, C.J., McClean, M.D., Furniss, C.S. and Kelsey, K.T. (2006) Epigenetic inactivation of the SFRP genes is associated with drinking, smoking and HPV in head and neck squamous cell carcinoma. *Int J Cancer*, **119**, 1761–1766.
Mathers, J.C. (2004) The biological revolution – towards a mechanistic understanding of the impact of diet on cancer risk. *Mutat Res*, **551**, 43–49.
Mazieres, J., He, B., You, L., Xu, Z., Lee, A.Y., Mikami, I., Reguart, N., Rosell, R., McCormick, F. and Jablons, D.M. (2004) Wnt inhibitory factor-1 is silenced by promoter hypermethylation in human lung cancer. *Cancer Res*, **64**, 4717–4720.
McKinsey, T.A. and Olson, E.N. (2004) Cardiac histone acetylation – therapeutic opportunities abound. *Trends Genet*, **20**, 206–213.
Mielnicki, L.M., Ying, A.M., Head, K.L., Asch, H.L. and Asch, B.B. (1999) Epigenetic regulation of gelsolin expression in human breast cancer cells. *Exp Cell Res*, **249**, 161–176.
Millar, D.S., Ow, K.K., Paul, C.L., Russell, P.J., Molloy, P.L. and Clark, S.J. (1999) Detailed methylation analysis of the glutathione S-transferase pi (GSTP1) gene in prostate cancer. *Oncogene*, **18**, 1313–1324.
Mittal, A., Piyathilake, C., Hara, Y. and Katiyar, S.K. (2003) Exceptionally high protection of photocarcinogenesis by topical application of (–)-epigallocatechin-3-gallate in hydrophilic

cream in SKH-1 hairless mouse model: relationship to inhibition of UVB-induced global DNA hypomethylation. *Neoplasia*, **5**, 555–565.
Mollemann, M., Wolter, M., Felsberg, J., Collins, V.P. and Reifenberger, G. (2005) Frequent promoter hypermethylation and low expression of the MGMT gene in oligodendroglial tumors. *Int J Cancer*, **113**, 379–385.
Morgan, H.D., Sutherland, H.G., Martin, D.I. and Whitelaw, E. (1999) Epigenetic inheritance at the agouti locus in the mouse. *Nat Genet*, **23**, 314–318.
Morris, M.R., Hesson, L.B., Wagner, K.J., Morgan, N.V., Astuti, D., Lees, R.D., Cooper, W.N., Lee, J., Gentle, D., Macdonald, F., Kishida, T., Grundy, R., Yao, M., Latif, F. and Maher, E.R. (2003) Multigene methylation analysis of Wilms' tumour and adult renal cell carcinoma. *Oncogene*, **22**, 6794–6801.
Morrissey, C., Martinez, A., Zatyka, M., Agathanggelou, A., Honorio, S., Astuti, D., Morgan, N.V., Moch, H., Richards, F.M., Kishida, T., Yao, M., Schraml, P., Latif, F. and Maher, E.R. (2001) Epigenetic inactivation of the RASSF1A 3p21.3 tumor suppressor gene in both clear cell and papillary renal cell carcinoma. *Cancer Res*, **61**, 7277–7281.
Muller, H.M., Widschwendter, A., Fiegl, H., Ivarsson, L., Goebel, G., Perkmann, E., Marth, C. and Widschwendter, M. (2003) DNA methylation in serum of breast cancer patients: an independent prognostic marker. *Cancer Res*, **63**, 7641–7645.
Murr, R., Loizou, J.I., Yang, Y.G., Cuenin, C., Li, H., Wang, Z.Q. and Herceg, Z. (2006) Histone acetylation by Trrap-Tip60 modulates loading of repair proteins and repair of DNA double-strand breaks. *Nat Cell Biol*, **8**, 91–99.
Murr, R., Vaissiere, T., Sawan, C., Shukla, V. and Herceg, Z. (2007) Orchestration of chromatin-based processes: mind the TRRAP. *Oncogene*, **26**, 5358–5372.
Nan, X., Ng, H.H., Johnson, C.A., Laherty, C.D., Turner, B.M., Eisenman, R.N. and Bird, A. (1998) Transcriptional repression by the methyl-CpG-binding protein MeCP2 involves a histone deacetylase complex. *Nature*, **393**, 386–389.
Nan, H.M., Song, Y.J., Yun, H.Y., Park, J.S. and Kim, H. (2005) Effects of dietary intake and genetic factors on hypermethylation of the hMLH1 gene promoter in gastric cancer. *World J Gastroenterol*, **11**, 3834–3841.
Niwa, Y., Kanda, H., Shikauchi, Y., Saiura, A., Matsubara, K., Kitagawa, T., Yamamoto, J., Kubo, T. and Yoshikawa, H. (2005) Methylation silencing of SOCS-3 promotes cell growth and migration by enhancing JAK/STAT and FAK signalings in human hepatocellular carcinoma. *Oncogene*, **24**, 6406–6417.
Nomoto, S., Kinoshita, T., Kato, K., Otani, S., Kasuya, H., Takeda, S., Kanazumi, N., Sugimoto, H. and Nakao, A. (2007) Hypermethylation of multiple genes as clonal markers in multicentric hepatocellular carcinoma. *Br J Cancer*, **97**, 1260–1265.
Oakey, R.J. and Beechey, C.V. (2002) Imprinted genes: identification by chromosome rearrangements and post-genomic strategies. *Trends Genet*, **18**, 359–366.
Oates, N.A., van Vliet, J., Duffy, D.L., Kroes, H.Y., Martin, N.G., Boomsma, D.I., Campbell, M., Coulthard, M.G., Whitelaw, E. and Chong, S. (2006) Increased DNA methylation at the AXIN1 gene in a monozygotic twin from a pair discordant for a caudal duplication anomaly. *Am J Hum Genet*, **79**, 155–162.
Ogama, Y., Ouchida, M., Yoshino, T., Ito, S., Takimoto, H., Shiote, Y., Ishimaru, F., Harada, M., Tanimoto, M. and Shimizu, K. (2004) Prevalent hyper-methylation of the CDH13 gene promoter in malignant B cell lymphomas. *Int J Oncol*, **25**, 685–691.
Ohtani-Fujita, N., Fujita, T., Aoike, A., Osifchin, N.E., Robbins, P.D. and Sakai, T. (1993) CpG methylation inactivates the promoter activity of the human retinoblastoma tumor-suppressor gene. *Oncogene*, **8**, 1063–1067.
Okoji, R.S., Yu, R.C., Maronpot, R.R. and Froines, J.R. (2002) Sodium arsenite administration via drinking water increases genome-wide and Ha-ras DNA hypomethylation in methyl-deficient C57BL/6 J mice. *Carcinogenesis*, **23**, 777–785.
Osada, H. and Takahashi, T. (2002) Genetic alterations of multiple tumor suppressors and oncogenes in the carcinogenesis and progression of lung cancer. *Oncogene*, **21**, 7421–7434.

Oshimo, Y., Oue, N., Mitani, Y., Nakayama, H., Kitadai, Y., Yoshida, K., Chayama, K. and Yasui, W. (2004) Frequent epigenetic inactivation of RIZ1 by promoter hypermethylation in human gastric carcinoma. *Int J Cancer*, **110**, 212–218.
Palmisano, W.A., Divine, K.K., Saccomanno, G., Gilliland, F.D., Baylin, S.B., Herman, J.G. and Belinsky, S.A. (2000) Predicting lung cancer by detecting aberrant promoter methylation in sputum. *Cancer Res*, **60**, 5954–5958.
Parkin, D.M., Bray, F.I. and Devesa, S.S. (2001) Cancer burden in the year 2000. The global picture. *Eur J Cancer*, **37 Suppl 8**, S4–66.
Paz, M.F., Wei, S., Cigudosa, J.C., Rodriguez-Perales, S., Peinado, M.A., Huang, T.H. and Esteller, M. (2003) Genetic unmasking of epigenetically silenced tumor suppressor genes in colon cancer cells deficient in DNA methyltransferases. *Hum Mol Genet*, **12**, 2209–2219.
Pembrey, M.E., Bygren, L.O., Kaati, G., Edvinsson, S., Northstone, K., Sjostrom, M. and Golding, J. (2006) Sex-specific, male-line transgenerational responses in humans. *Eur J Hum Genet*, **14**, 159–166.
Peterson, C.L. and Cote, J. (2004) Cellular machineries for chromosomal DNA repair. *Genes Dev*, **18**, 602–616.
Peto, J. (2001) Cancer epidemiology in the last century and the next decade. *Nature*, **411**, 390–395.
Petronis, A., Gottesman, I.I., Kan, P., Kennedy, J.L., Basile, V.S., Paterson, A.D. and Popendikyte, V. (2003) Monozygotic twins exhibit numerous epigenetic differences: clues to twin discordance? *Schizophr Bull*, **29**, 169–178.
Pfeifer, G.P., Denissenko, M.F., Olivier, M., Tretyakova, N., Hecht, S.S. and Hainaut, P. (2002) Tobacco smoke carcinogens, DNA damage and p53 mutations in smoking-associated cancers. *Oncogene*, **21**, 7435–7451.
Piva, R., Rimondi, A.P., Hanau, S., Maestri, I., Alvisi, A., Kumar, V.L. and del Senno, L. (1990) Different methylation of oestrogen receptor DNA in human breast carcinomas with and without oestrogen receptor. *Br J Cancer*, **61**, 270–275.
Poirier, L.A. (2002) The effects of diet, genetics and chemicals on toxicity and aberrant DNA methylation: an introduction. *J Nutr*, **132**, 2336S–2339S.
Poynard, T., Mathurin, P., Lai, C.L., Guyader, D., Poupon, R., Tainturier, M.H., Myers, R.P., Muntenau, M., Ratziu, V., Manns, M., Vogel, A., Capron, F., Chedid, A. and Bedossa, P. (2003) A comparison of fibrosis progression in chronic liver diseases. *J Hepatol*, **38**, 257–265.
Pufulete, M., Al-Ghnaniem, R., Leather, A.J., Appleby, P., Gout, S., Terry, C., Emery, P.W. and Sanders, T.A. (2003) Folate status, genomic DNA hypomethylation, and risk of colorectal adenoma and cancer: a case control study. *Gastroenterology*, **124**, 1240–1248.
Pulling, L.C., Vuillemenot, B.R., Hutt, J.A., Devereux, T.R. and Belinsky, S.A. (2004) Aberrant promoter hypermethylation of the death-associated protein kinase gene is early and frequent in murine lung tumors induced by cigarette smoke and tobacco carcinogens. *Cancer Res*, **64**, 3844–3848.
Puri, S.K., Si, L., Fan, C.Y. and Hanna, E. (2005) Aberrant promoter hypermethylation of multiple genes in head and neck squamous cell carcinoma. *Am J Otolaryngol*, **26**, 12–17.
Qiu, G., Fang, J. and He, Y. (2006) 5′ CpG island methylation analysis identifies the MAGE-A1 and MAGE-A3 genes as potential markers of HCC. *Clin Biochem*, **39**, 259–266.
Qu, G.Z., Grundy, P.E., Narayan, A. and Ehrlich, M. (1999) Frequent hypomethylation in Wilms tumors of pericentromeric DNA in chromosomes 1 and 16. *Cancer Genet Cytogenet*, **109**, 34–39.
Rakyan, V.K. and Beck, S. (2006) Epigenetic variation and inheritance in mammals. *Curr Opin Genet Dev*, **16**, 573–577.
Rakyan, V.K., Chong, S., Champ, M.E., Cuthbert, P.C., Morgan, H.D., Luu, K.V. and Whitelaw, E. (2003) Transgenerational inheritance of epigenetic states at the murine Axin(Fu) allele occurs after maternal and paternal transmission. *Proc Natl Acad Sci USA*, **100**, 2538–2543.
Rakyan, V.K., Hildmann, T., Novik, K.L., Lewin, J., Tost, J., Cox, A.V., Andrews, T.D., Howe, K.L., Otto, T., Olek, A., Fischer, J., Gut, I.G., Berlin, K. and Beck, S. (2004) DNA

methylation profiling of the human major histocompatibility complex: a pilot study for the human epigenome project. *PLoS Biol*, **2**, e405.

Rakyan, V. and Whitelaw, E. (2003) Transgenerational epigenetic inheritance. *Curr Biol*, **13**, R6.

Reik, W., Dean, W. and Walter, J. (2001) Epigenetic reprogramming in mammalian development. *Science*, **293**, 1089–1093.

Rice, J.C., Massey-Brown, K.S. and Futscher, B.W. (1998) Aberrant methylation of the BRCA1 CpG island promoter is associated with decreased BRCA1 mRNA in sporadic breast cancer cells. *Oncogene*, **17**, 1807–1812.

Rice, J.C., Ozcelik, H., Maxeiner, P., Andrulis, I. and Futscher, B.W. (2000) Methylation of the BRCA1 promoter is associated with decreased BRCA1 mRNA levels in clinical breast cancer specimens. *Carcinogenesis*, **21**, 1761–1765.

Richardson, B. (2003) Impact of aging on DNA methylation. *Ageing Res Rev*, **2**, 245–261.

Roberts, C.W. and Orkin, S.H. (2004) The SWI/SNF complex–chromatin and cancer. *Nat Rev Cancer*, **4**, 133–142.

Rowley, J.D. (1998) The critical role of chromosome translocations in human leukemias. *Annu Rev Genet*, **32**, 495–519.

Rubin, H. (2001) Synergistic mechanisms in carcinogenesis by polycyclic aromatic hydrocarbons and by tobacco smoke: a bio-historical perspective with updates. *Carcinogenesis*, **22**, 1903–1930.

Sakai, M., Hibi, K., Kanazumi, N., Nomoto, S., Inoue, S., Takeda, S. and Nakao, A. (2005) Aberrant methylation of the CHFR gene in advanced hepatocellular carcinoma. *Hepatogastroenterology*, **52**, 1854–1857.

Sakai, M., Hibi, K., Koshikawa, K., Inoue, S., Takeda, S., Kaneko, T. and Nakao, A. (2004) Frequent promoter methylation and gene silencing of CDH13 in pancreatic cancer. *Cancer Sci*, **95**, 588–591.

Sakai, T., Toguchida, J., Ohtani, N., Yandell, D.W., Rapaport, J.M. and Dryja, T.P. (1991) Allele-specific hypermethylation of the retinoblastoma tumor-suppressor gene. *Am J Hum Genet*, **48**, 880–888.

Sasaki, M., Tanaka, Y., Perinchery, G., Dharia, A., Kotcherguina, I., Fujimoto, S. and Dahiya, R. (2002) Methylation and inactivation of estrogen, progesterone, and androgen receptors in prostate cancer. *J Natl Cancer Inst*, **94**, 384–390.

Sato, F., Harpaz, N., Shibata, D., Xu, Y., Yin, J., Mori, Y., Zou, T.T., Wang, S., Desai, K., Leytin, A., Selaru, F.M., Abraham, J.M. and Meltzer, S.J. (2002) Hypermethylation of the p14(ARF) gene in ulcerative colitis-associated colorectal carcinogenesis. *Cancer Res*, **62**, 1148–1151.

Sato, N., Maitra, A., Fukushima, N., van Heek, N.T., Matsubayashi, H., Iacobuzio-Donahue, C.A., Rosty, C. and Goggins, M. (2003) Frequent hypomethylation of multiple genes overexpressed in pancreatic ductal adenocarcinoma. *Cancer Res*, **63**, 4158–4166.

Sato, N., Rosty, C., Jansen, M., Fukushima, N., Ueki, T., Yeo, C.J., Cameron, J.L., Iacobuzio-Donahue, C.A., Hruban, R.H. and Goggins, M. (2001) STK11/LKB1 Peutz-Jeghers gene inactivation in intraductal papillary-mucinous neoplasms of the pancreas. *Am J Pathol*, **159**, 2017–2022.

Schagdarsurengin, U., Pfeifer, G.P. and Dammann, R. (2007) Frequent epigenetic inactivation of cystatin M in breast carcinoma. *Oncogene*, **26**, 3089–3094.

Sheldon, C.C., Rouse, D.T., Finnegan, E.J., Peacock, W.J. and Dennis, E.S. (2000) The molecular basis of vernalization: the central role of FLOWERING LOCUS C (FLC). *Proc Natl Acad Sci USA*, **97**, 3753–3758.

Shukla, V., Vaissiere, T. and Herceg, Z. (2008) Histone acetylation and chromatin signature in stem cell identity and cancer. *Mutat Res*, **637**, 1–15.

Sirchia, S.M., Ren, M., Pili, R., Sironi, E., Somenzi, G., Ghidoni, R., Toma, S., Nicolo, G. and Sacchi, N. (2002) Endogenous reactivation of the RARbeta2 tumor suppressor gene epigenetically silenced in breast cancer. *Cancer Res*, **62**, 2455–2461.

Sollars, V., Lu, X., Xiao, L., Wang, X., Garfinkel, M.D. and Ruden, D.M. (2003) Evidence for an epigenetic mechanism by which Hsp90 acts as a capacitor for morphological evolution. *Nat Genet*, **33**, 70–74.

Song, M.J., Li, X., Brown, H.J. and Sun, R. (2002b) Characterization of interactions between RTA and the promoter of polyadenylated nuclear RNA in Kaposi's sarcoma-associated herpesvirus/human herpesvirus 8. *J Virol*, **76**, 5000–5013.

Song, J.Z., Stirzaker, C., Harrison, J., Melki, J.R. and Clark, S.J. (2002a) Hypermethylation trigger of the glutathione-S-transferase gene (GSTP1) in prostate cancer cells. *Oncogene*, **21**, 1048–1061.

Soppe, W.J., Jasencakova, Z., Houben, A., Kakutani, T., Meister, A., Huang, M.S., Jacobsen, S.E., Schubert, I. and Fransz, P.F. (2002) DNA methylation controls histone H3 lysine 9 methylation and heterochromatin assembly in Arabidopsis. *Embo J*, **21**, 6549–6559.

Strahl, B.D. and Allis, C.D. (2000) The language of covalent histone modifications. *Nature*, **403**, 41–45.

Sugiyama, A., Maruta, F., Ikeno, T., Ishida, K., Kawasaki, S., Katsuyama, T., Shimizu, N. and Tatematsu, M. (1998) Helicobacter pylori infection enhances N-methyl-N-nitrosourea-induced stomach carcinogenesis in the Mongolian gerbil. *Cancer Res*, **58**, 2067–2069.

Surani, M.A., Barton, S.C. and Norris, M.L. (1984) Development of reconstituted mouse eggs suggests imprinting of the genome during gametogenesis. *Nature*, **308**, 548–550.

Sutherland, J.E. and Costa, M. (2003) Epigenetics and the environment. *Ann NY Acad Sci*, **983**, 151–160.

Sutherland, K.D., Lindeman, G.J., Choong, D.Y., Wittlin, S., Brentzell, L., Phillips, W., Campbell, I.G. and Visvader, J.E. (2004) Differential hypermethylation of SOCS genes in ovarian and breast carcinomas. *Oncogene*, **23**, 7726–7733.

Suzuki, H., Gabrielson, E., Chen, W., Anbazhagan, R., van Engeland, M., Weijenberg, M.P., Herman, J.G. and Baylin, S.B. (2002) A genomic screen for genes upregulated by demethylation and histone deacetylase inhibition in human colorectal cancer. *Nat Genet*, **31**, 141–149.

Suzuki, H., Itoh, F., Toyota, M., Kikuchi, T., Kakiuchi, H. and Imai, K. (2000) Inactivation of the 14-3-3 sigma gene is associated with 5′ CpG island hypermethylation in human cancers. *Cancer Res*, **60**, 4353–4357.

Szaleczky, E., Pronai, L., Molnar, B., Berczi, L., Feher, J. and Tulassay, Z. (2000) Increased cell proliferation in chronic Helicobacter pylori positive gastritis and gastric carcinoma–correlation between immuno-histochemistry and Tv image cytometry. *Anal Cell Pathol*, **20**, 131–139.

Tada, Y., Wada, M., Taguchi, K., Mochida, Y., Kinugawa, N., Tsuneyoshi, M., Naito, S. and Kuwano, M. (2002) The association of death-associated protein kinase hypermethylation with early recurrence in superficial bladder cancers. *Cancer Res*, **62**, 4048–4053.

Takiguchi, M., Achanzar, W.E., Qu, W., Li, G. and Waalkes, M.P. (2003) Effects of cadmium on DNA-(Cytosine-5) methyltransferase activity and DNA methylation status during cadmium-induced cellular transformation. *Exp Cell Res*, **286**, 355–365.

Tamburini, B.A. and Tyler, J.K. (2005) Localized histone acetylation and deacetylation triggered by the homologous recombination pathway of double-strand DNA repair. *Mol Cell Biol*, **25**, 4903–4913.

Taniguchi, H., Yamamoto, H., Hirata, T., Miyamoto, N., Oki, M., Nosho, K., Adachi, Y., Endo, T., Imai, K. and Shinomura, Y. (2005) Frequent epigenetic inactivation of Wnt inhibitory factor-1 in human gastrointestinal cancers. *Oncogene*, **24**, 7946–7952.

Tchou, J.C., Lin, X., Freije, D., Isaacs, W.B., Brooks, J.D., Rashid, A., De Marzo, A.M., Kanai, Y., Hirohashi, S. and Nelson, W.G. (2000) GSTP1 CpG island DNA hypermethylation in hepatocellular carcinomas. *Int J Oncol*, **16**, 663–676.

Tischoff, I., Hengge, U.R., Vieth, M., Ell, C., Stolte, M., Weber, A., Schmidt, W.E. and Tannapfel, A. (2007) Methylation of SOCS-3 and SOCS-1 in the carcinogenesis of Barrett's adenocarcinoma. *Gut*, **56**, 1047–1053.

Tokumaru, Y., Nomoto, S., Jeronimo, C., Henrique, R., Harden, S., Trink, B. and Sidransky, D. (2003) Biallelic inactivation of the RIZ1 gene in human gastric cancer. *Oncogene*, **22**, 6954–6958.

Toyota, M., Ahuja, N., Suzuki, H., Itoh, F., Ohe-Toyota, M., Imai, K., Baylin, S.B. and Issa, J.P. (1999) Aberrant methylation in gastric cancer associated with the CpG island methylator phenotype. *Cancer Res*, **59**, 5438–5442.

Toyota, M., Shen, L., Ohe-Toyota, M., Hamilton, S.R., Sinicrope, F.A. and Issa, J.P. (2000) Aberrant methylation of the Cyclooxygenase 2 CpG island in colorectal tumors. *Cancer Res*, **60**, 4044–4048.

Trojan, J., Brieger, A., Raedle, J., Esteller, M. and Zeuzem, S. (2000) 5′-CpG island methylation of the LKB1/STK11 promoter and allelic loss at chromosome 19p13.3 in sporadic colorectal cancer. *Gut*, **47**, 272–276.

Turner, B.M. (2002) Cellular memory and the histone code. *Cell*, **111**, 285–291.

Uchida, T., Ohashi, H., Kinoshita, T., Saito, H., Taguchi, R., Hotta, T. and Murate, T. (1998) Hypermethylation of p15(INK4B) gene in a patient with acute myelogenous leukemia evolved from paroxysmal nocturnal hemoglobinuria. *Blood*, **92**, 2981–2983.

Umbricht, C.B., Evron, E., Gabrielson, E., Ferguson, A., Marks, J. and Sukumar, S. (2001) Hypermethylation of 14-3-3 sigma (stratifin) is an early event in breast cancer. *Oncogene*, **20**, 3348–3353.

Umetani, N., Mori, T., Koyanagi, K., Shinozaki, M., Kim, J., Giuliano, A.E. and Hoon, D.S. (2005) Aberrant hypermethylation of ID4 gene promoter region increases risk of lymph node metastasis in T1 breast cancer. *Oncogene*, **24**, 4721–4727.

van der Velden, P.A., Metzelaar-Blok, J.A., Bergman, W., Monique, H., Hurks, H., Frants, R.R., Gruis, N.A. and Jager, M.J. (2001) Promoter hypermethylation: a common cause of reduced p16(INK4a) expression in uveal melanoma. *Cancer Res*, **61**, 5303–5306.

van Doorn, R., Gruis, N.A., Willemze, R., van der Velden, P.A. and Tensen, C.P. (2005) Aberrant DNA methylation in cutaneous malignancies. *Semin Oncol*, **32**, 479–487.

van Engeland, M., Weijenberg, M.P., Roemen, G.M., Brink, M., de Bruine, A.P., Goldbohm, R.A., van den Brandt, P.A., Baylin, S.B., de Goeij, A.F. and Herman, J.G. (2003) Effects of dietary folate and alcohol intake on promoter methylation in sporadic colorectal cancer: the Netherlands cohort study on diet and cancer. *Cancer Res*, **63**, 3133–3137.

van Steensel, B. and Henikoff, S. (2003) Epigenomic profiling using microarrays. *Biotechniques*, **35**, 346–350, 352–354, 356–357.

Van Tine, B.A., Kappes, J.C., Banerjee, N.S., Knops, J., Lai, L., Steenbergen, R.D., Meijer, C.L., Snijders, P.J., Chatis, P., Broker, T.R., Moen, P.T., Jr. and Chow, L.T. (2004) Clonal selection for transcriptionally active viral oncogenes during progression to cancer. *J Virol*, **78**, 11172–11186.

Vasicek, T.J., Zeng, L., Guan, X.J., Zhang, T., Costantini, F. and Tilghman, S.M. (1997) Two dominant mutations in the mouse fused gene are the result of transposon insertions. *Genetics*, **147**, 777–786.

Velicescu, M., Weisenberger, D.J., Gonzales, F.A., Tsai, Y.C., Nguyen, C.T. and Jones, P.A. (2002) Cell division is required for de novo methylation of CpG islands in bladder cancer cells. *Cancer Res*, **62**, 2378–2384.

Virmani, A.K., Rathi, A., Sathyanarayana, U.G., Padar, A., Huang, C.X., Cunnigham, H.T., Farinas, A.J., Milchgrub, S., Euhus, D.M., Gilcrease, M., Herman, J., Minna, J.D. and Gazdar, A.F. (2001) Aberrant methylation of the adenomatous polyposis coli (APC) gene promoter 1A in breast and lung carcinomas. *Clin Cancer Res*, **7**, 1998–2004.

Virmani, A., Rathi, A., Sugio, K., Sathyanarayana, U.G., Toyooka, S., Kischel, F.C., Tonk, V., Padar, A., Takahashi, T., Roth, J.A., Euhus, D.M., Minna, J.D. and Gazdar, A.F. (2003) Aberrant methylation of TMS1 in small cell, non small cell lung cancer and breast cancer. *Int J Cancer*, **106**, 198–204.

Virmani, A.K., Rathi, A., Zochbauer-Muller, S., Sacchi, N., Fukuyama, Y., Bryant, D., Maitra, A., Heda, S., Fong, K.M., Thunnissen, F., Minna, J.D. and Gazdar, A.F. (2000) Promoter methylation and silencing of the retinoic acid receptor-beta gene in lung carcinomas. *J Natl Cancer Inst*, **92**, 1303–1307.

Wagner, K.J., Cooper, W.N., Grundy, R.G., Caldwell, G., Jones, C., Wadey, R.B., Morton, D., Schofield, P.N., Reik, W., Latif, F. and Maher, E.R. (2002) Frequent RASSF1A tumour suppressor gene promoter methylation in Wilms' tumour and colorectal cancer. *Oncogene*, **21**, 7277–7282.

Walsh, C.P., Chaillet, J.R. and Bestor, T.H. (1998) Transcription of IAP endogenous retroviruses is constrained by cytosine methylation. *Nat Genet*, **20**, 116–117.

Wang, S., Ding, Y.B., Chen, G.Y., Xia, J.G. and Wu, Z.Y. (2004) Hypermethylation of Syk gene in promoter region associated with oncogenesis and metastasis of gastric carcinoma. *World J Gastroenterol*, **10**, 1815–1818.

Wang, W., Huper, G., Guo, Y., Murphy, S.K., Olson, J.A., Jr. and Marks, J.R. (2005) Analysis of methylation-sensitive transcriptome identifies GADD45a as a frequently methylated gene in breast cancer. *Oncogene*, **24**, 2705–2714.

Waterland, R.A. (2006) Assessing the effects of high methionine intake on DNA methylation. *J Nutr*, **136**, 1706S–1710S.

Waterland, R.A. and Jirtle, R.L. (2003) Transposable elements: targets for early nutritional effects on epigenetic gene regulation. *Mol Cell Biol*, **23**, 5293–5300.

Weber, A., Hengge, U.R., Bardenheuer, W., Tischoff, I., Sommerer, F., Markwarth, A., Dietz, A., Wittekind, C. and Tannapfel, A. (2005) SOCS-3 is frequently methylated in head and neck squamous cell carcinoma and its precursor lesions and causes growth inhibition. *Oncogene*, **24**, 6699–6708.

Weksberg, R., Shuman, C., Caluseriu, O., Smith, A.C., Fei, Y.L., Nishikawa, J., Stockley, T.L., Best, L., Chitayat, D., Olney, A., Ives, E., Schneider, A., Bestor, T.H., Li, M., Sadowski, P. and Squire, J. (2002) Discordant KCNQ1OT1 imprinting in sets of monozygotic twins discordant for Beckwith-Wiedemann syndrome. *Hum Mol Genet*, **11**, 1317–1325.

Wheeler, J.M., Kim, H.C., Efstathiou, J.A., Ilyas, M., Mortensen, N.J. and Bodmer, W.F. (2001) Hypermethylation of the promoter region of the E-cadherin gene (CDH1) in sporadic and ulcerative colitis associated colorectal cancer. *Gut*, **48**, 367–371.

Widschwendter, A., Ivarsson, L., Blassnig, A., Muller, H.M., Fiegl, H., Wiedemair, A., Muller-Holzner, E., Goebel, G., Marth, C. and Widschwendter, M. (2004) CDH1 and CDH13 methylation in serum is an independent prognostic marker in cervical cancer patients. *Int J Cancer*, **109**, 163–166.

Wiley, D.J., Huh, J., Rao, J.Y., Chang, C., Goetz, M., Poulter, M., Masongsong, E., Chang, C.I. and Bernard, H.U. (2005) Methylation of human papillomavirus genomes in cells of anal epithelia of HIV-infected men. *J Acquir Immune Defic Syndr*, **39**, 143–151.

Wistuba, I.I., Mao, L. and Gazdar, A.F. (2002) Smoking molecular damage in bronchial epithelium. *Oncogene*, **21**, 7298–7306.

Wolffe, A.P. (2001) Chromatin remodeling: why it is important in cancer. *Oncogene*, **20**, 2988–2990.

Wright, T.L. (2006) Introduction to chronic hepatitis B infection. *Am J Gastroenterol*, **101 Suppl 1**, S1–6.

Wynder, E.L. and Graham, E.A. (1950) Tobacco smoking as a possible etiologic factor in bronchiogenic carcinoma; a study of 684 proved cases. *J Am Med Assoc*, **143**, 329–336.

Xing, M., Usadel, H., Cohen, Y., Tokumaru, Y., Guo, Z., Westra, W.B., Tong, B.C., Tallini, G., Udelsman, R., Califano, J.A., Ladenson, P.W. and Sidransky, D. (2003) Methylation of the thyroid-stimulating hormone receptor gene in epithelial thyroid tumors: a marker of malignancy and a cause of gene silencing. *Cancer Res*, **63**, 2316–2321.

Xu, X.L., Wu, L.C., Du, F., Davis, A., Peyton, M., Tomizawa, Y., Maitra, A., Tomlinson, G., Gazdar, A.F., Weissman, B.E., Bowcock, A.M., Baer, R. and Minna, J.D. (2001) Inactivation of human SRBC, located within the 11p15.5-p15.4 tumor suppressor region, in breast and lung cancers. *Cancer Res*, **61**, 7943–7949.

Xu, X.L., Yu, J., Zhang, H.Y., Sun, M.H., Gu, J., Du, X., Shi, D.R., Wang, P., Yang, Z.H. and Zhu, J.D. (2004) Methylation profile of the promoter CpG islands of 31 genes that may contribute to colorectal carcinogenesis. *World J Gastroenterol*, **10**, 3441–3454.

Yang, X.J. (2004) The diverse superfamily of lysine acetyltransferases and their roles in leukemia and other diseases. *Nucleic Acids Res*, **32**, 959–976.

Yoon, J.H., Dammann, R. and Pfeifer, G.P. (2001a) Hypermethylation of the CpG island of the RASSF1A gene in ovarian and renal cell carcinomas. *Int J Cancer*, **94**, 212–217.

Yoon, J.H., Smith, L.E., Feng, Z., Tang, M., Lee, C.S. and Pfeifer, G.P. (2001b) Methylated CpG dinucleotides are the preferential targets for G-to-T transversion mutations induced by benzo[a]pyrene diol epoxide in mammalian cells: similarities with the p53 mutation spectrum in smoking-associated lung cancers. *Cancer Res*, **61**, 7110–7117.

Yoshikawa, H., Matsubara, K., Qian, G.S., Jackson, P., Groopman, J.D., Manning, J.E., Harris, C.C. and Herman, J.G. (2001) SOCS-1, a negative regulator of the JAK/STAT pathway, is silenced by methylation in human hepatocellular carcinoma and shows growth-suppression activity. *Nat Genet*, **28**, 29–35.

Yuan, Y., Mendez, R., Sahin, A. and Dai, J.L. (2001) Hypermethylation leads to silencing of the SYK gene in human breast cancer. *Cancer Res*, **61**, 5558–5561.

Yuasa, Y., Nagasaki, H., Akiyama, Y., Sakai, H., Nakajima, T., Ohkura, Y., Takizawa, T., Koike, M., Tani, M., Iwai, T., Sugihara, K., Imai, K. and Nakachi, K. (2005) Relationship between CDX2 gene methylation and dietary factors in gastric cancer patients. *Carcinogenesis*, **26**, 193–200.

Zardo, G., Tiirikainen, M.I., Hong, C., Misra, A., Feuerstein, B.G., Volik, S., Collins, C.C., Lamborn, K.R., Bollen, A., Pinkel, D., Albertson, D.G. and Costello, J.F. (2002) Integrated genomic and epigenomic analyses pinpoint biallelic gene inactivation in tumors. *Nat Genet*, **32**, 453–458.

Zazula, M., Ferreira, A.M., Czopek, J.P., Kolodziejczyk, P., Sinczak-Kuta, A., Klimkowska, A., Wojcik, P., Okon, K., Bialas, M., Kulig, J. and Stachura, J. (2006) CDH1 gene promoter hypermethylation in gastric cancer: relationship to Goseki grading, microsatellite instability status, and EBV invasion. *Diagn Mol Pathol*, **15**, 24–29.

Zhang, Y.J., Ahsan, H., Chen, Y., Lunn, R.M., Wang, L.Y., Chen, S.Y., Lee, P.H., Chen, C.J. and Santella, R.M. (2002) High frequency of promoter hypermethylation of RASSF1A and p16 and its relationship to aflatoxin B1-DNA adduct levels in human hepatocellular carcinoma. *Mol Carcinog*, **35**, 85–92.

Zhang, Y.J., Chen, Y., Ahsan, H., Lunn, R.M., Lee, P.H., Chen, C.J. and Santella, R.M. (2003) Inactivation of the DNA repair gene O6-methylguanine-DNA methyltransferase by promoter hypermethylation and its relationship to aflatoxin B1-DNA adducts and p53 mutation in hepatocellular carcinoma. *Int J Cancer*, **103**, 440–444.

Zhang, J., Martins, C.R., Fansler, Z.B., Roemer, K.L., Kincaid, E.A., Gustafson, K.S., Heitjan, D.F. and Clark, D.P. (2005) DNA methylation in anal intraepithelial lesions and anal squamous cell carcinoma. *Clin Cancer Res*, **11**, 6544–6549.

Zhang, Y.J., Rossner, P., Jr., Chen, Y., Agrawal, M., Wang, Q., Wang, L., Ahsan, H., Yu, M.W., Lee, P.H. and Santella, R.M. (2006) Aflatoxin B1 and polycyclic aromatic hydrocarbon adducts, p53 mutations and p16 methylation in liver tissue and plasma of hepatocellular carcinoma patients. *Int J Cancer*, **119**, 985–991.

Zhao, C.Q., Young, M.R., Diwan, B.A., Coogan, T.P. and Waalkes, M.P. (1997) Association of arsenic-induced malignant transformation with DNA hypomethylation and aberrant gene expression. *Proc Natl Acad Sci USA*, **94**, 10907–10912.

Zhong, S., Tang, M.W., Yeo, W., Liu, C., Lo, Y.M. and Johnson, P.J. (2002) Silencing of GSTP1 gene by CpG island DNA hypermethylation in HBV-associated hepatocellular carcinomas. *Clin Cancer Res*, **8**, 1087–1092.

Zhou, L., Jiang, W., Ren, C., Yin, Z., Feng, X., Liu, W., Tao, Q. and Yao, K. (2005) Frequent hypermethylation of RASSF1A and TSLC1, and high viral load of Epstein-Barr Virus DNA in nasopharyngeal carcinoma and matched tumor-adjacent tissues. *Neoplasia*, **7**, 809–815.

Zochbauer-Muller, S., Fong, K.M., Geradts, J., Xu, X., Seidl, S., End-Pfutzenreuter, A., Lang, G., Heller, G., Zielinski, C.C., Gazdar, A.F. and Minna, J.D. (2005) Expression of the candidate tumor suppressor gene hSRBC is frequently lost in primary lung cancers with and without DNA methylation. *Oncogene*, **24**, 6249–6255.

Zoroddu, M.A., Kowalik-Jankowska, T., Kozlowski, H., Molinari, H., Salnikow, K., Broday, L. and Costa, M. (2000) Interaction of Ni(II) and Cu(II) with a metal binding sequence of histone H4: AKRHRK, a model of the H4 tail. *Biochim Biophys Acta*, **1475**, 163–168.

Chapter 8
Approaches to Identify Environmental and Epigenomic Components or Covariates of Cancer and Disease Susceptibility

Alok Deoraj and Deodutta Roy

Abstract A complex disease such as cancer is one of the major public health burdens for the United States and developing societies. A combination of variations in multiple genes and environmental factors contribute to the susceptibility and progression of different diseases. Comprehensive understanding of the interactions between multiple genetic and environmental factors will more accurately predict a risk of contracting a disease or a particular cancer and treatment response to explain the etiology than any single genetic or environmental factor. Although advances in the knowledge of measuring genetic variants and the amount of data available has steadily been increasing, a major barrier to further the success of molecular epidemiology studies, especially those with a environment-gene interactions, is to determine an appropriate methodological strategy for analysis and interpretation of results. Here we describe approaches to measure genome wide genetic variation and suggest resources to conduct gene × environment (G×E) interaction analysis. We also describe epigenomics that how it may play an important role in enhancing the risk for complex diseases such as cancer. Study of G×E interactions aim to describe how genetic and environmental factors jointly influence the risk of developing a disease. Analysis of G×E interactions take into account the various ways in which genetic effects are modified due to environmental exposures. The number of levels of these exposures and the model on which the genetic effects can be based are also discussed in this chapter. Choice of study design, sample size and genotyping technology influence the analysis and interpretation of observed G×E interactions. Current systems for reporting epidemiological studies make it difficult to assess whether the observed interactions are reproducible. Suggestions are made for improvements in this area.

Keywords Biomarkers of environmental and epigenomic components or covariates of cancer · Disease susceptibility · Interactions between multiple genetic and environmental factors · Genome wide genetic variation

---

A. Deoraj (✉)
Department of Environmental and Occupational Health, Florida International University, Miami, FL 33199, USA
e-mail: adeoraj@fiu.edu

D. Roy, M.T. Dorak (eds.), *Environmental Factors, Genes, and the Development of Human Cancers*, DOI 10.1007/978-1-4419-6752-7_8,

8.1 Introduction

Often a sibling suffers from cancer while the other is healthy and one alcoholic dies of liver cancer very young while another lives by his full life. The etiology of complex diseases such as cancer and asthma and many common diseases results from a complex interaction of our genetic makeup and the environment we live in. The subject—gene and environment (G×E) interactions has gained precedence over many available approaches to determine an individual or a population at risk for common and complex diseases. Evidence also suggests that macroenvironment—our lifestyle, the air we breathe, the food we eat, the chemicals we are exposed to, as well as viruses, radiation, and physical agents we come in contact with—that combines with the microenvironment of our cells influence our risk. A flow chart in Fig. 8.1 demonstrates a general pattern of G×E interactions. In recent years, the genomics revolution has inspired the genome wide scans to investigate G×E interactions. Concomitantly however, acquired and inherited epigenetic modifications cannot be overlooked. Epigenetic modifications at the levels of chromatin structure, including the higher order of chromatin folding and attachment to the nuclear matrix, packaging of DNA around nucleosomes, covalent modifications of

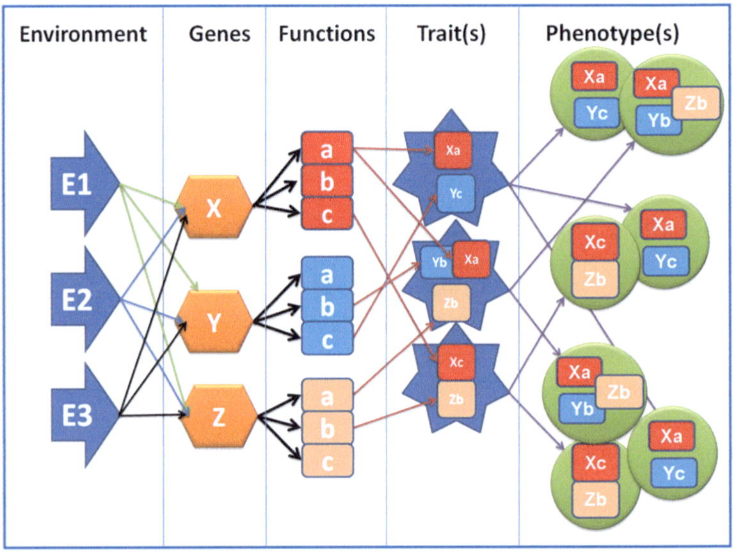

Fig. 8.1 Flow of G×E interaction. E1, E2 and E3 are the examples of environmental factors that influence gene activity (e.g., X, Y and Z). Genes can have different functions (e.g., a, b and c) in different molecular pathways of cellular and physiological homeostasis or disease etiology. Combinations of normal or aberrant gene functions due to genome wide SNP and haplotype differences and linkage disequilibrium (LD) can determine traits (e.g., Xa and Yc, Za, Yb, Xa etc.) of an individual to be susceptible or resistant to certain phenotypes

histone tails (acetylation, methylation, phosphorylation, ubiquitination), and DNA methylation provide a better appreciation of the environmental contributions that lead to various diseases.

Understanding the contribution of environmental factors to the development of disease has been a major concern of society. One of the earliest insights into the environment's contribution to the development of cancer was in 1775, when the British surgeon, Percival Pott, discovered a cluster of scrotal cancer among young chimney sweeps exposed to soot (Brown and Thronton, 1957). Subsequent research found that the soot contained mixtures of carcinogenic polycyclic hydrocarbons. Nonetheless, underlying premise of our individual response to the environmental factors is due to subtle changes at genetic level that determines the vulnerability or resistance to various diseases and certain type of cancer. Gene polymorphisms have been recognized as clues to individual susceptibility to diseases, explaining why individuals with shared environmental exposures do not always share cancer morbidity and mortality (Lobo, 2008). Thus, genetic polymorphisms are effect modifiers of environmental exposures. The ongoing genome wide discovery of single nucleotide polymorphisms (SNPs) and characterization of haplotypes in human populations is having a fundamental impact on molecular epidemiology. While likely common polymorphic variants interact with exposures to cause human diseases, the ability to evaluate the role of SNPs in human disease is limited by available methodologies. Identification of new genetic associations can be used to develop better strategies to detect, treat and prevent common, complex diseases, such as asthma, cancer, diabetes, heart disease and mental illnesses. Numerous association studies of SNPs or haplotypes have been published to elucidate the etiology of diseases, but there has been inconsistency in the ability to replicate results (Rebbeck et al., 2004; Tzu-Hao and Hsin-Shih, 2009; Chanock et al., 2007; Boffetta et al., 2008; Ioannidis, 2007). Therefore, an understanding of the analytical tools is needed to examine genomic information available for relating genetic variants to well-defined epidemiological end points. In this chapter we address methodological developments for association studies investigating complex interrelationships of SNPs, haplotypes, and environmental factors leading to various diseases and cancer.

8.2 Approaches to Identify Genetic Variance

The completion of human genome sequence and advancement in the technologies for genomic analysis has inspired the genetic variance investigation on a global scale rather than restricted to a single gene or a handful of single nucleotide polymorphic (SNP) markers. The basis of this evaluation is on the identification of the allelic variants of human genes. The process of identifying DNA variation that may be associated with disease or cancer is continuously being cataloged and mapped throughout the genome. Measurement of the frequency of these DNA variants in different populations, identification of diseases influenced by these variants and magnitude of the associated risk and their interactions with other genes and environment may aid in the identification of alterations that result in or contribute to disease states. Much of the work on identifying functional polymorphisms that influence an individual's risk has focused on gene products involved in the activation and detoxification of carcinogens and, more recently, on DNA repair (Wilson et al., 2002). Based on the current approach a general scheme of the identification of genetic variation at the genome level is shown in Fig. 8.2.

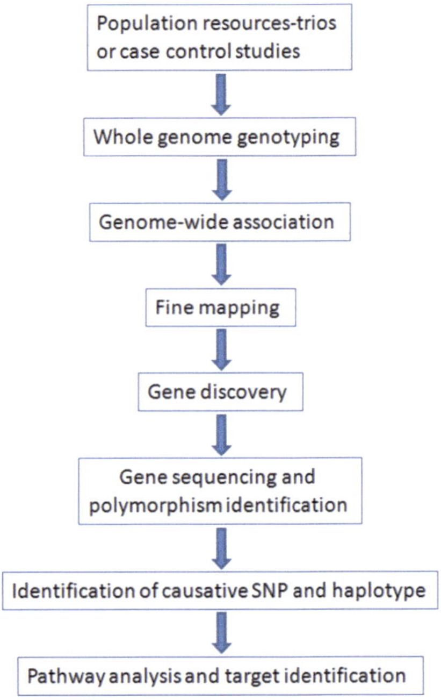

Fig. 8.2 Schematic of the process of genome wide association studies (GWAS). Modified from Keith (2007)

8.2.1 Candidate Gene

Candidate gene markers can be selected based on (a) prior information about biological pathways or linkage data (b) functional correlation for a SNP or haplotype, including pathway or the use of evolution-based approaches that shows sequence homology or belonging to a gene family; and (c) SNP haplotype studies that start with a "simple" haplotype (often including known non synonymous SNPs or regulatory SNPs). Later these SNPs can be expanded to increase the density of SNPs across the haplotype (Rebbeck et al., 2004). Regardless of the approach for choosing markers, validation of associations in both comparable and different genetic backgrounds is required. The working hypothesis becomes increasingly complex overtime as knowledge of interrelated pathways is included to account for relevant biological interactions. Pharmacogenetics and pharmacogenomics studies can extend beyond etiology to studies of treatment response, gene expression changes, survival, side effects or toxicities relating to specific agents, timing of later events, and dosing. With respect to candidate genes, paradigm for functional gene discovery began by using the distribution of phenotypic traits to infer genetic effects. More recently, it has been possible to relate functionally significant DNA sequence variation to clinically important variability. Both of these approaches are complementary and should be done to understand the functional significance of genes and SNPs. Gene expression profiling can be valuable to identify and characterize candidate genes (e.g., for treatment response). Genetic profiles can differ by exposure (i.e., where combinations of drug treatments did not evoke the same expression profile as each treatment individually). Therefore, expression profile approaches may be useful for identification of novel genes, characterizing function, novel disease classifications, and studying G×E interactions. Three independent studies found that macular degeneration is associated with variation in the gene for complement factor H, which produces a protein involved in regulating inflammation (Francis et al., 2007). Few previously thought that inflammation might contribute so significantly to age-related macular degeneration. Similar successes have been reported using genome-wide association studies to identify genetic variations that contribute to risk of type 2 diabetes, Parkinson disease, heart disorders, obesity, Crohn disease and prostate cancer, as well as genetic variations that influence response to anti-depressant medications. Examination of the mutational spectra of some of the cancer-related genes (e.g., p53, BRCA1, and p16INK4) has yielded molecular links between etiological agents and human cancer. In the 1970s and 1980s a set of genes, called tumor suppressor genes, was elucidated, one of which was called p53. The p53 gene recognizes the signal created by a precancerous condition and responds by killing the cell by a process called programmed cell death, or apoptosis. It has subsequently been shown that p53 mutations are common in diverse types of human cancer, where they are involved in genomic instability. The gene is involved in pathways of apoptosis and cell cycle control, and among its many functions, it is a transcription factor. It suppresses some genes and upregulates others. It is at the crossroads of multiple cellular stress response pathways, DNA damage of varying kinds, hypoxia, and oncogene activation. Other associations between the p53 mutational spectra and exposures to carcinogens have been observed. Candidate gene approaches have the advantage of maximizing inferences about biological plausibility and disease causality. However, candidate approaches are limited by the amount of information that is available about the function of the gene in a specific disease process.

8.2.2 Copy Number Variations (CNVs)

It was generally thought that genes were always present in two copies in a genome. However, recent discoveries have revealed that large segments of DNA, ranging in size from thousands to millions of DNA bases, can vary in copy-number. Such copy number variations (Carter, 2007) (or CNVs) can encompass genes leading to dosage imbalances. For example, genes that were thought to occur in two copies per genome have now been found to sometimes be present in one, three, or more than three copies (Sebat, 2007; Yoon et al., 2009). In rare instances, the genes are missing altogether. When CNV is taken into account, similarity between any two genomes is less than 99.9%. Thus, genomes of any two individuals in the human population differ more at the structural level than at the nucleotide sequence level. The discovery that structural variation of the genome including large insertions and deletions of DNA, collectively termed CNVs, as well as balanced chromosomal rearrangements, such as inversions, contribute to a major proportion of genetic difference in humans (Redon et al., 2006; Sebat, 2007; George et al., 2007).

8.2.3 Single Nucleotide Polymorphism (SNP)

Changes in a single base pair of the DNA sequence are the most frequently occurring form of variation in the human genome. Many genes have a large number of SNPs, and it is acknowledged that there are more than 10 million SNPs across the human genome, with an estimated two common missense variants per gene, making it impossible for cost-effective genotyping of all of them in studies of disease, even in very small samples (Rebbeck et al., 2004). New approaches, however, can reduce the genotyping burden by exploiting the strong correlation between some SNPs that are close together on the genome. This is due to the phenomenon of linkage disequilibrium (LD), or non-random association of SNP alleles at the population level, due to the sharing by multiple individuals of ancestral chromosomal segments. These segments, or haplotypes, are combinations of particular SNP alleles on the same chromosome that tend to segregate together. By choosing a subset of maximally informative SNPs, or "tag" SNPs, to represent these haplotypes, the number of SNPs to be genotyped in a larger sample can be reduced without losing the ability to capture most of the variation, and in particular any association between unmeasured "causal" alleles and the disease outcome (Constantine et al., 2008). The choice of tag SNPs becomes challenging when study subjects are from multiple populations, since the transferability of tag SNPs depends on similarity of linkage disequilibrium patterns. It is also desirable to incorporate resequencing data from local case and control samples generated during a "SNP discovery" phase. The NIEHS SNPinfo tool, has combined the power of three pipelines for SNP selection based on candidate genes, whole genome and linkage regions. The tools also incorporate functional predictions of protein structure, gene regulation, splicing and miRNA binding and the ability to consider whether the alternative alleles of a SNP are likely to have differential effects on function. A "snapshot" of gene-centric SNPs in the dbSNP database as of September 2003 suggest that distribution of these variants was 63% intronic, 11% untranslated region, 1% nonsynonymous, 1% synonymous, 24% locus region, <1% splice site, and <1% unknown coding variant. Recent surveys of human genetic diversity have estimated that there are about 100,000–300,000 SNPs in protein coding sequences (cSNPs) of the entire human genome. cSNPs are of particular interest because some of them, termed nonsynonymous SNPs (nsSNPs) or missense variants, introduce amino acid changes into their encoded proteins. Alterations in the regulation of genes by rSNPs may influence the kinetic parameters of enzymes, the DNA binding properties of proteins that regulate transcription, the signal transduction activities of transmembrane receptors, and the architectural roles of structural proteins are all susceptible to perturbation by nsSNPs. Similarly, the regulation of key elements of a pathway can alter the risk for cancer and disease outcomes either directly or through interacting pathways. Identification and characterization of such regulatory variants are projected to be a major challenge of future studies (Laumen et al., 2009). Researcher may have to ask whether the rSNP itself or the haplotype in which it may be imbedded is really the functional unit of interest. The identification of biologically meaningful, disease causing variants from among this large amount of genomic variability is a key challenge for association studies.

8.2.4 Haplotype Mapping

The HapMap is a catalog of common genetic variants that occur in human beings. It describes what these variants are, where they occur in our DNA, and how they are distributed among people within populations and among populations in different parts of the world (Deloukas and Bentley, 2004; Barnes, 2006; Manolio et al., 2008). Two unrelated people share about 99.5% of their DNA sequence. HapMap focuses only on common SNPs which are about 1% of the population. The International HapMap Project is not using the information in the HapMap to establish connections between particular genetic variants and diseases. Rather, the Project is designed to provide information that other researchers can use to link genetic variants to the risk for specific illnesses including cancer, which will lead to new methods of preventing, diagnosing, and treating disease. An additional assumption behind this approach is the idea of the "common variant common disease hypothesis". It is assumed that the variant and its haplotype are relatively common in the general population and will be ascertained using this approach. If, however, the disease is caused by a rare variant, this approach may fail to detect an association. Where haplotype diversity exists, particularly informative SNPs that best characterize a haplotype can be used to limit the amount of laboratory and analytical work in haplotype-based studies. Use of haplotype block information has been proposed to increase power 15–50% compared with a SNP-based analysis (Rebbeck et al., 2004; Huang et al., 2007).

8.2.5 Genome Wide Association Screen

A genome-wide association study is an approach that involves rapidly scanning markers (SNPs or haplotype) across the complete sets of DNA, or genomes, of many people to find genetic variations associated with a particular disease or cancer (Stranger et al., 2005). Candidate gene variants however may not be studied directly but that gene discovery studies can be accomplished using a strategy that relies on LD between genetic variants. This represents the underlying premise behind whole genome SNP scans. The impact on medical care from genome-wide association studies could potentially be substantial. Such research is laying the groundwork for the era of personalized medicine, in which the current one size-fits-all approach to medical care will give way to more customized strategies. In the future, after improvements are made in the cost and efficiency of genome-wide scans and other innovative technologies, health professionals will be able to use such tools to provide patients with individualized information about their risks of developing certain diseases and cancers. To carry out a genome-wide association study, researchers use two groups of participants: people with the disease being studied and similar people without the disease. Researchers obtain DNA from each participant, usually by drawing a blood sample or by rubbing a cotton swab along the inside of the mouth to harvest cells. Each person's complete set of DNA, or genome, is then purified from the blood or cells, placed on tiny chips and scanned on automated laboratory machines. The machines quickly survey each participant's genome for strategically selected markers of genetic variation. If certain genetic variations are found to be significantly more frequent in people with the disease compared to people without disease, the variations are said to be "associated" with the disease. The associated genetic variations can serve as powerful pointers to the region of the human genome where the disease-causing problem resides. However, the associated variants themselves may not directly cause the disease. They may just be "tagging along" with the actual causal variants. For this reason, researchers often need to take additional steps, such as sequencing a particular region of the genome, to identify the exact genetic change involved in the disease. The National Center for Biotechnology Information (NCBI), a part of NIH National Library of Medicine, is developing databases for use by the research community. Two genome-wide association studies on macular degeneration and Parkinson disease already can be accessed through an NCBI Web site, called the Database of Genotype and Phenotype (dbGaP). Over >150 million SNPs are expected to be analyzed. These data can be used to define haplotype block structures across the genome and thus facilitate selection of SNPs for whole genome analysis. Appropriate epidemiological study designs and adequate statistical power are essential and the number of samples and the number of SNPs required for these studies may be substantially higher than typical studies of the past. Results of genome-wide SNP association studies might not be easily replicated in subsequent studies but could still identify causative regions of the genome (Rebbeck et al., 2004). Similarly, large-scale genome-wide scans may find surrogate markers that will distinguish cases from controls but may not identify causative SNPs. Therefore, replication of associations is crucial for valid and causative associations.

8.3 Data Collection and Public Databases

With the completion of Human Genome Project in 2003 and the International HapMap Project in 2005, researchers now have a set of research tools that make it possible to find the genetic contributions to common diseases. Many researchers are turning to these large, publicly available databases of SNPs, HapMap and CNVs which provide a catalogue of human genetic variation to choose a set of informative "tag" SNPs for genotyping in association studies of diseases including cancer (please see the list of online resources at the end of the chapter). The tools include computerized databases that contain the reference human genome sequence, a map of human genetic variation and a set of new technologies that can quickly and accurately analyze whole-genome samples for genetic variations that contribute to the onset of a disease. The studies of G×E interactions require data on both elements of the relationship. Genetic predisposition can be inferred from family history, phenotype (for example, skin color), or direct analysis of DNA sequence (Hunter, 2005). Environmental and lifestyle factors are measured in epidemiological studies using self-reported information; this can be obtained by interview or questionnaire, from records or direct measures in participants (for example, anthropometry), or biomarker-based inference on environmental exposures. Until recently, many studies of genetic predisposition (for example, pedigree-based studies) obtained little information on environment and lifestyle. Similarly, many typical epidemiological association studies of unrelated individuals did not obtain blood samples or other sources of DNA that would allow direct assessment of genetic variation. More recently, in both family based and association studies, collection of both genetic and environmental data, so that the interaction between the two can be examined, is becoming more common. As studies of genetic susceptibility and environmental exposures have been largely pursued by different groups of investigators, multidisciplinary collaboration is necessary to generate the best studies in the field. The International HapMap Project and the Seattle SNPs project are complemented by several NIH initiatives including the National Institute of Environmental Health Sciences Environmental Genome Project (NIEHSEGP) and the National Heart Lung and Blood Institute Resequencing and Genotyping Project (Constantine et al., 2008). The "Data" section provides bulk downloads of data and analysis sets as well as interactive access to the HapMap and SNP database. Simultaneously it was also shown as a validation step that a very small panel of SNPs chosen may capture most of the SNPs subsequently shown to be associated with cancer. A variety of tools on the web sites allows investigators to easily see all SNPs in a gene, their frequency in different populations, linkage disequilibrium, predicted functional consequences and sequence context. To date, approximately 2000 CNVs have been described. There could be thousands more CNVs in the human population. About 100 CNVs were detected in each genome examined with the average size being 250,000 bases (an average gene is 60,000 bases). Additional CNVs will be discovered as technologies for detection improve and more DNA samples from worldwide populations are examined. Obtaining high-quality data on environment and lifestyle in conjunction with biological samples to assess these genetic variants will be crucial in the assessment of G×E interactions. The need for large sample sizes is the major challenge in a G×E study design. A longstanding rule for calculating sample sizes has been that the sample size required to detect a departure from the expectation that the joint effect of G×E variables is multiplicative is at least four times the sample size that is needed to evaluate the main effect of each of the variables (Teare and Barret, 2005; Hunter, 2005). If information on exposures is misclassified, then the power to detect interactions is attenuated, and even larger sample sizes are required. As many epidemiological studies are underpowered for main effects, this predicts that they will be seriously underpowered to detect interactions. Therefore, in the foreseeable future the occurrence of false-negative findings for interactions in individual studies is the major problem, unless the interactions are strong. It has been pointed out that most cohort studies will not accrue sufficient numbers of cases for rare cancers and might have only marginal power for common cancers (Hunter, 2005). Therefore, rigorously designed case-control studies will remain the only option for assessing G×E interactions for rare form of cancers. A potentially effective means of mitigating the lack of power in prospective studies is to pool data across these studies for meta-analysis. The emerging interest in assessing tagSNPs makes prior coordination particularly desirable, as it might not be possible to pool data from studies that have used different SNPs to capture haplotypes. Maximizing the power of ongoing prospective studies in this manner can mitigate the main weakness of prospective studies (that is, the limited number of incident cases) while capitalizing on the methodological strengths of the prospective design.

8.4 Environmental Epigenomics and Disease Susceptibility

The epigenome consists of the DNA methylation marks and histone modifications involved in controlling gene expression. It is accurately reproduced during mitosis and can be inherited transgenerationally. Imprinted genes and metastable epialleles represent two classes of genes that are particularly susceptible to environmental factors because their regulation is tightly linked to epigenetic mechanisms (Jirtle and Skinner, 2007). Understanding the complexity of human epigenome will need to be characterized to understand the etiology of devastating diseases (Foley et al., 2009). Three genomic targets that are likely to be susceptible to gene-expression changes owing to environmental influences on epigenetic marks are the promoter regions of some housekeeping genes, transposable elements that lie adjacent to genes with metastable epialleles, and regulatory elements of imprinted genes. These genomic targets contain regions that are rich in CpG dinucleotide sequences, which are normally unmethylated, methylated or differentially methylated in response to environmental exposures, respectively, and in some cases with the status of histone modifications in the same region, determining levels of gene expression (Fig. 8.3).

Microarray assays could be applied as a useful tool for mapping methylation changes in multiple CpG loci and for generating epigenetic profiles in various

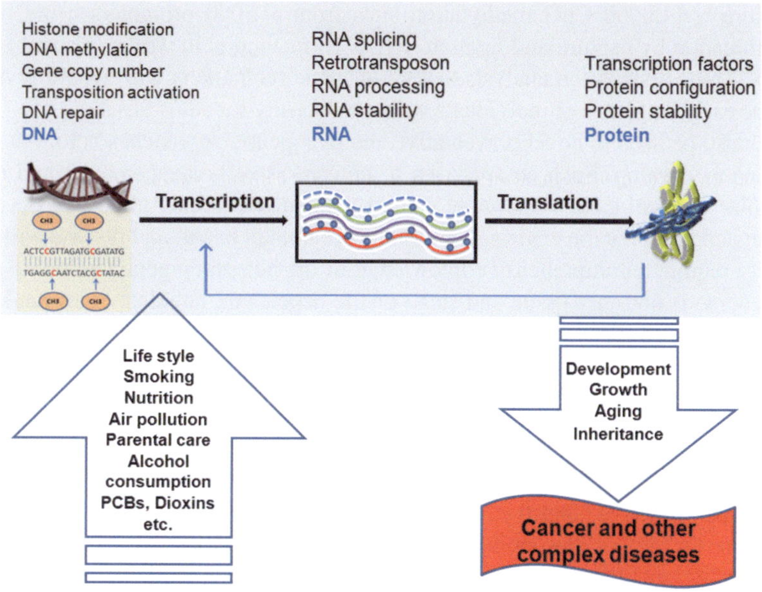

Fig. 8.3 Epigenomic targets of environmental exposures in gene regulatory mechanism with cancer and complex disease implications. Addition of a methyl group to a cytosine within C-G di-nucleotides, frequently present in the regulatory regions of the gene, is a lasting form of epigenomic modification. Methylation of cytosine in the regulatory region is a mechanism for gene silencing which prevents the binding of transcription factors and influence gene expression

diseases. It is important to identify imprinted genes and metastable epialleles as epigenetically labile genomic targets in the whole genome (Dolinoy et al., 2007a, b). The genome-wide identification of the full suite of epigenetically labile targets in human genomes have the potential to link the environment, through epigenetic changes, to early developmental influences on adult susceptibility to chronic diseases and behavioral disorders. Despite the different meaning of the environment to different people e.g., for sociologists and psychologists, social group interactions, family dynamics and maternal nurturing are environment while nutritionists envision food pyramids and dietary supplements as the environment, toxicologists think of water, soil and air pollutants, all environments are able to alter the gene expression. If these environmentally induced epigenetic adaptations occur at crucial stages of life, they can potentially change behavior, disease susceptibility and survival. Epigenetic modifications do not alter gene sequence but, rather, gene expression. Therefore, characterizing the expression profiles of epigenetically labile genes that are susceptible to environmental dysregulation will ultimately identify epigenetic biomarkers for disease and environmental exposure. Identification of methylation sites on large scale and other epigenetic phenomena hold enormous promise in expanding our knowledge of normal development and disease but the task present technological challenges. Development of high throughput assays to measure > 145,000 CpG methylation sites from > 5000 promoters using target amplification by capture and ligation (mTACL) method is in works (Nautial et al., 2010). Upon association analysis these epigenetic biomarkers will hopefully allow for the early diagnosis of individuals with a propensity for adult-onset disease. They could also be used in novel preventative and therapeutic approaches before disease symptoms develop. Such an approach to human disease management could revolutionize medical care, which now mainly treats diseases only after they develop. Understanding how the environment influences human health and disease will ultimately require a comprehensive knowledge of the human epigenome, because the epigenome is not only tissue and stage-of-life dependent, but also varies markedly between species (Jirtle and Skinner, 2007).

8.5 Analysis of G×E Interactions

G×E interactions explain that how genetic and environmental factors may jointly influence the risk of developing a disease. G×E interactions exist when observed effect of G and E together is not a simple function of their individual effects (Table 8.1). Although G×E interactions imply a specific relationship between genes and the environment, the existing disease models differ with respect to the statistical association between genes and the environment (Brennan, 2002). At least in part because of the many potential models of interactions, a G×E interaction will only be accepted if it can be reproduced and also seems plausible at the biological level (Fig. 8.4). Indeed, there are challenges in pinpointing and reproducibility of the data on G×E interactions before they can be incorporated into public-health and clinical practice. However, even with well-designed studies, there are many ways of declaring "success" in the search for interactions (Hunter, 2005). This is because of variability in the qualitative and statistical models of interaction and the difficulty of assessing biological plausibility (either a priori—that is, when trying to prioritize prior probabilities in these analyses—or once an interaction has been observed). This chapter provides a general background on the analytical models and study designs to uncover and confirm G×E interactions (Fig. 8.4). They are as follows.

Table 8.1 G×E interactions exist when observed effect of G and E together is not a simple function of their individual effects (Ho:$R_{GE} = R_G R_E$ vs. HA: $R_{GE} \neq R_G R_E$). R_E: Risk among exposed non-carriers, R_G: Risk among unexposed carriers, R_{GE}: Risk due to interaction

Exposure	Genotype	Case	Control	Odds ratio
No	No	A	B	1
No	Yes	C	D	$R_G = CB/AD$
Yes	No	E	F	$R_E = EB/AF$
Yes	Yes	G	H	$R_{GE} = GB/AH$

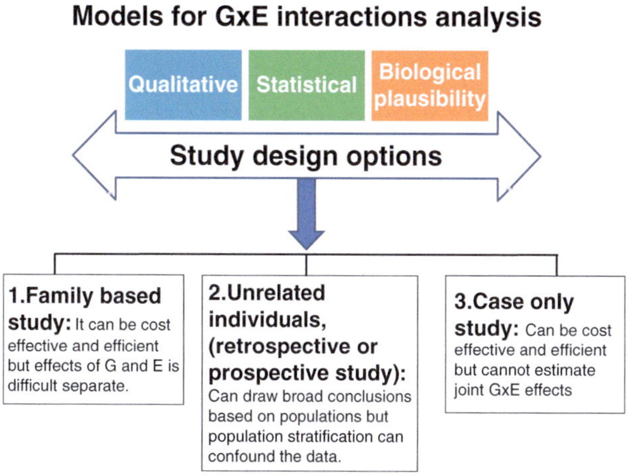

Fig. 8.4 Models and study design options for G×E interactions analysis. Study options can use different models to establish association. 1. Family based study option collect data on the Phenotype and risk factors are measured on individual family members. 2. In the study where unrelated individuals are considered (retrospective or prospective study) data on environmental and lifestyle factors, and samples for DNA and biomarker studies, are obtained after diagnosis of disease (Retrospective studies) or at baseline (the start of the study), and ideally at other points before diagnosis (Prospective studies) and 3. Case only studies where obtained data will ideally reveal the prevalence of the exposure in the genotype-positive cases would be expected to be the same as the prevalence of the exposure in the genotype-negative cases

8.5.1 Qualitative Models

In the simplest case of dichotomous genotype (such as carriers versus non-carriers of a gene variant) and dichotomous exposure (for example, exposed versus non-exposed), the four possible combinations of genotype and exposure can be displayed in a 2 × 4 table, and the relative risks can be ascertained (Botto and Khoury, 2001). However, even in this simplest case there are several models for describing interactions between genetic susceptibility and environmental exposures in different diseases. The possibilities are more numerous if there are many categories of environmental exposure and/or many genetic categories (as in the case of three genotypes for a biallelic system) or different genetic models (recessive, co-dominant and dominant). Therefore, many departures from the null result—where the risk of disease is the same in all cross-classified categories of exposure and genotype—might be compatible with the overall hypothesis of gene–environment interaction (Hunter, 2005). The "multiple comparisons" problem that is inherent in examining thousands or even hundreds of thousands of SNPs in association studies is relatively familiar. For gene–environment interactions, however, we face a comparison problem that arises from a model involving multiple genes, multiple exposures and multiple interactions. In addition to using statistical approaches to control the false-positive rate, the reproducibility of gene–environment interactions across two or more studies will be crucial.

8.5.2 Statistical Models

In true sense statistical interaction is absent when the effects of the two factors are additive with respect to some quantitative measure of response (Response = Gene effect + Environmental effect). Statistical interaction describes lack of fit of this simple statistical model for joint action. There are several methods of assessing the statistical significance of interactions. In the simplest case of dichotomous environmental exposure and genotype, perhaps the most commonly used procedure is to test departure from the multiplicative model of interaction (Hunter, 2005). This involves testing whether the relative risk for joint exposure is statistically significantly greater ("supermultiplicative") or smaller ("submultiplicative") than would be expected by multiplying the relative risks for environmental exposure or genetic predisposition alone. Another commonly used test for interaction uses rate differences rather than relative risks, and proposes that the joint effect of genes and the environment is different from the expectation. This additive model is often said to be of greater relevance to assessing the public-health impact of an interaction. Again, the option to use either of these two models adds further potential for multiple comparisons to the statistical analysis of G×E interactions. There are two approaches that have been proposed. The first is to compare haplotype frequencies in cases and controls separately where analysis must allow for error in estimates of haplotype frequencies and generally cannot control for covariates. Second models including regression substitution methods exist, in which an expected haplotype "score" is calculated as a predictor variable (e.g., using proc haplotype in SAS) as if it were equivalent to the true haplotype (Rebbeck et al., 2004). Under the alternative hypothesis, bias in estimates of effects can be evaluated and the degree of bias related to the formal measure of haplotype uncertainty. The development of these and other computational approaches to study haplotype data in samples of unrelated individuals (e.g., in case-control or cohort studies) will facilitate the evaluation of haplotypes in association studies.

8.5.2.1 Biological Plausibility

Screening a large number of potential gene–environment interactions in datasets with a large number of genotypes and many variables of exposure greatly increases the chance of finding false positive results at conventional levels of statistical significance. As most studies are not powerful enough to detect modest interactions, demanding small p values to counteract this problem will result in a lower probability of declaring true-positive interactions as "significant". Restricting the search for gene–environment interactions to those that involve gene products and exposures that plausibly interact in the same biological pathway is an attractive option. Furthermore, restricting analysis to gene variants that plausibly alter gene function is also attractive (Hunter, 2005). Indeed choice among theories of biological plausibility is enhanced hardly at all by the epidemiological assessment of interaction. What few causal systems can be rejected based on observed results would provide decidedly limited etiological insight.

8.6 Study Designs for Association Analyses

Genetic epidemiology has been dominated by the use of family-based designs from which inherited susceptibility can be inferred. However, with the advent of methods for assessing DNA-sequence variability directly, genome wide association studies using unrelated individuals are increasingly being used. Studies however, should be carefully designed to defeat their purpose to simply detect statistical interaction. Based on the analytical models, following are the common study design approaches for G×E interactions.

8.6.1 Family-Based Study

Family-based studies have been the cornerstone of identification and quantification of the familial risk and heritability of human diseases. The purpose of family based approach is to evaluate whether familial clustering among cases is greater than expected. By comparing disease concordance rates between monozygotic and dizygotic twins, twin studies can be used to partition components of variance between genetic and shared and non-shared environmental factors. Most reports of studies from twin registries do not include information on environmental exposures that could be shared (or different) between the twin siblings, precluding any inferences about specific gene–environment interactions. Analyses of multigenerational pedigrees might provide a preliminary assessment of the hypothesis that the penetrance of a mutation has changed over time, which would indicate that changes in lifestyle and environment have influenced gene penetrance (Hunter, 2005). This indicates the influence of environmental and lifestyle factors that are more prevalent in recent birth cohorts, although it does not provide direct clues about specific factors. A limitation of this approach is the assessments of this nature can only be made for relatively highly penetrant gene mutations (that is, where the penetrance is sufficiently high to cause clear familial aggregation). Incorporation of environmental data into pedigree or other family-based designs (for example, studies that use sib-pairs or case-parent designs) allows direct estimates of specific gene–environment interactions. In some cases, fewer matched sets might be required for these designs than for case-control studies using unrelated controls. Collection of adequate numbers of sibpairs, however, might take more effort than the use of unrelated controls and, for late-onset of cancers, the availability of living parents might limit case-parent accrual.

8.6.2 Unrelated Individuals

Epidemiology has been remarkably successful at identifying the main risk factors for many common diseases; use of the best available study designs and data-collection methods has been important in this success. The relative merits of population-based epidemiological studies are well established. It should also be noted that, under certain assumptions, G×E interactions can be estimated from case–case studies without controls. However, the search for G×E interactions imposes some further constraints on the use of these designs. In retrospective case-control studies, data on environmental and lifestyle factors, and samples for DNA and biomarker studies, are obtained after diagnosis of disease in the cases (Kraft and Hunter, 2005). In prospective cohort studies, environmental and lifestyle data are obtained at baseline (the start of the study), and ideally at other points before diagnosis. Samples for DNA and biomarker studies are also ideally obtained at baseline, although in prospective studies that do not have banked samples, DNA can be obtained after diagnosis from living cohort members.

8.6.2.1 Retrospective Design

The main limitation of retrospective studies, particularly case-control studies is the selection bias (in particular, the use of controls that do not represent the population in which the cases occurred). If the race or ethnicity of the controls is substantially different from that of the cases, then spurious associations with gene variants that differ by race or ethnicity (that is, population stratification) will occur (Hunter, 2005). The potential influence of population stratification can be substantially eliminated with attention to appropriate choice of controls and by controlling for self-reported ethnicity. Methods to assess the population substructure of cases and controls by genotyping non-causal gene variants ("genomic control") have been proposed, and can be used to correct for this phenomenon (Sham et al., 2009). With respect to G×E interactions, the principal problem is likely to consist of misclassified ("noisy") or biased information on environmental exposures. Bias can arise if cases report their pre-diagnosis exposure histories differently once they are diagnosed with the disease compared with what they would have reported before diagnosis (recall bias). Of more concern in retrospective studies is the possibility that poor recall (misclassification) of past exposures among both cases and controls might attenuate the estimates of risk to the point where any difference in risk according to genotype cannot be reliably detected. The potential for these biases and misclassification can be reduced, but rarely eliminated, by paying careful attention to best practices in enrollment and exposure assessment. The chief advantage of case-control studies is the potential for the sample size to be limited only by cost and by the number of cases of the disease that are available in the study area. Given the need for large sample sizes in gene-environment studies, this is a great potential advantage, which, when combined with the potential for increased detail of exposure assessment and disease phenotype, might make the case-control study the design of choice for complex diseases and some type of cancers.

8.6.2.2 Prospective Design

The problems of selection and recall bias in case-control studies can be minimized in prospective studies. Here, DNA samples and exposure information are obtained from participants in a longitudinal cohort who are followed up, usually for years or decades. If follow-up rates are high, then a virtually complete set of cases can be assembled and compared with a sample of individuals who did not develop the disease. The use of this "nested" case-control study minimizes selection bias because the population that gives rise to the cases is defined (Hunter, 2005). Because information on exposures is collected before diagnosis (in most cases, years to decades before), recall bias is eliminated as knowledge of diagnosis cannot influence the reporting of exposures. However, particularly in cohort studies that only have a baseline assessment and no repeated measurements during follow up, a single measure of an exposure might not be a good reflection of the pattern of exposure over time. A variant of the true nested case-control approach might be useful in studies that include prospectively collected environmental and lifestyle data, but that lack a source of DNA for genetic analyses. In this design, an attempt is made to obtain a DNA sample from cases arising in the cohort, and from matched or unmatched non-cases. Although the environmental data should be secure from recall bias in this design, failure to obtain DNA samples from a high proportion of cases and controls can result in selection bias in the same manner as in a conventional case-control study. Differential participation by cases and controls according to ethnicity could give rise to population stratification, particularly in populations whose ancestors have been recently mixed by intercontinental migration. However, again this bias can be minimized by collecting information on and controlling for ethnic background, or by using genomic control methods. The principal problem with prospective studies is that adequate sample sizes of cases will only be obtained for common conditions, such as hypertension, myocardial infarction and stroke, and common cancers, in the population that is being followed. Rare diseases, such as sarcomas, will not occur at sufficient frequency to provide statistical power. A typical cohort study might only accrue several hundred cases of a disease of moderate incidence (for example, Parkinson disease) over many years, and because most cohort studies enroll men and women in middle life, diseases with relatively early onset (for example, multiple sclerosis) will be under-represented. In addition, some of the special requirements for genomic analyses might only be met in case-control studies. For certain diseases, particularly cancers, expression-array analyses indicate that cancer types that look histologically similar might represent more than one disease process. Obtaining the fresh-frozen tissue or tumor blocks necessary to subtype these outcomes might be difficult in prospective studies, but more feasible in cases that are studied in a limited number of institutions. Phenotypic assays, such as assays that measure the activity of an enzyme or biochemical pathway by giving a test dose of a compound and measuring metabolites in blood, might be possible in a limited number of cases and controls, but are unlikely to be feasible in large prospective studies. Information on disease diagnosis and subtype from non-genomic tests, such as histology or imaging, might also be hard to obtain in a uniform manner in a prospective study, in which almost all cases might be diagnosed at different institutions, as opposed to a case-control study that operates in a limited number of hospitals.

8.6.2.3 Case-Only Designs

It has been shown that when a genotype is not correlated with an environmental factor and a disease is rare, then departure from multiplicative interaction can be tested by examining information from the cases only (Hunter, 2005). In this case-only design, the prevalence of the exposure in the genotype-positive cases would be expected to be the same as the prevalence of the exposure in the genotype-negative cases. Statistically significant departures from this expectation of equal prevalence indicate an interaction between genotype and exposure. The idea of dispensing with the need to identify appropriate controls and enroll them is attractive. Obtaining an estimate of the main effect of genotype (particularly given the genome wide potential candidate genotypes as our knowledge of gene function and common gene variants increases), is the primary interest and new, or as yet unproven, environmental hypotheses are always investigated. To estimate these, an appropriate control group is needed. In addition, for high-penetrance genes, the assumption that the disease is rare among exposed individuals is violated, leading to a distortion of the interaction estimates. It is possible that, as we identify the main genetic influences on common diseases and cancers, case–case methods might become more popular in assessing the interaction of established causal genotypes with environmental factors, particularly as these studies can form the baseline cohort for finding prognostic markers of disease outcomes. The small sample size increases the likelihood that case only study will be repeated.

8.7 Critical Parameters

8.7.1 Sample Size

The need for large sample sizes is the major challenge in a G×E study design. A longstanding rule for calculating sample sizes has been that the sample size required to detect a departure from the expectation that the joint effect of G×E variables is multiplicative is at least four times the sample size that is needed to evaluate the main effect of each of the variables (Teare and Barret, 2005; Hunter, 2005). If information on exposures is misclassified, then the power to detect interactions is attenuated, and even larger sample sizes are required. As many epidemiological studies are underpowered for main effects, this predicts that they will be seriously underpowered to detect interactions. Therefore, in the foreseeable future the occurrence of false-negative findings for interactions in individual studies is the major problem, unless the interactions are strong. It has been pointed out that most cohort studies will not accrue sufficient numbers of cases for rare cancers and might have only marginal power for common cancers (Hunter, 2005). Therefore, rigorously designed case-control studies will remain the only option for assessing G×E interactions for rare form of cancers. A potentially effective means of mitigating the lack of power in prospective studies is to pool data across these studies for meta-analysis. The emerging interest in assessing tagSNPs makes prior coordination particularly desirable, as it might not be possible to pool data from studies that have used different SNPs to capture haplotypes. Maximizing the power of ongoing prospective studies in this manner can mitigate the main weakness of prospective studies (that is, the limited number of incident cases) while capitalizing on the methodological strengths of the prospective design.

8.7.2 Complex Mixture of Covariates

Which components of "complex mixtures"—such as air pollution, diet or cigarette smoke—can cause disease is the most critical question to ask in any analysis of G×E interactions. This is difficult to study observationally as most components of complex mixtures are highly correlated, so that their effects cannot be statistically separated (Kraft and Hunter, 2005). If the effect of the environmental factor differs according to variation in one or more specific genes, then the function of the gene might help to isolate the causal components in the complex mixture. The related concept of "Mendelian randomization" has been used to argue that a reproducible effect on disease risk of a genotype that alters the level of an intermediate biomarker indicates that the relation of the biomarker to disease risk is unlikely to be confounded by other lifestyle variables, because in most cases, these other lifestyle variables would not be expected to correlate with genetic variation (Hunter, 2005; Schatzkin et al., 2009).

8.7.3 Coordination in Data Collection and Their Meta-analysis

Despite much information on both genetic and environmental disease-risk factors, there are relatively few examples of reproducible gene–environment interactions. The main reason is that many individual studies have been designed to examine the main effects of individual factors and do not have adequate power to examine interactions (Khoury et al., 2009). Even then, to convincingly show the main effect of a single factor might require meta-analysis of many studies, and it is uncommon for this level of detail to be available for interactions (Zeggini and Ioannidis, 2009; Richards et al., 2009). There are two approaches to mitigate this problem: (1) to facilitate web-based presentation of unpublished results in supplementary tables, and (2) to pre plan analyses across many studies so that the data are analysed and displayed in as uniform a format as possible. The latter approach is a prospective variant of the "meta-analysis of individual participants' data" approach. The extra advantage of this approach is that pre-planned analyses allow more consistent treatment of LD and haplotype definition. The study of G×E interactions has at least one advantage over that of conventional two-way environmental interactions because it should be possible to measure a defined functional genetic polymorphism almost without error. However, when several polymorphisms in a gene contribute to altered function, measuring a subset will result in misclassification and so will increase the sample size that is required to detect interactions. Furthermore, functional gene variants are not known—for example, if we are trying to detect genetic association through LD—it is likely that there will be substantial misclassification of the genetic variable, leading to dilution of the relative risk for the interaction. With the increasing use of haplotype-tagging or LD-tagging SNPs to explore genetic associations in candidate genes and regions, there is even more potential for incompatible information. Some degree of coordination of the main studies in each disease area would at least reduce the potential for incompatibility of information, and could hasten the confirmation of replication of both genetic effects and gene–environment interactions. The NCI Breast and Prostate Cancer and Hormone-Related Cohort Consortium (http://epi.grants.cancer.gov/BPC3/), for example, is a planned assessment of the same genetic variants in 53 candidate genes across 10 studies that collectively contribute more than 6,000 cases of breast cancer and 8,000 cases of prostate cancer. Consortia such as this have the potential to provide much more uniform data and analyses than are available through post-hoc or literature analyses.

8.8 Summary

A growing body of knowledge illustrates the influence of the G×E interactions in the disease incidence, susceptibility and progression. Genetic factors are known to be involved in the predisposition to and development of diseases. The interactions of multiple modifier genes with various environmental factors—that are G×E interactions—explain why rates of disease incidence vary across populations, among exposed groups, and even within families (Wilson et al., 2002). We have new tools available to analyze G×E interactions with an expanded and enhanced view of environmental health and exposures that include factors such as diet, lifestyle, metabolic alterations, socioeconomic status, and various environmental exposures. Genome-wide approaches have the advantage of scanning the entire genome for associations without having to rely on choosing a priori candidates. With advances in high-throughput technology and genome-wide association methods, these approaches will be more tractable in the future (Khoury et al., 2009) but present formidable challenges in throughput, databasing, and analysis. It will be necessary to establish mechanisms for collaboration across studies that operate within the boundaries of the original informed consent given by study participants, and to keep the environmental and lifestyle data confidential. New statistical methods are still in works to extract meaning from large data sets and to incorporate knowledge from other branches of science. Systems biology approaches to integrating "omics" information from many sources is predicted to lead to new insights about cellular and whole-organism function. This information will have to be integrated into the interpretation of studies of genes and the environment. Incorporating pharmacokinetic knowledge of specific biochemical pathways been proposed as the first step in this direction for carrying out epidemiological studies of gene variants in these pathways. Predicting the probability that a SNP alters function on the basis of phylogenetic or biochemical data, or from predicted effects on protein structure, might help to determine which SNPs to genotype, as well as the interpretation of subsequent results. Reporting of false-positive probability by incorporating the prior probability of an interaction might also be helpful for reducing false positives in the literature. Similarly, while knowledge of the functional significance of SNPs is key to understanding the biological basis of G×E association, function can be determined in advance for candidate gene studies or after the identification of novel genes from genome-wide association studies. The information will enable health professionals to tailor prevention programs to each person's unique genetic makeup. In addition, if an individual does become ill, the information can be used to select the treatments most likely to be effective and least likely to cause adverse reactions in that particular patient. Researchers already have reported considerable success using this new strategy. However, complete (and resource-intensive) studies of SNPs in a region are required to achieve sufficient statistical power. The alternative of studying incomplete sets of SNPs in a genomic region may result in less power but still identify causative loci. Increasingly in G×E studies the issues such as (a) level of genomic coverage (i.e., how many SNPs) to achieve an adequate result, (b) validity of tagSNP approaches, (c) characterization and validation of haplotype blocks in different populations will be addressed in the near future.

References

Barnes, M.R. 2006. Navigating the HapMap. Brief Bioinform. 7(3):211–24.

Boffetta, P., McLaughlin, J.K., La Vecchia, C., Tarone, R.E., Lipworth, L., Blot, W.J. 2008. False-positive results in cancer epidemiology: a plea for epistemological modesty. J. Natl. Cancer Inst. 100(14):988–95.

Botto, L.D., Khoury, M.J. 2001. Commentary: facing the challenge of gene-environment interaction: the two-by-four table and beyond. Am. J. Epidemiol. 153(10):1016–20.

Brennan, P. 2002. Gene-environment interaction and aetiology of cancer: what does it mean and how can we measure it? Carcinogenesis 23(3):381–7.

Brown, J.R., Thornton, J.L. 1957. Percivall Pott (1714–1788) and chimney sweepers' cancer of the scrotum. Br. J. Ind. 14(1):68–70.

Carter, N.P. 2007. Methods and strategies for analyzing copy number variation using DNA microarrays. Nat. Genet. 39:S16–21.

Chanock, S.J., Manolio, T., Boehnke, M., Boerwinkle, E., Hunter, D.J., Thomas, G., Hirschhorn, J.N., Abecasis, G., Altshuler, D., Bailey-Wilson, J.E., Brooks, L.D., Cardon, L.R., Daly, M., Donnelly, P., Fraumeni, J.F., Freimer, N.B., Gerhard, D.S., Gunter, C., Guttmacher, A.E., Guyer, M.S., Harris, E.L., Hoh, J., Hoover, R., Kong, C.A., Merikangas, K.R., Morton, C.C., Palmer, L.J., Phimister, E.G., Rice, J.P., Roberts, J., Rotimi, C., Tucker, M.A., Vogan, K.J., Wacholder, S., Wijsman, E.M., Winn, D.M., Collins, F.S. 2007. Replicating genotype-phenotype associations. Nature 447:655–60.

Constantine, C.C., Gurrin L.C., McLaren, C.E., Gurrin, L.C., McLaren, C.E., Bahlo, M., Anderson, G.J., Vulpe, C.D., Forrest, S.M., Allen, K.J., Gertig, D.M., The Health Iron Investigators. 2008. SNP selection for genes of iron metabolism in a study of genetic modifiers of hemochromatosis. BMC Med. Genet. 9:18.

Deloukas, P., Bentley, D. 2004. The HapMap project and its application to genetic studies of drug response. Pharmacogenom. J. 4(2):88–90.

Dolinoy, D.C., Weidman, J.R., Jirtle, R.L. 2007a. Epigenetic gene regulation: linking early developmental environment to adult disease. Reprod. Toxicol. 23(3):297–307.

Dolinoy, D.C., Das, R., Weidman, J.R., Jirtle, R.L. 2007b. Metastable epialleles, imprinting, and the fetal origins of adult diseases. Pediatr. Res. 61:30R–37R.

Foley, D.L., Craig, J.M., Morley, R., Olsson, C.A., Dwyer, T., Smith, K., Saffery, R. 2009. Prospects for epigenetic epidemiology. Am. J. Epidemiol. 169(4):389–400.

Francis, P.J., Schultz, D.W., Hamon, S., Ott, J., Weleber, R.G., Klein, M.L. 2007. Haplotypes in the complement factor H (CFH) gene: associations with drusen and advanced age-related macular degeneration. PloS One 2(11):e1197.

George, R.E., Attiyeh, E.F., Li, S., Moreau, L.A., Neuberg, D., Li, C., Fox, E.A., Meyerson, M., Diller, L., Fortina, P., Look, A.T., Maris, J.M. 2007. Genome-wide analysis of neuroblastomas using high-density single nucleotide polymorphism arrays. PLoS One, 2 (2):e255.

Hunter, D.J. 2005. Gene–environment interactions in human diseases. Nat. Rev. 6:287–298.

Huang, B.E., Amos, C.I., Lin, D.Y. 2007. Detecting haplotype effects in genomewide association studies. Genet. Epidemiol. 31(8):803–12.

Ioannidis, J.P. 2007. Non-replication and inconsistency in the genome-wide association setting. Hum. Hered. 64:203–13.

Jirtle, R.L., Skinner, M.K. 2007. Environmental epigenomics and disease susceptibility. Nat. Rev. Genet. 8:253–62.

Keith, T., 2007. Human genome-wide association studies, achieving a sufficient power to detect disease genes with the Quebec founder population. Genet. Eng. Biotechnol. 27:2.

Khoury, M.J., Feero, W.G., Reyes, M., Citrin, T., Freedman, A., Leonard, D., Burke, W., Coates, R., Croyle, R.T., Edwards, K., Kardia, S., McBride, C., Manolio, T., Randhawa, G., Rasooly, R., St Pierre, J., Terry, S. 2009. The genomic applications in practice and prevention network. Genet. Med. 11(7) 488–94.

Kraft, P., Hunter, D. 2005. Integrating epidemiology and genetic association: the challenge of gene–environment interaction. Philos. Trans. R. Soc. Lond. B. Biol. Sci. 360:1609–1616.

Laumen, H., Saningong, A.D., Heid, I.M., Hess, J., Herder, C., Claussnitzer, M., Baumert, J., Lamina, C., Rathmann, W., Sedlmeier, E.M., Klopp, N.,Thorand, B., Wichmann, H.E., Illig, T., Hauner, H. 2009. Functional characterization of promoter variants of the adiponectin gene complemented by epidemiological data. Diabetes 58(4):984–91.

Lobo, I. 2008. Epistasis: gene interaction and the phenotypic expression of complex diseases like Alzheimer's. Nat. Educ. 1(1).

Manolio, T.A., Brooks, L.D., Collins, F.S. 2008. A HapMap harvest of insights into the genetics of common disease. J. Clin. Invest. 118(5):1590–605.

Nautiyal, S., Carlton, V.E.H., Lu, Y., Iteland, J.S., Flaucher, D., Moorhead, M., Gray, J.W., Spellman, P., Mindrinos, M., Berg, P., Faham, M. 2010. High-throughput method for analyzing methylation of CpGs in targeted genomic regions. PNAS published ahead of print June 23, 2010, doi:10.1073/pnas.1005173107.

Rebbeck, T.R., Ambrosone, C.B., Bell, D.A., Chanock, S.J., Hayes, R.B., Kadlubar, F.F., Thomas, D.C. 2004. SNPs, haplotypes, and cancer: applications in molecular epidemiology. Cancer Epidemiol. Biomarkers Prev. 13(5):681–7.

Redon, R., Ishikawa, S., Fitch, K.R., Feuk, L., Perry, G.H., Andrews, T.D., Fiegler, H., Shapero, M.H., Carson, A.R., Chen, W., Cho, E.K., Dallaire, S., Freeman, J.L., Gonzalez, J.R., Gratacos, M., Huang, J., Kalaitzopoulos, D., Komura, D., MacDonald, J.R., Marshall, C.R., Mei, R., Montgomery, L., Nishimura, K., Okamura, K., Shen, F., Somerville, M.J., Tchinda, J., Valsesia, A., Woodwark, C., Yang, F., Zhang, J., Zerjal, T., Zhang, J., Armengol, L., Conrad, D.F., Estivill, X., Tyler-Smith, C., Carter, N.P., Aburatani, H., Lee, C., Jones, K.W., Scherer, S.W., Hurles, M.E. 2006. Global variation in copy number in the human genome. Nature 444(7118):444–54.

Richards, J.B., Kavvoura, F.K., Rivadeneira, F., Styrkarsdottir, U., Estrada, K., Halldorsson, B.V., Hsu, Y.H., Zillikens, M.C., Wilson, S.G., Mullin, B.H., Amin, N., Aulchenko, Y.S., Cupples, L.A., Deloukas, P., Demissie, S., Hofman, A., Kong, A., Karasik, D., van Meurs, J.B., Oostra, B.A., Pols, H.A., Sigurdsson, G., Thorsteinsdottir, U., Soranzo, N., Williams, F.M., Zhou, Y.,

Ralston, S.H., Thorleifsson, G., van Duijn, C.M., Kiel, D.P., Stefansson, K., Uitterlinden, A.G., Ioannidis, J.P., Spector, T.D. 2009. Collaborative meta-analysis: associations of 150 candidate genes with osteoporosis and osteoporotic fracture. Ann. Intern. Med. 151(8):528–37.

Stranger, B.E., Forrest, M.S., Clark, A.G., Stranger, B.E., Forrest, M.S., Clark, A.G., Minichiello, M.J., Deutsch, S., Lyle, R., Hunt, S., Kahl, B., Antonarakis, S.E., Tavare, S., Deloukas, P., Dermitzakis, E.T. 2005. Genome-wide associations of gene expression variation in humans. PLoS Genet. 1(6):e78.

Schatzkin, A., Abnet, C.C., Cross, A.J., Gunter, M., Pfeiffer, R., Gail, M., Lim, U., Davey-Smith, G. 2009. Mendelian randomization: how it can – and cannot – help confirm causal relations between nutrition and cancer. Cancer Prev. Res. (Phila. PA) 2(2):104–13.

Sebat, J. 2007. Major changes in our DNA lead to major changes in our thinking. Nature Genet. 39(Suppl.):53–55.

Sham, P.C., Cherny, S.S., Purcell, S. 2009. Application of genome-wide SNP data for uncovering pairwise relationships and quantitative trait loci. Genetica 136(2):237–43.

Wilson, S., Jones, L., Couseens, C., Hanna, K., eds. 2002. The links between environmental factors, genetics, and the development of Cancer. In Cancer and the Environment, Gene–Enviroment Interaction, pp 25–35. Washington, DC, National Academy Press.

Teare Dawn, M.D., Barrett, J.H., 2005. Genetic linkage studies. The Lancet 366(9490):1036–44.

Tzu-Hao, W., Hsin-Shih, W. 2009. A genome-wide association study primer for clinicians. Taiwan. J. Obstet. Gynecol. 48(2):89–95.

Yoon, S., Xuan, Z., Makarov, V., Ye, K., Sebat, J. 2009. Sensitive and accurate detection of copy number variants using read depth of coverage. Genome Res. 19(9):1586–92.

Zeggini, E, Ioannidis, J.P. 2009. Meta-analysis in genome-wide association studies. Pharmacogenomics. 10(2):191–201.

Online Resources

1. Glossary of terms: http://www.ornl.gov/sci/techresources/Human_Genome/glossary/glossary_a.shtml
2. Bioinformatic software site: http://helpdesk.genetics.ucla.edu/howtos/biosoft
3. SNPinfo from NIEHS: www.niehs.nih.gov/snpinfo(http://www.niehs.nih.gov/snpinfo)
4. GeneSNPs: http://www.genome.utah.edu/genesnps
5. HapMap site: http://hapmap.ncbi.nlm.nih.gov/index.html.en
6. Human Genome Project: http://www.ornl.gov/sci/techresources/Human_Genome/home.shtml
7. National Cancer Institute Breast and Prostate Cancer and Hormone-Related Gene: http://epi.grants.cancer.gov/BPC3
8. National Cancer Institute Cancer Genome Anatomy Project (SNP500Cancer Database): http://snp500cancer.nci.nih.gov
9. UK Biobank: http://www.ukbiobank.ac.uk
10. US National Institute of Environmental Health Sciences Environmental Genome Project: http://egp.gs.washington.edu
11. DECIPHER (Database of Chromosome Imbalances in Phenotypes Using Ensembl Resources): http://www.sanger.ac.uk/PostGenomics/decipher

Part II
Environment and Specific Types of Cancer

Chapter 9
Gene–Environment Interaction and Susceptibility to Pediatric Brain Tumors

Brian Kunkle, David Sandberg, Prasanna Jayakar, Quentin Felty, and Deodutta Roy

Abstract Many pediatric brain tumors (pBTs) may result from the interplay of environmental factors with biological mechanisms at critical developmental periods in a child's life. While several genetic disorders have been linked to development of pBTs, many pBTs may result from low-penetrant gene alterations in common pathways. Importantly, alterations and pathways that may be important to etiology in certain tumor types may not play a role in other pBT types. It is probable that heterogeneity in alterations, and possibly even pathways, exists within tumor groups as well. Identification of which pathways are most significant in the etiology of each pBT type will be critical in developing therapies for these tumors. While therapies for single gene mutations have been successful in the past for certain cancers, it is possible that therapies based on pathway inhibition will prove to be more successful in the treatment of tumors that have several mutations throughout a pathway such as pBTs. This chapter describes the current state of the research on environmental, genetic, and epigenetic factors possibly involved in the development of pBTs. It covers epidemiological research on environmental factors that have been investigated in relation to pBTs, the involvement of neural stem cells, progenitor cells, and developmental pathways in the etiology of pBTs, the genetic and epigenetic alterations that have been identified in common pBTs, and how these factors may interact with mitochondrial-nuclear signaling to increase individual susceptibility to pBTs.

Keywords Pediatric brain tumors (pBTs) · Gene–environment interactions · Mitochondrial-nuclear signaling · Environment · Individual susceptibility

D. Roy (✉)
Department of Environmental and Occupational Health, Robert Stempel College of Public Health & Social Work, Florida International University, Miami, FL 33199-0001, USA
e-mail: droy@fiu.edu

D. Roy, M.T. Dorak (eds.), *Environmental Factors, Genes, and the Development of Human Cancers*, DOI 10.1007/978-1-4419-6752-7_9,

9.1 Introduction

Pediatric brain tumors (pBT) are a genetically, biochemically, and clinically heterogeneous group of tumors located in both the central and peripheral nervous system. Collectively, they are the most common solid tumors of childhood and rank second to leukemias in both incidence and mortality for childhood cancers. Approximately 2,200 intracranial pBTs, or 16.6% of all childhood cancers are diagnosed each year in U.S. children under the age of 20, with 78% of these neoplasms being classified as malignant in nature and the remaining classified as benign or of unspecified behavior (Gurney et al., 1999a,b). Astrocytomas comprise 52% of these malignancies, primitive neuroectodermal tumor (PNET) comprise 21%, other gliomas 15%, and ependymomas an additional 9% (Gurney et al. 1999a,b). Neuroblastomas (NB), the most common solid extracranial nervous system tumor, arise in the adrenal medulla and sympathetic ganglia and account for another 6–10% of all childhood cancers, with approximately 650 new cases occurring in U.S. children each year (Brodeur and Castleberry, 1997). Nearly 50% of these extracranial tumors occur in children under the age of 2 years old (Brodeur and Castleberry, 1997). Given the early age of onset of a majority of pBTs, and the current dogma that most cancers have at least a 10 year period of formation, it appears that these tumors may have an etiology that contrasts with some of the traditionally accepted ideas on tumor formation. In fact, recent research is beginning to suggest an etiology focused on early life environmental factors interacting with dysregulated developmental mechanisms (e.g. signaling pathways and stem cell/progenitor cell growth and differentiation) and mitochondrial-nuclear signaling in pBTs.

While links between specific environmental exposures and pBTs are not yet fully established, several aspects of developmental biology increase the likelihood of their involvement in pBT etiology, including (1) the increased vulnerability of the fetus/neonatal nervous system to exposures, (2) the high rates of cellular proliferation and differentiation during development of the nervous system, and (3) the ability of environmental factors to produce and/or influence genetic and epigenetic alterations in pathways involved in both development and tumorigenesis. For instance, high rates of cell proliferation and differentiation during development and childhood increases susceptibility of cells to mutagenic and epigenetic alteration. In fact, in utero DNA damage resulting from environmental pollution has been associated with somatic gene mutation in newborns (Perera et al., 2002). Furthermore, it is becoming more evident that not only can drugs and environmental stressors interfere with normal fetal development by causing structural malformations, but that exposure to environmental stressors during development can also cause biochemical and functional abnormalities. Additionally, the blood-brain barrier, which acts as a barrier to potentially harmful substances, is not fully developed in the fetus and can allow harmful substances to reach sensitive organs such as the brain. Some suspected in utero carcinogens for pBT include pesticides, N-nitroso compounds, tobacco, and infectious biological agents. While evidence linking several of these exposures to pBTs is substantial, the only exposure known to clearly cause pBTs is ionizing radition. However, chemicals such as 1,3-Butadiene and N-Nitrosomethylurea have been shown to induce neurogenic tumors in animals, with both the fetus and neonatal animals being at dramatically increased susceptibility to brain tumor (BT) development compared to adults (Rice and Wilbourn, 2000). Furthermore, evidence showing that pesticides can influence glial development and differentiation well into childhood suggests that early life exposures may influence both pBT and adult BT (aBT) (Garcia et al., 2001). In fact, evidence from several other cancers suggests that susceptibility to adult tumor development may in fact be influenced by early life environmental exposures and their interaction with epigenetic mechanisms (Jirtle and Skinner, 2007). Given the above factors, it is probable that certain genetic, epigenetic, and environmental factors unique to a developing fetus/neonate, are part of a multifactorial cascade of differing events that lead to pBT development. It is likely that these factors exert influences on the growth and differentiation of neural stem cells/progenitor cells, leading to the production of genetic and epigenetic changes that increase an individual's susceptibility to pBTs (Fig. 9.1).

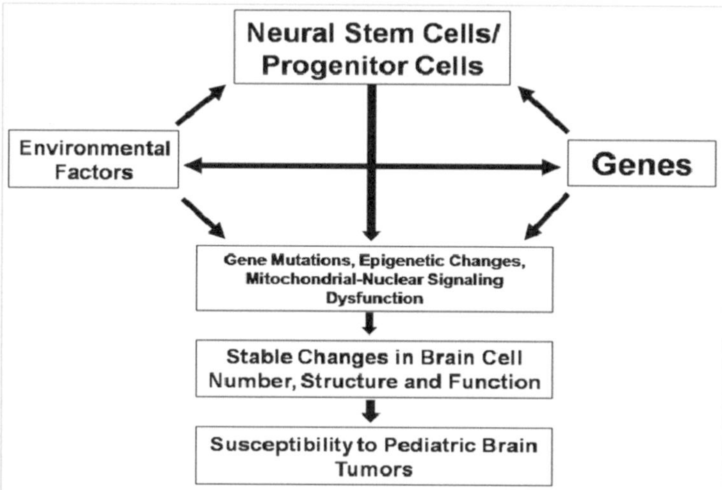

Fig. 9.1 A schematic representation of an early life gene-environment interaction model for development of pBT

The following is a review of the current state of the research on environmental, genetic, and epigenetic factors possibly involved in the development of pBTs. The first section of this review covers epidemiological research on environmental factors that have been investigated in relation to pBTs. Research supporting the involvement of neural stem cells, progenitor cells, and developmental pathways in the etiology of pBTs is then summarized. This section is followed by a brief review of the genetic and epigenetic alterations that have been identified in common pBTs, with the final section focusing on how these factors may interact with mitochondrial-nuclear signaling to increase individual susceptibility to pBTs.

9.2 Environmental Epidemiology of Pediatric Brain Tumors

9.2.1 Links Between the Environment and Traditional Epidemiology and Risk Factors

While the incidence of pBTs has been steadily increasing since the early 1980s, debate exists as to the reason for this rise, with some researchers suggesting diagnostic factors as a main cause, while others emphasize the importance of environmental factors (Hjalmars et al., 1999; McNeil et al., 2002). In the United States the recorded incidence of pBTs increased by 35% from 1973 to 1994 (Smith et al., 1998). Similar increases for these tumors were noted in Europe (Steliarova-Foucher et al., 2004) and in England (Birch et al., 2002; McNally et al., 2001). Considerable debate exists as to how much these large increases are due to an etiologic factor or the result of better diagnostic methods, improved reporting, and changes in classification (i.e. tumors earlier designated as benign being changed to malignant) (Kaiser, 1999). Supporting an increase due to better diagnostics and reporting, Smith et al. (1998) performed detailed statistical analysis which concluded that a statistical model with a "jump" in incidence in the mid 1980s fits the incidence data better than a model with a steady increase (Smith et al., 1998). A critical analysis of pBTs over this same period by Linet et al. (1999) also supported this view (Linet et al., 1999). However, some researchers remain doubtful that the increase is adequately explained with only this type of statistical analysis (Kaiser, 1999). Indeed, recent reports from Europe on childhood cancer incidence over this time period argue for a true increase in incidence over this time period (Magnani et al., 2003; Steliarova-Foucher et al., 2004), suggesting that environmental factors have played a role in this rise in incidence. Researchers have also pointed out that while incidence increases in some subgroups of pBTs can be attributed to better diagnostics and changes in classification, these changes do not explain increases in other pBTs (Jukich et al., 2001).

Although the etiology of pBTs is largely unknown, several genetic disorders are known risk factors for their development including neurofibromatosis type 1, Li-Fraumeni syndrome, basal cell nevus (Gorlin's) syndrome, Turcot syndrome, and ataxia telangiectasia. These single gene disorders are thought to play a part in less than 5% of all pBTs however. Still, epidemiological evidence does point to a genetic component in pBTs, as having a sibling or parent with brain cancer has been found to increase risk of pBTs from 3 to 9 times, while siblings of children with brain tumors have a greater risk of developing other cancers such as leukemia. These family patterns are likely due to multigenic inheritance patterns ("soft" but interacting mutations), modifiers that alter gene expression or penetrance, or epigenetic gene silencing, rather than the consequence of a highly penetrant gene (National Cancer Institute, 2000). It is also probable that common environmental factors among these family members contribute to this increased risk profile. Gender is another risk factor, as most pBTs have been found to occur at a higher frequency in males than in females, though the reason for this difference is unknown. This difference varies by tumor, as certain tumors including medulloblastoma and ependymoma show incidence rates in males 1.5–2 times that of females, while other tumor types such as astrocytoma show only small differences between these groups (Mealey and Hall, 1977; Preston-Martin et al., 2006; Schoenberg et al., 1976). While research on the subject is lacking, it is important to consider that gender-specific differences may in fact be related to gender-specific responses to a given toxicant. Other common risk factors for pBTs include race (they occur more often among Caucasians than other races) and age (they occur more often in children younger than 8 years old than in older children). Geographically, astrocytoma incidence is low in Asia, intermediate in Central and South America, and relatively higher in North America, Europe, Australia, and New Zealand. Additionally, astrocytoma is most common in Sweden, which has a rate 20% higher than any other reported rate. Similar to astrocytoma, PNET, a broad tumor group which includes medulloblastoma (MB), has incidence rates that are relatively low in Asia and higher in Europe and North America. Rates for PNET range from 2 to 12 per million year with the highest rates occurring in Hawaiians in Hawaii and Maori in New Zealand (IARC, 1998). Dietary patterns and other differences in environmental factors between these geographies could explain some of these patterns, as has been suggested in other cancers. Incidence patterns among developed and developing countries may not be comparable, as all brain tumors in developing countries may not come to medical attention and some of the low rates observed might be underestimates.

Studies in North Carolina, Japan, and Norway have found that medulloblastoma shows a statistically significant seasonal variation in incidence with a peak in October (Halperin et al., 2004; Manshande et al., 1985; Yamakawa et al., 1979). Researchers speculate that exposures during the Spring, when major fetal development would occur for these births, may be involved, including pesticide applications and use of allergic medications. Other tumor types including astrocytoma and ependymoma do not show this seasonal correlation (Hoffman et al., 2007) despite astrocytoma being the tumor most often linked with pesticide exposure. Studies have also assessed clinical parameters and their association with risk of pBTs. Findings on birthweight show only weak or null associations to pBTs, for most studies, although one study which looked at subtypes of tumors found high birthweight to cause an increased OR of 1.71 (95% CI: 1.01–2.90) for astrocytic tumors (Von and Reynolds, 2003). Head circumference has also been studied in relation to pBTs and is positively associated with their occurrence [OR = 1.27 (95% CI 1.16–1.38) per 1-cm increase in head circumference] (Samuelsen et al., 2006).

9.2.2 Epidemiologic Research on Specific Environmental Exposures and pBT

Whether specific environmental exposures cause pBTs remains unknown. Only high-intensity external ionizing radiation for therapy of childhood leukemia, tinea capitis and other malignancies is clearly associated with development of nervous system cancer (Meadows et al., 1985; Neglia et al., 1991; Ron et al., 1988); (Preston-Martin et al., 2006; Rice, 2006). Diagnostic radiography during pregnancy also appears to result in a small but significant increase in risk of pBT to the fetus, although this association is disputed (Doll and Wakeford, 1997). Neither of these exposures is thought to account for a significant number of pBTs today because diagnostic radiation has decreased in use and doseage in pregnant women (Bunin, 2004). Research over the past few decades does point to the relevancy of a few environmental exposures in pBT etiology however. A number of these exposures, including pesticides, N-nitroso compounds, and infection with polyomavirus, have been positively linked to pBT, although findings are inconclusive. While positive results have been found, the rarity of the disease, difficulty in assessing exposure during pregnancy and other critical time periods, assessment of diverse pBTs as a single type, and recall bias distort and confound results for these investigations. Several work-related exposures have been convincingly linked to aBTs however, providing support to the possibility that environmental exposures to a fetus or young child could produce pBTs. These work-related exposures include nuclear workers exposed to radiation, pathologists and embalmers exposed to formaldehyde, plastic workers exposed to vinyl chloride, and textile and plastic workers exposed to acrylonitrile (National Institutes of Health, 2002). A summary of the research on several environmental exposures and their relation to pBT is provided in Table 9.1. An overall "risk association level" for each exposure, and risk outcomes from select studies, is included.

Table 9.1 Summary of overall risk evaluation for selected environmental exposures in relation to pBT

Risk factors	Risk evaluation	Risks for exposures (OR/RR with 95% CI)
Ionizing radiation	Conclusive	– 33.1 (9.4–116.5) for benign nerve sheath tumors of head/neck (Ron et al., 1988) – 9.5 (3.5–25.7) for meningiomas (Ron et al., 1988) – 2.6 (0.8–8.6) for malignant gliomas (Ron et al., 1988) – 21.7-fold increase in central nervous system neoplasms in a large cohort of 9,720 children who had undergone radiation for leukemia (Neglia et al., 1991) – Atomic bomb exposure followed a dose-response curve [excess relative risk (ERR) = 1.2 (0.6–2.1), with the highest ERR found in relation to schwannoma 4.5 (1.9–9.2)] (Preston et al., 2002).
Pesticides	Suggestive but not conclusive	– Agricultural pesticide use and pBT risk in children aged 0–14 years [RR = 3.37 (1.63–6.94)] (Kristensen et al., 1996). – Increased risk of astrocytoma for exposure to herbicides from residential use [OR = 1.9 (1.2–3.0)] (Shim Y.K. et al., 2009)

Table 9.1 (continued)

Risk factors	Risk evaluation	Risks for exposures (OR/RR with 95% CI)
N-nitroso	Suggestive but not conclusive	– Four of eight studies on cured meat exposure found 2–2.5 times increased risk of pBT (Kuijten et al. 1990; McCredie et al. 1994; Preston-Martin et al. 1982; Preston-Martin et al., 1996) – Mother's frequent ingestion of hot dogs [RR = 1.33 (1.08–1.66)] and sausage [RR = 1.44 (1.01–2.06)] during pregnancy (Huncharek and Kupelnick 2004) – Meta-analysis of cured meat consumption [RR = 1.68 (1.30–2.17)] (Huncharek and Kupelnick 2004) – Use of metronidazole and neuroblastoma [RR = 2.60 (0.89–7.59)] (Thapa et al., 1998). – Use of narcotics [OR = 1.3 (1.0–1.6)] and the anasthic penthrane [OR = 1.5 (1.1–2.0)] during delivery (Linet et al., 1996). – Anticonvulsant use during pregnancy [OR = 1.4 (0.6–3.2)] (Gurney et al., 1997)
Infectious agents	Inconsistent or limited	– Viral infection during pregnancy [OR = 10.6 (1.1–503.2)] (Fear et al., 2001) – Influenza during gestation [OR = 3.15 (CI = 1.13–8.77)] (Linos et al., 1998) – Three siblings, or younger siblings increased risk for astrocytoma (RR = 1.34), medulloblastoma (RR = 2.30), ependymoma (RR = 2.61), meningioma (RR = 3.71), and neuroblastoma (RR = 2.31) (Altieri et al., 2006).
Tobacco	Inconsistent or limited	– Meta-analysis of 12 observational studies on maternal smoking during pregnancy [RR = 1.05 (0.90–1.21)] (Huncharek et al., 2002) – Paternal smoking exposure [RR = 1.22 (1.05–1.40)] (Huncharek et al., 2002) – Second meta-analysis on maternal smoking during pregnancy [RR = 1.04 (CI: 0.92–1.18)] (Boffetta et al., 2000).
Electro-magnetic frequencies	Inconsistent or limited	Electromagnetic frequencies and childhood exposure [OR = 0.97 (0.46–2.05)] (UK Childhood Cancer Study Investigators, 1999).
Trauma	Inconsistent or limited	Medical attention for head injury [OR = 1.4 (1.0–1.9)] (Gurney et al., 1996)
Vitamins	Inconsistent or limited	Children of mothers who used multivitamins [OR = 0.7 (0.4–1.0)] and had a diet high in iron and folate [OR for iron, 0.5 (1.3–0.9); OR for folate, 0.5 (0.3–0.9)] (Bunin et al., 2006)

9.3 Origin and Neurobiology of Pediatric Brain Tumors

Many pBTs are embryonal in nature, while carcinomas in epithelial tissues, the most frequent type of cancer in adults, are rare in children. A large amount of pediatric gliomas, the most frequent pBTs, arise in the cerebellum and brainstem (infratentorial), though gliomas located in the cerebrum (supratentorial) are also fairly common. This is in contrast to aBTs, the majority of which are located in the cerebrum. Gliomas arise from glia, non-neural cells that provide support and nutrition and participate in signal transmission in the nervous system. These tumors are usually broken down into more specific subtypes based on their predicted cell type of origin. The most common glial tumors in patients under 20 years of age are astrocytoma (from astrocytes), oligodendroglioma (from oligodendrocytes), and ependymoma (from ependymal cells). Some pBTs are composed of primitive or undifferentiated cells, as would be expected given their origin during early life when the nervous system is still developing. These include the primitive neuroectodermal tumors (PNETs) of the brain, notably medulloblastoma (MB), ependymoblastoma, and neuroblastoma (NB). One other common brain tumor, type in childhood, germ cell tumors (germinomas, embryonal cell carcinomas, choriocarcinomas, and teratomas), arise from germ cells, which are very primitive cells in the developing brain. Mixed forms of brain tumors also exist. For instance, mixed gliomas (aka oligoastrocytomas) have both an astrocytic and an oligodendroglial cell component. Additionally, mixed glio-neuronal tumors (tumors displaying a neuronal, as well as a glial component, e.g. gangliogliomas, disembryoplastic neuroepithelial tumors) and tumors originating from neuronal cells (e.g. gangliocytoma, central gangliocytoma) can also develop in the central nervous system (CNS). Other varieties of primary brain tumors include: tumors of the pineal parenchyma (e.g. pineocytoma, pineoblastoma), choroid plexus tumors, and neuroepithelial tumors of uncertain origin (e.g. gliomatosis cerebri, astroblastoma). Additionally, many subtypes of these tumors also exist and are often grouped by histological grade (i.e. Astrocytoma grades I–IV).

9.3.1 Cellular Origins of pBTs

One of the critical issues involving BT biology has been the inability to determine a definitive cell of origin of each individual tumor type, including the three most prevalent tumors of the pediatric CNS: pilocytic astrocytoma, MB, and NB. Identification of these cell types would allow for better comparisons to normal cell counterparts, and a more definitive genomic profile of the tumor cells involved. Currently, tumors are classified by the World Health Organization (WHO) according to the cell type that tumor cells resemble most in the developing embryo or adult. The three main cell types from which tumor cells are thought to arise are neural stem cells, progenitor cells, or differentiated cells, and genetic changes in each cell type have been associated with BT development (Read et al., 2006). It is likely these genetic changes, which may be either inherited or somatic in nature, deregulate normal proliferation and differentiation and initiate tumor formation. Many pBTs (which are predominantly immature tumors) may arise from neural stem cells (which produce both glial and neuronal cells) or progenitor cells in their respective precursor cell type (i.e. granule cell precursors for MBs), while most adult tumors probably form from differentiated cell types (i.e. astrocytes in astroctyoma) that have acquired stem cell-like or progenitor cell-like properties (Read et al., 2006). Recent research on MBs in mice models does in fact suggest that alterations in either cell type can produce MB, with the critical determinant of tumorigenesis being neuronal lineage commitment of the cell (Schuller et al., 2008; Yang et al., 2008). Additionally, alterations in genes such as Bmi1, an oncogene involved in proliferation of differentiated cells and self renewal of stem cells, likely lead to different phenotypic outcomes of BT (Bruggeman et al., 2007; Dirks, 2007). Also, tumors arising in different regions of the brain retain distinct patterns of gene expression, though cells in different parts of the brain carry the same genes. This is a result of factors that have modified the use of these genes differently in distinct parts of the brain, suppressing some genes and activating others to allow the cells to take on specialized characteristics as the brain matures.

Extensive debate exists within this framework however, as evidence for differing points of view exists in the literature. For example, MB having a neuronal cell of origin as suggested by Wright et al. is in contrast to a view by Bailey and Cushing, who suggested that because MBs generate both glial and neuronal cells, they may originate from a cell they termed as embryonic neuroepithelial (Bailey and Cushing, 1925; Wright, 1910). For a complete review of the current information on cell of origin in brain tumors the reader is referred to a review by Read et al. (Read et al., 2006). While the cellular origins of these tumors is still debated, recent research is beginning to elucidate how the deregulation of developmental pathways within these cells contributes to pBT etiology, and an overview of this research is provided below.

9.3.2 Disruption of Developmental Pathways, "Tumor Precursor Cells", and pBTs

Some pBTs are embryonal tumors that arise from abnormal development of nervous system tissue. Embryonal development is marked by organogenesis from stem cell populations producing "precursor" cells that give rise to lineage-committed progenitor cells. These progenitor cells then undergo stages of proliferation and differentiation to produce tissue. Several cellular pathways that regulate these developmental processes have been implicated in the development of pBT, including the Sonic Hedgehog (SHh) pathway, the WNT-wingless (WNT) pathway, Mycn signaling, and the NOTCH signaling pathway. During normal nervous system development, these signaling pathways regulate growth and differentiation of progenitor cells, including granule cell precursors (GCPs) in the cerebellum and neural crest cells in the peripheral neural system (PNS). These cell populations ultimately form the cerebellum, peripheral neural crest, and other nervous system components. In cerebellar development, SHh accomplishes regulatation of GCPs in part via expression of N-myc, a commonly expressed tumor suppressor gene thought to be an essential downstream target of Shh signaling in both normal and neoplastic cerebellar growth (Hatton et al., 2006). Mutations that dysregulate the SHh pathway can cause excessive growth and failure in cell differentiation, producing "tumor precursor cells" that predispose an individual to MB (Marino, 2005). Note that we use the term "tumor precursor cells" as a generic term for all forms of stem, precursor, or progenitor cells that have acquired tumor producing alterations. Similar to dysregulation of SHh pathway in MB, N-myc signaling appears to direct proliferation and differentiation of neural crest cells in PNS development, and its dysregulation appears to make a large contribution to development of neuroblastoma (Maris, 2005). Finally, several alterations identified in astrocytic tumors are located in genes important for normal differentiation of astroglial cells during development, including changes in several SHh pathway proteins (Katayam et al., 2002; Kinzler et al., 1988; Ligon et al., 2004). Figure 9.2 provides a schematic showing commonly mutated genes in these and other developmentally regulated pathways thought to be involved in pBT tumorigenesis. There are possible roles for environmental regulation within these pathways. For instance, regulation of N-myc by Shh is thought to occur through activation of phosphoinositide 3-kinase (PI3K), which, through downstream activation of Akt, and inactivation of glycogen synthase kinase-3β (GSK-3β) leads to stabilization of N-myc. High levels of N-myc, which are linked to cellular transformation and aggressive tumors, lead to proliferation, migration, and cell cycle activation, while reduced levels produce cell cycle exit and differentiation. Thus, when Shh signaling is activated, Akt signaling and amplification of N-myc, promotes cell survival and growth, and possibly tumor initation and promotion (Grimmer and Weiss, 2006). Interestingly, the PI3K/Akt pathway

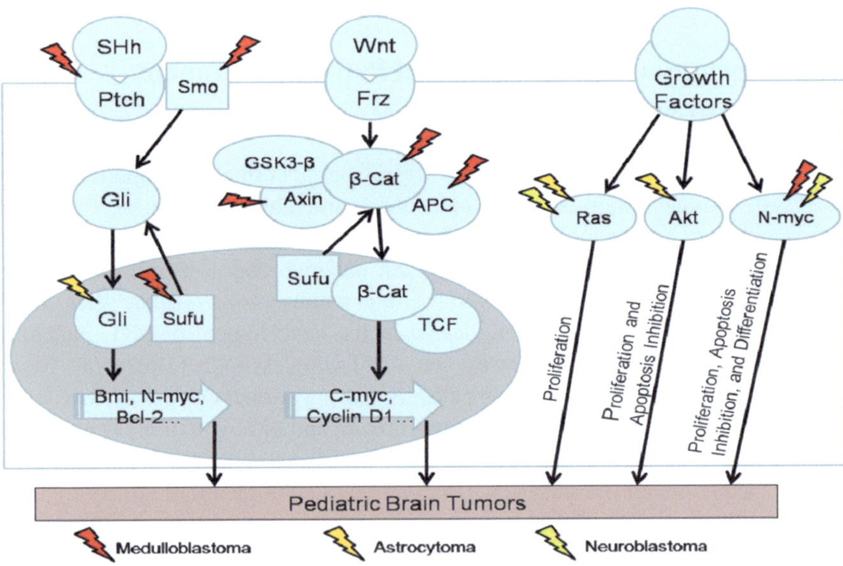

Fig. 9.2 Dysregulation of developmental pathway in pBTs. Alterations in pathways important to cellular growth, proliferation and differentiation during development appear to be important in pBT etiology. Cross-talk between these pathways has also been shown. Lightning bolts signify alterations in genes linked to development of their respective pBT

is implicated in ROS related disorders and has been linked to control of nuclear-receptor factor 1 (NRF-1) signaling in mitochondrial biogenesis (Suliman et al., 2003), linking two biological mechanisms thought to be important in environmental disease.

9.4 Genetic and Epigenetic Alterations in Pediatric Brain Tumors

The differing demographic profiles and heterogeneity within and between types of pBT suggests differing etiologies for these tumors, with genetic alterations possibly playing a more substantial role in some tumor types than in others, and individual cell types perhaps being more vulnerable to toxins at different stages of development (Baldwin and Preston-Martin, 2004). Additionally, this heterogeneity suggests the probable involvement of epigenetic and mitochondrial mechanisms of disease, both of which have been shown to interact with the environment to produce heterogeneous disease profiles (Jirtle and Skinner, 2007). Despite these probable etiologic differences, the research highlighted above suggests that many pBTs may have a common origin through in utero and early life disruption of developmental pathways. Alterations in developmental pathways do not currently account for a majority of pBTs however, and few other significant genetic changes in these tumors have been established. However, when taken as a whole, the collective alterations identified within some of the common pBTs fit a model where environmental factors interacting with numerous genetic and epigenetic changes influences cellular proliferation and function to produce tumorigenesis. As referenced in Part II, several genetic disorders have been linked to development of pBTs. Several mutations in genes causing these familial forms of pBT have been identified (Table 9.2). These genes, most of which are tumor suppressors, also appear altered in sporadic cases

Table 9.2 Disorders and mutations in genes causing familial forms of pBTs

Disorder	pNT type	Germline mutation	Locus	Signaling pathway
Neurofibromatosis type 1	Astrocytoma	NF1	17q11.2	Ras
Li-Fraumeni syndrome	Astroctyoma, PNET	p53	17p13	p53
Basal cell nevus (Gorlin's) syndrome	Medulloblastoma	PTCH	9q22.3–q31	SHh
Turcot syndrome	Medulloblastoma Malignant Glioma	APC	5q21	Wnt
Ataxia telangiectasia	Medulloblastoma Pilocytic Astrocytoma	ATM	11q22–23	ATM/p53

of their respective brain tumor types. Moreover, some also function in the developmental processes discussed above. For instance, the ataxia telangiectasia gene ATM has been shown to be pivotal for stem cell differentiation in neurodevelopment. Additionally, through interaction with the proapoptotic factor Bax, it appears to play a critical role in elimination of damaged neuronal cells in the developing CNS. Along with these predisposing genes, numerous alterations in susceptibility genes have been discovered for the sporadic forms of pBTs. Importantly, these alterations may be produced and/or influenced by environmental factors acting on the susceptible child through several different exposure routes and time periods. These include: (1) parental exposure prior to conception causing genetic alterations; (2) in utero exposure causing genetic or teratogenic effects to the fetus; (3) postnatal exposure via the mother's breast milk; (4) direct exposure of the child. Importantly, these alteration may be either a result of the exposure, or may be influenced by the exposure, and may be genetic (including chromosomal) or epigenetic in nature.

9.5 Environment, Mitochondrial-Nuclear Interactions, and Development of Pediatric Brain Tumors

Given that mutations in mtDNA have been reported in most cancers (reviewed in (Modica-Napolitano and Singh, 2002)), it appears important to consider their effect on tumorigenesis. A key argument in cancer initiation to date however, has been "what comes first, mitochondrial dysfunction or tumor formation?". Until recently, most reports have suggested that mitochondrial dysfunction occurs after tumor formation. However, research in 2000 and 2001 showing that inherited and sporadic cases of neuroendocrine tumors (paraganglioma and pheochromocytoma) are caused by mutation of succinate dehydrogenase, a mitochondrial-specific protein of the Krebs cycle, provided support to the idea that mitochondria (mt) may control tumorigenesis. Subsequently, mutations in another mitochondrial Krebs cycle protein, fumarase, were associated with the development of uterine fibroids, skin leiomyomata and renal cell cancer. Though the specific mechanisms for tumor formation in these instances are yet to be determined, it has been suggested that accumulation of these proteins in mitochondria could lead to a decrease in the ROS-scavenging activity of the respiratory chain, causing excess superoxide and tumor initiation (Rustin, 2002). Importantly, it appears mutations in either the mitochondrial or nuclear genomes could lead to tumorigenesis, as alterations in both genomes have been shown to lead to mitochondrial diseases (Enns and Criddle, 1977; Larsson and Luft, 1999). Alterations in the epigenome of both the nucleus and mitochondria may also play a role in tumorigenesis, as recent research demonstrating that depletion of mtDNA can regulate epigenetic modification in the nucleus suggests (Smiraglia et al., 2008). These tumorigenic scenarios described above fit well with a model where both cell death and proliferation are in large part controlled by the functioning state of the mitochondria. In this model, the redox state of the cell would be of ultimate importance to development of disease. While a low level of ROS would allow for normal cellular function, increasing ROS amounts would signal increased cell proliferation, and an overwhelming excess of ROS would trigger apoptosis. Importantly, research showing that mtDNA-depleted cells increased antioxidant levels (MnSOD) and resisted apoptosis even in an elevated ROS environment, suggest that mitochondrial apoptosis pathways may often be blocked even in dysregulated mitochondria, allowing for cellular transformation to occur (Park et al., 2004). Given that interaction between mitochochdrial and nuclear genomes is essential for normal cellular function, variations in the mitochondrial redox state could be of tremendous importance for the fate of the cell, and ROS signaling could have a central role in communication between mitochondria and the nucleus.

Because mitochondria play a large part in brain development (Erecinska et al., 2004) and are abundant in brain tissue (Lerman-Sagie et al., 2005), their health is critical to the wellbeing of the pediatric brain. The pediatric brain is at high risk of oxidative stress and very susceptible to free radical oxidative damage (Buonocore et al., 2001). The electron transport chain (ETC) found in brain mitochondria can be impaired by both inherited and acquired mutations. An impaired ETC leads to decreased ATP production, increased ROS formation, and altered calcium homeostasis. Thus, mutations in mitochondrial DNA (mtDNA) and nuclear DNA (nDNA) could affect cellular energy levels, increase oxidative stress, cause ROS-mediated damage to both the mitochondrial and nuclear genome, affect cellular differentiation, and alter the cellular response to apoptosis (Carew and Huang, 2002; Copeland et al., 2002; Delsite et al., 2003; Penta et al., 2001). Figure 9.3 provides a schematic overview of how environmental factors could interact with dysfunction in mitochondrial-nuclear signaling pathways and developmental pathways to produce pBTs.

9.5.1 *Effects of Early Life Exposures on Mitochondria and the Pediatric Brain*

There is a growing body of evidence suggesting that there are critical periods of time extending from conception to puberty when the reproductive (Lemasters et al., 2000), immune (Dietert et al., 2000), nervous (Lemasters et al., 2000), and endocrine (Sadler, 2000) systems in children may be more affected by chemical exposures. In fact, a consensus group has concluded that there is sufficient evidence to support the hypothesis that in utero and early life exposures can lead to cancer in both children and adults (Olshan et al., 2000). Evidence supporting this conclusion includes experimental findings that suggests tumors initiated in utero can be promoted postnatally, resulting in cancerous growths (Autrup, 1993). Additionally, the ability of environmental exposures to cause micronuclei, chromosomal aberrations, sister chromatic exchanges, DNA adducts, DNA single-strand breaks, and somatic mutations in the DNA of a fetus has been demonstrated (reviewed in Neri et al., 2003; 2006).

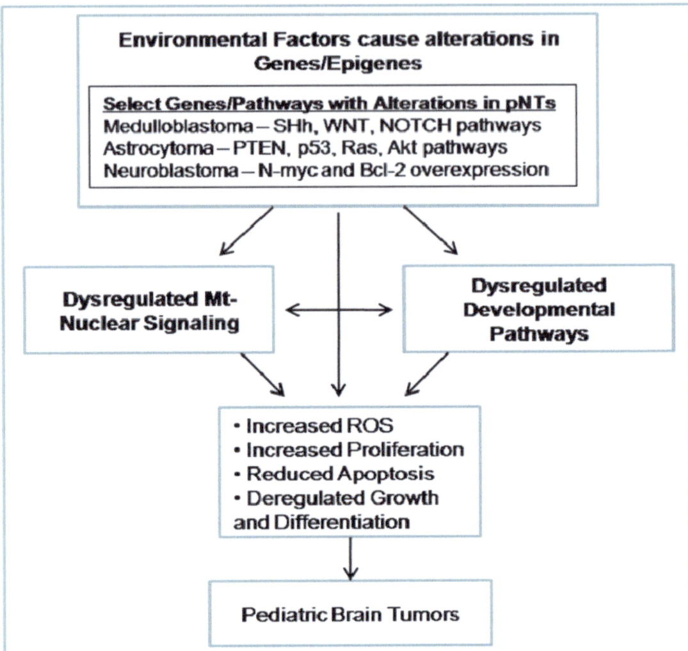

Fig. 9.3 Interaction of environmental factors, dysregulation of mt-nuclear signaling and developmental pathways, and development of pBT

Several characteristics of the developing brain in pediatrics may make agents normally thought not to target the central nervous system harmful to the brain during these critical time periods. These include the blood-brain barrier of the fetus being incompletely developed, the immune system being compromised due to its immaturity, and the increased vulnerability of the developing nervous system to carcinogenosis (Rice and Ward, 1982). Furthermore, several factors including high rates of cell division, lowered detoxification capabilities, and clonal expansion of initiated cells are thought to explain the increased sensitivity of embryos, fetuses, and newborns to chemical carcinogens (reviewed in Anderson et al., 2000). Many carcinogens, including ENU, cadmium, and monosodium glutamate, have been shown to freely traverse the blood-brain barrier of a developing fetus in experimental animals, while being blocked from entering the mature brain (Branstetter et al., 1987; Rodier, 1995). Furthermore, numerous agents including rubella virus, lead, methylmercury, retinoids and thalidomide have been shown to be neurotoxic when exposure occurs during gestation. These same agents show no neurotoxicity after adult exposures (Rodier, 1995). Though few quantitative studies on this topic have been completed, one study assessing the blood-brain barrier of sheep during the last 2 months of gestation and the first month of neonatal compared to adult animals found that the influx of radioactive compounds in all regions of the brain decreased significantly with maturation ($p < 0.0001$). A more in depth review on this topic has been published by Adinolfi, 1985. (Adinolfi, 1985)

9.5.2 Experimental Evidence Linking Early Life Exposures to Mitochondrial Dysfunction and pBT Development

The effects of environmental exposures on BT development have been studied both in vitro and in animal models. Several studies have investigated manganese toxicity in brain tumor cell lines. Manganese (Mn) exposure in humans is rare but can occur through occupational pathways. Mn targets brain mitochondria and interferes with energy metabolism in both astrocyoma and neuroblastoma cells through reduction of activity of glycolytic and TCA enzymes such as hexokinase, pyruvate kinase, lactate dehydrogenase, citrate synthase, and malate dehydrogenase (Malthankar et al., 2004). As a result of this metabolic change, Mn exposure may increase oxidative stress via activation of the mitochondrial permeability transition pore (mPTP), a result found in Mn exposed astrocytes (Rao et al., 2004). Manganese-induced cell death in both astroctyoma and neuroblastoma cells is primarily necrotic in nature and is enhanced by glutathione depletion (Dukhande et al., 2006). Interestingly, neuroblastoma cells are more susceptible to Mn toxicity than GBM cells, possibly because of Mn treatments effects on apoptosis in GBM cells. When used to treat GBM cells, Mn increases apoptosis and has differential effects on proliferation pathways as it induces down-regulation of MAPK pathway, but does not significantly affect the AKT pathway. Furthermore, Mn reduces levels of c-Jun, c-Fos, and MMP-2 (an extracellular matrix degrading enzyme), which are all associated with invasiveness of GBM (Malthankar et al., 2004).

An in vitro study investigating the effect of chlorpyrifos exposure on glioma cells found that the cell signaling interference produced by chlorpyrifos exposure was greater in undifferentiated cells compared to differentiating cells, though effects were still noticed on this cell type as well. However, differentiation enhanced reactive oxygen species (ROS) production from chlorpyrifos exposure and provoked shortage of the nuclear transcription factor Sp1, an essential molecule in differentiation (Garcia et al., 2001). Other in vitro studies include a report which found selenium levels in the cerebrospinal fluid of patients with malignant brain tumors to be lower than those with benign tumors. Furthermore, selenium's anticancer effects are seen in its ability to preferentially target human glioma cells for cell death through induction of superoxide and its subsequent disruption of mitochondria (Kim et al., 2007).

In vivo studies showing environmental exposure effects on BT have been performed on several animal species. Studies in rats and mice showing transplacental induction of BT from chemical exposures have mainly produced glial tumors (most commonly oligodendrogliomas), with some meningeal tumors being induced as well, and peripheral nervous tumors only rare occurences. Significant incidences of BTs in rats using long-term bioassays have also been produced through exposure to acrylonitrile, acrylamide, 1,3-butadiene, ethylene oxide, glycidol, and isoprene; the alkylating agents1,3-propane sultone and 2-methylaziridine; and several hydrazine derivatives including 1,2-diethylhydrazine (Rice and Wilbourn, 2000). Studies in mice show increased susceptibility to brain mutations for prenatal and neonatal (N-ethyl-N-nitrosourea) ENU-exposed mice over adult ENU-exposed mice (Slikker et al., 2004). It should be noted that while numerous tumor types have been produced from transplacental exposure of rodents, most tumors are not of embryonal origin, but instead are of glial origin and only become clinically evident in adult rats. Other in vivo studies have found that phenothiazine chlorpromazine can cause CNS abnormalities in the fetus while cadmium has been shown to be toxic to sensory ganglia in many animal species.

Experiments on mitochondrial function in the nervous system point to their involvement in environmentally-induced BTs. Because mitochondria are the main source of superoxide in physiologic conditions, the detoxification of superoxide by mitochondrial MnSOD plays an important role in neuroprotection and ROS homeostasis (Robertson et al., 2006). Even a modest increase in endogenous ROS could damage both mtDNA and nDNA, leading to cancer development, genetic instability, and disease progression. MnSOD has been shown to have high activity in mice brain when compared to other tissues such as lungs (Van et al., 1999). Because the MnSOD by-product H_2O_2 is itself a ROS, it is interesting to note that overexpression of MnSOD in rat glioma cells increased risk for oxidative damage (Zhong et al., 1996). However, loss of MnSOD also produces neurodegeneration, DNA oxidative damage and mitochondrial respiratory chain abnormalities, indicating that both overexpression and underexpression of MnSOD can be harmful (Melov et al., 1995). A more focused discussion on mitochondrial ROS production and its effects on the pediatric nervous system is provided below.

9.5.3 Mitochondrial ROS, Electron Transport Chain Defects, and Pediatric Susceptibility

Mitochondrial ETC disorders are believed to occur with an incidence of 1/10,000 live births and research correlates increases in mitochondrial ROS production with both neurodegenerative disease and cancer in animal models (Aleardi et al., 2005; Kontush, 2001). In fact, the importance of ROS levels and pBT development can be seen in the fact that numerous genes and signal transduction pathways important to normal fetal brain development (i.e. myc) can be influenced by ROS (Calabrese et al., 2000; Thannickal and Fanburg, 2000). While no studies to date have been published on age-dependent differences in brain mitochondrial ROS production in immature animals, research has documented developmental disparities in antioxidant defense systems. Both Mavelli et al. (Mavelli et al., 1982) and Khan et al. (Khan et al., 2003) reported increases in mitochondrial MnSOD in the first weeks of life in mice. Mavelli et al. reported no significant changes with age for Cu,Zn-SOD or GPX activity, while catalase activities were inconclusive. On the contrary,

Khan et al. did report an increase in GPX activity near birth. One report also noted a developmental lag in SOD-1 and SOD-2 when compared with GPX and catalase levels present in prenatal telecephalic white matter (Folkerth et al., 2004). On the whole, the above studies describe a profile where a newborn brain must be protected from oxidative stress through increased activity of antioxidant enzymes in utero and around birth.

The large transmembrane protein cytochrome *c* oxidase (aka complex IV or COX) is the last enzyme in the ETC of mitochondria. This complex catalyzes the transfer of electrons from reduced COX to molecular oxygen to form water, and ultimately, ATP through the coupled process of oxidative phosphorylation. The importance of COX to neurons is seen in this enzyme's reduced expression in neurodegenerative diseases, such as Alzheimer disease (Manczak et al., 2006). This is because neurons, which are highly dependent upon ATP for their activity and functions (Wong-Riley, 1989), receive roughly 90% of their ATP from mitochondria via oxidative phosphorylation (Gunter and Gunter, 1994). MtDNA diseases exhibit low COX activity and evidence points to clonal expansion of individual mtDNA deletions within single cells as a reason for this decreased action (Cottrell et al., 2000). Moreover, COX deficiency most often manifests in high energy demand organs, such as the brain (Lerman-Sagie et al., 2005), and is the most prominent ETC defect in infancy and early childhood (Rahman et al., 2001).

Finally, Tfam, a key regulator of mtDNA copy number and mitochondrial transcription, and a gene associated with a moderate risk for Alzheimer's disease (Gunther et al., 2004), may play a key role in mtDNA-related disease. Evidence suggests Tfam protects against mtDNA damage by preventing a decrease in mtDNA copy number and ETC function. This action may ultimately protect against oxidative stress and its effects on lipid peroxidation, apoptosis, and mtDNA (Kang et al., 2007). Importantly, Tfam, appears to accomplish much of these actions through interaction with NRF-1 and other nuclear genes controlling mitochondrial biogenesis and function (Roy et al., 2007; Scarpulla, 2008; Taanman, 1999). While these while nuclear proteins contribute to mitochondrial regulation, mitochondria can also modulate the expression of nuclear cell cycle genes (Roy et al., 2007), suggesting the importance of cross-talk between the cell nucleus and mitochondria in the apoptosis, proliferation, and differentiation of both normal and malignant cells. We now discuss possible implications of this cross-talk on pBT development.

9.5.4 Evidence of Mitochondrial-Nuclear Interactions and Mitochondrial Dysfunction in pBTs

Recent evidence is beginning to provide support for a model of mitchochondrial-nuclear signaling dysfunction in formation of tumors, including pBTs. Studies in yeast models and human cancer cell models showed that depletion of mtDNA increased oxidative stress which then produced extensive damage to the nuclear genome (Delsite et al., 2003; Rasmussen et al., 2003). Additionally, it appears that expression of certain nuclear genes may play a key role in mitochondrial mediated tumorigenesis. In fact, APE1, a nuclear encoded gene involved in redox regulation, apoptosis, and DNA repair (both independently and through interaction with p53), may be one such gene, as it was shown to be underexpressed in 68% (13 of 19) of CNS tumors (Singh et al., 2005). It appears mitochondrial defects can lead to down regulation of APE1 to produce tumors. Restoration of expression of APE1 in mtDNA depleted cells reversed the tumorigenic feature of anchorage independence, suggesting that restoration of mtDNA could reverse tumorigenesis in these cells. Significantly, DNA binding activity of genes regulated by APE1 is sensitive to reduction-oxidation (redox). Proteins for which APE1 functions as a transcriptional cofactor include AP-1 (Fos, Jun) proteins, nuclear factor-κB (NF-κB), polyoma virus enhancer-binding protein, early growth response-1, Myb members of the ATF/CREB family, HIF-1α, HIF-like factor, Oak5 and Pax-8 (Evans et al., 2000; Singh et al., 2005). Interestingly, AP1 and NF-κB have been shown to mediate the expression of proteins involved in neuronal function and survival (Evans et al., 2000; Xanthoudakis and Curran, 1996). APE1 itself has been shown to promote survival of neurons after oxidative stress (Vasko et al., 2005) and to be essential for proper embryonic development (Xanthoudakis and Curran, 1996). Additionally, APE1 has been shown to repair DNA, influence apoptosis, and interact with p53, a protein found upregulated in many cancers, including many pBTs.

The above evidence highlights a nuclear protein (APE1) and its links to redox signaling in pBT development. We now present other evidence of mitochondrial dysfunction in pBT, first on mitochondrial genome alterations, and then on mitochondrial apoptotic pathways.

Identified alterations in the mitochondrial genome of BTs. Several features distinguish the mitochondrial and nuclear genomes, some of which allow mtDNA to be far more vulnerable to mutations than nDNA. mtDNA's lack of histone protection, limited repair capacity, and close proximity to the electron transport chain (and hence superoxide radicals), are a few major reasons for this increased susceptibility to damage. While mtDNA is more vulnerable to damage, the fact that only a small percentage of its proteins are coded by mtDNA increases the chances that a mutation that affects mitochondrial function will occur in chromosomal DNA. In fact, of over 3,000 mitochondrial proteins, mtDNA only encodes (1) 13 subunits of respiratory chain complexes: seven subunits (ND 1–6 and 4L) of complex I, cytochrome b (Cyt b) of complex III, the COX I–III subunits of cytochrome oxidase or complex IV, ATPase 6 and 8 subunits of F_OF_1 ATP synthase; (2) the 12S and 16S rRNA genes; and (3) 22 tRNA genes. The remainder of the proteins are encoded by nDNA and imported into the mitochondria by chaperones. Still, somatic mtDNA mutations have been linked to several cancers, and while their contribution to tumorigenesis has been debated, recent studies have concluded that mutant mitochondria positively and directly contribute to tumorigenesis by preventing apoptosis (Ohta, 2006). Additionally, novel research showing depletion of mtDNA encoded OXPHOS genes plays a role in tumor cell transformation supports the involvement of mtDNA alterations and depletion in tumorigenesis (Kulawiec et al., 2008). Here we review alterations in mtDNA that have been observed in the mitochondrial genome of both pediatric and adult BTs.

The D-loop region of mitochondria is a region important for replication and mt nucleoid organization found mutated in many cancers. Several BTs, including meningiomas, schwannomas, gliomatosis cerebri, neurofibroma and astrocytoma, including GBMs, have been shown to have mitochondrial genome instability in the hypervariable regions of the D-loop. Somatic mtDNA mutations of this region have been found in tumors of NF1, a familial disease which predisposes to development of pilocytic astrocytoma (Kurtz et al., 2004). Astrocytic tumors themselves, in fact contain mutations in this region. A recent study of 42 cases of malignant astrocytomas (39 GBMs, two anaplastic astrocytomas, and one anaplastic oligoastrocytoma) showed alterations in 36% of the cases in the D-loop region, including 16 different somatic alterations [three in the hypervariable 1 region (HV1) and thirteen in the D310 region] (Montanini et al., 2005). This frequency is comparable to other reports of mtDNA instability in malignant gliomas (Kirches et al., 1999; Vega et al., 2004). These alterations do not appear to be associated with increased aggressiveness (Montanini et al., 2005). Furthermore, somatic mtDNA mutations have been observed in a series of chemically induced and spontaneous mouse brain tumors in regions that correspond to the hypervariable regions of human mtDNA, though they do not appear to alter the amino acid sequence and therefore may not affect disease status (Kiebish and Seyfried, 2005).

Studies have also found mitochondrial mutations in other regions of the mitochondria as well. One study which analyzed the entire mitochondrial genome of 15 cases of MB and the cerebrospinal fluid (CSF) of eight of these 15 cases, found that 40% (6 of 15) of the tumors and 87.5% (7 of 8) of the CSF samples had at least one mtDNA mutation. The somatic mutations identified in this study, which were located primarily in regions of mononucleotide repeats, but also in respiratory chain related genes, include: three coding region mutations (1) G7521A mutation in tRNA aspartate that changes a GT base pairing to an AT base pairing at the amino acyl stem region, (2) the T15904C mutation in tRNA threonine at the loop region, and (3) the A15937G mutation at the first bp next to the loop, all of which may affect tRNA structure and stability; two missense mutations that can alter mt structure and function: (1) Y496H in cytochrome c oxidase and (2) L96P in NADH subunit 4, which are involved in the substitution of the hydrophobic aromatic tyrosine with positively charged histidine, and the hydrophobic leucine residue with helix destabilizing secondary amino acid proline; and several noncoding region mutations in areas such as transcription factor binding sites and replication primer sites that can affect mtDNA replication, transcription, and expression. Five (29.4%) mutations were located in the np 303–315 polyC tract region and 11 (61%) were in the previously discussed D-loop region.

Studies have also identified other alterations in BTs, with the most frequent observation involving changes in the copy number of mtDNA. A study that examined 45 glioma specimens found that mtDNA was highly amplified in 87% of the cases. In comparison, a nuclear-encoded reference gene (erb-b) that is frequently amplified in human cancers, increased in only 18% of the tumor specimens, indicating that mtDNA alterations may be much more frequent in gliomas than nuclear-encoded gene alterations. In addition, a high frequency of mtDNA copy number changes has been found in comparison to normal control tissue in both low and high grade gliomas. Furthermore, the mt content of gliomas is significantly lower than normal rat brain tissue, as is activity levels of cytochrome c oxidase and citrate synthase. Differential hybridization experiments have also revealed decreased expression of seven mt genes in GBM tumors. Genes downregulated were mt NADH dehydrogenase subunits 1 and 4 (ND1; ND4); mt cytochrome oxidase subunits I, II, and III (COXI; COXII; COXIII); mt ATP synthase subunit 6 (ATP6); and mt 12S rRNA. Regardless of their functional significance, the above studies clearly show that mtDNA alterations are a frequent event in the development and progression of brain disease pathologies and warrant further investigation.

Mitochondrial-directed apoptosis and pBTs. Defects in the regulation of apoptosis (programmed cell death) can contribute to development of cancer by a failure to eliminate harmful cells. The mitochondria's link to control of apoptosis could play an important role in pBT etiology, as most tumors are often relatively resistant to the induction of the mPTP, the rate-limiting step of the intrinsic pathway of apoptosis. Mitochondria play a large role in apoptosis, with their intermembrane space acting as a storage site for numerous proapoptotic proteins, including cytochrome c and apoptosis-inducing factor (AIF). Both oxidative stress and mitochondrial calcium (Ca^{2+}) overload can favor activation of the mPTP leading to release of cytochrome c and the induction of caspase-mediated apoptosis (Stavrovskaya and Kristal, 2005). In addition, as mentioned above, a more specific pathway to apoptosis exists in which Bcl-2 family proteins (e.g. Bax, Bid) regulate cytochrome c release by binding to the outer mitochondrial membrane. Other proteins involved in apoptosis, such as AIF, endonuclease G, and Smac/Diablo are also released in this process (Robertson et al., 2004). It appears environmental factors may be important in determining which apoptotic pathway is chosen; as research on the ERK signaling pathway shows that H_2O_2-induced apoptosis in glioma cells may be initiated upstream of the mitochondria (Lee et al., 2005). In contrast, a study investigating exposure of neuroblastoma cells to thimerosal, an organomercury compound used in vaccines, found that apoptosis was induced through the cytochrome c/capsase mitochondrial cascade described above (Humphrey et al., 2005). Additionally, experiments on the proapoptotic Apoptosis Related Protein in TGF beta Signaling Pathway (ARTS) using astrocytic tumors also point to mitochondrial-mediated apoptosis in brain tumors (Gottfried et al., 2004).

Selective programmed apoptosis is an important part of normal brain development. In fact, more than 50% of some neuronal populations actually die during the pre- and postnatal period (Raff et al., 1993). Several major apoptotic pathways, working through the mitochondria, play a major role in these early developmental processes, and their dysregulation may affect risk of pBT development. The Bcl-2/Bax, cytochrome c complex governs apoptosis by controlling the cytochrome c levels via the mitochondrial permeability transition pore (mPTP) of the mitochondria. The anti-apoptotic Bcl-2 protein strongly protects against free radical-mediated cell death by preventing release of cytochrome c, while other members of the bcl family (i.e. Bax) promote apoptosis (Reed, 1997). Studies have shown Bcl-2 expression levels in the neocortex and hippocampus of the developing rat to be extremely elevated during development and the first week of life. These levels then show a rapid decrease to low levels in childhood and relatively non-existent levels in adulthood (Ferrer et al., 1994). Caspases, which can be activated by the Bcl-2/cytochrome c complex, also regulate many aspects of apoptosis during development. It appears the interplay between these systems during development may be important in the etiology of brain-related disorders as deletion of caspase-3, -9, or Apaf-1 in mice results in gross malformations specific to the brain because of defective apoptosis and hyperplasia (Marks and Berg, 1999). Furthermore, recent evidence shows that SHh signaling promotes survival of medulloblastoma cells via up-regulation of Bcl-2, linking a developmental pathway and mitochondrial-mediated apoptosis to pBT development (Bar et al., 2007).

9.6 Population Studies on Gene–Environment Interactions in Pediatric Brain Tumors

Very few epidemiological studies to date have investigated GEI in relation to BT development, especially in pediatric populations. To date, only one epidemiologic study has assessed the affect of environmental interactions with gene mutations on development of pBT. In this study, two frequent polymorphisms in Paraoxonase (PON1), a gene that metabolizes two residential insecticides (chlorpyrifos and diazinon), were investigated in relation to BT [n = astrocytoma (37), PNET (15), other (14)]. A nonsignificantly increased risk of pBT in relation to the inefficient PON1 promoter allele was found [$PON1_{-108T}$ allele, relative to $PON1_{-108CC}$: odds ratio (OR) = 1.4; 95% CI, 1.0–2.2; p-value for trend = 0.07] was found. However, this association was strongest, and reached statistical significance, among children whose mothers reported chemical treatment of the home for pests during pregnancy or childhood ($PON1_{-108T}$ allele: among exposed, OR = 2.6; 95% CI, 1.2–5.5; among unexposed, OR = 0.9; 95% CI, 0.5–1.6) and when PNETs were assessed alone (per $PON1_{-108T}$ allele: OR = 2.4; 95% CI, 1.1–5.4) (Searles et al., 2005).

In addition to the above GEI study on pBT, two studies have assessed GEI in adult glioma. A case-control study on lead exposure, the lead toxicity associated gene δ-aminolevulinic acid dehydratase (ALAD), and risk of brain tumors found increased risk of meningioma with occupational lead exposure. Risk of meningioma, a tumor present mainly in later life, was markedly increased in individuals with the ALAD2 variant allele, for whom risks increased in a dose dependent fashion from 1.1 (0.3–4.5) to 5.6 (0.7–45.5) and 12.8 (1.4–120.8) compared to unexposed persons. Risk for glioma was not associated with occupational lead exposure (Rajaraman et al., 2006). A second adult GEI study on glutathione transferases (GST) polymorphisms, cigarette smoke exposure, and development of adult glioma failed to find any significant GEI (Schwartzbaum et al., 2007). Several other studies have investigated genes involved in detoxification of carcinogens and their relation to both pBT and aBT development, but exposures were not considered in these studies. Polymorphisms in the carcinogen metabolizing genes GSTM1, GSTP1, and GSTT1 have been investigated for their effect on risk of pBT. The frequency of the GSTM1 null allele was found to be significantly lower in high-grade pediadtric astrocytomas ($p < 0.002$). Additionally, a significant increase in the frequency of the rare GSTP1 variant Val114/Val114 was found in all pediatric astrocytomas combined ($p < 0.002$) and all pediatric brain tumor types that displayed microsatellite instability (MSI) from mismatch repair (MMR) defects (0.003), suggesting this genotype may define a population susceptible to pBT development. This same study assessed these polymorphisms in relation to aBT and found no relation of GST polymorphisms to tumor development (Ezer et al., 2002). Another study found the relative risk of pBT to be increased 4.9-fold for patients carrying one nonnull (GSTM1*A) allele of GSTM1 compared to patients with two null alleles (95% confidence interval 1.5–16, $P = 0.009$) (Barnette et al., 2004). Finally, a meta-analysis on GST polymorphisms and aBT tumor risk also failed to find any association between GST and tumor development, though the GSTT1 null genotype was associated with meningioma development (OR = 1.95; 95% CI, 1.02–3.76) (Lai et al., 2005).

Population studies on folate involvement in BT development have also been performed. Folate is an important micronutrient molecule involved in DNA synthesis and methylation. Studies have linked folate deficiency with both pediatric cancer (Krajinovic et al., 2004; Thompson et al., 2001) and genomic damage (Duthie and Dobson, 1999). Disturbances in DNA synthesis, methylation, and repair of this pathway may be involved in BT development (Cadieux et al., 2006). An investigation of single nucleotide polymorphisms (SNPs) in the folate pathway [methylenetetrahydrofolate reductase (MTHFR) C677Tand A1298C, methionine synthase (MTR) A2756G, thymidylate synthase (TS) 28-bp tandem repeat, and reduced folate carrier (RFC) G80A] and their relation to NT susceptibility in pediatrics found that the homozygous CC allele of MTHFR A1298C, which reduces MTHFR activity, conferred an increased risk of BT (medulloblastoma, pinealoblastoma, and PNETs) (OR: 3.9; 95% CI: 1.3–11.4, $p = 0.02$). SNPs in glial tumors (astrocytoma, oligodendroglioma, and ependymoma) were not related to development of disease (Sirachainan et al., 2008). A recent report on folate pathway SNPs in adult meningioma and high grade glioma found that MTHFR C677T and A1298C genotypes associated with increased 5,10 methylenetetrahydrofolate levels elevated disease risk while another report on these tumors failed to associate the MTHFR 677T SNP with tumor development (Kafadar et al., 2006). Dietary influence on brain tumors also find support in animal models as incidence and degree of aggressiveness of gliomas has been shown to be influenced by dietary supplementation of rats with phytochemicals. Rats fed a diet high in phytochemicals show both reduced incidence and aggressiveness of tumors, and are associated with an increase in bcl-II and catalase and a decrease in ki-67, sod-1 and sod-2 transcripts (Pouliquen et al., 2008). This result correlates with an epidemiologal study on adult glioma which showed reduced risk of glioma for those consuming a diet high in phytoestrogens (Tedeschi-Blok et al., 2006).

9.7 Conclusions

There is a growing body of scientific evidence suggesting that there are critical periods of time extending from conception to puberty when the central nervous system in children may be more affected by toxic exposures. While only 1% of pediatric brain tumors are diagnosed at birth or in the first few months of life, the majority of pBTs occur early in childhood, strongly suggesting that both prenatal and postnatal exposures may be involved in their etiology. These exposures likely interact with the genome/epigenome of the fetus or young child to produce alterations in their genetic makeup which can predispose to development of disease including pBTs. Importantly, the ability of environmental exposures to cause micronuclei, chromosomal aberrations, sister chromatic exchanges, DNA adducts, DNA single-strand breaks, and somatic mutations in the DNA of a fetus has been demonstrated. Furthermore, many of these alterations have been shown to predispose to tumor development, and it is likely they play a role in pBT etiology. We have also highlighted a role for both developmental pathway alteration and mitochondrial dysfunction in the etiology of these tumors. It is likely, that pBTs result from the interplay of environmental factors with these biological mechanisms at critical developmental periods in a child's life.

Although past research has elucidated several potentially significant environmental, genetic and epigenetic factors in pBTs, evidence linking a majority of pBTs to specific genetic or environmental exposures is limited. Factors such as the relatively low numbers of accessible tumor tissue for pBTs and the heterogeneity of these tumors have contributed to the considerable difficulty involved with determining their etiologies. Moreover, most epidemiological research on these tumors has not considered important factors such as timing of exposure, gene–environment interaction, and gene–gene interaction within their design. Additionally, the ability to appropriately measure levels of exposure at time of development or predisposition to disease through molecular biomarkers has been limited. Improved research methods and tools, combined with larger studies involving homogenous tumor types, should help answer questions on the etiology of pBTs in the future.

While several genetic disorders have been linked to development of pBTs, it is possible that many pBTs are a result of low-penetrant gene alterations in common pathways. Importantly, alterations and pathways that may be important to etiology in certain tumor types may not play a role in other pBT types. It is possible that heterogeneity in alterations and even pathways exists within tumor groups as well. Identification of which pathways are most significant in the etiology of each pBT type may contribute to the development of novel therapies for these tumors. While therapies for single gene mutations have been successful in the past for certain cancers, it appears that therapies based on pathway inhibition will prove to be more successful in the treatment of tumors that have several mutations throughout a pathway such as pBTs.

References

Adinolfi M. 1985. The development of the human blood-CSF-brain barrier. Dev Med Child Neurol 27: 532–537.

Aleardi AM, Benard G, Augereau O, Malgat M, Talbot JC, Mazat JP, et al. 2005. Gradual alteration of mitochondrial structure and function by beta-amyloids: importance of membrane viscosity changes, energy deprivation, reactive oxygen species production, and cytochrome c release. J Bioenerg Biomembr 37: 207–225.

Anderson LM, Diwan BA, Fear NT, Roman E. 2000. Critical windows of exposure for children's health: cancer in human epidemiological studies and neoplasms in experimental animal models. Environ Health Perspect 108(Suppl 3): 573–594.

Autrup H. 1993. Transplacental transfer of genotoxins and transplacental carcinogenesis. Environ Health Perspect 101(Suppl 2): 33–38.

Bailey P, Cushing H. 1925. Medulloblastoma cerebelli: a common type of midcerebellar glioma of childhood. Arch Neurol Psychiatry 14: 192–223.

Baldwin RT, Preston-Martin S. 2004. Epidemiology of brain tumors in childhood–a review. Toxicol Appl Pharmacol 199: 118–131.

Bar EE, Chaudhry A, Farah MH, Eberhart CG. 2007. Hedgehog signaling promotes medulloblastoma survival via Bc/II. Am J Pathol 170: 347–355.

Barnette P, Scholl R, Blandford M, Ballard L, Tsodikov A, Magee J, et al. 2004. High-throughput detection of glutathione s-transferase polymorphic alleles in a pediatric cancer population. Cancer Epidemiol Biomarkers Prev 13: 304–313.

Birch JM, Alston RD, Kelsey AM, Quinn MJ, Babb P, McNally RJ. 2002. Classification and incidence of cancers in adolescents and young adults in England 1979–1997. Br J Cancer 87: 1267–1274.

Branstetter DG, Stoner GD, Schut HA, Senitzer D, Conran PB, Goldblatt PJ. 1987. Ethylnitrosourea-induced transplacental carcinogenesis in the mouse: tumor response, DNA binding, and adduct formation. Cancer Res 47: 348–352.

Brodeur GM, Castleberry RP. 1997. Neuroblastoma. In: Principles and practice of pediatric oncology (Pizzo PA, Poplack DG, eds.). Philadelphia, PA: Lippincott, 761–797.

Bruggeman SW, Hulsman D, Tanger E, Buckle T, Blom M, Zevenhoven J, et al. 2007. Bmi1 controls tumor development in an Ink4a/Arf-independent manner in a mouse model for glioma. Cancer Cell 12: 328–341.

Bunin GR. 2004. Nongenetic causes of childhood cancers: evidence from international variation, time trends, and risk factor studies. Toxicol Appl Pharmacol 199: 91–103.

Buonocore G, Perrone S, Bracci R. 2001. Free radicals and brain damage in the newborn. Biol Neonate 79: 180–186.

Cadieux B, Ching TT, VandenBerg SR, Costello JF. 2006. Genome-wide hypomethylation in human glioblastomas associated with specific copy number alteration, methylenetetrahydrofolate reductase allele status, and increased proliferation. Cancer Res 66: 8469–8476.

Calabrese V, Copani A, Testa D, Ravagna A, Spadaro F, Tendi E, et al. 2000. Nitric oxide synthase induction in astroglial cell cultures: effect on heat shock protein 70 synthesis and oxidant/antioxidant balance. J Neurosci Res 60: 613–622.

Carew JS, Huang P. 2002. Mitochondrial defects in cancer. Mol Cancer 1: 9.

Copeland WC, Wachsman JT, Johnson FM, Penta JS. 2002. Mitochondrial DNA alterations in cancer. Cancer Invest 20: 557–569.

Cottrell DA, Ince PG, Blakely EL, Johnson MA, Chinnery PF, Hanna M, et al. 2000. Neuropathological and histochemical changes in a multiple mitochondrial DNA deletion disorder. J Neuropathol Exp Neurol 59: 621–627.

Delsite RL, Rasmussen LJ, Rasmussen AK, Kalen A, Goswami PC, Singh KK. 2003. Mitochondrial impairment is accompanied by impaired oxidative DNA repair in the nucleus. Mutagenesis 18: 497–503.

Dietert RR, Etzel RA, Chen D, Halonen M, Holladay SD, Jarabek AM, et al. 2000. Workshop to identify critical windows of exposure for children's health: immune and respiratory systems work group summary. Environ Health Perspect 108(Suppl 3): 483–490.

Dirks P. 2007. Bmi1 and cell of origin determinants of brain tumor phenotype. Cancer Cell 12: 295–297.

Doll R, Wakeford R. 1997. Risk of childhood cancer from fetal irradiation. Br J Radiol 70: 130–139.

Dukhande VV, Malthankar-Phatak GH, Hugus JJ, Daniels CK, Lai JC. 2006. Manganese-induced neurotoxicity is differentially enhanced by glutathione depletion in astrocytoma and neuroblastoma cells. Neurochem Res 31: 1349–1357.

Duthie SJ, Dobson VL. 1999. Dietary flavonoids protect human colonocyte DNA from oxidative attack in vitro. Eur J Nutr 38: 28–34.

Enns R, Criddle RS. 1977. Investigation of the structural arrangement of the protein subunits of mitochondrial ATPase. Arch Biochem Biophys 183: 742–752.

Erecinska M, Cherian S, Silver IA. 2004. Energy metabolism in mammalian brain during development. Prog Neurobiol 73: 397–445.

Evans AR, Limp-Foster M, Kelley MR. 2000. Going APE over ref-1. Mutat Res 461: 83–108.

Ezer R, Alonso M, Pereira E, Kim M, Allen JC, Miller DC, et al. 2002. Identification of glutathione S-transferase (GST) polymorphisms in brain tumors and association with susceptibility to pediatric astrocytomas. J Neurooncol 59: 123–134.

Fear NT, Roman E, Ansell P, Bull D. 2001. Malignant neoplasms of the brain during childhood: the role of prenatal and neonatal factors (United Kingdom). Cancer Causes Control 12: 443–449.

Ferrer I, Tortosa A, Condom E, Blanco R, Macaya A, Planas A. 1994. Increased expression of bcl-2 immunoreactivity in the developing cerebral cortex of the rat. Neurosci Lett 179: 13–16.

Folkerth RD, Haynes RL, Borenstein NS, Belliveau RA, Trachtenberg F, Rosenberg PA, et al. 2004. Developmental lag in superoxide dismutases relative to other antioxidant enzymes in premyelinated human telencephalic white matter. J Neuropathol Exp Neurol 63: 990–999.

Garcia SJ, Seidler FJ, Crumpton TL, Slotkin TA. 2001. Does the developmental neurotoxicity of chlorpyrifos involve glial targets? Macromolecule synthesis, adenylyl cyclase signaling, nuclear transcription factors, and formation of reactive oxygen in C6 glioma cells. Brain Res 891: 54–68.

Gottfried Y, Voldavsky E, Yodko L, Sabo E, Ben-Itzhak O, Larisch S. 2004. Expression of the pro-apoptotic protein ARTS in astrocytic tumors: correlation with malignancy grade and survival rate. Cancer 101: 2614–2621.

Grimmer MR, Weiss WA. 2006. Childhood tumors of the nervous system as disorders of normal development. Curr Opin Pediatr 18: 634–638.

Gunter KK, Gunter TE. 1994. Transport of calcium by mitochondria. J Bioenerg Biomembr 26: 471–485.

Gunther C, von Hadeln K, Muller-Thomsen T, Alberici A, Binetti G, Hock C, et al. 2004. Possible association of mitochondrial transcription factor A (TFAM) genotype with sporadic Alzheimer disease. Neurosci Lett 369: 219–223.

Gurney JG, Smith MA, Bunin GR. 1999a. CNS and miscellaneous intracranial and intraspinal neoplasms (ICCC III). Online NIH Pub. no. 99-4649. Bethesda, MD: Cancer Statistics Branch, Cancer Surveillance Research Program, Division of Cancer Control and Population Sciences, National Cancer Institute.

Gurney JG, Wall DA, Jukich PJ, Davis FG. 1999b. The contribution of nonmalignant tumors to CNS tumor incidence rates among children in the United States. Cancer Causes Control 10: 101–105.
Halperin EC, Miranda ML, Watson DM, George SL, Stanberry M. 2004. Medulloblastoma and birth date: evaluation of 3 U.S. datasets. Arch Environ Health 59: 26–30.
Hatton BA, Knoepfler PS, Kenney AM, Rowitch DH, de Alboran IM, Olson JM, et al. 2006. N-myc is an essential downstream effector of Shh signaling during both normal and neoplastic cerebellar growth. Cancer Res 66: 8655–8661.
Hjalmars U, Kulldorff M, Wahlqvist Y, Lannering B. 1999. Increased incidence rates but no space-time clustering of childhood astrocytoma in Sweden, 1973–1992: a population-based study of pediatric brain tumors. Cancer 85: 2077–2090.
Hoffman S, Schellinger KA, Propp JM, McCarthy BJ, Campbell RT, Davis FG. 2007. Seasonal variation in incidence of pediatric medulloblastoma in the United States, 1995–2001. Neuroepidemiology 29: 89–95.
Humphrey ML, Cole MP, Pendergrass JC, Kiningham KK. 2005. Mitochondrial mediated thimerosal-induced apoptosis in a human neuroblastoma cell line (SK-N-SH). Neurotoxicology 26: 407–416.
IARC. 1998. In: International incidence of childhood cancer (Parkin DM, Kramarova E, Draper GJ, Masuyer E, Michaelis J, Neglia JP, et al., eds.). Lyon: International Agency for Research on Cancer.
Jirtle RL, Skinner MK. 2007. Environmental epigenomics and disease susceptibility. Nat Rev Genet 8: 253–262.
Jukich PJ, McCarthy BJ, Surawicz TS, Freels S, Davis FG. 2001. Trends in incidence of primary brain tumors in the United States, 1985–1994. Neuro Oncol 3: 141–151.
Kafadar AM, Yilmaz H, Kafadar D, Ergen A, Zeybek U, Bozkurt N, et al. 2006. C677T gene polymorphism of methylenetetrahydrofolate reductase (MTHFR) in meningiomas and high-grade gliomas. Anticancer Res 26: 2445–2449.
Kaiser J. 1999. No meeting of minds on childhood cancer. Science 286: 1832–1834.
Kang D, Kim SH, Hamasaki N. 2007. Mitochondrial transcription factor A (TFAM): roles in maintenance of mtDNA and cellular functions. Mitochondrion 7: 39–44.
Katayam M, Yoshida K, Ishimori H, Katayama M, Kawase T, Motoyama J, et al. 2002. Patched and smoothened mRNA expression in human astrocytic tumors inversely correlates with histological malignancy. J Neurooncol 59: 107–115.
Khan MA, Van DJ, Yeung IW, Hill RP. 2003. Partial volume rat lung irradiation; assessment of early DNA damage in different lung regions and effect of radical scavengers. Radiother Oncol 66: 95–102.
Kiebish MA, Seyfried TN. 2005. Absence of pathogenic mitochondrial DNA mutations in mouse brain tumors. BMC Cancer 5: 102.
Kim EH, Sohn S, Kwon HJ, Kim SU, Kim MJ, Lee SJ, et al. 2007. Sodium selenite induces superoxide-mediated mitochondrial damage and subsequent autophagic cell death in malignant glioma cells. Cancer Res 67: 6314–6324.
Kinzler KW, Ruppert JM, Bigner SH, Vogelstein B. 1988. The GLI gene is a member of the Kruppel family of zinc finger proteins. Nature 332: 371–374.
Kirches E, Michael M, Woy C, Schneider T, Warich-Kirches M, Schneider-Stock R, et al. 1999. Loss of heteroplasmy in the displacement loop of brain mitochondrial DNA in astrocytic tumors. Genes Chromosomes Cancer 26: 80–83.
Kontush A. 2001. Amyloid-beta: an antioxidant that becomes a pro-oxidant and critically contributes to Alzheimer's disease. Free Radic Biol Med 31: 1120–1131.
Krajinovic M, Lamothe S, Labuda D, Lemieux-Blanchard E, Theoret Y, Moghrabi A, et al. 2004. Role of MTHFR genetic polymorphisms in the susceptibility to childhood acute lymphoblastic leukemia. Blood 103: 252–257.
Kulawiec M, Safina A, Desouki MM, Still I, Matsui SI, Bakin A, et al. 2008. Tumorigenic transformation of human breast epithelial cells induced by mitochondrial DNA depletion. Cancer Biol Ther 7(11): 1732–1743.

Kurtz A, Lueth M, Kluwe L, Zhang T, Foster R, Mautner VF, et al. 2004. Somatic mitochondrial DNA mutations in neurofibromatosis type 1-associated tumors. Mol Cancer Res 2: 433–441.
Lai R, Crevier L, Thabane L. 2005. Genetic polymorphisms of glutathione S-transferases and the risk of adult brain tumors: a meta-analysis. Cancer Epidemiol Biomarkers Prev 14: 1784–1790.
Larsson NG, Luft R. 1999. Revolution in mitochondrial medicine. FEBS Lett 455: 199–202.
Lee WC, Choi CH, Cha SH, Oh HL, Kim- YK. 2005. Role of ERK in hydrogen peroxide induced cell death of human glioma cells. Neurochem Res 30: 263–270.
Lemasters GK, Perreault SD, Hales BF, Hatch M, Hirshfield AN, Hughes CL, et al. 2000. Workshop to identify critical windows of exposure for children's health: reproductive health in children and adolescents work group summary. Environ Health Perspect 108(Suppl 3): 505–509.
Lerman-Sagie T, Leshinsky-Silver E, Watemberg N, Luckman Y, Lev D. 2005. White matter involvement in mitochondrial diseases. Mol Genet Metab 84: 127–136.
Ligon KL, Alberta JA, Kho AT, Weiss J, Kwaan MR, Nutt CL, et al. 2004. The oligodendroglial lineage marker OLIG2 is universally expressed in diffuse gliomas. J Neuropathol Exp Neurol 63: 499–509.
Linet MS, Ries LA, Smith MA, Tarone RE, Devesa SS. 1999. Cancer surveillance series: recent trends in childhood cancer incidence and mortality in the United States. J Natl Cancer Inst 91: 1051–1058.
Magnani C, Dalmasso P, Pastore G, Terracini B, Martuzzi M, Mosso ML, et al. 2003. Increasing incidence of childhood leukemia in Northwest Italy, 1975–98. Int J Cancer 105: 552–557.
Malthankar GV, White BK, Bhushan A, Daniels CK, Rodnick KJ, Lai JC. 2004. Differential lowering by manganese treatment of activities of glycolytic and tricarboxylic acid (TCA) cycle enzymes investigated in neuroblastoma and astrocytoma cells is associated with manganese-induced cell death. Neurochem Res 29: 709–717.
Manczak M, Anekonda TS, Henson E, Park BS, Quinn J, Reddy PH. 2006. Mitochondria are a direct site of A beta accumulation in Alzheimer's disease neurons: implications for free radical generation and oxidative damage in disease progression. Hum Mol Genet 15: 1437–1449.
Manshande JP, Van TJ, Coppens M, Casaer P. 1985. Seasonal variation in incidence of cerebellar medulloblastoma. Brain Dev 7: 525–526.
Marino S. 2005. Medulloblastoma: developmental mechanisms out of control. Trends Mol Med 11: 17–22.
Maris JM. 2005. The biologic basis for neuroblastoma heterogeneity and risk stratification. Curr Opin Pediatr 17: 7–13.
Marks N, Berg MJ. 1999. Recent advances on neuronal caspases in development and neurodegeneration. Neurochem Int 35: 195–220.
Mavelli I, Rigo A, Federico R, Ciriolo MR, Rotilio G. 1982. Superoxide dismutase, glutathione peroxidase and catalase in developing rat brain. Biochem J 204: 535–540.
McNally RJ, Kelsey AM, Cairns DP, Taylor GM, Eden OB, Birch JM. 2001. Temporal increases in the incidence of childhood solid tumors seen in Northwest England (1954–1998) are likely to be real. Cancer 92: 1967–1976.
McNeil DE, Cote TR, Clegg L, Rorke LB. 2002. Incidence and trends in pediatric malignancies medulloblastoma/primitive neuroectodermal tumor: a SEER update. Surveillance Epidemiology and End Results. Med Pediatr Oncol 39: 190–194.
Meadows AT, Baum E, Fossati-Bellani F, Green D, Jenkin RD, Marsden B, et al. 1985. Second malignant neoplasms in children: an update from the Late Effects Study Group. J Clin Oncol 3: 532–538.
Mealey J Jr., Hall PV. 1977. Medulloblastoma in children. Survival and treatment. J Neurosurg 46: 56–64.
Melov S, Lithgow GJ, Fischer DR, Tedesco PM, Johnson TE. 1995. Increased frequency of deletions in the mitochondrial genome with age of Caenorhabditis elegans. Nucleic Acids Res 23: 1419–1425.

Modica-Napolitano JS, Singh KK. 2002. Mitochondria as targets for detection and treatment of cancer. Expert Rev Mol Med 4: 1–19.

Montanini L, Regna-Gladin C, Eoli M, Albarosa R, Carrara F, Zeviani M, et al. 2005. Instability of mitochondrial DNA and MRI and clinical correlations in malignant gliomas. J Neurooncol 74: 87–89.

National Cancer Institute NIoNDaS. 2000. Report of the Brain Tumor Progress Review Group. NIH Publication Number 01-4902.

National Institutes of Health. 2002. What you need to know about brain tumors. Bethesda, MD: National Cancer Institute.

Neglia JP, Meadows AT, Robison LL, Kim TH, Newton WA, Ruymann FB, et al. 1991. Second neoplasms after acute lymphoblastic leukemia in childhood. N Engl J Med 325: 1330–1336.

Neri M, Fucic A, Knudsen LE, Lando C, Merlo F, Bonassi S. 2003. Micronuclei frequency in children exposed to environmental mutagens: a review. Mutat Res 544: 243–254.

Neri M, Ugolini D, Bonassi S, Fucic A, Holland N, Knudsen LE, et al. 2006. Children's exposure to environmental pollutants and biomarkers of genetic damage. II. Results of a comprehensive literature search and meta-analysis. Mutat Res 612: 14–39.

Ohta S. 2006. Contribution of somatic mutations in the mitochondrial genome to the development of cancer and tolerance against anticancer drugs. Oncogene 25: 4768–4776.

Olshan AF, Anderson L, Roman E, Fear N, Wolff M, Whyatt R, et al. 2000. Workshop to identify critical windows of exposure for children's health: cancer work group summary. Environ Health Perspect 108(Suppl 3): 595–597.

Park SY, Chang I, Kim J, Kang SW, Park S, Singh K, et al. 2004. Resistance of mitochondrial DNA-depleted cells against cell death. J Biol Chem 279: 7512–7520.

Penta JS, Johnson FM, Wachsman JT, Copeland WC. 2001. Mitochondrial DNA in human malignancy. Mutat Res 488: 119–133.

Perera F, Hemminki K, Jedrychowski W, Whyatt R, Campbell U, Hsu Y, et al. 2002. In utero DNA damage from environmental pollution is associated with somatic gene mutation in newborns. Cancer Epidemiol Biomarkers Prev 11: 1134–1137.

Pouliquen D, Olivier C, Hervouet E, Pedelaborde F, Debien E, Le Cabellec MT, et al. 2008. Dietary prevention of malignant glioma aggressiveness, implications in oxidant stress and apoptosis. Int J Cancer 123: 288–295.

Preston-Martin S, Munir R, Chakrabarti I. 2006. Neoplasms of the nervous system. In: Cancer Epidemiology and Prevention (Schottenfield D, Fraumeni JF, eds.). New York, NY: Oxford University Press.

Raff MC, Barres BA, Burne JF, Coles HS, Ishizaki Y, Jacobson MD. 1993. Programmed cell death and the control of cell survival: lessons from the nervous system. Science 262: 695–700.

Rahman S, Hargreaves I, Clayton P, Heales S. 2001. Neonatal presentation of coenzyme Q10 deficiency. J Pediatr 139: 456–458.

Rajaraman P, Stewart PA, Samet JM, Schwartz BS, Linet MS, Zahm SH, et al. 2006. Lead, genetic susceptibility, and risk of adult brain tumors. Cancer Epidemiol Biomarkers Prev 15: 2514–2520.

Rao G, Pedone CA, Del VL, Reiss K, Holland EC, Fults DW. 2004. Sonic hedgehog and insulin-like growth factor signaling synergize to induce medulloblastoma formation from nestin-expressing neural progenitors in mice. Oncogene 23: 6156–6162.

Rasmussen AK, Chatterjee A, Rasmussen LJ, Singh KK. 2003. Mitochondria-mediated nuclear mutator phenotype in Saccharomyces cerevisiae. Nucleic Acids Res 31: 3909–3917.

Read TA, Hegedus B, Wechsler-Reya R, Gutmann DH. 2006. The neurobiology of neurooncology. Ann Neurol 60: 3–11.

Reed JC. 1997. Bcl-2 family proteins and the hormonal control of cell life and death in normalcy and neoplasia. Vitam Horm 53: 99–138.

Rice JM. 2006. Inducible and transmissible genetic events and pediatric tumors of the nervous system. J Radiat Res (Tokyo) 47(Suppl B): B1–B11.

Rice JM, Ward JM. 1982. Age dependence of susceptibility to carcinogenesis in the nervous system. Ann N Y Acad Sci 381: 274–289.
Rice JM, Wilbourn JD. 2000. Tumors of the nervous system in carcinogenic hazard identification. Toxicol Pathol 28: 202–214.
Robertson JD, Gogvadze V, Kropotov A, Vakifahmetoglu H, Zhivotovsky B, Orrenius S. 2004. Processed caspase-2 can induce mitochondria-mediated apoptosis independently of its enzymatic activity. EMBO Rep 5: 643–648.
Robertson CL, Soane L, Siegel ZT, Fiskum G. 2006. The potential role of mitochondria in pediatric traumatic brain injury. Dev Neurosci 28: 432–446.
Rodier PM. 1995. Developing brain as a target of toxicity. Environ Health Perspect 103(Suppl 6): 73–76.
Ron E, Modan B, Boice JD Jr., Alfandary E, Stovall M, Chetrit A, et al. 1988. Tumors of the brain and nervous system after radiotherapy in childhood. N Engl J Med 319: 1033–1039.
Roy D, Cai Q, Felty Q, Narayan S. 2007. Estrogen-induced generation of reactive oxygen and nitrogen species, gene damage, and estrogen-dependent cancers. J Toxicol Environ Health B Crit Rev 10: 235–257.
Rustin P. 2002. Mitochondria, from cell death to proliferation. Nat Genet 30: 352–353.
Sadler TW. 2000. Susceptible periods during embryogenesis of the heart and endocrine glands. Environ Health Perspect 108(Suppl 3): 555–561.
Samuelsen SO, Bakketeig LS, Tretli S, Johannesen TB, Magnus P. 2006. Head circumference at birth and risk of brain cancer in childhood: a population-based study. Lancet Oncol 7: 39–42.
Scarpulla RC. 2008. Nuclear control of respiratory chain expression by nuclear respiratory factors and PGC-1-related coactivator. Ann N Y Acad Sci 1147: 321–334.
Schoenberg BS, Schoenberg DG, Christine BW, Gomez MR. 1976. The epidemiology of primary intracranial neoplasms of childhood. A population study. Mayo Clin Proc 51: 51–56.
Schuller U, Heine VM, Mao J, Kho AT, Dillon AK, Han YG, et al. 2008. Acquisition of granule neuron precursor identity is a critical determinant of progenitor cell competence to form Shh-induced medulloblastoma. Cancer Cell 14: 123–134.
Schwartzbaum JA, Ahlbom A, Lonn S, Warholm M, Rannug A, Auvinen A, et al. 2007. An international case-control study of glutathione transferase and functionally related polymorphisms and risk of primary adult brain tumors. Cancer Epidemiol Biomarkers Prev 16: 559–565.
Searles NS, Mueller BA, De Roos AJ, Viernes HM, Farin FM, Checkoway H. 2005. Risk of brain tumors in children and susceptibility to organophosphorus insecticides: the potential role of paraoxonase (PON1). Environ Health Perspect 113: 909–913.
Singh KK, Kulawiec M, Still I, Desouki MM, Geradts J, Matsui S. 2005. Inter-genomic cross talk between mitochondria and the nucleus plays an important role in tumorigenesis. Gene 354: 140–146.
Sirachainan N, Wongruangsri S, Kajanachumpol S, Pakakasama S, Visudtibhan A, Nuchprayoon I, et al. 2008. Folate pathway genetic polymorphisms and susceptibility of central nervous system tumors in Thai children. Cancer Detect Prev 32: 72–78.
Slikker W III, Mei N, Chen T. 2004. N-ethyl-N-nitrosourea (ENU) increased brain mutations in prenatal and neonatal mice but not in the adults. Toxicol Sci 81: 112–120.
Smiraglia DJ, Kulawiec M, Bistulfi GL, Gupta SG, Singh KK. 2008. A novel role for mitochondria in regulating epigenetic modification in the nucleus. Cancer Biol Ther 7: 1182–1190.
Smith MA, Freidlin B, Ries LA, Simon R. 1998. Trends in reported incidence of primary malignant brain tumors in children in the United States. J Natl Cancer Inst 90: 1269–1277.
Stavrovskaya IG, Kristal BS. 2005. The powerhouse takes control of the cell: is the mitochondrial permeability transition a viable therapeutic target against neuronal dysfunction and death? Free Radic Biol Med 38: 687–697.
Steliarova-Foucher E, Stiller C, Kaatsch P, Berrino F, Coebergh JW, Lacour B, et al. 2004. Geographical patterns and time trends of cancer incidence and survival among children and adolescents in Europe since the 1970s (the ACCISproject): an epidemiological study. Lancet 364: 2097–2105.

Suliman HB, Carraway MS, Welty-Wolf KE, Whorton AR, Piantadosi CA. 2003. Lipopolysaccharide stimulates mitochondrial biogenesis via activation of nuclear respiratory factor-1. J Biol Chem 278: 41510–41518.
Taanman JW. 1999. The mitochondrial genome: structure, transcription, translation and replication. Biochim Biophys Acta 1410: 103–123.
Tedeschi-Blok N, Lee M, Sison JD, Miike R, Wrensch M. 2006. Inverse association of antioxidant and phytoestrogen nutrient intake with adult glioma in the San Francisco Bay Area: a case-control study. BMC Cancer 6: 148.
Thannickal VJ, Fanburg BL. 2000. Reactive oxygen species in cell signaling. Am J Physiol Lung Cell Mol Physiol 279: L1005–L1028.
Thompson JR, Gerald PF, Willoughby ML, Armstrong BK. 2001. Maternal folate supplementation in pregnancy and protection against acute lymphoblastic leukaemia in childhood: a case-control study. Lancet 358: 1935–1940.
Van RH, Salvador C, Yang H, Huang TT, Epstein CJ, Richardson A. 1999. Characterization of the antioxidant status of the heterozygous manganese superoxide dismutase knockout mouse. Arch Biochem Biophys 363: 91–97.
Vasko MR, Guo C, Kelley MR. 2005. The multifunctional DNA repair/redox enzyme Ape1/Ref-1 promotes survival of neurons after oxidative stress. DNA Repair (Amst) 4: 367–379.
Vega A, Salas A, Gamborino E, Sobrido MJ, Macaulay V, Carracedo A. 2004. mtDNA mutations in tumors of the central nervous system reflect the neutral evolution of mtDNA in populations. Oncogene 23: 1314–1320.
Von BJ, Reynolds P. 2003. Birth characteristics and brain cancers in young children. Int J Epidemiol 32: 248–256.
Wong-Riley MT. 1989. Cytochrome oxidase: an endogenous metabolic marker for neuronal activity. Trends Neurosci 12: 94–101.
Wright J. 1910. Neurocytoma and neuroblastomas, a kind of tumor not generally recognized. J Exp Med 12: 556–561.
Xanthoudakis S, Curran T. 1996. Redox regulation of AP-1: a link between transcription factor signaling and DNA repair. Adv Exp Med Biol 387: 69–75.
Yamakawa Y, Fukui M, Kinoshita K, Ohgami S, Kitamura K. 1979. Seasonal variation in incidence of cerebellar medulloblastoma by month of birth. Fukuoka Igaku Zasshi 70: 295–300.
Yang ZJ, Ellis T, Markant SL, Read TA, Kessler JD, Bourboulas M, et al. 2008. Medulloblastoma can be initiated by deletion of Patched in lineage-restricted progenitors or stem cells. Cancer Cell 14: 135–145.
Zhong W, Oberley LW, Oberley TD, Yan T, Domann FE, St Clair DK. 1996. Inhibition of cell growth and sensitization to oxidative damage by overexpression of manganese superoxide dismutase in rat glioma cells. Cell Growth Differ 7: 1175–1186.

Chapter 10
Genetic Polymorphisms Predisposing Individuals to Breast Cancer Via Gene–Environment Interaction

Keun-Young Yoo, Sue K. Park, and Aesun Shin

Abstract Breast cancer incidence varies considerably between Western and non Western countries. Breast cancer incidence and mortality rates are highest in North America and Northern Europe, intermediate in Southern Europe and Latin America, and lowest in Asia and Africa. In recent years, however, a dramatic increase in breast cancer incidence has been reported in several Asian countries, including Korea. Immigrant studies have suggested that environmental rather than genetic factors are primarily responsible for the international variability and secular trend of breast cancer rates. This chapter presents current findings on environmental risk factors for breast cancer, specifically in terms of gene–environment interactions. The scope of environmental factors encompasses obesity, hormonal factors, including menstrual and reproductive history, and dietary factors, including alcohol, folate, fruits, vegetables, antioxidant vitamins, and meats and their metabolic mutagens. For each environmental factor, we reviewed articles that assessed genetic polymorphisms that have a plausible biological mechanism for breast cancer risk modification.

Keywords Genetic polymorphisms · Gene–environment interaction · Predisposition of individuals to breast cancer

K.-Y. Yoo (✉)
Department of Preventive Medicine, Seoul National University College of Medicine, Seoul, Korea
e-mail: kyyoo@plaza.snu.ac.kr

S.K. Park (✉)
Department of Preventive Medicine and Cancer Research Institute, Seoul National University College of Medicine, Seoul, Korea

A. Shin (✉)
Cancer Epidemiology Branch, Research Institute, National Cancer Center, Goyang-si, Korea

D. Roy, M.T. Dorak (eds.), *Environmental Factors, Genes, and the Development of Human Cancers*, DOI 10.1007/978-1-4419-6752-7_10,

10.1 Introduction

Breast cancer incidence varies considerably between Western and non-Western countries. Breast cancer incidence and mortality rates are highest in North America and Northern Europe, intermediate in Southern Europe and Latin America, and lowest in Asia and Africa (Yoo et al., 2002). Nevertheless, in recent years, a dramatic increase in breast cancer incidence has been reported in several Asian countries, including Korea. Immigrant studies have suggested that environmental rather than genetic factors are primarily responsible for the international variability and secular trend of breast cancer rates (Kelsey and Horn-Ross, 1993).

In recent years, thousands of SNPs in single genes have been identified through advances in genetic techniques and knowledge, and the results from whole genome association studies (WGA) are now being published. Nevertheless, results from WGA studies related to gene–environment interactions are still limited. Therefore, our review focused mainly on candidate-gene studies that included a substantial number of papers on candidate gene–environment interactions with breast cancer risk.

This chapter presents environmental risk factors for breast cancer, specifically in terms of gene–environment interaction. The scope of environmental factors encompasses obesity, hormonal factors, including menstrual and reproductive history, and dietary factors, including alcohol, folate, fruits, vegetables, antioxidant vitamins, and meats and their metabolic mutagens. For each environmental factor, we reviewed articles that assessed genetic polymorphisms that have a plausible biological mechanism for breast cancer risk modification. Readers who are interested in the effect modification of genes on the association between smoking and breast cancer risk can refer to a review by Terry and Goodman (Terry and Goodman, 2006).

10.2 Obesity

The International Agency for Research on Cancer estimates that 25% of breast cancer cases worldwide are due to overweight/obesity and sedentary lifestyle (IARC Working Group 2002). Overweight or obese postmenopausal women had a 30-50% greater risk for breast cancer development than leaner women, whereas overweight or obese premenopausal women had a lower risk (IARC Working Group 2002). This difference in risk according to menopausal status suggests a hormonal influence on breast cancer risk. Because fat tissue is the primary non-ovarian site for estrogen production after menopause, obese postmenopausal women have higher levels of circulating estrogen and thus, an elevated risk for breast cancer.

The estrogen receptor (ER), one of the most important mediators of estrogenic response in estrogen-sensitive tissues, including the breast, plays a crucial role in breast growth and differentiation, as well as in the development of cancer. The ER is known to exist in two forms, estrogen receptor alpha (ESR1) and estrogen receptor beta (ESR2), the latter having been discovered more recently. Although the role of *ER* polymorphisms in breast cancer etiology is biologically plausible, most studies (Yaich et al., 1992; Southey et al., 1998; Curran et al., 2001; Kang et al., 2002; Comings et al., 2003) have reported a null effect for *ESR*1 genetic variants on breast cancer risk. Some studies have reported a weakly increased risk (Shin et al., 2003 for the *G* allele in *c*.454–351*A*>*G*; Cai et al., 2003 for the *C* allele in *c*.454–397*C*>*T*; Iwase et al., 1996 and Vasconcelos et al., 2002 for the *G* allele in *c*.975*C*>*G*), while other studies have shown non-significant results (Comings et al., 2003, and Cai et al., 2003 for the *G* allele in *c*.454–351*A*>*G*; Yaich et al., 1992; Shin et al., 2003 for the *C* allele in *c*.454–397*C*>*T*; Southey et al., 1998; Schubert et al., 1999; Curran et al., 2001; Kang et al., 2002 for the *G* allele in *c*.975*C*>*G*) due to small sample sizes. However, in multi-SNP studies, a moderately increased risk of 2.5-fold for both *ESR*1 *PvuII* (*rs*2234693) and *XbaI* (*rs*9340799) (Shin et al., 2003) and a weakly increased risk of 1.2–1.5 fold for *ESR*1 haplotypes have been found (Wedrén et al., 2004; Einarsdóttir et al., 2008). Additionally, the interactive effect between haplotype variants with obesity modified breast cancer risk, and the risk for the haplotypes was stronger in heavier women (Wedrén et al., 2004).

The progesterone receptor (PR), a member of the steroid receptor superfamily, mediates the physiologic effects of progesterone and can play a role in the growth and differentiation of breast tumors. The *PGR* 331*G*>*A* (*rs*10895068) polymorphism demonstrated an interactive effect with obesity to increase breast cancer risk up to 2.3-fold (De Vivo et al., 2003).

Subjects with the *SHBG Asp*327*Asn* (*rs*6259) polymorphism had a 2-fold higher breast cancer risk through an interactive effect with overweight (BMI> = 24 kg/m^2) or higher WHR (waist-hip ratio) (WHR> = 0.81) relative to subjects with the Asp/Asn or Asn/Asn genotypes and who were not overweight and had lower WHR (Cui et al., 2005).

The sulfotransferase SULT1A1 is involved in the inactivation and elimination of estrogens and catechol estrogens (Weinshilboum et al., 1997). In most studies (Tang et al., 2003, Han et al., 2004a; Chacko et al., 2004, Sillanpää et al., 2005; Yang et al., 2005; Han et al., 2005; Seth et al., 2000), the *SULT*1*A*1 *His* allele in the 638*G*>*A* (*Arg*213*His*) polymorphism (*rs*9282861) was associated with a 1.4 to 4-fold increased risk for postmenopausal breast cancer. Conversely, some studies have found a null association with overall or postmenopausal breast cancer risk relative to the *Arg/Arg* genotype (Sparks et al., 2004, Jerevall et al., 2005; Le Marchand et al., 2005; Shatalova et al., 2006; Rebbeck et al., 2007a). Additionally, the increased risk of the *SULT*1*A*1 genetic variant was more prominent in overweight (BMI$\geq$25 kg/m^2) postmenopausal women (Yang et al., 2005; Zheng et al., 2001).

The enzyme cytochrome P450 17*a* hydroxylase (CYP17) controls two successive early steps of endogenous estrogen biosynthesis by converting pregnenolone and progesterone to precursors of androgen and estrogen (Brentano et al., 1990). The *CYP*17*A*1 *c*.27*T*>*C* (*rs*743572) and *CYP*17*A*2 *c*.-34 *T*>*C* (*rs*2486758) polymorphisms were not associated with breast cancer risk in most studies (for *CYPA*1 *c*.-27*T*>*C*, Setiawan et al., 2007; Silva et al., 2006; Piller et al., 2006; Verla-Tebit et al., 2005; Shin et al., 2005; Ambrosone et al., 2003; Wu et al., 2003, Feigelson et al., 2001; Mitrunen et al., 2000; Hamajima et al., 2000; Haiman et al., 1999; Huang et al., 1999; Dunning et al., 1998; Weston et al., 1998; Helzlsouer et al., 1998, for *CYPA*2 *c.-34T>C*, Chen et al., 2008; Ahsan et al., 2005, Hefler et al., 1998). However, the interaction between the *C* alleles in these *CYP*17 polymorphisms and obesity (BMI>25 kg/m^2) significantly increased the risk of breast cancer relative to non-obese counterparts with the *TT* genotype (Chen et al., 2008; Setiawan et al., 2007).

ERCC2 (*XPD*) is one of seven nucleotide excision repair enzymes that cause xeroderma pigmentosum when mutated in the germ line (Coin et al., 1998). *ERCC2* polymorphisms have been associated with breast cancer risk (Lunn et al., 2000; Tang et al., 2002). The *ERCC*2 *Asp*312*Asn* (*rs*1799793) polymorphism had an interactive effect with WHR and subjects with the Asn/Asn genotype and higher WHR (>0.85) had a 4-fold increased risk for breast cancer relative to subjects with the Asp/Asp genotype and lower WHR (Bernard-Gallon et al., 2008).

Subjects with $\leq$18 repeats for the VDR gene fragment and with a BMI>28 kg/m^2 had a 1.3-fold marginally significantly increased risk of breast cancer, compared with subjects with 2 alleles with $\geq$19 repeats (Wedren et al., 2007).

The main role of *STK*15 is to control chromosome segregation during mitosis in tumor development (Bischoff and Plowman, 1999). The *STK*15 *F*31*I* or *V*57*I* gene encodes a serine/threonine kinase, which acts as a key regulator of mitotic chromosome segregation (Hirota et al., 2003). No effect on breast cancer risk was observed in a recent meta-analysis (Fletcher et al., 2006), but the *STK*15 *Ile/Ile* variant of codon 31 showed a 4-fold (95% CI 1.7–9.8) increased breast cancer risk for subjects with a BMI greater than 25 kg/m^2, especially among postmenopausal women (Dai et al., 2004). In addition, the *STK*15 *Ile/Ile* variant was associated with a 2-fold increased risk for subjects with higher WHR (> = 0.835) (Dai et al., 2004). The association of breast cancer risk with obesity was not modified by an interaction with *ERCC*4 (*rs*1799801), (Lee et al., 2005b), *IGF*1 CA repeat genotypes (*rs*10665874), *IGFBP*3 -202*A>C* (*rs*2854744) (Slattery et al., 2007b), *IL*1*b* -31*C>T* (*rs*1143627) (Lee et al., 2005), or *FGFR*2 (*rs*2420946) (Kawase et al., 2009).

10.3 Hormonal Factors

Women who experience early onset of menarche and late onset of menopause have an increased risk of developing breast cancer. The *CYP*17 *c*.27*T>C* (rs743572) and *c*.34*T>C* (*rs*2486758) genetic polymorphisms modify breast cancer risk up to twofold to threefold through menarche or menopause (Einarsdóttir et al., 2005; Ambrosone et al., 2003), although no overall association has been found (Chen et al., 2008; Einarsdóttir et al., 2005; Ahsan et al., 2005; Hefler et al., 1998). In contrast, other studies have not observed an interactive effect with *CYP*17 (*rs*743572; *rs*2486758) (Verla-Tebit et al., 2005; Chang et al., 2005).

Mutations of the human RecQ helicase genes such as WRN have been linked to Werner syndrome, a rare autosomal recessive disease characterized by premature aging and predisposed to cancer (Chakraverty and Hickson, 1999). RecQ helicases are involved in interactions with several important cancer-related proteins, including the tumor suppressor BRCA1 (Futaki and liu, 2001). The *WRN* gene polymorphisms 46729*A*>*C* (*rs*9649886), 83316*T*>*G* (*rs*2725362), and 46729*A*>*C* (*rs*9649886) have been shown to increase breast cancer risk up to 4-fold among women with a longer menarche-first full-term pregnancy (FFTP) interval (>16 years) relative to women with a shorter menarche-FFTP interval (<9 years) (Ding et al., 2007).

The association of breast cancer risk with early age at menarche, late age at menopause, and duration of estrogen exposure was not modified by interaction with *FGFR*2 (*rs*2420946), *SHBG* (*rs*6259) (Cui et al., 2005), *STK*15 codon 31 (Dai et al., 2004), or *STK*15 *F*31*I* genotypes (Kawase et al., 2009; Egan et al., 2004b).

The positive association of the *SULT*1*A*1 *His* allele of the 638*G*>*A* (*Arg*213*His*) (*rs*9282861) polymorphism with breast cancer risk in combination with factors related to high endogenous estrogen exposure, including early age at menarche, late age at menopause, and longer duration of menstruation was further increased by interactive effects (Zheng et al., 2001; Yang et al., 2005).

"High-risk birth factors", such as nulliparity and late age at FFTP, both increased the lifetime incidence of breast cancer relative to "low-risk birth ", such as early age at FFTP (aged <30 years). The *GSTM*1 and *T*1 polymorphisms had a synergistic effect on breast cancer risk (2.2-fold; 95% CI 1.13–4.45), and the combined interactive effect with "high-risk birth factor" increased moderately up to 2.4-fold (Park et al., 2003).

Estrogen can induce breast cancer through the initiation of an estrogen metabolite, catechol estrogen. One study investigated the five genes involved in catechol estrogen detoxification and metabolism, including *COMT Val*108*Met* (*rs*4680), *GSTM*1, and *GSTT*1 (Chen et al., 2005). The combined effect of the *GSTM*1 and *T*1 null genotypes and the *COMT Val*108*Met* (*rs*4680) genotype increased risk for breast cancer 2.0-fold, whereas the interaction between the combined effect of the *GSTM*1, *T*1, and *COMT* polymorphisms and high-risk birth factors increased risk a more notable 3.0-fold (95% CI 1.1–8.2) (Park et al., 2004). The interaction between one or more high-risk catechol estrogen detoxification and metabolism genotypes with high-risk birth factors and longer estrogen exposure before FFTP was found to be statistically significant (Chen et al., 2005).

Among women with high-risk birth factors, the *ESR*1 *XbaI* (rs9340799) *xx* genetic variant modified breast cancer risk up to 4-fold relative to women with low-risk birth factors (parous women who experienced FFTP at <29 years) and carried the *ESR* genotype with the *X* allele (Shin et al., 2003). The *C* alleles in the *CYP*17 *c*.34*T*>*C* (*rs*2486758) and *FGFR*2 (*rs*2420946) polymorphisms have been associated with an increased risk of breast cancer through interaction with high-risk birth factors (Ambrosone et al., 2003; Wu et al., 2003; Kawase et al., 2009). In contrast, the *SULT*1*A*1 *2 allele (*rs*9282861) has been shown to reduce breast cancer risk through interaction with parity factors and among women with high parity (>3 pregnancies) (Sillanpää et al., 2005).

The *WRN* gene, a genetic determinant of Werner syndrome, which is thought to act through defective DNA repair and cell growth enhancement is associated with cancer (Li and Comai, 2000). The interaction between a *WRN* haplotype (46729*A*>*C* *rs*9649886 and 83316*T*>*G* *rs*2725362) and number of full-term pregnancies reduced breast cancer risk (OR = 0.4 for premenopausal women; 0.5 for postmenopausal women (Ding et al., 2007).

The vitamin D receptor (VDR) is a mediator for vitamin D that plays a role in modulating gene transcription involved in breast and prostate cellular differentiation and proliferation James et al., (1996; Habuchi et al., 2000) and calcium and phosphorus homeostasis Hannah and Norman, (1994). The *VDR* gene fragment repeats ≤ 18 in combination with parity factors, was associated with a significant 0.5-fold reduced risk of breast cancer compared with presence of 2 alleles with ≥ 19 repeats, although neither the number of repeats (Wedren et al., 2007) nor the *VDR* gene itself were significantly associated with breast cancer risk (for the *Fok*1 polymorphism, Abbas et al., 2008; John et al., 2007; McCullough et al., 2007; Guy et al., 2003; Bretherton-Watt et al., 2001; Ingles et al., 2000; Curran et al., 1999, For *Apa*1 polymorphism, McCullough et al., 2007; Hou et al., 2002, for the *Bsm*1 polymorphism, McCullough et al., 2007; Lowe et al., 2005; Hou et al., 2002, for the *TaqI* polymorphism, John et al., 2007; McCullough et al., 2007; Sillanpää et al., 2004; Hou et al., 2002; Dunning et al., 1999; Lundin et al., 1999, for *VDR*-5132 *C* and *Cdx*2 *A*, Abbas et al., 2008, for *BglI*, John et al., 2007). However, neither *CYP*17 polymorphisms (*rs*743572; *rs*2486758) nor AR gene fragment lengths modified breast cancer risk through interaction with parity factors (Chang et al., 2005; Wedren et al., 2007).

The *CYP3A4* 729*A*>*C* (*rs*2740574) and *PGR* 331 *G/A* (*rs*10895068) polymorphisms modify breast cancer risk through interaction with hormone replacement therapy (HRT), (Chang et al., 2005; Feigelson et al., 1997; Rebbeck et al., 2007b; Kotsopoulos et al., 2009) and use of oral contraceptives (Ambrosone et al., 2003). Both genes modify risk through interaction with duration of HRT use (MARIE-GENICA Consortium, 2010; Kotsopoulos et al., 2009). The *HSD*17*B*1_937*A*>*G* (*rs*605059) polymorphism was associated with a 1.2-fold marginally significantly increased risk (1.1-fold) for duration of estrogen monotherapy (MARIE-GENICA Consortium, 2010). In contrast, carriers of the *G* allele of the *IVS*1 +896*A*>*G* polymorphism of the *ADH*1*B* gene through interaction with HRT reduced the risk of breast cancer (Visvanathan et al., 2007).

The *ERCC*2 *Lys*751*Gln* (*rs*13181) polymorphism has shown an interactive effect with oral contraceptive use. Subjects with the *Gln/Gln* genotype who used oral contraceptives had a 0.3-fold reduced risk for breast cancer relative to subjects with the *Lys/Lys* genotype who did not use oral contraceptives (Bernard-Gallon et al., 2008). In contrast, *ERCC*2 *Asp*312*Asn* (*rs*1799793) showed no interactive effect with oral contraceptive use in the modification of breast cancer risk (Bernard-Gallon et al., 2008).

Interleukins (IL) are inflammatory and anti-inflammatory cytokines. IL-6 is a pro-inflammatory cytokine secreted by adipose tissue. Inflammation is accepted as a key component of the carcinogenic process, and IL-6 may affect breast cancer risk through modification of associations with obesity and diabetes mellitus (Bennermo et al., 2004; Mohlig et al., 2004; Lu et al., 2006). *IL*-6 polymorphisms (*rs*1800797/-596*A>G, rs*1800796/-572*G>C, rs*1800795/-174*G>C, rs*2069832/*IVS*2*G>A,* and *rs*2069849 *exon* 5 *C>T*) have been shown to modify breast cancer risk through interactive effects with HRT in non-Hispanic women (Slattery et al., 2008).

In summary, none of the following genetic variants have been shown to modify breast cancer risk through interaction with HRT or oral contraceptive use, *CYP*17 polymorphisms (*rs*743572; *rs*2486758) (Einarsdóttir et al., 2005; Verla-Tebit et al., 2005, Chang et al., 2005; Haiman et al., 2002, 2003), *HSD*17*B*1 (*rs*605059) and *HSD*3*B*1 (*rs*1047303) (Haiman et al., 2002), *COMT Met/Val* (*rs*4680), (Haiman et al., 2002, 2003), *UGT*1*A*1 (*rs*8175347), *CYP*1*B*1 (*rs*59472972) and *CYP*19 (TTTA)*n* microsatellite (*rs*57921193) (Haiman et al., 2003), *STK*15 *F*31*I* (Egan et al., 2004), *FGFR*2 (*rs*2981582, *rs*11200014, *rs*2981579, *rs*1219648 and *rs*2420946) (Kawase et al., 2009), *IGF*1 *CA* repeat genotypes (*rs*10665874) and *IGFBP*3 -202*A>C* (*rs*2854744) (Slattery et al., 2007), and *AR* and *VDR* gene fragment lengths (Wedren et al., 2007).

10.4 Dietary Factors

The second report from the World Cancer Research Fund and American Institute for Cancer Research (WCRF/AICR) on Food, Nutrition, Physical Activity, and the Prevention of Cancer: a Global Perspective provided extensive systematic reviews on the existing epidemiologic evidence between diet and cancer risk (WCRF/AICR, 2007). The second report concluded that alcoholic beverages were convincing risk factors for both premenopausal and postmenopausal breast cancer and that total fat intake was a suggestive risk factor for postmenopausal breast cancer with limited evidence (WCRF/AICR, 2007). However, food groups or nutrients such as vegetables and fruits, animal fat, meat, fiber, and carotenoids that were classified as probable or possible factors in the first report were reclassified into the no conclusion category in the second report (WCRF/AICR, 1997; WCRF/AICR, 2007).

10.5 Alcohol

Alcohol may induce breast cancer by putative mechanisms, which include the following: increase of total estrogen and free estradiol; formation of free radicals and a rise of lipid peroxidation; change of cell membrane infiltration; altered liver function leading to interference in carcinogen detoxification or hormone metabolism; and production of cytotoxic compounds (Park et al., 2000). The oxidation of alcohol in the liver is catalyzed by alcohol dehydrogenases (ADHs) and aldehyde dehydrogenases (ALDHs) (Bosron and Li, 1986). Most studies reported no main effect of *ADH*1*B* or *ADH*1*C* polymorphisms on the risk of breast cancer (Freudenheim et al., 1999; Hines et al., 2000; Lilla et al., 2005; Terry et al., 2006; 2007), while one study suggested a reduction in breast cancer risk among *G* allele carriers of the *IVS*1 +896*A*>*G* (*rs*1353621) polymorphism of the *ADH*1*B* gene (Visvanathan et al., 2007). Two studies reported a highest risk of premenopausal breast cancer among those with higher alcohol intake and the *1/*1 genotype of the *ADH*1*C* gene, which exhibited fast enzyme activity (Freudenheim et al., 1999; Terry et al., 2006). No effect modification of the *ALDH*2 *Glu*487*Lys* (*rs*671) or *FGFR*2 (*rs*2420946) polymorphisms were reported with regard to the association of alcohol with breast cancer risk (Choi et al., 2003; Kawase et al., 2009).

Xenobiotic metabolizing enzymes, including glutathione S-transferases (GSTs), cytochrome p450 (CYP) isoenzymes, and SULT1A1 also metabolize alcohol and alcohol metabolites. The low activity allele of the detoxification enzyme *GSTT*1, in combination with alcohol consumption, presented an increased risk of breast cancer (Helzlsouer et al., 1998; Park et al., 2000; Zheng et al., 2003). Among alcohol drinkers, Park et al. (2000) reported a 5.3-fold increase of premenopausal breast cancer risk in women lacking both the *GSTT*1 and *GSTM*1 genes compared to women who possessed both genes (Park et al., 2000). One study reported that women who possessed the *Val* allele of the *Ile*105*Val* polymorphism (*rs*1695) of the *GSTP*1 gene and consumed alcohol showed the highest risk for breast cancer (Kim et al., 2004). In contrast, another study (Helzlsouer et al., 1998) did not show the same findings. The low activity *His* allele of *Arg*213*His* polymorphism (*rs*9282861) of the *SULT*1*A*1 gene was associated with breast cancer risk, especially among women who regularly consumed alcohol (Zheng et al., 2001).

Chronic alcohol consumption may induce CYP2E1 enzymes, which lead to an increased production of acetaldehyde and reactive oxygen species (ROS), such as superoxide anions and hydroxyl radicals. These ROS can damage DNA by producing oxidized bases such as 8-hydroxy-2′-deoxyguanine and thymine glycol, which have mutagenic or cytotoxic consequences for cells (Choi et al., 2003). In a Korean study (Choi et al., 2003), female ever alcohol drinkers who carried the *c*2 allele of *CYP*2*E*1 had a 1.9-fold higher risk of breast cancer compared to non-drinkers with the *c*1/*c*1 genotype. A similar interactive effect was observed between the *CYP*19 genotype and alcohol consumption. Female ever drinkers who carried the *Cys* allele of the *Arg*264*Cys* (*rs*700519) polymorphism of the *CYP*19 gene showed a 3.3-fold increased risk of breast cancer compared with female never drinkers who were homozygous for the *Arg* allele (Lee et al., 2003). No significant interactive effect between *CYP*1*B*1 polymorphisms and alcohol consumption on breast cancer risk was observed (Lee et al., 2003).

Alcohol is known to act as a folate antagonist and therefore, the possible modifying effect of alcohol intake on the association between genes involved in one-carbon metabolism and breast cancer risk was evaluated. Stevens et al. (2007) observed a significant interaction between alcohol intake and the *A*1298*C* polymorphism (*rs*1801131) of the *methylenetetrahydrofolate reductase* (*MTHFR*) gene in a case-control dataset from the Cancer Prevention II Nutritional Cohort (Stevens et al., 2007), whereas Le Marchand et al. (2004) did not find any effect modification between ethanol intake level and the *C*677*T* polymorphism (*rs*1801133) among ever users of HRT in a nested case-control study within the Multiethnic Cohort Study (Le Marchand et al., 2004). The interaction between the C677T polymorphism and alcohol consumption in another case-control study (Semenza et al., 2003) was not statistically significant. Lissowska et al. (2007) did not find an effect modification of ethanol intake level on the main effect of the *methionine synthase* (*MTR*) *D919G* (*rs*1805087) polymorphism (Lissowska et al., 2007).

Mitochondrial manganese superoxide dismutase (MnSOD) catalyzes superoxide radicals to hydrogen peroxide and thereby protects cells from oxidative stress. *Ala* allele carriers of the *Ala9Val* polymorphism (*rs*4880) who consumed alcohol (Mitrunen et al., 2001) or who consumed $\geq$19 g/day of alcohol (Slanger et al., 2006) showed the highest risk of breast cancer, although the interaction terms did not reach statistical significance. The possible effect modification was not replicated in other studies (Egan et al., 2003; Gaudet et al., 2005; Millikan et al., 2004; Tamimi et al., 2004). The results of a few studies (Ravn-Haren et al., 2006; Rossner et al., 2006) that evaluated other genes encoding antioxidant enzymes, including *glutathione peroxidase* (*GPX*1) and *OGG*1, and their effect modification regarding alcohol consumption, were inconclusive.

Peroxisome proliferator-activated receptor-γ2 (PPARG2) is a transcription factor and member of the nuclear hormone receptor subfamily that modulates intracellular insulin-signaling events. The *Ala* allele of the *Pro*12*Ala* (*rs*1801282) polymorphism reduces promoter affinity by approximately 50% and also reduces ligand-independent and -dependent activities (Deeb et al., 1998). Alcohol intake increased the risk of breast cancer among homozygous carriers of the *Pro* allele, and a statistically significant interaction level was found by Vogel et al. (2007). However, that study did not find any effect modification between alcohol and the *IL*-6 *G*-174*C* (*rs*1800795), *IL*-8 *T*-251*A* (*rs*4073), *COX*2 *T*8473C (rs5275) polymorphisms involved in inflammatory response (Vogel et al., 2007).

10.6 Folate

Folate, vitamin B_6, and vitamin B_{12} have several roles in cancer development (Zhang et al., 2003). They function as coenzymes in one-carbon metabolism, which is critical for the production of purines and thymidylate in DNA synthesis. Folate and vitamin B_{12} are also involved in DNA methylation. Additionally, the conversion of homocysteine into cysteine is facilitated by two pyridoxal 5′-phosphate (the principal active form of vitamin B_6)-dependent enzymes, cystathionine β-synthase, and γ-cystathionate. Lastly, high intracellular levels of pyridoxal 5′-phosphate may lead to decreased steroid hormone-induced gene expression (Zhang et al., 2003).

MTHFR catalyzes the biologically irreversible reduction of 5, 10-methylenetetrahydrofolate to 5-methylatetrahydrofolate, which acts as a methyl donor for methionine synthesis from homocysteine (Bailey and Gregory, 1999). A meta-analysis of the *MTHFR C677T* (*rs*1801133) polymorphism and breast cancer risk reported no main effect of this polymorphism (Lewis et al., 2006; Lissowska et al., 2007), whereas an increased risk for postmenopausal breast cancer was observed among *TT* genotype carriers (Lissowska et al., 2007). However, when the interaction between *MTHFR* genotypes and dietary folate intake was examined, three studies reported the highest risk of breast cancer among women with the *TT* genotype and low folate intake, although none of the studies showed a statistically significant interaction (Chen et al., 2005; Shrubsole et al., 2004; Suzuki et al., 2008). Other studies also did not find evidence of an interaction between this polymorphism and folate intake level (Le Marchand et al., 2004; Sharp et al., 2002; Stevens et al., 2007). The combination of the 677*TT* genotype, which has lower enzymatic activity, and low intake of folate leads to less available 5-methylatetrahydrofolate, which is required for DNA methylation. The *MTHFR A*1298*C* polymorphism and folate intake showed a significant interaction in one study (Stevens et al., 2007), but not in others (Chen et al., 2005; Le Marchand et al., 2004; Shrubsole et al., 2004). Chou et al., observed a reduction in breast cancer risk for compound heterozygote and homozygote variants (677 *CT/TT* and 1298 *AA/AA*) among women with lower plasma folate levels (Chou et al., 2006).

Methionine synthase (MTR) and methionine synthase reductase (MTRR) transfer a methyl group from 5-methyltetrahydrofolate to methionine, which is a precursor for the universal methyl donor, *S*-adenosylmethionine (SAM) (Shrubsole et al., 2006). The *A*2756*G* (*rs*1805087) polymorphism of the *MTR* gene did not show a significant interaction when combined with dietary intake of folate (Lissowska et al., 2007; Shrubsole et al., 2006; Suzuki et al., 2008), methionine, vitamin B_6, or B_{12} (Lissowska et al., 2007; Shrubsole et al., 2006). Suzuki et al. (2008) reported the highest risk of postmenopausal breast cancer among women with the *GG* genotype of the *A*66*G* (*rs*1801394) polymorphism of the *MTRR* gene and the lowest tertile of folate intake (Suzuki et al., 2008).

In studies that assessed the possible interaction between plasma folate levels and genetic polymorphisms of genes involved in DNA repair, the results suggested interactions between plasma folate levels and the *XRCC*1 *Arg*194*Trp* (*rs*1799782) and *XRCC*2 *Arg*188*His* (*rs*3218536) polymorphisms (Han et al., 2004). Since SAM, the necessary methyl donor for catechol-O-methyltransferase (COMT), detoxifys catechol estrogens by methylation to methoxyestrogens, an association between the *COMT Val*108*Met* (*rs*4680) polymorphism and breast cancer risk was observed among subjects with lower plasma folate or higher plasma homocysteine levels (Goodman et al., 2001).

10.7 Fruits, Vegetables, and Antioxidant Vitamins

Reactive oxygen species (ROS) generated through normal oxidative metabolism have the potential to cause oxidative damage to DNA (WCRF/AICR, 2007). The first line of defense against oxidative stress includes enzymes such as MnSOD, glutathione peroxidase (GPX), and catalase (Gago-Dominguez et al., 2007). The resultant secondary oxidation products can still damage DNA, proteins, lipids, and therefore require further detoxification by enzymes such as GSTs (Gago-Dominguez et al., 2007).

The *Ala* allele of the *Ala9Val* (*rs*4880) polymorphism of the *MnSOD* gene has been found to generate 30–40% more enzymatic activity. Therefore, overexpression of MnSOD can increase hydrogen peroxide production, which can contribute to further production of ROS, if it is not subsequently neutralized and converted to H_2O and O_2 (Ambrosone et al., 2005). Premenopausal women who were homozygous for the *Ala* allele had a 4-fold increased risk of breast cancer compared to women with one or two *Val* alleles. Additionally, the increased risk was more pronounced among women who consumed fruits, vegetables, dietary ascorbic acid, and α-tocopherol below the median level (Ambrosone et al., 1999b). Similar interactions were found between genotypes and low intake of fruits, vegetables, vitamin supplements, selenium, and antioxidant vitamins among premenopausal Chinese women (Cai et al., 2004). However, these modifications of the gene's main effect by intake levels of fruits, vegetables, dietary antioxidants, vitamin supplements, and plasma antioxidant levels were not replicated in other studies (Egan et al., 2003; Gaudet et al., 2005; Millikan et al., 2004; Mitrunen et al., 2001; Slanger et al., 2006; Tamimi et al., 2004).

The high activity *CC* genotype of the *C-262T* (*rs*1001179) polymorphism of the *catalase* gene was associated with a 17% reduction in risk of breast cancer, and the association was more pronounced among women who consumed high amounts of fruit and did not consume vitamin supplements in the Long Island Breast Cancer Study Project (Ahn et al., 2005b). In the same study population, a reduced risk for premenopausal breast cancer among *A* allele carriers of the *G-463A* (*rs*2333227)polymorphism of the *myeloperoxidase* (*MPO*) gene was most pronounced in women who consumed higher amounts of total fruits and vegetables (Ahn et al., 2004). This study did not find evidence for a main genetic effect or effect modification by antioxidant intake in relation to the *GPX*1 *Pro*198*Leu* (*rs*1050450) polymorphism (Ahn et al., 2005a).

A genetic polymorphism of the phase II detoxifying enzyme *GSTM*1 did not show an association with breast cancer risk regardless of dietary antioxidant level (Ambrosone et al., 1999a). Since multiple phase II enzymes are induced by isothiocyanates, which are abundant in cruciferous vegetables, the interactive effects between cruciferous vegetable intake and genetic polymorphism of *GSTs* were evaluated. Two studies found no evidence of an effect modification of genetic polymorphisms of *GSTs* on the preventive effect of cruciferous vegetable intake (Ambrosone et al., 2004; Steck et al., 2007). Ahn et al. (2006) found that among women in the two lowest tertiles of cruciferous vegetable intake, those who possessed the **B/*B* genotypes of the *GSTA*1 gene had an increased risk of breast cancer compared to women with the **A/*A* genotypes (Ahn et al., 2006). Lee et al. (2008) observed the highest risk for breast cancer among women with the *Val/Val* genotype of the *GSTP*1 *Ile*105*Val* (*rs*1695) polymorphism and low cruciferous vegetable intake, although no significant interaction was found (Lee et al., 2008).

10.8 Iron Overload

Iron overload has been linked to an increased risk of breast cancer. Free iron catalyzes the generation of potential free-radical species, which are highly toxic to cells (Kallianpur et al., 2004). Therefore, genetic variance in genes related to hemochromatosis, an iron overload disorder, have been assessed for their role in cancer. Several studies have assessed the association of the hemochromatosis gene *HFE*, the ferroprotein 1 gene *FPN*1, and trensferrin receptor gene *TFR*2 and breast cancer risk, however, the results have been inconclusive (Kallianpur et al., 2004; Abraham et al., 2005; Beckman et al., 1999).

10.9 Meat and Meat Mutagens

When cooking meat at high temperatures, heterocyclic amines (HCAs) and polycyclic aromatic hydrocarbons (PAHs) are formed, and these amine compounds have been shown to be mutagenic in animal studies (Sinha and Rothman, 1999). HCAs exert their mutagenic action through an enzyme-catalyzed activation consisting of *N*-oxidation by hepatic CYP1A2 and other extrahepatic P450 isozymes, followed by *O*-acetylation by N-acetyltransferase 1 (NAT1) and 2 (NAT2) (Nowell et al., 2004). Deitz et al. (2000) observed a higher risk of breast cancer in women who had higher scores for well-done meat only when women possessed rapid or intermediate acetylator genotypes for *NAT*2 (Deitz et al., 2000). Similarly, Egeberg et al. (2008) found a positive association between total meat intake and red meat intake and breast cancer risk that was confined to intermediate or rapid NAT2 acetylators. Additionally, they reported a statistically significant interaction (Egeberg et al., 2008). However, other studies did not find effect modifications by meat intake levels, cooking methods, doneness levels, or HCA intake levels (Ambrosone et al., 1998; Delfino et al., 2000; Gertig et al., 1999; Krajinovic et al., 2001; van der Hel et al., 2004; Zheng et al. (1999)) reported that a positive association of breast cancer with the *NAT*1 *11 allele was more evident among those who consumed high levels of red meat or consistently consumed well-done red meat (Zheng et al., 1999). Krajinovic et al. (2001) also reported that women who possessed the rapid acetylator allele *10 of *NAT*1 and consumed well-done meat were at a 4-fold increased risk for breast cancer compared to those with the *10 allele who did not consume well-done meat (Krajinovic et al., 2001). An interactive effect between meat intake and *NAT*1 genotypes, however, was not found in other studies (Egeberg et al., 2008; van der Hel et al., 2004).

SULT1A1 is involved in the bioactivation of HCAs and PAHs, and the low activity *His* allele of the *Arg*213*His* (*rs*9282861) polymorphism is related to lower risk of meat mutagen-related carcinogenesis. Zheng et al. (2001) observed a dose-response relationship between meat doneness levels and breast cancer risk among women with the *Arg* allele but not among those with the His/His genotype (Zheng et al., 2001). Carcinogenic compounds from meat are detoxified by GSTs, and an elevated risk of breast cancer in women who were null for both *GSTM*1 and *GSTT*1 was mainly observed among women who consistently consumed well-done meat (Zheng et al., 2002). No apparent interactions between *GSTM*1, *T*1, *P*1 polymorphisms, and meat or meat doneness levels were found in other studies (Egan et al., 2004; Krajinovic et al., 2001; van der Hel et al., 2004; Zhao et al., 2001).

10.10 Other Environmental Factors

10.10.1 Circadian Disruption

Nurses and flight attendants who work evening or overnight shifts exhibit a consistently higher risk of breast cancer in epidemiological studies. This finding lead to the circadian disruption hypothesis, which suggests that exposure to light at night disrupts the endogenous circadian rhythm and consequently suppresses nocturnal melatonin production (Stevens, 2005). Melatonin has been recognized as a strong inhibitor of mammary tumorigenesis in rodents.

Eight core circadian genes have been identified and their functional effects have been tested in mice: *Clock, casein kinase* 1*e* (*CK*1*e*), *cryptochrome* 1 (*Cry*1) and *cryptochrome* 2 (*Cry*2), *Period* 1 (*PER*1), *Period* 2 (*PER*2) and *Period* 3 (*PER*3), and *Bmal*1 (Stevens, 2005). Expression of the *PER*1, *PER*2, and *PER*3 genes has also been shown to be lower in breast cancer tissues (Winter et al., 2007) and breast cancer cell lines (Chen et al., 2005). However, the role of genetic polymorphisms of these genes in circardian rhythm disruption has not yet been assessed.

10.11 Conclusions

It is generally accepted that neither genetic factors nor environmental factors are solely responsible for breast cancer development and that differences in genetic factors result in different responses to the same environmental exposures. These are the main reasons for the investigation of gene–environment interactions. Unfortunately, evidence of statistical interaction between genes and environmental factors is still limited, although this may change in the near future with recent advances in genetic techniques and knowledge. International collaboration through multicenter consortia which encompass information not only on genetic but also environmental risk factors would contribute greatly to the production of more solid knowledge on the role of gene–environment interactions and their effect on breast carcinogenesis.

Acknowledgments The authors would like to thank Kwang-Pil Ko, M.D., Ph.D., Eun Ha Lee, M.D. and Eorin Cho, Ph.D. for their contributions to the literature review.

References

Abbas, S., Nieters, A., Linseisen, J., Slanger, T., Kropp, S., Mutschelknauss, E. J., lesch-Janys, D., Chang-Claude, J. 2008. Vitamin D receptor gene polymorphisms and haplotypes and postmenopausal breast cancer risk. Breast Cancer Res 10(2):R31.

Abraham, B. K., Justenhoven, C., Pesch, B., Harth, V., Weirich, G., Baisch, C., Rabstein, S., Ko, Y. D., Bruning, T., Fischer, H. P., Haas, S., Brod, S., Oberkanins, C., Hamann, U., Brauch, H. 2005. Investigation of genetic variants of genes of the hemochromatosis pathway and their role in breast cancer. Cancer Epidemiol Biomarkers Prev 14:1102–1107.

Ahn, J., Gammon, M. D., Santella, R. M., Gaudet, M. M., Britton, J. A., Teitelbaum, S. L., Terry, M. B., Neugut, A. I., Ambrosone, C. B. 2005a. No association between glutathione peroxidase Pro198Leu polymorphism and breast cancer risk. Cancer Epidemiol Biomarkers Prev 14: 2459–2461.

Ahn, J., Gammon, M. D., Santella, R. M., Gaudet, M. M., Britton, J. A., Teitelbaum, S. L., Terry, M. B., Neugut, A. I., Eng, S. M., Zhang, Y., Garza, C., Ambrosone, C. B. 2006. Effects of glutathione S-transferase A1 (GSTA1) genotype and potential modifiers on breast cancer risk. Carcinogenesis 27:1876–1882.

Ahn, J., Gammon, M. D., Santella, R. M., Gaudet, M. M., Britton, J. A., Teitelbaum, S. L., Terry, M. B., Neugut, A. I., Josephy, P. D., Ambrosone, C. B. 2004. Myeloperoxidase genotype, fruit and vegetable consumption, and breast cancer risk. Cancer Res 64:7634–7639.

Ahn, J., Gammon, M. D., Santella, R. M., Gaudet, M. M., Britton, J. A., Teitelbaum, S. L., Terry, M. B., Nowell, S., Davis, W., Garza, C., Neugut, A. I., Ambrosone, C. B. 2005b. Associations between breast cancer risk and the catalase genotype, fruit and vegetable consumption, and supplement use. Am J Epidemiol 162:943–952.

Ahsan, H., Whittemore, A. S., Chen, Y., Senie, R. T., Hamilton, S. P., Wang, Q., Gurvich, I., Santella, R. M. 2005. Variants in estrogen-biosynthesis genes CYP17 and CYP19 and breast cancer risk: a family-based genetic association study. Breast Cancer Res 7(1):R71–R81.

Ambrosone, C. B., Ahn, J., Singh, K. K., Rezaishiraz, H., Furberg, H., Sweeney, C., Coles, B., Trovato, A. 2005. Polymorphisms in genes related to oxidative stress (MPO, MnSOD, CAT) and survival after treatment for breast cancer. Cancer Res 65:1105–1111.

Ambrosone, C. B., Coles, B. F., Freudenheim, J. L., Shields, P. G. 1999a. Glutathione-S-transferase (GSTM1) genetic polymorphisms do not affect human breast cancer risk, regardless of dietary antioxidants. J Nutr 129:565S–568S.

Ambrosone, C. B., Freudenheim, J. L., Thompson, P. A., Bowman, E., Vena, J. E., Marshall, J. R., Graham, S., Laughlin, R., Nemoto, T., Shields, P. G. 1999b. Manganese superoxide dismutase (MnSOD) genetic polymorphisms, dietary antioxidants, and risk of breast cancer. Cancer Res 59:602–606.

Ambrosone, C. B., Freudenheim, J. L., Sinha, R., Graham, S., Marshall, J. R., Vena, J. E., Laughlin, R., Nemoto, T., Shields, P. G. 1998. Breast cancer risk, meat consumption and N-acetyltransferase (NAT2) genetic polymorphisms. Int J Cancer 75:825–830.

Ambrosone, C. B., McCann, S. E., Freudenheim, J. L., Marshall, J. R., Zhang, Y., Shields, P. G. 2004. Breast cancer risk in premenopausal women is inversely associated with consumption of broccoli, a source of isothiocyanates, but is not modified by GST genotype.

Ambrosone, C. B., Moysich, K. B., Furberg, H., Freudenheim, J. L., Bowman, E. D., Ahmed, S., Graham, S., Vena, J. E., Shields, P. G. 2003. CYP17 genetic polymorphism, breast cancer, and breast cancer risk factors. Breast Cancer Res 5(2):R45–R51.

Bailey, L. B., Gregory, J. F., 3rd. 1999. Polymorphisms of methylenetetrahydrofolate reductase and other enzymes: metabolic significance, risks and impact on folate requirement. J Nutr 129: 919–922.

Beckman, L. E., Van Landeghem, G. F., Sikstrom, C., Wahlin, A., Markevarn, B., Hallmans, G., Lenner, P., Athlin, L., Stenling, R., Beckman, L. 1999. Interaction between haemochromatosis and transferrin receptor genes in different neoplastic disorders. Carcinogenesis 20:1231–1233.

Bennermo, M., Held, C., Stemme, S., Ericsson, C. G., Silveira, A., Green, F., Tornvall, P. 2004. Genetic predisposition of the interleukin-6 response to inflammation: implications for a variety of major diseases? Clin Chem 50:2136–2140.

Bernard-Gallon, D., Bosviel, R., Delort, L., Fontana, L., Chamoux, A., Rabiau, N., Kwiatkowski, F., Chalabi, N., Satih, S., Bignon, Y. J. 2008. DNA repair gene ERCC2 polymorphisms and associations with breast and ovarian cancer risk. Mol Cancer 7:36.

Bischoff, J. R., Plowman, G. D. 1999. The Aurora/Ipl1p kinase family: regulators of chromosome segregation and cytokinesis. Trends Cell Biol 9:454–459.

Bosron, W. F., Li, T. K. 1986. Genetic polymorphism of human liver alcohol and aldehyde dehydrogenases, and their relationship to alcohol metabolism and alcoholism. Hepatology 6:502–510.

Brentano, S. T., Picado-Leonard, J., Mellon, S. H., Moore, C. C., Miller, W. L. 1990. Tissue-specific, cyclic adenosine 3#,5#-monophosphate-induced, and phorbol ester-repressed transcription from the human P450c17 promoter in mouse cells. Mol Endocrinol 4(12):1972–1979.

Bretherton-Watt, D., Given-Wilson, R., Mansi, J. L., Thomas, V., Carter, N., Colston, K. W. 2001. Vitamin D receptor gene polymorphisms are associated with breast cancer risk in a UK Caucasian population. Br J Cancer 85(2):171–175.

Cai, Q., Shu, X. O., Jin, F., Dai, Q., Wen, W., Cheng, J. R., Gao, Y. T., Zheng, W. 2003. Genetic polymorphisms in the estrogen receptor alpha gene and risk of breast cancer: results from the Shanghai Breast Cancer Study. Cancer Epidemiol Biomarkers Prev 12:853–859.

Cai, Q., Shu, X. O., Wen, W., Cheng, J. R., Dai, Q., Gao, Y. T., Zheng, W. 2004. Genetic polymorphism in the manganese superoxide dismutase gene, antioxidant intake, and breast cancer risk: results from the Shanghai Breast Cancer Study. Breast Cancer Res 6:R647–R655.

Chacko, P., Rajan, B., Mathew, B. S., Joseph, T., Pillai, M. R. 2004. CYP17 and SULT1A1 gene polymorphisms in Indian breast cancer. Breast Cancer 11(4):380–388.

Chakraverty, R. K., Hickson, I. D. 1999. Defending genome integrity during DNA replication: a proposed role for RecQ family helicases. Bioessays 21:286–294.

Chang, J. H., Gertig, D. M., Chen, X., Dite, G. S., Jenkins, M. A., Milne, R. L., Southey, M. C., McCredie, M. R., Giles, G. G., Chenevix-Trench, G., Hopper, J. L., Spurdle, A. B. 2005. CYP17 genetic polymorphism, breast cancer, and breast cancer risk factors: Australian Breast Cancer Family Study. Breast Cancer Res 7(4):R513–R521.

Chang, J. H., Gertig, D. M., Chen, X., Dite, G. S., Jenkins, M. A., Milne, R. L., Southey, M. C., McCredie, M. R., Giles, G. G., Chenevix-Trench, G., Hopper, J. L., Spurdle, A. B. 2005. CYP17 genetic polymorphism, breast cancer, and breast cancer risk factors: Australian Breast Cancer Family Study. Breast Cancer Res 7(4):R513–R521.

Chen, S. T., Choo, K. B., Hou, M. F., Yeh, K. T., Kuo, S. J., Chang, J. G. 2005b. Deregulated expression of the *PER*1, *PER*2, and *PER*3 genes in breast cancers. Carcinogenesis 26: 1241–1246.

Chen, J., Gammon, M. D., Chan, W., Palomeque, C., Wetmur, J. G., Kabat, G. C., Teitelbaum, S. L., Britton, J. A., Terry, M. B., Neugut, A. I., Santella, R. M. 2005a. One-carbon metabolism, MTHFR polymorphisms, and risk of breast cancer. Cancer Res 65:1606–1614.

Chen, Y., Gammon, M. D., Teitelbaum, S. L., Britton, J. A., Terry, M. B., Shantakumar, S., Eng, S. M., Wang, Q., Gurvich, I., Neugut, A. I., Santella, R. M., Ahsan, H. 2008. Estrogen-biosynthesis gene CYP17 and its interactions with reproductive, hormonal and lifestyle factors in breast cancer risk: results from the Long Island Breast Cancer Study Project. Carcinogenesis 29(4):766–771.

Cheng, T. C., Chen, S. T., Huang, C. S., Fu, Y. P., Yu, J. C., Cheng, C. W., Wu, P. E., Shen, C. Y. 2005. Breast cancer risk associated with genotype polymorphism of the catechol estrogen-metabolizing genes: a multigenic study on cancer susceptibility. Int J Cancer 113(3):345–353.

Choi, J. Y., Abel, J., Neuhaus, T., Ko, Y., Harth, V., Hamajima, N., Tajima, K., Yoo, K. Y., Park, S. K., Noh, D. Y., Han, W., Choe, K. J., Ahn, S. H., Kim, S. U., Hirvonen, A., Kang, D. 2003. Role of alcohol and genetic polymorphisms of CYP2E1 and ALDH2 in breast cancer development. Pharmacogenetics 13:67–72.

Chou, Y. C., Wu, M. H., Yu, J. C., Lee, M. S., Yang, T., Shih, H. L., Wu, T. Y., Sun, C. A. 2006. Genetic polymorphisms of the methylenetetrahydrofolate reductase gene, plasma folate levels and breast cancer susceptibility: a case-control study in Taiwan. Carcinogenesis 27:2295–2300.

Coin, F., Marinoni, J. C., Rodolfo, C., Fribourg, S., Pedrini, A. M., Egly, J. M. 1998. Mutations in the XPD helicase gene result in XP and TTD phenotypes, preventing interaction between XPD and the p44 subunit of TFIIH. Nat Genet 20:184–188.

Comings, D. E., Gade-Andavolu, R., Cone, L. A., Muhleman, D., MacMurray, J. P. 2003. A multigene test for the risk of sporadic breast carcinoma. Cancer 97:2160–2170.

Cui, Y., Shu, X. O., Cai, Q., Jin, F., Cheng, J. R., Cai, H., Gao, Y. T., Zheng, W. 2005. Association of breast cancer risk with a common functional polymorphism (Asp327Asn) in the sex hormone-binding globulin gene. Cancer Epidemiol Biomarkers Prev 14(5):1096–1101.

Curran, J. E., Lea, R. A., Rutherford, S., Weinstein, S. R., Griffiths, L. R. 2001. Association of estrogen receptor and glucocorticoid receptor gene polymorphisms with sporadic breast cancer. Int J Cancer 95:271–275.

Curran, J. E., Vaughan, T., Lea, R. A., Weinstein, S. R., Morrison, N. A., Griffiths, L. R. 1999. Association of A vitamin D receptor polymorphism with sporadic breast cancer development. Int J Cancer 83(6):723–726.

Dai, Q., Cai, Q. Y., Shu, X. O., Ewart-Toland, A., Wen, W. Q., Balmain, A., Gao, Y. T., Zheng, W. 2004. Synergistic effects of STK15 gene polymorphisms and endogenous estrogen exposure in the risk of breast cancer. Cancer Epidemiol Biomarkers Prev 13:2065–2070.

De Vivo, I., Hankinson, S. E., Colditz, G. A., Hunter, D. J. 2003. A functional polymorphism in the progesterone receptor gene is associated with an increase in breast cancer risk. Cancer Res 63:5236–5238.

Deeb, S. S., Fajas, L., Nemoto, M., Pihlajamaki, J., Mykkanen, L., Kuusisto, J., Laakso, M., Fujimoto, W., Auwerx, J. 1998. A Pro12Ala substitution in PPARgamma2 associated with decreased receptor activity, lower body mass index and improved insulin sensitivity. Nat Genet 20:284–287.

Deitz, A. C., Zheng, W., Leff, M. A., Gross, M., Wen, W. Q., Doll, M. A., Xiao, G. H., Folsom, A. R., Hein, D. W. 2000. N-Acetyltransferase-2 genetic polymorphism, well-done meat intake, and breast cancer risk among postmenopausal women. Cancer Epidemiol Biomarkers Prev 9:905–910.

Delfino, R. J., Sinha, R., Smith, C., West, J., White, E., Lin, H. J., Liao, S. Y., Gim, J. S., Ma, H. L., Butler, J., Anton-Culver, H. 2000. Breast cancer, heterocyclic aromatic amines from meat and N-acetyltransferase 2 genotype. Carcinogenesis 21:607–615.

Ding, S. L., Yu, J. C., Chen, S. T., Hsu, G. C., Shen, C. Y. 2007. Genetic variation in the premature aging gene WRN: a case-control study on breast cancer susceptibility. Cancer Epidemiol Biomarkers Prev 16(2):263–269.

Dunning, A. M., Healey, C. S., Pharoah, P. D., Foster, N. A., Lipscombe, J. M., Redman, K. L., Easton, D. F., Day, N. E., Ponder, B. A. 1998. No association between a polymorphism in the steroid metabolism gene CYP17 and risk of breast cancer. Br J Cancer 77:2045–2047.

Dunning, A. M., McBride, S., Gregory, J., Durocher, F., Foster, N. A., Healey, C. S., Smith, N., Pharoah, P. D., Luben, R. N., Easton, D. F., Ponder, B. A. 1999. No association between androgen or vitamin D receptor gene polymorphisms and risk of breast cancer. Carcinogenesis 20(11):2131–2135.

Egan, K. M., Cai, Q., Shu, X. O., Jin, F., Zhu, T. L., Dai, Q., Gao, Y. T., Zheng, W. 2004a. Genetic polymorphisms in GSTM1, GSTP1, and GSTT1 and the risk for breast cancer: results from the Shanghai Breast Cancer Study and meta-analysis. Cancer Epidemiol Biomarkers Prev 13: 197–204.

Egan, K. M., Newcomb, P. A., Ambrosone, C. B., Trentham-Dietz, A., Titus-Ernstoff, L., Hampton, J. M., Kimura, M. T., Nagase, H. 2004b. STK15 polymorphism and breast cancer risk in a population-based study. Carcinogenesis 25:2149–2153.

Egan, K. M., Thompson, P. A., Titus-Ernstoff, L., Moore, J. H., Ambrosone, C. B. 2003. MnSOD polymorphism and breast cancer in a population-based case-control study. Cancer Lett 199: 27–33.
Egeberg, R., Olsen, A., Autrup, H., Christensen, J., Stripp, C., Tetens, I., Overvad, K., Tjonneland, A. 2008. Meat consumption, N-acetyl transferase 1 and 2 polymorphism and risk of breast cancer in Danish postmenopausal women. Eur J Cancer Prev 17:39–47.
Einarsdóttir, K., Darabi, H., Li, Y., Low, Y. L., Li, Y. Q., Bonnard, C., Sjölander, A., Czene, K., Wedrén, S., Liu, E. T., Hall, P., Humphreys, K., Liu, J. 2008. ESR1 and EGF genetic variation in relation to breast cancer risk and survival. Breast Cancer Res 10(1):R15.
Einarsdóttir, K., Rylander-Rudqvist, T., Humphreys, K., Ahlberg, S., Jonasdottir, G., Weiderpass, E., Chia, K. S., Ingelman-Sundberg, M., Persson, I., Liu, J., Hall, P., Wedrén, S. 2005. CYP17 gene polymorphism in relation to breast cancer risk: a case-control study. Breast Cancer Res 7(6):R890–R896.
Feigelson, H. S., Coetzee, G. A., Kolonel, L. N., Ross, R. K., Henderson, B. E. 1997. A polymorphism in the CYP17 gene increases the risk of breast cancer. Cancer Res 57:1063–1065.
Fletcher, O., Johnson, N., Palles, C., dos Santos Silva, I., McCormack, V., Whittaker, J., Ashworth, A., Peto, J. 2006. Inconsistent association between the STK15 F31I genetic polymorphism and breast cancer risk. J Natl Cancer Inst 98(14):1014–1018.
Freudenheim, J. L., Ambrosone, C. B., Moysich, K. B., Vena, J. E., Graham, S., Marshall, J. R., Muti, P., Laughlin, R., Nemoto, T., Harty, L. C., Crits, G. A., Chan, A. W., Shields, P. G. 1999. Alcohol dehydrogenase 3 genotype modification of the association of alcohol consumption with breast cancer risk. Cancer Causes Control 10:369–377.
Futaki, M., Liu, J. M. 2001. Chromosomal breakage syndromes and the BRCA1 genome surveillance complex. Trends Mol Med 7:560–565.
Gago-Dominguez, M., Jiang, X., Castelao, J. E. 2007. Lipid peroxidation, oxidative stress genes and dietary factors in breast cancer protection: a hypothesis. Breast Cancer Res 9:201.
Gaudet, M. M., Gammon, M. D., Santella, R. M., Britton, J. A., Teitelbaum, S. L., Eng, S. M., Terry, M. B., Bensen, J. T., Schroeder, J., Olshan, A. F., Neugut, A. I., Ambrosone, C. B. 2005. MnSOD Val-9Ala genotype, pro- and anti-oxidant environmental modifiers, and breast cancer among women on Long Island, New York. Cancer Causes Control 16:1225–1234.
Gertig, D. M., Hankinson, S. E., Hough, H., Spiegelman, D., Colditz, G. A., Willett, W. C., Kelsey, K. T., Hunter, D. J. 1999. N-acetyl transferase 2 genotypes, meat intake and breast cancer risk. Int J Cancer 80:13–17.
Goodman, J. E., Lavigne, J. A., Wu, K., Helzlsouer, K. J., Strickland, P. T., Selhub, J., Yager, J. D. 2001. COMT genotype, micronutrients in the folate metabolic pathway and breast cancer risk. Carcinogenesis 22:1661–1665.
Guy, M., Lowe, L. C., Bretherton-Watt, D., Mansi, J. L., Colston, K. W. 2003. Approaches to evaluating the association of vitamin D receptor gene polymorphisms with breast cancer risk. Recent Results Cancer Res 164:43–54.
Habuchi, T., Suzuki, T., Sasaki, R., Wang, L., Sato, K., Satoh, S., Akao, T., Tsuchiya, N., Shimoda, N., Wada, Y., Koizumi, A., Chihara, J., Ogawa, O., Kato, T. 2000. Association of vitamin D receptor gene polymorphism with prostate cancer and benign prostatic hyperplasia in a Japanese population. Cancer Res 60:305–308.
Haiman, C. A., Bernstein, L., Berg, D., Ingles, S. A., Salane, M., Ursin, G. 2002. Genetic determinants of mammographic density. Breast Cancer Res 4:R5.
Haiman, C. A., Hankinson, S. E., De Vivo, I., Guillemette, C., Ishibe, N., Hunter, D. J., Byrne, C. 2003. Polymorphisms in steroid hormone pathway genes and mammographic density. Breast Cancer Res Treat 77:27–36.
Haiman, C. A., Hankinson, S. E., Spiegelman, D., Colditz, G. A., Willett, W. C., Speizer, F. E., Kelsey, K. T., Hunter, D. J. 1999. The relationship between a polymorphism in CYP17 with plasma hormone levels and breast cancer. Cancer Res 59:1015–1020.
Hamajima, N., Iwata, H., Obata, Y., Matsuo, K., Mizutani, M., Iwase, T., Miura, S., Okuma, K., Ohashi, K., Tajima, K. 2000. No association of the 5′promoter region polymorphism of CYP17 with breast cancer risk in Japan. Jpn J Cancer Res 91:880–885.

Han, J., Hankinson, S. E., Zhang, S. M., De Vivo, I., Hunter, D. J. 2004b. Interaction between genetic variations in DNA repair genes and plasma folate on breast cancer risk. Cancer Epidemiol Biomarkers Prev 13:520–524.
Han, D. F., Zhou, X., Hu, M. B., Wang, C. H., Xie, W., Tan, X. D., Zheng, F., Liu, F. 2004a. Sulfotransferase 1A1 (SULT1A1) polymorphism and breast cancer risk in Chinese women. Toxicol Lett 150(2):167–177.
Han, D. F., Zhou, X., Hu, M. B., Xie, W., Mao, Z. F., Chen, D. E., Liu, F., Zheng, F. 2005. Polymorphisms of estrogen-metabolizing genes and breast cancer risk: a multigenic study. Chin Med J (Engl) 118(18):1507–1516.
Hannah, S. S., Norman, A. W. 1994. 1a, 25(OH)2 vitamin D3-regulated expression of the eukaryotic genome. Nutr Rev 52:376–382.
Hefler, L. A., Tempfer, C. B., Grimm, C., Lebrecht, A., Ulbrich, E., Heinze, G., Leodolter, S., Helzlsouer, K. J., Huang, H. Y., Strickland, P. T., Hoffman, S., Alberg, A. J., Comstock, G. W., Bell, D. A. 1998. Association between CYP17 polymorphisms and the development of breast cancer. Cancer Epidemiol Biomarkers Prev 7:945–949.
Helzlsouer, K. J., Selmin, O., Huang, H. Y., Strickland, P. T., Hoffman, S., Alberg, A. J., Watson, M., Comstock, G. W., Bell, D. 1998. Association between glutathione S-transferase M1, P1, and T1 genetic polymorphisms and development of breast cancer. J Natl Cancer Inst 90: 512–518.
Hines, L. M., Hankinson, S. E., Smith-Warner, S. A., Spiegelman, D., Kelsey, K. T., Colditz, G. A., Willett, W. C., Hunter, D. J. 2000. A prospective study of the effect of alcohol consumption and ADH3 genotype on plasma steroid hormone levels and breast cancer risk. Cancer Epidemiol Biomarkers Prev 9:1099–1105.
Hirota, T., Kunitoku, N., Sasayama, T., Marumoto, T., Zhang, D., Nitta, M., Hatakeyama, K., Saya, H. 2003. Aurora-A and an interacting activator, the LIM protein Ajuba, are required for mitotic commitment in human cells. Cell 114:585–598.
Hou, M. F., Tien, Y. C., Lin, G. T., Chen, C. J., Liu, C. S., Lin, S. Y., Huang, T. J. 2002. Association of vitamin D receptor gene polymorphism with sporadic breast cancer in Taiwanese patients. Breast Cancer Res Treat 74(1):1–7.
Huang, C. S., Chern, H. D., Chang, K. J., Cheng, C. W., Hsu, S. M., Shen, C. Y. 1999. Breast cancer risk associated with genotype polymorphism of the estrogen-metabolizing genes CYP17, CYP1A1, and COMT: a multigenic study on cancer susceptibility. Cancer Res 59:4870–4875.
IARC Working Group on the Evaluation of Cancer-Preventive Agents. 2002. Weight Control and Physical Activity, IARC Handbooks of Cancer Prevention, Volume 6. Lyon, France: IARC.
Ingles, S. A., Garcia, D. G., Wang, W., Nieters, A., Henderson, B. E., Kolonel, L. N., Haile, R. W., Coetzee, G. A. 2000. Vitamin D receptor genotype and breast cancer in Latinas (United States). Cancer Causes Control 11(1):25–30.
Iwase, H., Greenman, J. M., Barnes, D. M., Hodgson, S., Bobrow, L., Mathew, C. G. 1996. Sequence variants of the estrogen receptor (ER) gene found in breast cancer patients with ER negative and progesterone receptor positive tumors. Cancer Lett 108:179–184; J Nutr 134:1134–8.
James, S. Y., Mackay, A. G., Colston, K. W. 2006. Effects of 1, 25 dihydroxyvitamin D3 and its analogues on induction of apoptosis in breast cancer cells. J Steroid Biochem Mol Biol 58:395–401.
Jerevall, P. L., Ahmadi, A., Bergman, M., Stål, O., Wingren, S. 2005. Sulfotransferase1A1 and risk of postmenopausal breast cancer. Anticancer Res 25(3c):2515–2517.
John, E. M., Schwartz, G. G., Koo, J., Wang, W., Ingles, S. A. 2007. Sun exposure, vitamin D receptor gene polymorphisms, and breast cancer risk in a multiethnic population. Am J Epidemiol 166(12):1409–1419.
Kallianpur, A. R., Hall, L. D., Yadav, M., Christman, B. W., Dittus, R. S., Haines, J. L., Parl, F. F., Summar, M. L. 2004. Increased prevalence of the HFE C282Y hemochromatosis allele in women with breast cancer. Cancer Epidemiol Biomarkers Prev 13:205–212.

Kang, H. J., Kim, S. W., Kim, H. J., Ahn, S. J., Bae, J. Y., Park, S. K., Kang, D., Hirvonen, A., Choe, K. J., Noh, D. Y. 2002. Polymorphisms in the estrogen receptor-alpha gene and breast cancer risk. Cancer Lett 178:175–180.

Kawase, T., Matsuo, K., Suzuki, T., Hiraki, A., Watanabe, M., Iwata, H., Tanaka, H., Tajima, K. 2009. FGFR2 intronic polymorphisms interact with reproductive risk factors of breast cancer: results of a case control study in Japan. Int J Cancer 125:1946–1952.

Kelsey, J. L., Horn-Ross, P. L. 1993. Breast cancer: magnitude of the problem and descriptive epidemiology. Epidemiol Rev 15:7–16.

Kim, S. U., Lee, K. M., Park, S. K., Yoo, K. Y., Noh, D. Y., Choe, K. J., Ahn, S. H., Hirvonen, A., Kang, D. 2004. Genetic polymorphism of glutathione S-transferase P1 and breast cancer risk. J Biochem Mol Biol 37:582–585.

Kotsopoulos, J., Tworoger, S. S., De Vivo, I., Hankinson, S. E., Hunter, D. J., Willett, W. C., Chen, W. Y. 2009. +331G/A variant in the progesterone receptor gene, postmenopausal hormone use and risk of breast cancer. Int J Cancer 125:1685–1691.

Krajinovic, M., Ghadirian, P., Richer, C., Sinnett, H., Gandini, S., Perret, C., Lacroix, A., Labuda, D., Sinnett, D. 2001. Genetic susceptibility to breast cancer in French-Canadians: role of carcinogen-metabolizing enzymes and gene-environment interactions. Int J Cancer 92:220–225.

Le Marchand, L., Donlon, T., Kolonel, L. N., Henderson, B. E., Wilkens, L. R. 2005. Estrogen metabolism-related genes and breast cancer risk: the multiethnic cohort study. Cancer Epidemiol Biomarkers Prev 14(8):1998–2003.

Le Marchand, L., Haiman, C. A., Wilkens, L. R., Kolonel, L. N., Henderson, B. E. 2004. MTHFR polymorphisms, diet, HRT, and breast cancer risk: the multiethnic cohort study. Cancer Epidemiol Biomarkers Prev 13:2071–2077.

Lee, K. M., Abel, J., Ko, Y., Harth, V., Park, W. Y., Seo, J. S., Yoo, K. Y., Choi, J. Y., Shin, A., Ahn, S. H., Noh, D. Y., Hirvonen, A., Kang, D. 2003. Genetic polymorphisms of cytochrome P450 19 and 1B1, alcohol use, and breast cancer risk in Korean women. Br J Cancer 88: 675–678.

Lee, K. M., Choi, J. Y., Kang, C., Kang, C. P., Park, S. K., Cho, H., Cho, D. Y., Yoo, K. Y., Noh, D. Y., Ahn, S. H., Park, C. G., Wei, Q., Kang, D. 2005a. Genetic polymorphisms of selected DNA repair genes, estrogen and progesterone receptor status, and breast cancer risk. Clin Cancer Res 11:4620–4626.

Lee, S. A., Fowke, J. H., Lu, W., Ye, C., Zheng, Y., Cai, Q., Gu, K., Gao, Y. T., Shu, X. O., Zheng, W. 2008. Cruciferous vegetables, the GSTP1 Ile105Val genetic polymorphism, and breast cancer risk. Am J of Clin Nutr 87:753–760.

Lee, S. A., Lee, K. M., Park, W. Y., Kim, B., Nam, J., Yoo, K. Y., Noh, D. Y., Ahn, S. H., Hirvonen, A., Kang, D. 2005b. Obesity and genetic polymorphism of ERCC2 and ERCC4 as modifiers of risk of breast cancer. Exp Mol Med 37:86–90.

Lewis, S. J., Harbord, R. M., Harris, R., Smith, G. D. 2006. Meta-analyses of observational and genetic association studies of folate intakes or levels and breast cancer risk. J Natl Cancer Inst 98:1607–1622.

Li, B., Comai, L. 2000. Functional interaction between Ku and the werner syndrome protein in DNA end processing. J Biol Chem 275(37):28349–28352.

Lilla, C., Koehler, T., Kropp, S., Wang-Gohrke, S., Chang-Claude, J. 2005. Alcohol dehydrogenase 1B (ADH1B) genotype, alcohol consumption and breast cancer risk by age 50 years in a German case-control study. Br J Cancer 92:2039–2041.

Lissowska, J., Gaudet, M. M., Brinton, L. A., Chanock, S. J., Peplonska, B., Welch, R., Zatonski, W., Szeszenia-Dabrowska, N., Park, S., Sherman, M., Garcia-Closas, M. 2007. Genetic polymorphisms in the one-carbon metabolism pathway and breast cancer risk: a population-based case-control study and meta-analyses. Int J Cancer 120:2696–2703.

Lowe, L. C., Guy, M., Mansi, J. L., Peckitt, C., Bliss, J., Wilson, R. G., Colston, K. W. 2005. Plasma 25-hydroxy vitamin D concentrations, vitamin D receptor genotype and breast cancer risk in a UK Caucasian population. Eur J Cancer 41(8):1164–1169.

Lu, H., Ouyang, W., Huang, C. 2006. Inflammation, a key event in cancer development. Mol Cancer Res 4:221–233.

Lundin, A. C., Söderkvist, P., Eriksson, B., Bergman-Jungeström, M., Wingren, S. 1999. Association of breast cancer progression with a vitamin D receptor gene polymorphism. South-East Sweden Breast Cancer Group. Cancer Res 59(10):2332–2334.

Lunn, R. M., Helzlsouer, K. J., Parshad, R., Umbach, D. M., Harris, E. L., Sanford, K. K., Bell, D. A. 2000. XPD polymorphisms: effects on DNA repair proficiency. Carcinogenesis 21:551–555.

McCullough, M. L., Stevens, V. L., Diver, W. R., Feigelson, H. S., Rodriguez, C., Bostick, R. M., Thun, M. J., Calle, E. E. 2007. Vitamin D pathway gene polymorphisms, diet, and risk of postmenopausal breast cancer: a nested case-control study. Breast Cancer Res 9(1):R9.

Millikan, R. C., Player, J., de Cotret, A. R., Moorman, P., Pittman, G., Vannappagari, V., Tse, C. K., Keku, T. 2004. Manganese superoxide dismutase Ala-9Val polymorphism and risk of breast cancer in a population-based case-control study of African Americans and whites. Breast Cancer Res 6:R264–R274.

Mitrunen, K., Jourenkova, N., Kataja, V., Eskelinen, M., Kosma, V. M., Benhamou, S., Vainio, H., Uusitupa, M., Hirvonen, A. 2000. Steroid metabolism gene CYP17 polymorphism and the development of breast cancer. Cancer Epidemiol Biomarkers Prev 9(12):1343–1348.

Mitrunen, K., Sillanpaa, P., Kataja, V., Eskelinen, M., Kosma, V. M., Benhamou, S., Uusitupa, M., Hirvonen, A. 2001. Association between manganese superoxide dismutase (MnSOD) gene polymorphism and breast cancer risk. Carcinogenesis 22:827–829.

Mohlig, M., Boeing, H., Spranger, J., Osterhoff, M., Kroke, A., Fisher, E., Bergmann, M. M., Ristow, M., Hoffmann, K., Pfeiffer, A. F. 2004. Body mass index and C-174G interleukin-6 promoter polymorphism interact in predicting type 2 diabetes. J Clin Endocrinol Metab 89:1885–1890.

Nowell, S. A., Ahn, J., Ambrosone, C. B. 2004. Gene-nutrient interactions in cancer etiology. Nutr Rev 62:427–438.

Park, S. K., Kang, D., Noh, D. Y., Lee, K. M., Kim, S. U., Choi, J. Y., Choi, I. M., Ahn, S. H., Choe, K. J., Hirvonen, A., Strickland, P. T., Yoo, K. Y. 2003. Reproductive factors, glutathione S-transferase M1 and T1 genetic polymorphism and breast cancer risk. Breast Cancer Res Treat 78(1):89–96.

Park, S. K., Yim, D. S., Yoon, K. S., Choi, I. M., Choi, J. Y., Yoo, K. Y., Noh, D. Y., Choe, K. J., Ahn, S. H., Hirvonen, A., Kang, D. 2004. Combined effect of GSTM1, GSTT1, and COMT genotypes in individual breast cancer risk. Breast Cancer Res Treat 88(1):55–62.

Park, S. K., Yoo, K. Y., Lee, S. J., Kim, S. U., Ahn, S. H., Noh, D. Y., Choe, K. J., Strickland, P. T., Hirvonen, A., Kang, D. 2000. Alcohol consumption, glutathione S-transferase M1 and T1 genetic polymorphisms and breast cancer risk. Pharmacogenetics 10:301–309.

Piller, R., Verla-Tebit, E., Wang-Gohrke, S., Linseisen, J., Chang-Claude, J. 2006. CYP17 genotype modifies the association between lignan supply and premenopausal breast cancer risk in humans. J Nutr 136(6):1596–1603.

Ravn-Haren, G., Olsen, A., Tjonneland, A., Dragsted, L. O., Nexo, B. A., Wallin, H., Overvad, K., Raaschou-Nielsen, O., Vogel, U. 2006. Associations between GPX1 Pro198Leu polymorphism, erythrocyte GPX activity, alcohol consumption and breast cancer risk in a prospective cohort study. Carcinogenesis 27:820–825.

Rebbeck, T. R., Troxel, A. B., Norman, S., Bunin, G., DeMichele, A., Schinnar, R., Berlin, J. A., Strom, B. L. 2007b. Pharmacogenetic modulation of combined hormone replacement therapy by progesterone-metabolism genotypes in postmenopausal breast cancer risk. Am J Epidemiol 166:1392–1399.

Rebbeck, T. R., Troxel, A. B., Walker, A. H., Panossian, S., Gallagher, S., Shatalova, E. G., Blanchard, R., Norman, S., Bunin, G., DeMichele, A., Berlin, M., Schinnar, R., Berlin, J. A., Strom, B. L. 2007a. Pairwise combinations of estrogen metabolism genotypes in postmenopausal breast cancer etiology. Cancer Epidemiol Biomarkers Prev 16(3):444–450.

Rossner, P., Jr., Terry, M. B., Gammon, M. D., Zhang, F. F., Teitelbaum, S. L., Eng, S. M., Sagiv, S. K., Gaudet, M. M., Neugut, A. I., Santella, R. M. 2006. OGG1 polymorphisms and breast cancer risk. Cancer Epidemiol Biomarkers Prev 15:811–815.

Schubert, E. L., Lee, M. K., Newman, B., King, M. C. 1999. Single nucleotide polymorphisms (SNPs) in the estrogen receptor gene and breast cancer susceptibility. J Steroid Biochem Mol Biol 71:21–27.

Semenza, J. C., Delfino, R. J., Ziogas, A., Anton-Culver, H. 2003. Breast cancer risk and methylenetetrahydrofolate reductase polymorphism. Breast Cancer Res Treat 77:217–223.

Seth, P., Lunetta, K. L., Bell, D. W., Gray, H., Nasser, S. M., Rhei, E., Kaelin, C. M., Iglehart, D. J., Marks, J. R., Garber, J. E., Haber, D. A., Polyak, K. 2000. Phenol sulfotransferases: hormonal regulation, polymorphism, and age of onset of breast cancer. Cancer Res 60(24):6859–6863.

Setiawan, V. W., Schumacher, F. R., Haiman, C. A., Stram, D. O., Albanes, D., Altshuler, D., Berglund, G., Buring, J., Calle, E. E., Clavel-Chapelon, F., Cox, D. G., Gaziano, J. M., Hankinson, S. E., Hayes, R. B., Henderson, B. E., Hirschhorn, J., Hoover, R., Hunter, D. J., Kaaks, R., Kolonel, L. N., Kraft, P., Ma, J., Le Marchand, L., Linseisen, J., Lund, E., Navarro, C., Overvad, K., Palli, D., Peeters, P. H., Pike, M. C., Riboli, E., Stampfer, M. J., Thun, M. J., Travis, R., Trichopoulos, D., Yeager, M., Ziegler, R. G., Spencer Feigelson, H., Chanock, S. J. 2007. CYP17 genetic variation and risk of breast and prostate cancer from the National Cancer Institute Breast and Prostate Cancer Cohort Consortium (BPC3). Cancer Epidemiol Biomarkers Prev 16(11):2237–2246.

Sharp, L., Little, J., Schofield, A. C., Pavlidou, E., Cotton, S. C., Miedzybrodzka, Z., Baird, J. O., Haites, N. E., Heys, S. D., Grubb, D. A. 2002. Folate and breast cancer: the role of polymorphisms in methylenetetrahydrofolate reductase (MTHFR). Cancer Lett 181:65–71.

Shatalova, E. G., Loginov, V. I., Braga, E. A., Kazubskaia, T. P., Sudomoina, M. A., Blanchard, R. L., Favorova, O. O. 2006. Association of polymorphisms in SULT1A1 and UGT1A1 Genes with breast cancer risk and phenotypes in Russian women. Mol Biol (Mosk) 40(2):263–270.

Shin, A., Kang, D., Nishio, H., Lee, M. J., Park, S. K., Kim, S. U., Noh, D. Y., Choe, K. J., Ahn, S. H., Hirvonen, A., Kim, J. H., Yoo, K. Y. 2003. Estrogen receptor alpha gene polymorphisms and breast cancer risk. Breast Cancer Res Treat 80:127–131.

Shin, M. H., Lee, K. M., Yang, J. H., Nam, S. J., Kim, J. W., Yoo, K. Y., Park, S. K., Noh, D. Y., Ahn, S. H., Kim, B., Kang, D. 2005. Genetic polymorphism of CYP17 and breast cancer risk in Korean women. Exp Mol Med 37(1):11–17.

Shrubsole, M. J., Gao, Y. T., Cai, Q., Shu, X. O., Dai, Q., Hebert, J. R., Jin, F., Zheng, W. 2004. MTHFR polymorphisms, dietary folate intake, and breast cancer risk: results from the Shanghai Breast Cancer Study. Cancer Epidemiol Biomarkers Prev 13:190–196.

Shrubsole, M. J., Gao, Y. T., Cai, Q., Shu, X. O., Dai, Q., Jin, F., Zheng, W. 2006. MTR and MTRR polymorphisms, dietary intake, and breast cancer risk. Cancer Epidemiol Biomarkers Prev 15:586–588.

Sillanpää, P., Hirvonen, A., Kataja, V., Eskelinen, M., Kosma, V. M., Uusitupa, M., Vainio, H., Mitrunen, K. 2004. Vitamin D receptor gene polymorphism as an important modifier of positive family history related breast cancer risk. Pharmacogenetics 14(4):239–245.

Sillanpää, P., Kataja, V., Eskelinen, M., Kosma, V. M., Uusitupa, M., Vainio, H., Mitrunen, K., Hirvonen, A. 2005. Sulfotransferase 1A1 genotype as a potential modifier of breast cancer risk among premenopausal women. Pharmacogenet Genomics 15(10):749–752.

Silva, S. N., Cabral, M. N., Bezerra de Castro, G., Pires, M., Azevedo, A. P., Manita, I., Pina, J. E., Rueff, J., Gaspar, J. 2006. Breast cancer risk and polymorphisms in genes involved in metabolism of estrogens (CYP17, HSD17beta1, COMT and MnSOD): possible protective role of MnSOD gene polymorphism Val/Ala and Ala/Ala in women that never breast fed. Oncol Rep 16(4):781–788.

Sinha, R., Rothman, N. 1999. Role of well-done, grilled red meat, heterocyclic amines (HCAs) in the etiology of human cancer. Cancer Lett 143:189–194.

Slanger, T. E., Chang-Claude, J., Wang-Gohrke, S. 2006. Manganese superoxide dismutase Ala-9Val polymorphism, environmental modifiers, and risk of breast cancer in a German population. Cancer Causes Control 17:1025–1031.

Slattery, M. L., Curtin, K., Sweeney, C., Wolff, R. K., Baumgartner, R. N., Baumgartner, K. B., Giuliano, A. R., Byers, T. 2008. Modifying effects of IL-6 polymorphisms on body size-associated breast cancer risk. Obesity (Silver Spring) 16:339–347.

Slattery, M. L., Sweeney, C., Herrick, J., Wolff, R., Baumgartner, K., Giuliano, A., Byers, T. 2007a. ESR1, AR, body size, and breast cancer risk in Hispanic and non-Hispanic white women living in the Southwestern United States. Breast Cancer Res Treat 105:327–335.

Slattery, M. L., Sweeney, C., Wolff, R., Herrick, J., Baumgartner, K., Giuliano, A., Byers, T. 2007b. Genetic variation in IGF1, IGFBP3, IRS1, IRS2 and risk of breast cancer in women living in Southwestern United States. Breast Cancer Res Treat 104:197–209.

Southey, M. C., Batten, L. E., McCredie, M. R., Giles, G. G., Dite, G., Hopper, J. L., Venter, D. J. 1998. Estrogen receptor polymorphism at codon 325 and risk of breast cancer in women before age forty. J Natl Cancer Inst 90:532–536.

Sparks, R., Ulrich, C. M., Bigler, J., Tworoger, S. S., Yasui, Y., Rajan, K. B., Porter, P., Stanczyk, F. Z., Ballard-Barbash, R., Yuan, X., Lin, M. G., McVarish, L., Aiello, E. J., McTiernan, A. 2004. UDP-glucuronosyltransferase and sulfotransferase polymorphisms, sex hormone concentrations, and tumor receptor status in breast cancer patients. Breast Cancer Res 6(5):R488–R498.

Steck, S. E., Gaudet, M. M., Britton, J. A., Teitelbaum, S. L., Terry, M. B., Neugut, A. I., Santella, R. M., Gammon, M. D. 2007. Interactions among GSTM1, GSTT1 and GSTP1 polymorphisms, cruciferous vegetable intake and breast cancer risk. Carcinogenesis 28:1954–1959.

Stevens, R. G. 2005. Circadian disruption and breast cancer from melatonin to clocl genes. Epidemiology 16:254–258.

Stevens, V. L., McCullough, M. L., Pavluck, A. L., Talbot, J. T., Feigelson, H. S., Thun, M. J., Calle, E. E. 2007. Association of polymorphisms in one-carbon metabolism genes and postmenopausal breast cancer incidence. Cancer Epidemiol Biomarkers Prev 16: 1140–1147.

Suzuki, T., Matsuo, K., Hirose, K., Hiraki, A., Kawase, T., Watanabe, M., Yamashita, T., Iwata, H., Tajima, K. 2008. One-carbon metabolism-related gene polymorphisms and risk of breast cancer. Carcinogenesis 29:2142–2147.

Tamimi, R. M., Hankinson, S. E., Spiegelman, D., Colditz, G. A., Hunter, D. J. 2004. Manganese superoxide dismutase polymorphism, plasma antioxidants, cigarette smoking, and risk of breast cancer. Cancer Epidemiol Biomarkers Prev 13:989–996.

Tang, D., Cho, S., Rundle, A., Chen, S., Phillips, D., Zhou, J., Hsu, Y., Schnabel, F., Estabrook, A., Perera, F. P. 2002. Polymorphisms in the DNA repair enzyme XPD are associated with increased levels of PAH-DNA adducts in a case-control study of breast cancer. Breast Cancer Res Treat 75:159–166.

Tang, D., Rundle, A., Mooney, L., Cho, S., Schnabel, F., Estabrook, A., Kelly, A., Levine, R., Hibshoosh, H., Perera, F. 2003. Sulfotransferase 1A1 (SULT1A1) polymorphism, PAH-DNA adduct levels in breast tissue and breast cancer risk in a case-control study. Breast Cancer Res Treat 78(2):217–222.

Terry, M. B., Gammon, M. D., Zhang, F. F., Knight, J. A., Wang, Q., Britton, J. A., Teitelbaum, S. L., Neugut, A. I., Santella, R. M. 2006. ADH3 genotype, alcohol intake and breast cancer risk. Carcinogenesis 27:840–847.

Terry, P. D., Goodman, M. 2006. Is the association between cigarette smoking and breast cancer modified by genotype? A review of epidemiologic studies and meta-analysis. Cancer Epidemiol Biomarkers Prev 15:602–611.

Terry, M. B., Knight, J. A., Zablotska, L., Wang, Q., John, E. M., Andrulis, I. L., Senie, R. T., Daly, M., Ozcelik, H., Briollais, L., Santella, R. M. 2007. Alcohol metabolism, alcohol intake, and breast cancer risk: a sister-set analysis using the Breast Cancer Family Registry. Breast Cancer Res Treat 106:281–288.

The MARIE-GENICA Consortium on Genetic Susceptibility for Menopausal Hormone Therapy Related Breast Cancer Risk. 2010. Postmenopausal estrogen monotherapy-associated breast cancer risk is modified by CYP17A1_-34_T>C polymorphism. Breast Cancer Res Treat 120(3):737–744.

van der Hel, O. L., Peeters, P. H., Hein, D. W., Doll, M. A., Grobbee, D. E., Ocke, M., Bueno de Mesquita, H. B. 2004. GSTM1 null genotype, red meat consumption and breast cancer risk (The Netherlands). Cancer Causes Control 15:295–303.

Vasconcelos, A., Medeiros, R., Veiga, I., Pereira, D., Carrilho, S., Palmeira, C., Azevedo, C., Lopes, C. S. 2002. Analysis of estrogen receptor polymorphism in codon 325 by PCR-SSCP in breast cancer: association with lymph node metastasis. Breast J 8:226–229.

Verla-Tebit, E., Wang-Gohrke, S., Chang-Claude, J. 2005. CYP17 5′-UTR MspA1 polymorphism and the risk of premenopausal breast cancer in a German population-based case-control study. Breast Cancer Res 7(4):R455–R464.

Visvanathan, K., Crum, R. M., Strickland, P. T., You, X., Ruczinski, I., Berndt, S. I., Alberg, A. J., Hoffman, S. C., Comstock, G. W., Bell, D. A., Helzlsouer, K. J. 2007. Alcohol dehydrogenase genetic polymorphisms, low-to-moderate alcohol consumption, and risk of breast cancer. Alcohol Clin Exp Res 31:467–476.

Vogel, U., Christensen, J., Nexo, B. A., Wallin, H., Friis, S., Tjonneland, A. 2007. Peroxisome proliferator-activated receptor-gamma2 Pro12Ala, interaction with alcohol intake and NSAID use, in relation to risk of breast cancer in a prospective study of Danes. Carcinogenesis 28: 427–434.

WCRF/AICR. 1997. Food, Nutrition and the Prevention of Cancer: a global Perspective. Washington, DC: AICR.

WCRF/AICR. 2007. Food, Nutrition, Physical Activity, and the Prevention of Cancer: a Global Perspective. Washington DC: AICR.

Wedren, S., Magnusson, C., Humphreys, K., Melhus, H., Kindmark, A., Stiger, F., Branting, M., Persson, I., Baron, J., Weiderpass, E. 2007. Associations between androgen and Vitamin D receptor microsatellites and postmenopausal breast cancer. Cancer Epidemiol Biomarkers Prev 16(9):1775–1783.

Wedrén, S., Lovmar, L., Humphreys, K., Magnusson, C., Melhus, H., Syvänen, A. C., Kindmark, A., Landegren, U., Fermér, M. L., Stiger, F., Persson, I., Baron, J., Weiderpass, E. 2004. Oestrogen receptor alpha gene haplotype and postmenopausal breast cancer risk: a case control study. Breast Cancer Res 6(4):R437–R449.

Weinshilboum, R. M., Otterness, D. M., Aksoy, I. A., Wood, T. C., Her, C., Raftogianis, R. B. 1997. Sulfation and sulfotransferases 1: sulfotransferase molecular biology: cDNAs and genes. FASEB J 11:3–14.

Weston, A., Pan, C. F., Bleiweiss, I. J., Ksieski, H. B., Roy, N., Maloney, N., Wolff, M. S. 1998. CYP17 genotype and breast cancer risk. Cancer Epidemiol Biomarkers Prev 7:941–944.

Winter, S. L., Bosnoyan-Collins, L., Pinnaduwage, D., Andrulis, I. L. 2007. Expression of the circadian clock genes Per1 and Per2 in sporadic and familial breast tumors. Neoplasia 9: 797–800.

Wu, A. H., Seow, A., Arakawa, K., Van Den Berg, D., Lee, H. P., Yu, M. 2003. HSD17B1 and CYP17 polymorphisms and breast cancer risk among Chinese women in Singapore. Int J Cancer 104:450–457.

Yaich, L., Dupont, W. D., Cavener, D. R., Parl, F. F. 1992. Analysis of the PvuII restriction fragment-length polymorphism and exon structure of the estrogen receptor gene in breast cancer and peripheral blood. Cancer Res 52:77–83.

Yang, G., Gao, Y. T., Cai, Q. Y., Shu, X. O., Cheng, J. R., Zheng, W. 2005. Modifying effects of sulfotransferase 1A1 gene polymorphism on the association of breast cancer risk with body mass index or endogenous steroid hormones. Breast Cancer Res Treat 94(1):63–70.

Yoo, K. Y., Kang, D., Park, S. K., Kim, S. U., Kim, S. U., Shin, A., Yoon, H., Ahn, S. H., Noh, D. Y., Choe, K. J. 2002. Epidemiology of breast cancer in Korea: occurrence, high-risk groups, and prevention. J Korean Med Sci 17:1–6.

Zhang, S. M., Willett, W. C., Selhub, J., Hunter, D. J., Giovannucci, E. L., Holmes, M. D., Colditz, G. A., Hankinson, S. E. 2003. Plasma folate, vitamin B6, vitamin B12, homocysteine, and risk of breast cancer. J Natl Cancer Inst 95:373–380.

Zhao, M., Lewis, R., Gustafson, D. R., Wen, W. Q., Cerhan, J. R., Zheng, W. 2001. No apparent association of GSTP1 A(313)G polymorphism with breast cancer risk among postmenopausal Iowa women. Cancer Epidemiol Biomarkers Prev 10:1301–2.

Zheng, W., Deitz, A. C., Campbell, D. R., Wen, W. Q., Cerhan, J. R., Sellers, T. A., Folsom, A. R., Hein, D. W. 1999. N-acetyltransferase 1 genetic polymorphism, cigarette smoking, well-done meat intake, and breast cancer risk. Cancer Epidemiol Biomarkers Prev 8:233–239.

Zheng, T., Holford, T. R., Zahm, S. H., Owens, P. H., Boyle, P., Zhang, Y., Zhang, B., Wise, J. P., Sr., Stephenson, L. P., Ali-Osman, F. 2003. Glutathione S-transferase M1 and T1 genetic polymorphisms, alcohol consumption and breast cancer risk. Br J Cancer 88:58–62.

Zheng, W., Wen, W. Q., Gustafson, D. R., Gross, M., Cerhan, J. R., Folsom, A. R. 2002. GSTM1 and GSTT1 polymorphisms and postmenopausal breast cancer risk. Breast Cancer Res Treat 74:9–16.

Zheng, W., Xie, D., Cerhan, J. R., Sellers, T. A., Wen, W., Folsom, A. R. 2001. Sulfotransferase 1A1 polymorphism, endogenous estrogen exposure, well-done meat intake, and breast cancer risk. Cancer Epidemiol Biomarkers Prev 10:89–94.

Chapter 11
Environment, Genetic Immunology and Childhood Cancer

Esma Ucisik-Akkaya and M. Tevfik Dorak

Abstract Childhood cancers make up 1% of the total cancer burden. Despite their rarity, they cause highest disease mortality in childhood. Research on the etiology of childhood cancers has been hampered by small sample sizes, lack of appropriate controls, reliance on case-control studies and difficulties with the definition of environment and measurement of environmental exposures. Only few and small studies have explored gene and environment interactions in childhood cancers. Consistent epidemiologic associations with male sex, birth weight, maternal reproductive history, allergic and autoimmune disorders, and infection frequency in early childhood as well as HLA associations may be exploited to gain further insight into the etiology. Currently available data suggest the involvement of immune surveillance in the development of childhood leukemia. Genetic epidemiologic approach should provide clues for the genetic risk factors when larger national and international cohort studies are completed. These studies should ideally consider the strong sex effect, potential parental effects and environmental factors including prenatal environment.

Keywords Gender effect · Potential parental effects and environmental factors including prenatal environment · Genetics · Immune surveillance in the development of childhood leukemia

11.1 Childhood Cancer Epidemiology, Genes and Environment

Childhood cancers include a heterogeneous group consisting of leukemia and lymphomas, and solid tumors. Overall they are rare; cancer in children under 15 years of age accounts for less than 1% of total cancer burden in developed countries (Linet et al., 2003; Lightfoot and Roman, 2004). However rare, cancer is still the biggest killer disease of childhood and ranks only second to accidents (Jemal et al., 2008). The most common childhood cancers are leukemias and brain tumors. Among

---

M.T. Dorak (✉)
Department of Environmental and Occupational Health, Robert Stempel College of Public Health & Social Work, Florida International University, Miami, FL 33199-0001, USA
e-mail: mdorak@fiu.edu

D. Roy, M.T. Dorak (eds.), *Environmental Factors, Genes, and the Development of Human Cancers*, DOI 10.1007/978-1-4419-6752-7_11,

leukemias, childhood acute lymphoblastic leukemia (ALL) is the most common and consists of almost 25% of all childhood cancers. This is the reason that most childhood cancer studies have been on childhood ALL. Both North American (Linabery and Ross, 2008) and European data (Steliarova-Foucher et al., 2004) suggest a small increase in the incidence rates of all childhood cancers in recent decades. If this increase is real and not entirely due to improvements in diagnosis, it implies environmental changes in the etiology of childhood cancers. This chapter will cover the aspects of childhood cancer epidemiology related to genetic immunology of childhood cancer. The descriptive epidemiology and general risk factors of childhood cancer have been extensively reviewed elsewhere (Reynolds, 1998a, b; Linet et al., 2003; Lightfoot and Roman, 2004; Stiller, 2004; Buffler et al., 2005; McNally and Parker, 2006; Belson et al., 2007).

11.1.1 Study Design Issues

Studies in childhood cancer epidemiology are constrained by a number of issues in epidemiologic study design (Table 11.1). Perhaps the most important one is the rarity of the disease as a whole and significant etiologic and clinical heterogeneity

Table 11.1 Most common problems in childhood cancer genetic epidemiology research

Issue	Difficulty encountered	Possible solution
Rare disease	Low power studies	National and international consortia
No common familial form	Low power studies, no linkage or segregation studies	Case-control or cohort studies
Reliance on retrospective case-control study design	Bias is possible	Careful design, record based study, family-based study
Twin studies	Spread of leukemia through shared circulation in utero and deficit for male twins with leukemia	Careful interpretation in leukemia
Control selection	Hard to obtain blood samples from age- and sex-matched healthy children	Newborn control group (cord blood samples) or buccal swab from healthy children, case-only design, family-based study
Prenatal environmental exposure	No specific marker, timing of critical windows unknown	Proxy markers, animal experiments
Parental effects	Parental samples not routinely collected	Family-based association studies
Sex effects	Frequently neglected	Stratified analysis (not adjustment), frequency matching of cases and controls rather than individual matching

in individual childhood cancers. Specific studies even on brain tumors or leukemias, the most common types, are usually restricted to small studies with insufficient statistical power. Most studies have had to use retrospective designs and inevitably suffer from their inherent flaws, recall bias being the most recognized one (Stiller, 2004). Other unique problems include lack of information on critical windows of exposure (Dutz et al., 1976; Ghavami et al., 1979; Anderson et al., 2000; Ma et al., 2002) and the effect modification by sex which may have its origin in prenatal period where cell proliferation rates differ between male and female fetuses (Mittwoch, 1993; Kochhar et al., 2001) (increased cell proliferation rate itself is a risk factor for cancer development (Albanes and Winick, 1988; Preston-Martin et al., 1990)).

In gene and environment interaction (GEI) studies of childhood cancer, it may be important to consider parental genotypes (Labuda et al., 2002). Parental biologic samples may not be readily available although easier to obtain compared with adult-onset diseases. Given the rarity of childhood cancers, single-center studies are unlikely to provide sufficient statistical power. Multi-center studies or large studies in national or international reference centers suffer from the genetic heterogeneity problem. Family-based association studies overcome this problem and also have the additional advantage of providing information on parental genotypes to assess parental, especially maternal effects.

In recent years, national and international consortiums have been trying to address the problem caused by rarity of childhood cancer. The established consortia include Children's Oncology Group (COG), United Kingdom Childhood Cancer Study (UKCCS), Childhood Leukemia International Consortium (CLIC) with participation of USA, Canada, Brazil, United Kingdom, France, Italy, Germany, South Korea, Australia and New Zealand. The CLIC has recruited around 9,000 cases and 14,000 controls so far (Buffler, 2008). Likewise International Childhood Cancer Cohort Consortium (I4C) is another large consortium aiming to study genetic and environmental factors in the etiology of childhood cancers (Brown et al., 2007). These efforts are expected to contribute to better understanding of risk factors for all childhood cancers.

Familial forms of childhood cancers are extremely rare. Only a few syndromic forms occur in families. The lack of a common familial form hampers the efforts of making use of traditional genetic epidemiology methods such as parametric linkage, non-parametric linkage allele-sharing (affected sib-pair/relative-pair) studies, twin studies or segregation studies. Twin studies are not informative as in adult cancers for two reasons: (1) shared circulation may cause spread of leukemia initiated in utero and causing concordant leukemia in twin pairs which may be confused with shared genetic susceptibility (Macmahon and Levy, 1964; Ford et al., 1997; Wiemels et al., 1999b; Greaves et al., 2003; Maia et al., 2003) and (2) there is a deficit of male twins with leukemia which is attributed to prenatal selection against males destined to develop leukemia (Inskip et al., 1991; Rodvall et al., 1992). Another implication of the lack of familial forms is that childhood cancer research does not benefit from the opportunity to increase statistical power to detect genetic associations by oversampling cases with a family history (Le Marchand, 2005).

The most common design in genetic studies of childhood cancer is retrospective case-control studies. Even this design is not ideal because of the difficulties in obtaining comparable healthy children as controls. Ethical and other obvious issues restrict the collection of age- and sex-matched controls from the same study base. This difficulty has led to the use of either adults or newborn controls in genetic studies. Either approach has problems but in the absence of a better alternative, they have been tried with some success. A newborn control group is likely to provide an advantage at least for leukemia studies. Childhood leukemia has a consistent association with maternal history of repeated miscarriages and even with threatened miscarriages (Stewart et al., 1958; van Steensel-Moll et al., 1985; Smulevich et al., 1999). No mechanism is known for this association but a shared genetic susceptibility is one possibility. Thus, children who have narrowly escaped the elimination by miscarriage may have a higher risk for developing childhood leukemia (and this connection is stronger for boys) (Dorak et al., 2007b). If the same genotype is a shared marker for prenatal selection and childhood leukemia risk, using a newborn control group increases the statistical power to detect a genetic association. Given the sex effect in miscarriage association, using sex as an environmental factor and looking for GEI may be a productive approach to identify shared genetic susceptibility factors for miscarriages and childhood leukemia. It is only natural that a childhood leukemia association study uses a newborn control group to be able to estimate the approximate risk for a newborn to develop a childhood disease. This may introduce an error since some newborns will develop leukemia later on. Given the frequency of childhood leukemia or cancer in general, this is unlikely to distort the results and can be tolerated as a minor conservative error.

In the absence of an age- and sex-matched control group or a newborn control group, a case-only design or family trios are valid alternative approaches to explore GEI in childhood cancers. Both types of designs are capable of examining GEI. Case-only design in the study of GEI has been used successfully in cancer (Hamajima et al., 1999) and more specifically in childhood leukemia (Goodman and Dana Flanders, 2007). However, if the assumptions of the case-only design regarding the presence of GxE correlation in the population or population mixture are not met, the validity of this design is questionable (Liu et al., 2004).

11.1.2 Environment and Childhood Cancer

In the context of GEI studies, environmental risk factors are defined as exposure (physical, chemical, biological), behavior pattern or a life event (Ottman, 1996). Examples for each category include exposure to sunshine, N-nitrosamines, viruses, day care attendance or injuries. This definition does not cover all possibilities for childhood cancer. Prenatal origin of adult disease has been an active field of research lately (Gluckman et al., 2008) and it also applies to childhood leukemias (Macmahon and Levy, 1964; Wiemels et al., 1999a; 2002; Greaves and Wiemels,

2003; Taub and Ge, 2004; Gruhn et al., 2008). It has long been known that the molecular origin of childhood leukemia extends to prenatal period (Wasserman et al., 1992; Steenbergen et al., 1994) and has been documented using the screening of blood samples taken at birth of leukemic children (Greaves and Wiemels, 2003; Taub and Ge, 2004). There are good reasons to think that this may be a general phenomenon for other childhood cancers. Prenatal origin of childhood leukemia has two important implications. Firstly, it emphasizes the need to include prenatal environmental exposures into genetic association studies. Secondly, not every child born with a leukemia-specific chromosomal translocation goes on to develop leukemia (Mori et al., 2002) and postnatal environmental exposures must also play a role in leukemogenesis.

Exposures during prenatal development pose a few problems in their measurement and timing. The evidence for exposures occurring during the preconceptional period that have an association with childhood or adulthood cancers is equivocal. In terms of GEI, one problem is that the most important environment for childhood cancer is the intra-uterine environment. This poses a difficulty since there is a complex interplay among intra-uterine events and the dynamics continuously change as pregnancy progresses. For example, iron measurements in maternal blood during pregnancy or in cord blood at birth are heavily confounded (Dorak et al., 2009). Only real-time monitoring of fetal iron levels, which is not possible, would provide reliable information. Possible confounders are the rate of materno-fetal iron transport, fetal growth rate that differs by sex (Mittwoch, 1993; Kochhar et al., 2001), maternal body iron content and background iron levels in the population. It is therefore hard to assess the prenatal environment accurately in GEI studies of childhood cancer.

Agents definitely related to cancer in children, and adulthood if exposure occurs in utero, include: maternal exposure to ionizing radiation during pregnancy and childhood leukemia and certain other cancers (Bithell and Stewart, 1975), and maternal use of diethylstilbestrol (DES) during pregnancy and clear-cell adenocarcinoma of the vagina in their daughters (Anderson et al., 2000). Male progeny also suffer the effects of in utero exposure to DES. These effects include epididymal cysts, small penis size, cryptorchidism and subsequent testicular cancer (Niculescu, 1985). The demonstration of cancers induced by transplacental exposure to DES has confirmed the speculation that the prenatal environment may influence subsequent carcinogenesis. Many other prenatal exposures including chemicals with estrogenic effects have been implicated in the etiology of childhood cancer (Anderson et al., 2000; McNally and Parker, 2006). Most studies of estrogen exposure have used proxy markers that are not necessarily highly correlated with fetal or maternal estrogen levels (Peck et al., 2003). Birth weight is one of the proxy markers used as a cumulative index of prenatal exposures in disease association studies but it has very little predictive value for steroid hormone levels during pregnancy (Peck et al., 2003) and its use as a surrogate marker for other exposures may also be doubtful.

An important route of postnatal environmental exposure for a child is breast-feeding. Breast-feeding is generally found weakly protective in childhood cancers

(Martin et al., 2005). The latest truly population-based UKCCS study did not find any statistically significant association with breast-feeding in childhood ALL or AML (Hughes et al., 2007). The weak and generally inconsistent findings may be due to an intriguing possibility. The first-born status, breast-feeding and environmental pollution may interact to have different associations if stratified analysis is used. The clues come from wildlife observations. Along the west coast of Florida, a majority of first-born bottlenose dolphin calves die before they separate from their mothers. This is attributed to high levels of environmental toxins in the fat tissue of marine mammals. Mother dolphins unload as much as 80% of pollutants accumulated in their bodies into their calves, probably through nursing. In general, excess risk of reproductive failure measured in terms of stillbirth or neonatal mortality for primiparous females was estimated as 60% (Beaufort), 79% (Sarasota), and 78% (Matagorda Bay). Females of higher parity, who have previously off-loaded their polychlorinated biphenyls burden, exhibit a much lower risk (Schwacke et al., 2002). The first-born gets the highest dose by far, as the mother has been accumulating toxins for many years while subsequent siblings receive the toxins accumulated over shorter periods of time. Similar observations have also been made in orcas and Northern fur seals suggesting that first-born babies are exposed to milk with higher concentrations of pollutants than the offspring of mothers who have previously given birth, and that first-borns may have significantly higher pollutant blood concentrations.

These observations in natural world may contribute to the understanding of the first-born effect in humans. Human milk is not pristine and may contain fat-soluble toxic material acquired from the environment throughout mother's life span (Sonawane, 1995; Anderson and Wolff, 2000; Landrigan et al., 2002). It reflects environmental levels of pollutants (Albers et al., 1996; Hooper and McDonald, 2000) and exposures through breast milk can be substantial compared to environmental exposure (Anderson and Wolff, 2000). Human milk may contain very high levels of toxic chemicals and breast-feeding increases their transfer to infants (Yakushiji et al., 1984; Koopman-Esseboom et al., 1994; Patandin et al., 1999; Boersma and Lanting, 2000; Nickerson, 2006). Maternal age and length of previous lactation show positive and inverse correlations, respectively, with the level of contaminants in human milk (Albers et al., 1996). It is therefore plausible that in polluted parts of the world, mainly the developed countries, human milk may be a source of carcinogenic compounds, especially for the first-born. No study has examined the effect modification by birth order of the breast-feeding association in childhood cancer in environmentally polluted areas. Such a study may uncover an environmental factor as a modifier of childhood cancer risk and can also be extended to study GEI using xenobiotic gene polymorphisms.

In terms of environmental factors, an important concept in childhood cancer epidemiology is developmental immunotoxicity (DIT) (Dietert, 2009). DIT refers to environmentally-induced disruption of developing immune system producing postnatal immune dysfunction. Exposure to certain toxicants as well as maternal infections and other pregnancy stressors is known to induce postnatal immune dysfunction, the former being called xenobiotically-induced developmental immunotoxicity. It has been proposed that increased risk in childhood cancer risk following xenobiotic exposure during pregnancy may be contributed by the toxic effects on the immune system besides the genotoxic damage. According to the DIT concept, exposures during critical windows of immune system development result in skewed, incomplete or misregulated childhood immune responses and inappropriate inflammatory responses that increase the risk for childhood cancer, asthma, allergies and infections as well as later-life autoimmunity (Dietert, 2008, 2009). This attractive hypothesis will be more convincing with the identification of critical windows, immunotoxicants and specific nature of the immune dysregulation.

11.1.3 Gene and Environment Interaction, and Childhood Cancer

To uncover genetic influences on disease susceptibility, interactions between genotypes and environmental factors should be evaluated using epidemiologic research designs (Khoury et al., 1988; Ottman, 1990; Khoury and Wagener, 1995; Ottman, 1996). Genetic models of complex diseases need to take into account both gene–gene and gene–environment interactions (Table 11.2). The most plausible scenario of genetic susceptibility is the co-occurrence of the genetic and non-genetic factors that would augment the disease risk. Purely genetic or environmental studies may fail to unravel effects of genetic or environmental factors that may not show any effect individually but increase the risk substantially in the presence of each other. When present, GEI may be exploited to detect genetic associations (Kraft and

Table 11.2 Gene and environment interactions examined in childhood cancer

Gene/polymorphism	Environmental effect	References
HFE (C282Y)	Enhanced with alcohol consumption	Waalen et al. (2005)
MDR1	Indoor air pollution	Urayama et al. (2007)
MTHFR	Folate intake	Krajinovic et al. (2004)
Xenobiotic enzyme polymorphism	Maternal use of tobacco, coffee and alcohol	Clavel et al. (2005)
Hepatic lipase polymorphism	Dietary fat intake	Ordovas et al. (2002)
NQO1	potential topoisomerase II inhibitors i.e. benzene and maternal smoking	Infante-Rivard (2007) and Guha (2008)
CYP1A1	pesticide exposure & parental smoking	Infante-Rivard et al. (1999) and Infante-Rivard et al. (2000)
Chromosomal aberrations in cord blood	prenatal exposure to airborne carcinogenic polycyclic aromatic hydrocarbons	Bocskay et al. (2005)
AML-associated t(8;21)	prenatal pesticide exposures	Lafiura et al. (2007)

Hunter, 2005; Kraft et al., 2007) and it is often used to denote that both genes and environmental factors are important in disease development. While this is true, GEI means more than that and comes in different shapes and forms (Khoury et al., 1988; Ottman, 1990; Khoury and Wagener, 1995; Ottman, 1996).

We are born with genetic risk markers and they cannot be changed. For effective prevention from a disease, GEI should be recognized so that public health measures can be implemented to reduce exposure to the environmental risk factors. It is important to recognize that genetic polymorphisms mainly act as effect modifiers for environmental exposures but their own main effects may be small. A simple example is that iron loading genotypes would have no detectable effect on individuals in iron-deficient populations but those with high iron intake would be at very high risk for iron overload disorders. Such genetic markers can only be discovered in populations at high risk for exposure (Le Marchand, 2005). The iron-loading mutation of the HFE gene, C282Y, has relatively low penetrance, which is enhanced with alcohol consumption (Waalen et al., 2005). This is due to facilitation of intestinal iron absorption by alcohol. A well-documented example of GEI depending on the nutrient intake is the effect modification by dietary fat intake of a hepatic lipase polymorphism association with high-density lipoprotein cholesterol concentration (Ordovas et al., 2002). In one of the rare GEI studies in childhood cancer, the protection conferred by methylene tetrahydrofolate reductase (MTHFR) gene variants that modify folate usage was detectable only in the time period previous to the beginning of folate supplementation of food stuff in Canada (Krajinovic et al., 2004). When there is no folate deficiency, the genetic variant on its own cannot protect. Even these few examples are sufficient to show that exclusive studies of genetic variants or environmental factors are unlikely to be fully informative.

11.2 Genetic Immunology and Childhood Cancer

The genetically determined variation in immune response capability plays roles in infectious diseases, allergic and autoimmune disorders, and cancer. Besides modifying cancer susceptibility directly, such variation is also relevant through its effect on susceptibility to infections, allergy and autoimmune disorders since these conditions show associations with cancer. There is a well-established sex effect in all of these conditions and it is likely that genetic and hormonal mechanisms mediate this effect. In childhood, most cancers (Ashley, 1969; Pearce and Parker, 2001; Johnson et al., 2008) and infections (Washburn et al., 1965; Schlegel and Bellanti, 1969; Green, 1992; Read et al., 1997) are more common in boys, the prevalence of asthma is higher in boys before adolescence (Almqvist et al., 2008) and autoimmune disorders are more common in girls (Lo et al., 1999). The interactions among these conditions and the involvement of sex in the interplay are clear indications of genetic and environmental multifactor etiology of childhood cancers. Surprisingly, sex effect is rarely considered in susceptibility studies in childhood but may provide important clues when taken into account (Dorak et al., 1999a; 2002; Do et al., 2010; Ucisik-Akkaya et al., 2010).

11.2.1 Infections and Childhood Cancer

The immune system is intimately related to protection from cancer. Cancer immunosurveillance has recently gained more support with identification of molecular mechanisms involved. Since the immune system is primarily evolved to defend the body against infections, parallels between immunity to cancer and infection exist. The simplest idea connecting the two major roles of the immune system is that when the immune system is not working as efficient as it should, susceptibility to infections and cancer increases. If cancer immune surveillance exists and its failure increases the risk for cancer, the risk for infections should also increase at the same time. This intuitive connection is simply exemplified by increased risk for cancer in immunodeficient (congenital immunodeficiencies or AIDS) or immunosuppressed subjects (transplant recipients) (Dunn et al., 2004; Kinlen, 2004a; Nakachi et al., 2004; Zitvogel et al., 2006).

The last few decades have witnessed emergence of several hypotheses putting forward an infectious etiology for the most common childhood cancer, childhood ALL. The best known hypotheses are those of Greaves and Kinlen, respectively known as the "delayed infection" and "population mixing" hypotheses. Neither hypothesis requires an infection with a specific agent but rather a lack of common infections in early infancy or lack of herd immunity and mixing of this population with outsiders are blamed to invoke an abnormal immune response. Another hypothesis by Smith (Smith et al., 1998), attributes ALL to an in utero exposure to infection that occurs as a result of improved hygiene conditions. Smith has suggested JC virus (JCV), a member of the polyoma family of viruses, as a candidate agent. However, polyoma virus sequences including JCV were not detected in children with ALL but this does not rule out their involvement in the pathogenesis of ALL (Smith et al., 1999; Priftakis et al., 2003). On the other hand, Dorak postulated that the male-specific HLA class II association with childhood ALL (Dorak et al., 1999a) may be due to increased susceptibility to persistent adenovirus infections in lymphocytes and facilitation of leukemia development due to immune evasive roles of adenoviruses (Dorak, 1996).

Of these hypotheses, only the Dorak hypothesis has some direct support. It primarily relies on the immune surveillance theory, which is widely recognized (Dunn et al., 2004; Kinlen, 2004a; Nakachi et al., 2004; Zitvogel et al., 2006). It has support from early serologic studies which suggested increased exposure of leukemic children to adenovirus (Dorak et al., 1999a). Most recently, two studies of blood spots obtained at birth on Guthrie cards, showed opposite results on the presence of adenoviral sequences in leukemic children (Gustafsson et al., 2007; Vasconcelos et al., 2008). Studies of clinical specimens also showed occasional but inconclusive presence of adenoviral sequences in leukemia and lymphoma (Fernandez-Soria et al., 2002; Kosulin et al., 2007). Thus, adenovirus is the only virus whose involvement in leukemia development may have any direct evidence. Other viruses or other microorganisms have been sought by various investigators with no positive results (see Refs. (McNally and Eden, 2004; O'Connor and Boneva, 2007)). Most of these studies attempted to detect viral nucleic acids. Studies designed to detect the protein products may represent an improvement.

The population mixing hypothesis as put forward by Kinlen has some support from research in recently mixed populations and clustering studies (reviewed in Refs. (Greaves, 2006; O'Connor and Boneva, 2007)). Kinlen suggested that in rural areas, which experienced an influx of residents from other areas, a situation referred to as population mixing, there would be an increased level of contacts between susceptible and infected individuals (impaired herd immunity hypothesis). Non-exposed individuals living where the relevant infection is not endemic, subsequently become at risk when exposed by mixing with an incoming population of infected carriers. Such mixing will increase the level of contacts between susceptible (more prevalent in rural areas) and infected individuals, promoting localized (frequently subclinical) epidemics of infections. If childhood leukemia is a rare response to a common—but unidentified—infection, then these localized epidemics will produce excess cases of the unusual complication, childhood leukemia. Kinlen tested these ideas in a number of areas and population groups in the UK and in each situation an increased relative risk (about 2-fold) of childhood acute leukemia was observed in the period after the mixing had occurred (Kinlen, 1995). The support to the population mixing hypothesis has not been universal. In at least two studies, high levels of population mixing were associated with lower risks (Parslow et al., 2002; Law et al., 2003) (see also Kinlen, 2004b). There is yet no infectious agent shown to be responsible for observed increases in leukemia incidence following documented population mixing events.

The Greaves hypothesis, which proposes an abnormal immune response to a delayed infection, has gained some indirect support from epidemiologic studies of the connection between daycare attendance and decreased risk for leukemia development (Greaves, 2006; O'Connor and Boneva, 2007). Here, daycare attendance is a surrogate marker for infectious exposure. Likewise, being first-born is also used as a surrogate marker for reduced infectious exposure (for the lack of older siblings to bring home infections) and its association with leukemia risk is often cited as supporting evidence (Greaves, 2001) although the UKCCS study failed to show any association with being first-born (Hughes et al., 2007). In most studies, being first-born is not separated from being the only child or the possibility of confounding by maternal miscarriage history is not considered. Some of the risk association found with being the first-born child may be due to being the only child that in turn, may be a reflection of the well-known association with the maternal history of miscarriage (Dorak et al., 2007b).

The daycare attendance studies indeed show a relatively consistent protective association with childhood ALL but it may well be confounded by an unknown factor. It is best to investigate the connection between delayed infection and subsequent leukemia risk using actual infection records. This has recently been possible. Two studies in the UK have now reported results of such explorations (Roman et al., 2007; Cardwell et al., 2008). When medical records of actual infection occurrence in infancy were used, neither study showed any correlation. If anything, the study by Roman et al suggested a positive correlation between the number of infectious diseases and leukemia risk (Roman et al., 2007). It has already been pointed out that these results are against the delayed infection hypothesis and only provide support for the cancer immune surveillance concept (Dorak et al., 2007a). Another negative result between scarcity of infections in infancy and childhood leukemia risk was reported in a population-based study in New York (Rosenbaum et al., 2005). These recent and large studies basically confirmed earlier studies. One such study was the inter-regional epidemiological study of childhood cancer (IRESCC) (McKinney et al., 1987). In the IRESCC study (234 children with leukemia or lymphoma and 468 age- and sex-matched controls), it was found that viral illnesses in the first 6 months of life increased the risk for childhood leukemia and lymphoma (RR = 4.1, 95% CI = 1.5 to 11.3, $P < 0.01$). In fact, increasing number of viral illnesses elevates the risk for adult AML (Cooper et al., 1996) and hospital admissions for infections during infancy increase the risk for adult non-Hodgkin lymphoma (Paltiel et al., 2006). These findings may help with better interpretation of studies of childhood infections and cancer connection and appear to support the simple immune surveillance concept, which was proposed specifically for childhood leukemia by Till et al in 1975 in the immunologic study of parents and grandparents of leukemic children (Till et al., 1975).

Children born with suboptimal immune functions are now treated with antibiotics and supportive treatment to survive early childhood. There is therefore an increased number of susceptibles surviving infancy for later leukemia development. The increase in childhood leukemia incidence in the developed countries may have been contributed by improved child care.

11.2.2 Autoimmune Diseases and Childhood Cancer

A risk association of autoimmune disorders in the family with childhood leukemia was first reported in 1979 (Till et al., 1979). Later, Woods *et al* found that cases had a history of autoimmune disease among their maternal relatives more often than did controls, but the association was not statistically significant (relative risk, 1.76; $P = 0.10$) (Woods et al., 1987). Following studies confirmed the association between childhood leukemia and parental autoimmune disorders (Bernard et al., 1987; Buckley et al., 1989; Mellemkjaer et al., 2000; Perillat-Menegaux et al., 2003). No such effect has been shown in infantile leukemia (Wen et al., 1998).

A specific autoimmune disorder, multiple sclerosis shows an association with adult leukemia/ lymphoma (Bernard et al., 1987). More specifically, an increased risk of ALL in children of women with MS has been observed (relative risk = 4.0; 95% CI = 1.3 to 9.3) (Buckley et al., 1989). As an autoimmune disorder, MS susceptibility shows a strong association with the HLA class II haplotype DRB1*1501-DQB1*0602 for which the proxy marker rs3135388 in the HLA-DRA gene is the strongest risk marker in a genome-wide association study (Hafler et al., 2007). A case-control study confirmed the same association in childhood ALL but in females only (Morrison et al., 2010). This connection and its possible sex effect require further exploration.

11.2.3 Atopic Diseases and Childhood Cancer

One of the most consistent findings in childhood leukemia is its negative association with asthma and allergic diseases (Wen et al., 2000; Schuz et al., 2003; Jourdan-Da Silva et al., 2004; Rosenbaum et al., 2005; Hughes et al., 2007). Although there is no study in childhood brain tumors, the negative association has been observed for adult gliomas (Brenner et al., 2002; Schwartzbaum et al., 2003). A general inverse relationship with cancer in adults has also been reported (Vena et al., 1985). Hygiene hypothesis has been put forward as an etiologic possibility for both childhood leukemia (Smith et al., 1998) and allergies (Strachan, 1989; Romagnani, 2004). It is important to note that childhood allergies are more common in boys (until adolescence) (Almqvist et al., 2008) and since childhood cancers are also more common in boys, analysis of effect modification by sex (by stratification) is particularly important in the analysis of association studies between allergies and cancer in childhood.

One prenatal environmental exposure class associated with later development of childhood allergic disorders is maternal exposure to farm animals (Ege et al., 2006). Exposure to microbial compounds in the environment during early childhood is known to be protective from allergic disorders and a molecular basis has been demonstrated for the effects of prenatal (maternal) exposure to farm environment on the innate immune system (Ege et al., 2006). Likewise, prenatal (maternal) exposure to organic toxins (polycyclic aromatic hydrocarbons and polychlorinated biphenyl) results in altered lymphocyte immunophenotypic distributions in cord blood, changes in cord serum immunoglobulin E levels and smaller thymus size (Hertz-Picciotto et al., 2008). Exposure to the same organic compounds is linked to the increased risk for childhood cancer (Perera et al., 2006). Thus, these observations are relevant to childhood leukemia susceptibility because of its correlation with immune functions. Similarly, the slight but beneficial association of breastfeeding for subsequent childhood cancer development may be due to the immune system promoting effect of human milk (Hosea Blewett et al., 2008).

The inverse association of allergic disorders with childhood leukemia is generally interpreted as the protective effect of a hyperactive immune system, thus this association lends support to the immune surveillance concept. The UKCCS study showed the same association (Hughes et al., 2007) but the observed reciprocal relationship between allergy and childhood ALL is interpreted as "a dysregulated immune response is a critical determinant of childhood ALL". Particularly because the same UKCCS study has already shown a positive association with the number of infections and subsequent ALL risk (Roman et al., 2007), it is more likely that the results further strengthen the immune surveillance concept in the development of childhood ALL.

11.2.4 HLA Associations and Childhood Cancer

The HLA complex is the major regulator of the immune response as it harbors the HLA genes directly involved in antigen presentation and genes for tumor necrosis factor (TNF), complement components as well as many other relevant ones (Horton et al., 2004). HLA genes are highly polymorphic and account for most of the variation in the magnitude of immune response among individuals. Most autoimmune disorders and infectious diseases show strong associations with HLA polymorphisms. There have been attempts to suggest an HLA gene association as the evidence for infectious etiology for childhood leukemia (Taylor et al., 1998; 2002; Taylor et al., 2008). While this may be true and more data other than statistical associations may strengthen this proposal in the future, more plausible alternative explanations exist. What needs to be better appreciated in HLA research is that the HLA complex and its extension towards the telomere on chromosome 6p are the two most gene-dense regions in the human genome (Xie et al., 2003). The HLA complex contains genes encoding transcription factors (including RXRB), DNA repair molecules (including MDC1), cell cycle and apoptosis-related molecules (for example, DDR1) as well as homologues of known proto-oncogenes (PBX2, NOTCH4). There are, therefore, many other candidate genes for leukemia susceptibility, which are no doubt in linkage disequilibrium with HLA genes, and it would be premature to conclude that an HLA association necessarily means evidence for infectious etiology.

One of the first genetic markers for leukemia susceptibility was HLA homozygosity (Von Fliedner et al., 1983). HLA homozygosity increases the risk for infectious diseases as the opposite of heterozygote advantage for resistance to infection (Penn et al., 2002) however alternative explanations are possible (Dorak and Burnett, 1992). A consistent HLA association in all leukemias is having two copies of HLA-DRB4 (-DR53) family haplotypes (Dorak et al., 1994; 1996; Dorak et al., 1999a). In childhood ALL, the association is male-specific (Dorak et al., 1999a). As discussed elsewhere (Dorak et al., 2002), the HLA-DRB4 haplotypes have unfavorable features like lower expression levels as opposed to other HLA haplotypes. Having two copies of DRB4 haplotypes is expected to result in suboptimal immune response capability. Since males already have lower levels of immune response (Purtilo and Sullivan, 1979; Grossman, 1989; Verthelyi, 2001), the interaction between the HLA-DRB4 association and sex (that is, its male-specificity) further suggests that the mechanism of the association is probably lower immune response capacity of the people who have two copies of DRB4 haplotypes. According to a preliminary report of the ongoing studies covering the whole of the HLA complex (Dorak et al., 2008), the HLA-DRB4 association is not confounded by a neighboring locus (i.e., not due to linkage disequilibrium). In fact, even the HSPA1B locus SNP rs1061581, which is in linkage disequilibrium with HLA-DRB4, shows an independent protective association with childhood ALL (Ucisik-Akkaya et al., 2010). Larger systematic studies incorporating past medical (infectious disease frequency) and autoimmune or allergic disorder history in the family are required to have more conclusive interpretations of the HLA associations in childhood leukemia.

Associations with homozygous HLA genotypes, stronger in males and in earlier ages would support the modification of immune surveillance as the mechanism of an HLA association.

11.2.5 Iron and Immune Surveillance

Since the demonstration of an HFE association in childhood ALL in 1999 (Dorak et al., 1999b), more cancers have shown associations with HFE or other iron-related gene variants [Beckman, 1999; Kallianpur, 2004; Hartikainen, 2006] (reviewed in (Dorak et al., 2005; Dorak, 2006)). The HFE gene is involved in iron homeostasis and its variants associated with cancer increase body iron levels. These associations are interpreted as evidence for iron's genotoxic effect that increases the risk for cancer development (Dorak et al., 2005). This is an active area of research and ultimate demonstration of the iron-cancer connection is awaited (see the Iron Excess & Cancer chapter). The birth weight association in childhood ALL may also be related to iron-related gene variants as proposed (Dorak et al., 2007b), which is supported by experimental data (Dorak et al., 2009). In this scenario, iron-related gene variants increase the risk for childhood leukemia by increasing materno-fetal iron transfer and subsequently, fetal iron levels. Birth weight is also increased due to excess iron, which induces cell proliferation (Bergeron, 1986), as an epiphenomenon resulting in the observed association with childhood ALL (Caughey and Michels, 2009; Samuelsen et al., 2009).

Since iron excess has deleterious effects on the immune system (Walker and Walker, 2000; Porto and De Sousa, 2007), this may also contribute to associations between iron levels and cancer (see the Iron Excess and Cancer chapter). It has damaging effects on lymphocytes (de Sousa and Porto, 1998; Walker and Walker, 2000) and the cell-mediated immunity overall (Weiss et al., 1995). One of the immune disturbances in iron overload is the higher average CD4:CD8 ratios and this is not related to the mutations in HFE but directly to iron (de Sousa and Porto, 1998). A molecular mechanism for the deleterious effect on T-lymphocytes has been shown (Regis et al., 2005). Two of the iron-related genes, the master regulator of iron homeostasis hepcidin anti-microbial peptide (HAMP) (Ganz, 2006), and natural resistance-associated macrophage protein 2 (NRAMP2, SLC11A2) (Wardrop et al., 2002) are well-known members of innate immunity. It is therefore plausible that iron-related gene variants may be directly involved in genetic regulation of immune surveillance and this may be another mechanism for iron and cancer connection.

11.2.6 Sex Effect in Predisposition to Childhood Cancer

Childhood cancers (Ashley, 1969; Pearce and Parker, 2001; Johnson et al., 2008) and infections (Washburn et al., 1965; Schlegel and Bellanti, 1969; Green, 1992;

Read et al., 1997) are more common in boys. It is customary to attribute this sex-differential to hormonal or genetic factors but none has been shown to be responsible for increased susceptibility of males to cancer and infection in childhood. The sex effect is most likely to be due to multiple mechanisms. Some observations relevant to the sex effect in cancer include the higher penetrance of mutations in DNA mismatch repair genes MLH1/MSH2 in males (Mitchell et al., 2002), greater susceptibility of male animals to oxidative damage (Ma et al., 1998) with similar observations in humans (Loft et al., 1992; Proteggente et al., 2002), greater sensitivity of males to mutagenic carcinogens and to radiation carcinogenesis in animals (Hattis et al., 2004), and higher radiosensitivity of lymphocytes from males (Wang et al., 2000).

In recent years, much progress has been made in understanding the molecular mechanisms of sex-differential in cancer susceptibility. The well-established male predominance in liver cancer has been shown to be due to estrogen-mediated inhibition of interleukin-6 production in the liver in females (Lawrence et al., 2007; Naugler et al., 2007). In thyroid cancer that is more common in females including childhood (Steliarova-Foucher et al., 2006), again, sex hormones are involved in the sex-differential. Female predominance in thyroid cancer may be due to androgen receptor expression in thyroid follicular cells through which androgens reduce proliferation of follicular cells (Rossi et al., 1996). Lacking this effect, females may be at higher risk of developing thyroid follicular cancer. Furthermore, 17ß-estradiol is a potent mitogen for thyroid cells (Manole et al., 2001). Estrogens also have general carcinogenic properties due to their effects on oxidant formation and oxidative DNA damage (Cavalieri et al., 2000). More recently reported sex-specific associations in childhood ALL appear to be related to interactions with sex hormones presumably during fetal development (Do et al., 2009, 2010; Ucisik-Akkaya et al., 2010).

Besides organ-specific roles and effects on oxidative stress, sex hormones are at least partially responsible for sexual dimorphism in the strength of the immune response (Purtilo and Sullivan, 1979; Grossman, 1989; Verthelyi, 2001). Since children do not have sex hormones at appreciable levels till puberty, sex hormones may be considered irrelevant in childhood cancer development. Prenatal exposures to sex hormones, however, may have long-lasting effects on post-natal immunity. Evidence for this suggestion comes mainly from animal experiments (Martin, 2000). Most strikingly, when pregnant rats are exposed to the adrenal sex steroid dehydroepiandrosterone, their male offspring develop cellular immune defects (Shelat et al., 1997). Likewise, if pregnant rhesus monkeys are administered adrenocorticotropic hormone, there is a deleterious effect on the immune system in male offspring (Coe et al., 1996). The sex effect observed in cancer prevalence therefore may be partially attributed to sex hormones. Their stronger effect in males who already have lower cancer immune surveillance capacity may contribute to the increased male-to-female ratio in childhood cancers. This well-known sex effect in most cancers is not taken into account in most studies. If considered, however, it may help better understand cancer pathogenesis.

11.3 Future Prospects

The disproportionate emphasis on the genetic factors following the completion of human genome mapping project is evolving to a more fair assessment of individual and joint roles by genes and environment in cancer etiology (Le Marchand, 2005; Hemminki et al., 2006). The concept of environment and critical windows of exposure in the development of childhood cancer are better defined. The importance of combined analysis of environment and genetics, consideration of potential confounders and effect modifiers (including sex) are better appreciated. These conceptual improvements are soon going to couple with availability of large, population-based cohorts for more meaningful and conclusive studies of all childhood cancers with results less affected by selection and recall bias. If these developments are accompanied with a more flexible interpretation of the overall results rather than being tests of whether they fit one of the existing hypotheses, it may not be long before we have results that are useful for preventive purposes. Childhood cancers may constitute only 1% of total cancer burden but they are still the main killer disease in childhood. Progress in this field is possible and overdue. Fortunately, there are reasons for being optimistic. Genetic immunology is an important field in cancer epidemiology because of its role in cancer immune surveillance. The results of few studies in this field and many more of those related to this field have been generally interpreted with prejudice and even bias towards a specific hypothesis. The immune surveillance concept is currently the most plausible explanation for most findings. Larger genetic immunology studies of the near future will unravel the contribution of genetic immunology to childhood cancer susceptibility if they take into account the effect modification by sex, exposure to infections, and possible connections with autoimmunity, allergic disorders, birth order and maternal reproductive history. The studies of the HLA complex will only yield useful information if the gene content of the HLA complex is better appreciated and possible confounding by locus is considered in the design, analysis and interpretation. It is most important to recognize that single gene studies of the HLA complex are unlikely to generate conclusive findings unless many other genes in the vicinity are also included. Genetic epidemiology is a powerful tool to probe disease biology when used appropriately and it is time to apply the cumulative experience of the past decades to childhood cancer epidemiology.

References

Albanes, D., Winick, M., 1988. Are cell number and cell proliferation risk factors for cancer? J Natl Cancer Inst 80, 772–774.

Albers, J.M., Kreis, I.A., Liem, A.K., van Zoonen, P., 1996. Factors that influence the level of contamination of human milk with poly-chlorinated organic compounds. Arch Environ Contam Toxicol 30, 285–291.

Almqvist, C., Worm, M., Leynaert, B., 2008. Impact of gender on asthma in childhood and adolescence: a GA2LEN review. Allergy 63, 47–57.

Anderson, L.M., Diwan, B.A., Fear, N.T., Roman, E., 2000. Critical windows of exposure for children's health: cancer in human epidemiological studies and neoplasms in experimental animal models. Environ Health Perspect 108 (Suppl 3), 573–594.

Anderson, H.A., Wolff, M.S., 2000. Environmental contaminants in human milk. J Expo Anal Environ Epidemiol 10, 755–760.

Ashley, D.J., 1969. A male-female differential in tumour incidence. Br J Cancer 23, 21–25.

Beckman, L.E., Van Landeghem, G.F., Sikström, C., Wahlin, A., Markevärn, B., Hallmans, G., Lenner, P., Athlin, L., Stenling, R., Beckman, L., 1999. Interaction between haemochromatosis and transferrin receptor genes in different neoplastic disorders. Carcinogenesis 20, 1231–1233.

Belson, M., Kingsley, B., Holmes, A., 2007. Risk factors for acute leukemia in children: a review. Environ Health Perspect 115, 138–145.

Bergeron, R.J., 1986. Iron: A controlling nutrient in proliferative processes. Trends Biochem Sci 11, 133–136.

Bernard, S.M., Cartwright, R.A., Darwin, C.M., Richards, I.D., Roberts, B., O'Brien, C., Bird, C.C., 1987. A possible epidemiological association between multiple sclerosis and lymphoma/leukaemia. Br J Haematol 65, 122–123.

Bithell, J.F., Stewart, A.M., 1975. Pre-natal irradiation and childhood malignancy: a review of British data from the Oxford Survey. Br J Cancer 31, 271–287.

Bocskay, K.A., Tang, D., Orjuela, M.A., Liu, X., Warburton, D.P., Perera, F.P., 2005. Chromosomal aberrations in cord blood are associated with prenatal exposure to carcinogenic polycyclic aromatic hydrocarbons. Cancer Epidemiol Biomarkers Prev 14, 506–511.

Boersma, E.R., Lanting, C.I., 2000. Environmental exposure to polychlorinated biphenyls (PCBs) and dioxins. Consequences for longterm neurological and cognitive development of the child lactation. Adv Exp Med Biol 478, 271–287.

Brenner, A.V., Linet, M.S., Fine, H.A., Shapiro, W.R., Selker, R.G., Black, P.M., Inskip, P.D., 2002. History of allergies and autoimmune diseases and risk of brain tumors in adults. Int J Cancer 99, 252–259.

Brown, R.C., Dwyer, T., Kasten, C., Krotoski, D., Li, Z., Linet, M.S., Olsen, J., Scheidt, P., Winn, D.M., 2007. Cohort profile: the International Childhood Cancer Cohort Consortium (I4C). Int J Epidemiol 36, 724–730.

Buckley, J.D., Gilchrist, G.S., Ruccione, K., Sather, H.N., Woods, W.G., Hammond, G.D., 1989. Multiple sclerosis in mothers of children with acute lymphoblastic leukemia. Leukemia 3, 736–739.

Buffler, P.A., 2008. Childhood Leukemia International Consortium (CLIC), National Cancer Institute, Grant No: 5R03CA132172–02.

Buffler, P.A., Kwan, M.L., Reynolds, P., Urayama, K.Y., 2005. Environmental and genetic risk factors for childhood leukemia: appraising the evidence. Cancer Invest 23, 60–75.

Cardwell, C.R., McKinney, P.A., Patterson, C.C., Murray, L.J., 2008. Infections in early life and childhood leukaemia risk: a UK case-control study of general practitioner records. Br J Cancer 99, 1529–1533.

Caughey, R.W., Michels, K.B., 2009. Birth weight and childhood leukemia: A meta-analysis and review of the current evidence. Int J Cancer 124, 2658–2670.

Cavalieri, E., Frenkel, K., Liehr, J.G., Rogan, E., Roy, D., 2000. Estrogens as endogenous genotoxic agents–DNA adducts and mutations. J Natl Cancer Inst Monogr, 2000(27) 75–93.

Clavel, J., Bellec, S., Rebouissou, S., Menegaux, F., Feunteun, J., Bonaiti-Pellie, C., Baruchel, A., Kebaili, K., Lambilliotte, A., Leverger, G., Sommelet, D., Lescoeur, B., Beaune, P., Hemon, D., Loriot, M.A., 2005. Childhood leukaemia, polymorphisms of metabolism enzyme genes, and interactions with maternal tobacco, coffee and alcohol consumption during pregnancy. Eur J Cancer Prev 14, 531–540.

Coe, C.L., Lubach, G.R., Karaszewski, J.W., Ershler, W.B., 1996. Prenatal endocrine activation alters postnatal cellular immunity in infant monkeys. Brain Behav Immun 10, 221–234.

Cooper, G.S., Kamel, F., Sandler, D.P., Davey, F.R., Bloomfield, C.D., 1996. Risk of adult acute leukemia in relation to prior immune-related conditions. Cancer Epidemiol Biomarkers Prev 5, 867–872.
de Sousa, M., Porto, G., 1998. The immunological system in hemochromatosis. J Hepatol 28 Suppl 1, 1–7.
Dietert, R.R., 2008. Developmental immunotoxicology (DIT): windows of vulnerability, immune dysfunction and safety assessment. J Immunotoxicol 5, 401–412.
Dietert, R.R., 2009. Developmental immunotoxicity (DIT), postnatal immune dysfunction and childhood leukemia. Blood Cells Mol Dis 42, 108–112.
Do, T.N., Ucisik-Akkaya, E., Davis, C.F., Morrison, B.A., Dorak, M.T., 2009. TP53 R72P and MDM2 SNP309 polymorphisms in modification of childhood acute lymphoblastic leukemia susceptibility. Cancer Genet Cytogenet 195, 31–36.
Do, T.N., Ucisik-Akkaya, E., Davis, C.F., Morrison, B.A., Dorak, M.T., 2010. An intronic polymorphism of IRF4 gene influences gene transcription in vitro and shows a risk association with childhood acute lymphoblastic leukemia in males. Biochim Biophys Acta 1802(2): 292–300.
Dorak, M.T., 1996. The implications for childhood leukemia of infection with adenovirus. Trends Microbiol 4, 60–63.
Dorak, M.T., 2006. HFE H63D variant and leukemia susceptibility. Leuk Lymphoma 47, 2269–2270.
Dorak, M.T., Burnett, A.K., 1992. Major histocompatibility complex, t-complex, and leukemia. Cancer Causes Control 3, 273–282.
Dorak, M.T., Burnett, A.K., Worwood, M., 2005. HFE gene mutations in susceptibility to childhood leukemia: HuGE review. Genet Med 7, 159–168.
Dorak, M.T., Chalmers, E.A., Gaffney, D., Wilson, D.W., Galbraith, I., Henderson, N., Worwood, M., Mills, K.I., Burnett, A.K., 1994. Human major histocompatibility complex contains several leukemia susceptibility genes. Leuk Lymphoma 12, 211–222.
Dorak, M.T., Lawson, T., Machulla, H.K., Darke, C., Mills, K.I., Burnett, A.K., 1999a. Unravelling an HLA-DR association in childhood acute lymphoblastic leukemia. Blood 94, 694–700.
Dorak, M.T., Machulla, H.K., Hentschel, M., Mills, K.I., Langner, J., Burnett, A.K., 1996. Influence of the major histocompatibility complex on age at onset of chronic lymphoid leukaemia. Int J Cancer 65, 134–139.
Dorak, M.T., Mackay, R.K., Relton, C.L., Worwood, M., Parker, L., Hall, A.G., 2009. Hereditary hemochromatosis gene (HFE) variants are associated with birth weight and childhood leukemia risk. Pediatr Blood Cancer 53, 1242–1248.
Dorak, M.T., McNally, R.J., Parker, L., 2007a. Re: "Childhood acute lymphoblastic leukemia and infections in the first year of life: a report from the United Kingdom childhood cancer study". Am J Epidemiol 166, 364–365.
Dorak, M.T., Oguz, F.S., Yalman, N., Diler, A.S., Kalayoglu, S., Anak, S., Sargin, D., Carin, M., 2002. A male-specific increase in the HLA-DRB4 (DR53) frequency in high-risk and relapsed childhood ALL. Leuk Res 26, 651–656.
Dorak, M.T., Pearce, M.S., Hammal, D.M., McNally, R.J., Parker, L., 2007b. Examination of gender effect in birth weight and miscarriage associations with childhood cancer (United Kingdom). Cancer Causes Control 18, 219–228.
Dorak, M.T., Sproul, A.M., Gibson, B.E., Burnett, A.K., Worwood, M., 1999b. The C282Y mutation of *HFE* is another male-specific risk factor for childhood ALL. Blood 94, 3957–3958.
Dorak, M.T., Ucisik-Akkaya, E., Davis, C., Morrison, B.A., Do, D., 2008. Genetic associations in childhood leukemia and interactions with sex. 58th Annual Meeting of the American Society for Human Genetics. Philadelphia, PA. November 11–15, 2008.
Dunn, G.P., Old, L.J., Schreiber, R.D., 2004. The immunobiology of cancer immunosurveillance and immunoediting. Immunity 21, 137–148.
Dutz, W., Rossipal, E., Ghavami, H., Vessal, K., Kohout, E., Post, C., 1976. Persistent cell mediated immune-deficiency following infantile stress during the first 6 months of life. Eur J Pediatr 122, 117–130.

Ege, M.J., Bieli, C., Frei, R., van Strien, R.T., Riedler, J., Ublagger, E., Schram-Bijkerk, D., Brunekreef, B., van Hage, M., Scheynius, A., Pershagen, G., Benz, M.R., Lauener, R., von Mutius, E., Braun-Fahrlander, C., 2006. Prenatal farm exposure is related to the expression of receptors of the innate immunity and to atopic sensitization in school-age children. J Allergy Clin Immunol 117, 817–823.

Fernandez-Soria, V., Bornstein, R., Forteza, J., Parada, C., Sanchez-Prieto, R., Ramon y Cajal, S., 2002. Inconclusive presence of adenovirus sequences in human leukemias and lymphomas. Oncol Rep 9, 897–902.

Ford, A.M., Pombo-de-Oliveira, M.S., McCarthy, K.P., MacLean, J.M., Carrico, K.C., Vincent, R.F., Greaves, M., 1997. Monoclonal origin of concordant T-cell malignancy in identical twins. Blood 89, 281–285.

Ganz, T., 2006. Hepcidin–a peptide hormone at the interface of innate immunity and iron metabolism. Curr Top Microbiol Immunol 306, 183–198.

Ghavami, H., Dutz, W., Mohallattee, M., Rossipal, E., Vessal, K., 1979. Immune disturbances after severe enteritis during the first six months of life. Isr J Med Sci 15, 364–368.

Gluckman, P.D., Hanson, M.A., Cooper, C., Thornburg, K.L., 2008. Effect of in utero and early-life conditions on adult health and disease. N Engl J Med 359, 61–73.

Goodman, M., Dana Flanders, W., 2007. Study design options in evaluating gene-environment interactions: practical considerations for a planned case-control study of pediatric leukemia. Pediatr Blood Cancer 48, 375–379.

Greaves, M.F., 2001. Commentary: Birth order and risk of childhood acute lymphoblastic leukaemia (ALL). Int J Epidemiol 30, 1438–1439.

Greaves, M., 2006. Infection, immune responses and the aetiology of childhood leukaemia. Nat Rev Cancer 6, 193–203.

Greaves, M.F., Maia, A.T., Wiemels, J.L., Ford, A.M., 2003. Leukemia in twins: lessons in natural history. Blood 102, 2321–2333.

Greaves, M.F., Wiemels, J., 2003. Origins of chromosome translocations in childhood leukaemia. Nat Rev Cancer 3, 639–649.

Green, M.S., 1992. The male predominance in the incidence of infectious diseases in children: a postulated explanation for disparities in the literature. Int J Epidemiol 21, 381–386.

Grossman, C., 1989. Possible underlying mechanisms of sexual dimorphism in the immune response, fact and hypothesis. J Steroid Biochem 34, 241–251.

Gruhn, B., Taub, J.W., Ge, Y., Beck, J.F., Zell, R., Hafer, R., Hermann, F.H., Debatin, K.M., Steinbach, D., 2008. Prenatal origin of childhood acute lymphoblastic leukemia, association with birth weight and hyperdiploidy. Leukemia 22, 1692–1697.

Guha, N., Chang, J.S., Chokkalingam, A.P., Wiemels, J.L., Smith, M.T., Buffler, P.A., 2008. NQO1 polymorphisms and de novo childhood leukemia: a HuGE review and meta-analysis. Am J Epidemiol 168, 1221–1232.

Gustafsson, B., Huang, W., Bogdanovic, G., Gauffin, F., Nordgren, A., Talekar, G., Ornelles, D.A., Gooding, L.R., 2007. Adenovirus DNA is detected at increased frequency in Guthrie cards from children who develop acute lymphoblastic leukaemia. Br J Cancer 97, 992–994.

Hafler, D.A., Compston, A., Sawcer, S., Lander, E.S., Daly, M.J., De Jager, P.L., de Bakker, P.I., Gabriel, S.B., Mirel, D.B., Ivinson, A.J., Pericak-Vance, M.A., Gregory, S.G., Rioux, J.D., McCauley, J.L., Haines, J.L., Barcellos, L.F., Cree, B., Oksenberg, J.R., Hauser, S.L., 2007. Risk alleles for multiple sclerosis identified by a genomewide study. N Engl J Med 357, 851–862.

Hamajima, N., Yuasa, H., Matsuo, K., Kurobe, Y., 1999. Detection of gene-environment interaction by case-only studies. Jpn J Clin Oncol 29, 490–493.

Hartikainen, J.M., Tuhkanen, H., Kataja, V., Eskelinen, M., Uusitupa, M., Kosma, V.M., Mannermaa, A., 2006. Refinement of the 22q12-q13 breast cancer-associated region: evidence of TMPRSS6 as a candidate gene in an eastern Finnish population. Clin Cancer Res 12, 1454–1462.

Hattis, D., Goble, R., Russ, A., Chu, M., Ericson, J., 2004. Age-related differences in susceptibility to carcinogenesis: a quantitative analysis of empirical animal bioassay data. Environ Health Perspect 112, 1152–1158.
Hemminki, K., Lorenzo Bermejo, J., Forsti, A., 2006. The balance between heritable and environmental etiology of human disease. Nat Rev Genet 7, 958–965.
Hertz-Picciotto, I., Park, H.Y., Dostal, M., Kocan, A., Trnovec, T., Sram, R., 2008. Prenatal exposures to persistent and non-persistent organic compounds and effects on immune system development. Basic Clin Pharmacol Toxicol 102, 146–154.
Hooper, K., McDonald, T.A., 2000. The PBDEs: an emerging environmental challenge and another reason for breast-milk monitoring programs. Environ Health Perspect 108, 387–392.
Horton, R., Wilming, L., Rand, V., Lovering, R.C., Bruford, E.A., Khodiyar, V.K., Lush, M.J., Povey, S., Talbot, C.C., Wright, M.W., Wain, H.M., Trowsdale, J., Ziegler, A., Beck, S., 2004. Gene map of the extended human MHC. Nat Rev Genet 5, 889–899.
Hosea Blewett, H.J., Cicalo, M.C., Holland, C.D., Field, C.J., 2008. The immunological components of human milk. Adv Food Nutr Res 54, 45–80.
Hughes, A.M., Lightfoot, T., Simpson, J., Ansell, P., McKinney, P.A., Kinsey, S.E., Mitchell, C.D., Eden, T.O., Greaves, M., Roman, E., 2007. Allergy and risk of childhood leukaemia: results from the UKCCS. Int J Cancer 121, 819–824.
Infante-Rivard, C., Vermunt, J.K., Weinberg, C.R., 2007. Excess transmission of the NAD(P)H:quinone oxidoreductase 1 (NQO1) C609T polymorphism in families of children with acute lymphoblastic leukemia. Am J Epidemiol 165, 1248–1254.
Infante-Rivard, C., Krajinovic, M., Labuda, D., Sinnett, D., 2000. Parental smoking, CYP1A1 genetic polymorphisms and childhood leukemia (Quebec, Canada). Cancer Causes Control 11, 547–553.
Infante-Rivard, C., Labuda, D., Krajinovic, M., Sinnett, D., 1999. Risk of childhood leukemia associated with exposure to pesticides and with gene polymorphisms. Epidemiology 10, 481–487.
Inskip, P.D., Harvey, E.B., Boice, J.D., Jr., Stone, B.J., Matanoski, G., Flannery, J.T., Fraumeni, J.F., Jr., 1991. Incidence of childhood cancer in twins. Cancer Causes Control 2, 315–324.
Jemal, A., Siegel, R., Ward, E., Hao, Y., Xu, J., Murray, T., Thun, M.J., 2008. Cancer statistics, 2008. CA Cancer J Clin 58, 71–96.
Johnson, K.J., Soler, J.T., Puumala, S.E., Ross, J.A., Spector, L.G., 2008. Parental and infant characteristics and childhood leukemia in Minnesota. BMC Pediatr 8, 7.
Jourdan-Da Silva, N., Perel, Y., Mechinaud, F., Plouvier, E., Gandemer, V., Lutz, P., Vannier, J.P., Lamagnere, J.L., Margueritte, G., Boutard, P., Robert, A., Armari, C., Munzer, M., Millot, F., De Lumley, L., Berthou, C., Rialland, X., Pautard, B., Hemon, D., Clavel, J., 2004. Infectious diseases in the first year of life, perinatal characteristics and childhood acute leukaemia. Br J Cancer 90, 139–145.
Kallianpur, A.R., Hall, L.D., Yadav, M., Christman, B.W., Dittus, R.S., Haines, J.L., Parl, F.F., Summar, M.L., 2004. Increased prevalence of the HFE C282Y hemochromatosis allele in women with breast cancer. Cancer Epidemiol Biomarkers Prev 13, 205–212.
Khoury, M.J., Adams, M.J., Jr., Flanders, W.D., 1988. An epidemiologic approach to ecogenetics. Am J Hum Genet 42, 89–95.
Khoury, M.J., Wagener, D.K., 1995. Epidemiological evaluation of the use of genetics to improve the predictive value of disease risk factors. Am J Hum Genet 56, 835–844.
Kinlen, L.J., 1995. Epidemiological evidence for an infective basis in childhood leukaemia. Br J Cancer 71, 1–5.
Kinlen, L., 2004a. Infections and immune factors in cancer: the role of epidemiology. Oncogene 23, 6341–6348.
Kinlen, L.J., 2004b. Re: "Childhood cancer and population mixing". Am J Epidemiol 159, 716–717; author reply 717.
Kochhar, H.P., Peippo, J., King, W.A., 2001. Sex related embryo development. Theriogenology 55, 3–14.

Koopman-Esseboom, C., Huisman, M., Weisglas-Kuperus, N., Boersma, E.R., de Ridder, M.A., Van der Paauw, C.G., Tuinstra, L.G., Sauer, P.J., 1994. Dioxin and PCB levels in blood and human milk in relation to living areas in The Netherlands. Chemosphere 29, 2327–2338.

Kosulin, K., Haberler, C., Hainfellner, J.A., Amann, G., Lang, S., Lion, T., 2007. Investigation of adenovirus occurrence in pediatric tumor entities. J Virol 81, 7629–7635.

Kraft, P., Hunter, D., 2005. Integrating epidemiology and genetic association: the challenge of gene-environment interaction. Philos Trans R Soc Lond B Biol Sci 360, 1609–1616.

Kraft, P., Yen, Y.C., Stram, D.O., Morrison, J., Gauderman, W.J., 2007. Exploiting gene-environment interaction to detect genetic associations. Hum Hered 63, 111–119.

Krajinovic, M., Lamothe, S., Labuda, D., Lemieux-Blanchard, E., Theoret, Y., Moghrabi, A., Sinnett, D., 2004. Role of MTHFR genetic polymorphisms in the susceptibility to childhood acute lymphoblastic leukemia. Blood 103, 252–257.

Labuda, D., Krajinovic, M., Sabbagh, A., Infante-Rivard, C., Sinnett, D., 2002. Parental genotypes in the risk of a complex disease. Am J Hum Genet 71, 193–197.

Lafiura, K.M., Bielawski, D.M., Posecion, N.C., Jr., Ostrea, E.M., Jr., Matherly, L.H., Taub, J.W., Ge, Y., 2007. Association between prenatal pesticide exposures and the generation of leukemia-associated T(8;21). Pediatr Blood Cancer 49, 624–628.

Landrigan, P.J., Sonawane, B., Mattison, D., McCally, M., Garg, A., 2002. Chemical contaminants in breast milk and their impacts on children's health: an overview. Environ Health Perspect 110, A313–A315.

Law, G.R., Parslow, R.C., Roman, E., 2003. Childhood cancer and population mixing. Am J Epidemiol 158, 328–336.

Lawrence, T., Hageman, T., Balkwill, F., 2007. Cancer. Sex, cytokines, and cancer. Science 317, 51–52.

Le Marchand, L., 2005. The predominance of the environment over genes in cancer causation: implications for genetic epidemiology. Cancer Epidemiol Biomarkers Prev 14, 1037–1039.

Lightfoot, T.J., Roman, E., 2004. Causes of childhood leukaemia and lymphoma. Toxicol Appl Pharmacol 199, 104–117.

Linabery, A.M., Ross, J.A., 2008. Trends in childhood cancer incidence in the U. S. (1992–2004). Cancer, 112, 416–432.

Linet, M.S., Wacholder, S., Zahm, S.H., 2003. Interpreting epidemiologic research: lessons from studies of childhood cancer. Pediatrics 112, 218–232.

Liu, X., Fallin, M.D., Kao, W.H., 2004. Genetic dissection methods: designs used for tests of gene-environment interaction. Curr Opin Genet Dev 14, 241–245.

Lo, J.T., Tsai, M.J., Wang, L.H., Huang, M.T., Yang, Y.H., Lin, Y.T., Liu, J., Chiang, B.L., 1999. Sex differences in pediatric systemic lupus erythematosus: a retrospective analysis of 135 cases. J Microbiol Immunol Infect 32, 173–178.

Loft, S., Vistisen, K., Ewertz, M., Tjonneland, A., Overvad, K., Poulsen, H.E., 1992. Oxidative DNA damage estimated by 8-hydroxydeoxyguanosine excretion in humans: influence of smoking, gender and body mass index. Carcinogenesis 13, 2241–2247.

Ma, X., Buffler, P.A., Gunier, R.B., Dahl, G., Smith, M.T., Reinier, K., Reynolds, P., 2002. Critical windows of exposure to household pesticides and risk of childhood leukemia. Environ Health Perspect 110, 955–960.

Ma, Y., Kawabata, T., Hamazaki, S., Ogino, T., Okada, S., 1998. Sex differences in oxidative damage in ddY mouse kidney treated with a renal carcinogen, iron nitrilotriacetate. Carcinogenesis 19, 1983–1988.

Macmahon, B., Levy, M.A., 1964. Prenatal origin of childhood leukemia. Evidence from twins. N Engl J Med 270, 1082–1085.

Maia, A.T., van der Velden, V.H., Harrison, C.J., Szczepanski, T., Williams, M.D., Griffiths, M.J., van Dongen, J.J., Greaves, M.F., 2003. Prenatal origin of hyperdiploid acute lymphoblastic leukemia in identical twins. Leukemia 17, 2202–2206.

Manole, D., Schildknecht, B., Gosnell, B., Adams, E., Derwahl, M., 2001. Estrogen promotes growth of human thyroid tumor cells by different molecular mechanisms. J Clin Endocrinol Metab 86, 1072–1077.

Martin, J.T., 2000. Sexual dimorphism in immune function: the role of prenatal exposure to androgens and estrogens. Eur J Pharmacol 405, 251–261.

Martin, R.M., Gunnell, D., Owen, C.G., Smith, G.D., 2005. Breast-feeding and childhood cancer: A systematic review with metaanalysis. Int J Cancer 117, 1020–1031.

McKinney, P.A., Cartwright, R.A., Saiu, J.M., Mann, J.R., Stiller, C.A., Draper, G.J., Hartley, A.L., Hopton, P.A., Birch, J.M., Waterhouse, J.A., et al., 1987. The inter-regional epidemiological study of childhood cancer (IRESCC): a case control study of aetiological factors in leukaemia and lymphoma. Arch Dis Child 62, 279–287.

McNally, R.J., Eden, T.O., 2004. An infectious aetiology for childhood acute leukaemia: a review of the evidence. Br J Haematol 127, 243–263.

McNally, R.J., Parker, L., 2006. Environmental factors and childhood acute leukemias and lymphomas. Leuk Lymphoma 47, 583–598.

Mellemkjaer, L., Alexander, F., Olsen, J.H., 2000. Cancer among children of parents with autoimmune diseases. Br J Cancer 82, 1353–1357.

Mitchell, R.J., Farrington, S.M., Dunlop, M.G., Campbell, H., 2002. Mismatch repair genes hMLH1 and hMSH2 and colorectal cancer: a HuGE review. Am J Epidemiol 156, 885–902.

Mittwoch, U., 1993. Blastocysts prepare for the race to be male. Hum Reprod 8, 1550–1555.

Mori, H., Colman, S.M., Xiao, Z., Ford, A.M., Healy, L.E., Donaldson, C., Hows, J.M., Navarrete, C., Greaves, M., 2002. Chromosome translocations and covert leukemic clones are generated during normal fetal development. Proc Natl Acad Sci USA 99, 8242–8247.

Morrison, B.A., Ucisik-Akkaya, E., Flores, H., Gorodezky, C., Dorak, M.T., 2010. The HLA-DRA and HLA-C-linked multiple sclerosis risk markers are shared by childhood ALL with sex effect. Autoimmunity (in press)

Nakachi, K., Hayashi, T., Imai, K., Kusunoki, Y., 2004. Perspectives on cancer immuno-epidemiology. Cancer Sci 95, 921–929.

Naugler, W.E., Sakurai, T., Kim, S., Maeda, S., Kim, K., Elsharkawy, A.M., Karin, M., 2007. Gender disparity in liver cancer due to sex differences in MyD88-dependent IL-6 production. Science 317, 121–124.

Nickerson, K., 2006. Environmental contaminants in breast milk. J Midwifery Womens Health 51, 26–34.

Niculescu, A.M., 1985. Effects of in utero exposure to DES on male progeny. J Obstet Gynecol Neonatal Nurs 14, 468–470.

O'Connor, S.M., Boneva, R.S., 2007. Infectious etiologies of childhood leukemia: plausibility and challenges to proof. Environ Health Perspect 115, 146–150.

Ordovas, J.M., Corella, D., Demissie, S., Cupples, L.A., Couture, P., Coltell, O., Wilson, P.W., Schaefer, E.J., Tucker, K.L., 2002. Dietary fat intake determines the effect of a common polymorphism in the hepatic lipase gene promoter on high-density lipoprotein metabolism: evidence of a strong dose effect in this gene-nutrient interaction in the Framingham Study. Circulation 106, 2315–2321.

Ottman, R., 1990. An epidemiologic approach to gene-environment interaction. Genet Epidemiol 7, 177–185.

Ottman, R., 1996. Gene-environment interaction: definitions and study designs. Prev Med 25, 764–770.

Paltiel, O., Laniado, D.E., Yanetz, R., Deutsch, L., Calderon-Margalit, R., Harlap, S., Friedlander, Y., 2006. The risk of cancer following hospitalization for infection in infancy: a population-based cohort study. Cancer Epidemiol Biomarkers Prev 15, 1964–1968.

Parslow, R.C., Law, G.R., Feltbower, R., Kinsey, S.E., McKinney, P.A., 2002. Population mixing, childhood leukaemia, CNS tumours and other childhood cancers in Yorkshire. Eur J Cancer 38, 2033–2040.

Patandin, S., Dagnelie, P.C., Mulder, P.G., Op de Coul, E., van der Veen, J.E., Weisglas-Kuperus, N., Sauer, P.J., 1999. Dietary exposure to polychlorinated biphenyls and dioxins from infancy until adulthood: A comparison between breast-feeding, toddler, and long-term exposure. Environ Health Perspect, 107, 45–51.

Pearce, M.S., Parker, L., 2001. Childhood cancer registrations in the developing world: still more boys than girls. Int J Cancer 91, 402–406.

Peck, J.D., Hulka, B.S., Savitz, D.A., Baird, D., Poole, C., Richardson, B.E., 2003. Accuracy of fetal growth indicators as surrogate measures of steroid hormone levels during pregnancy. Am J Epidemiol 157, 258–266.

Penn, D.J., Damjanovich, K., Potts, W.K., 2002. MHC heterozygosity confers a selective advantage against multiple-strain infections. Proc Natl Acad Sci USA 99, 11260–11264.

Perera, F., Viswanathan, S., Whyatt, R., Tang, D., Miller, R.L., Rauh, V., 2006. Children's environmental health research–highlights from the Columbia Center for Children's Environmental Health. Ann N Y Acad Sci 1076, 15–28.

Perillat-Menegaux, F., Clavel, J., Auclerc, M.F., Baruchel, A., Leverger, G., Nelken, B., Philippe, N., Sommelet, D., Vilmer, E., Hemon, D., 2003. Family history of autoimmune thyroid disease and childhood acute leukemia. Cancer Epidemiol Biomarkers Prev 12, 60–63.

Porto, G., De Sousa, M., 2007. Iron overload and immunity. World J Gastroenterol 13, 4707–4715.

Preston-Martin, S., Pike, M.C., Ross, R.K., Jones, P.A., Henderson, B.E., 1990. Increased cell division as a cause of human cancer. Cancer Res 50, 7415–7421.

Priftakis, P., Dalianis, T., Carstensen, J., Samuelsson, U., Lewensohn-Fuchs, I., Bogdanovic, G., Winiarski, J., Gustafsson, B., 2003. Human polyomavirus DNA is not detected in Guthrie cards (dried blood spots) from children who developed acute lymphoblastic leukemia. Med Pediatr Oncol 40, 219–223.

Proteggente, A.R., England, T.G., Rehman, A., Rice-Evans, C.A., Halliwell, B., 2002. Gender differences in steady-state levels of oxidative damage to DNA in healthy individuals. Free Radic Res 36, 157–162.

Purtilo, D.T., Sullivan, J.L., 1979. Immunological bases for superior survival of females. Am J Dis Child 133, 1251–1253.

Read, J.S., Troendle, J.F., Klebanoff, M.A., 1997. Infectious disease mortality among infants in the United States, 1983 through 1987. Am J Public Health 87, 192–198.

Regis, G., Bosticardo, M., Conti, L., De Angelis, S., Boselli, D., Tomaino, B., Bernabei, P., Giovarelli, M., Novelli, F., 2005. Iron regulates T-lymphocyte sensitivity to the IFN-gamma/STAT1 signaling pathway in vitro and in vivo. Blood 105, 3214–3221.

Reynolds, T., 1998a. Causes of childhood leukemia beginning to emerge. J Natl Cancer Inst 90, 8–10.

Reynolds, T., 1998b. Researchers hunt for elusive environmental causes of leukemia. J Natl Cancer Inst 90, 90–92.

Rodvall, Y., Hrubec, Z., Pershagen, G., Ahlbom, A., Bjurman, A., Boice, J.D., Jr., 1992. Childhood cancer among Swedish twins. Cancer Causes Control 3, 527–532.

Romagnani, S., 2004. The increased prevalence of allergy and the hygiene hypothesis: missing immune deviation, reduced immune suppression, or both? Immunology 112, 352–363.

Roman, E., Simpson, J., Ansell, P., Kinsey, S., Mitchell, C.D., McKinney, P.A., Birch, J.M., Greaves, M., Eden, T., 2007. Childhood acute lymphoblastic leukemia and infections in the first year of life: a report from the United Kingdom Childhood Cancer Study. Am J Epidemiol 165, 496–504.

Rosenbaum, P.F., Buck, G.M., Brecher, M.L., 2005. Allergy and infectious disease histories and the risk of childhood acute lymphoblastic leukaemia. Pediatr Perinat Epidemiol 19, 152–164.

Rossi, R., Zatelli, M.C., Franceschetti, P., Maestri, I., Magri, E., Aguiari, G., Cavazzini, P., degli Uberti, E.C., del Senno, L., 1996. Inhibitory effect of dihydrotestosterone on human thyroid cell growth. J Endocrinol, 151, 185–194.

Samuelsen, S.O., Bakketeig, L.S., Tretli, S., Johannesen, T.B., Magnus, P., 2009. Birth weight and childhood cancer. Epidemiology 20, 484–487.
Schlegel, R.J., Bellanti, J.A., 1969. Increased susceptibility of males to infection. Lancet 2, 826–827.
Schuz, J., Morgan, G., Bohler, E., Kaatsch, P., Michaelis, J., 2003. Atopic disease and childhood acute lymphoblastic leukemia. Int J Cancer 105, 255–260.
Schwacke, L.H., Voit, E.O., Hansen, L.J., Wells, R.S., Mitchum, G.B., Hohn, A.A., Fair, P.A., 2002. Probabilistic risk assessment of reproductive effects of polychlorinated biphenyls on bottlenose dolphins (Tursiops truncatus) from the Southeast United States Coast. Environ Toxicol Chem 21, 2752–2764.
Schwartzbaum, J., Jonsson, F., Ahlbom, A., Preston-Martin, S., Lonn, S., Soderberg, K.C., Feychting, M., 2003. Cohort studies of association between self-reported allergic conditions, immune-related diagnoses and glioma and meningioma risk. Int J Cancer 106, 423–428.
Shelat, S.G., Aird, F., Redei, E., 1997. Exposure to dehydroepiandrosterone in utero affects T-cell function in males only. Neuroimmunomodulation 4, 154–162.
Smith, M.A., Simon, R., Strickler, H.D., McQuillan, G., Ries, L.A., Linet, M.S., 1998. Evidence that childhood acute lymphoblastic leukemia is associated with an infectious agent linked to hygiene conditions. Cancer Causes Control 9, 285–298.
Smith, M.A., Strickler, H.D., Granovsky, M., Reaman, G., Linet, M., Daniel, R., Shah, K.V., 1999. Investigation of leukemia cells from children with common acute lymphoblastic leukemia for genomic sequences of the primate polyomaviruses JC virus, BK virus, and simian virus 40. Med Pediatr Oncol 33, 441–443.
Smulevich, V.B., Solionova, L.G., Belyakova, S.V., 1999. Parental occupation and other factors and cancer risk in children: I. Study methodology and non-occupational factors. Int J Cancer 83, 712–717.
Sonawane, B.R., 1995. Chemical contaminants in human milk: an overview. Environ Health Perspect 103 Suppl 6, 197–205.
Steenbergen, E.J., Verhagen, O.J., van Leeuwen, E.F., Behrendt, H., Merle, P.A., Wester, M.R., von dem Borne, A.E., van der Schoot, C.E., 1994. B precursor acute lymphoblastic leukemia third complementarity-determining regions predominantly represent an unbiased recombination repertoire: leukemic transformation frequently occurs in fetal life. Eur J Immunol, 24 900–908.
Steliarova-Foucher, E., Stiller, C., Kaatsch, P., Berrino, F., Coebergh, J.W., Lacour, B., Parkin, M., 2004. Geographical patterns and time trends of cancer incidence and survival among children and adolescents in Europe since the 1970s (the ACCISproject): an epidemiological study. Lancet 364, 2097–2105.
Steliarova-Foucher, E., Stiller, C.A., Pukkala, E., Lacour, B., Plesko, I., Parkin, D.M., 2006. Thyroid cancer incidence and survival among European children and adolescents (1978–1997): report from the Automated Childhood Cancer Information System project. Eur J Cancer 42, 2150–2169.
Stewart, A., Webb, J., Hewitt, D., 1958. A survey of childhood malignancies. BMJ 1, 1495–1508.
Stiller, C.A., 2004. Epidemiology and genetics of childhood cancer. Oncogene 23, 6429–6444.
Strachan, D.P., 1989. Hay fever, hygiene, and household size. BMJ 299, 1259–1260.
Taub, J.W., Ge, Y., 2004. The prenatal origin of childhood acute lymphoblastic leukemia. Leuk Lymphoma 45, 19–25.
Taylor, G.M., Dearden, S., Payne, N., Ayres, M., Gokhale, D.A., Birch, J.M., Blair, V., Stevens, R.F., Will, A.M., Eden, O.B., 1998. Evidence that an HLA-DQA1-DQB1 haplotype influences susceptibility to childhood common acute lymphoblastic leukaemia in boys provides further support for an infection-related aetiology. Br J Cancer 78, 561–565.
Taylor, G.M., Dearden, S., Ravetto, P., Ayres, M., Watson, P., Hussain, A., Greaves, M., Alexander, F., Eden, O.B., 2002. Genetic susceptibility to childhood common acute lymphoblastic leukaemia is associated with polymorphic peptide-binding pocket profiles in HLA-DPB1*0201. Hum Mol Genet 11, 1585–1597.

Taylor, G.M., Hussain, A., Lightfoot, T.J., Birch, J.M., Eden, T.O., Greaves, M.F., 2008. HLA-associated susceptibility to childhood B-cell precursor ALL: definition and role of HLA-DPB1 supertypes. Br J Cancer 98, 1125–1131.
Till, M.M., Jones, L.H., Pentycross, C.R., Hardisty, R.M., Lawler, S.D., Harvey, B.A., Soothill, J.F., 1975. Leukaemia in children and their grandparents: studies of immune function in six families. Br J Haematol 29, 575–586.
Till, M., Rapson, N., Smith, P.G., 1979. Family studies in acute leukaemia in childhood: a possible association with autoimmune disease. Br J Cancer 40, 62–71.
Ucisik-Akkaya, E., Davis, C.F., Gorodezky, C., Alaez, C., Dorak, M.T., 2010. HLA complex-linked heat shock protein genes and childhood acute lymphoblastic leukemia susceptibility. Cell Stress Chaperones (in press)
Urayama, K.Y., Wiencke, J.K., Buffler, P.A., Chokkalingam, A.P., Metayer, C., Wiemels, J.L., 2007. MDR1 gene variants, indoor insecticide exposure, and the risk of childhood acute lymphoblastic leukemia. Cancer Epidemiol Biomarkers Prev 16, 1172–1177.
van Steensel-Moll, H.A., Valkenburg, H.A., Vandenbroucke, J.P., van Zanen, G.E., 1985. Are maternal fertility problems related to childhood leukaemia? Int J Epidemiol 14, 555–559.
Vasconcelos, G.M., Kang, M., Pombo-de-Oliveira, M.S., Schiffman, J.D., Lorey, F., Buffler, P., Wiemels, J.L., 2008. Adenovirus detection in Guthrie cards from paediatric leukaemia cases and controls. Br J Cancer 99, 1668–1672.
Vena, J.E., Bona, J.R., Byers, T.E., Middleton, E., Jr., Swanson, M.K., Graham, S., 1985. Allergy-related diseases and cancer: an inverse association. Am J Epidemiol 122, 66–74.
Verthelyi, D., 2001. Sex hormones as immunomodulators in health and disease. Int Immunopharmacol 1, 983–993.
Von Fliedner, V.E., Merica, H., Jeannet, M., Barras, C., Feldges, A., Imbach, P., Wyss, M., 1983. Evidence for HLA-linked susceptibility factors in childhood leukemia. Hum Immunol 8, 183–193.
Waalen, J., Nordestgaard, B.G., Beutler, E., 2005. The penetrance of hereditary hemochromatosis. Best Pract Res Clin Haematol 18, 203–220.
Walker, E.M., Jr., Walker, S.M., 2000. Effects of iron overload on the immune system. Ann Clin Lab Sci 30, 354–365.
Wang, L.E., Bondy, M.L., de Andrade, M., Strom, S.S., Wang, X., Sigurdson, A., Spitz, M.R., Wei, Q., 2000. Gender difference in smoking effect on chromosome sensitivity to gamma radiation in a healthy population. Radiat Res 154, 20–27.
Wardrop, S.L., Wells, C., Ravasi, T., Hume, D.A., Richardson, D.R., 2002. Induction of Nramp2 in activated mouse macrophages is dissociated from regulation of the Nramp1, classical inflammatory genes, and genes involved in iron metabolism. J Leukoc Biol 71, 99–106.
Washburn, T.C., Medearis, D.N., Jr., Childs, B., 1965. Sex differences in susceptibility to infections. Pediatrics 35, 57–64.
Wasserman, R., Galili, N., Ito, Y., Reichard, B.A., Shane, S., Rovera, G., 1992. Predominance of fetal type DJH joining in young children with B precursor lymphoblastic leukemia as evidence for an in utero transforming event. J Exp Med 176, 1577–1581.
Weiss, G., Wachter, H., Fuchs, D., 1995. Linkage of cell-mediated immunity to iron metabolism. Immunol Today 16, 495–500.
Wen, W., Shu, X.O., Linet, M.S., Neglia, J.P., Potter, J.D., Trigg, M.E., Robison, L.L., 2000. Allergic disorders and the risk of childhood acute lymphoblastic leukemia (United States). Cancer Causes Control 11, 303–307.
Wen, W.Q., Shu, X.O., Sellers, T., Bhatia, S., Lampkin, B., Robison, L.L., 1998. Family history of cancer and autoimmune disease and risk of leukemia in infancy: a report from the Children's Cancer Group (United States and Canada). Cancer Causes Control 9, 161–171.
Wiemels, J.L., Cazzaniga, G., Daniotti, M., Eden, O.B., Addison, G.M., Masera, G., Saha, V., Biondi, A., Greaves, M.F., 1999a. Prenatal origin of acute lymphoblastic leukaemia in children. Lancet 354, 1499–1503.
Wiemels, J.L., Ford, A.M., Van Wering, E.R., Postma, A., Greaves, M., 1999b. Protracted and variable latency of acute lymphoblastic leukemia after TEL-AML1 gene fusion in utero. Blood 94, 1057–1062.

Wiemels, J.L., Xiao, Z., Buffler, P.A., Maia, A.T., Ma, X., Dicks, B.M., Smith, M.T., Zhang, L., Feusner, J., Wiencke, J., Pritchard-Jones, K., Kempski, H., Greaves, M., 2002. In utero origin of t(8;21) AML1-ETO translocations in childhood acute myeloid leukemia. Blood 99, 3801–3805.
Woods, W.G., Robison, L.L., Kim, Y., Schuman, L.M., Heisel, M., Smithson, A., Finlay, J., Hutchinson, R., Gibson, R.W., 1987. Association of maternal autoimmunity with childhood acute lymphocytic leukemia (ALL). Proc Am Assoc Cancer Res 28, 251.
Xie, T., Rowen, L., Aguado, B., Ahearn, M.E., Madan, A., Qin, S., Campbell, R.D., Hood, L., 2003. Analysis of the gene-dense major histocompatibility complex class III region and its comparison to mouse. Genome Res 13, 2621–2636.
Yakushiji, T., Watanabe, I., Kuwabara, K., Tanaka, R., Kashimoto, T., Kunita, N., Hara, I., 1984. Postnatal transfer of PCBs from exposed mothers to their babies: influence of breast-feeding. Arch Environ Health 39, 368–375.
Zitvogel, L., Tesniere, A., Kroemer, G., 2006. Cancer despite immunosurveillance: immunoselection and immunosubversion. Nat Rev Immunol 6, 715–727.

Internet Links

National Cancer Institute Childhood Cancers: http://www.cancer.gov/cancertopics/types/childhoodcancers

SEER (Surveillance, Epidemiology and End Results Program), Cancer Incidence and Survival among Children and Adolescents, 1975–1995 (USA): http://seer.cancer.gov/publications/childhood

ACCIS (Automated Childhood Cancer Information System), Cancer Incidence and Survival among Children and Adolescents, (Europe): http://www-dep.iarc.fr/accis/data.htm

CLIC: http://cancercontrol.cancer.gov/grants/abstract.asp?ApplID=7502115

I4C: http://www.nationalchildrensstudy.gov/research/internationalinvolvement/pages/default.aspx#i4c

COG: http://www.childrensoncologygroup.org

UKCCS: http://www.ukccs.org

Review of Childhood Cancer Epidemiology: http://www.dorak.info/epi/ccepi.html

Chapter 12
Exposure to Environmental Mutagens: APC and Colorectal Carcinogenesis

Aruna S. Jaiswal, Melissa L. Armas, Shahnjayla K. Connors, Harekrushna Panda, and Satya Narayan

Abstract Environmental mutagens are global health hazards and a major risk factor for colon cancer development. Environmental mutagens include a variety of genotoxic carcinogenic compounds including polycyclic aromatic hydrocarbons, heterocyclic amines, nitrosamines, and aromatic amines. Their sources are pollution, diet, alcohol and cigarette smoke. These mutagens come in contact with large bowel through blood circulation or direct ingestion. Once these mutagens are in contact with DNA of the gut epithelial cells, they form DNA-adducts. If the damage exceeds the repair capacity of the epithelial cells, then the persistence of mutations can lead to the transformation of these cells. Mutations in *adenomatous polyposis coli* (*APC*) gene is considered to be one of the earliest events in the genesis of colorectal cancer, and its role has been well documented in a broad spectrum of functions ranging from cell adhesion to cell migration, regulation of Wnt/β-catenin-signaling pathway, cell cycle control, apoptosis, and chromosomal segregation at mitosis. The contribution of environmental mutagens on the *APC* gene mutations is very scanty in the literature. In the past several years, we have initiated studies to examine the interaction of APC with pathways induced by environmental mutagens. We showed that APC can be transcriptionally upregulated after DNA damage subsequent to the exposure of environmental mutagens including cigarette smoking. In addition, we recently discovered a novel role of APC in base excision repair (BER) pathway. APC interacts with DNA polymerase β and Fen-1 and blocks Pol-β-directed BER. Thus, APC-mediated block of BER in response to environmental mutagens, especially the DNA-alkylating agents, can be detrimental to the cell.

Keywords Environmental mutagens · DNA damage · Adenomatous polyposis coli · DNA repair · Colorectal carcinogenesis

---

S. Narayan (✉)
Department of Anatomy and Cell Biology, UF Shands Cancer Center, University of Florida, Gainesville, FL 32610, USA
e-mail: snarayan@ufl.edu

D. Roy, M.T. Dorak (eds.), *Environmental Factors, Genes, and the Development of Human Cancers*, DOI 10.1007/978-1-4419-6752-7_12,

12.1 Introduction

Exposure to environmental pollutants are primarily responsible for many diseases inclusive of cancers. The toxic chemicals present in the hazardous environmental pollutants come in contact with humans through the air, soil, water, food, tobacco smoke, and combustion emissions, and are a serious threat to human health. Tobacco smoking is associated with the increased risk of cancers in organs that are not in direct contact with the smoke, such as the stomach, kidney, bladder, pancreas (IARC, 2004; ACS, 2007a). Smoking is also proposed to be an initiator of colorectal carcinogenesis (Giovannucci et al., 1994a, b; Giovannucci and Martinez, 1996). It is estimated that 21% of microsatellite instability (MIN) in colon tumors may be attributed to cigarette smoke (Slattery et al. 2000). Burning tobacco produces a variety of genotoxic carcinogenic compounds including polycyclic aromatic hydrocarbons, heterocyclic amines, nitrosamines, and aromatic amines (IARC, 1986; Manabe et al., 1991; Alexandrov et al., 1996; Hoffman and Hoffman, 1997). The large bowel is exposed to these compounds either through the circulatory system (Yamaski and Ames, 1977) or by direct ingestion (Kune et al., 1992). The contribution of dietary carcinogens is another major concern to colorectal carcinogenesis. It has been well documented that the surface of charcoal-broiled fish or meat contains heterocyclic amines which are powerful mutagens. Similar environmental mutagens accumulate on the surface of other types of fried and broiled foods. These heterocyclic amines are capable of inducing colorectal carcinomas in animal models. The pollutants present in the complex mixtures generally up-regulate the expression of a variety of genes. In addition, some of the environmental pollutants damage the genomic DNA resulting in the mutations, which if not repaired in a timely fashion, could lead to catastrophic consequences. The incidence of colorectal cancer is greatest in industrialized countries where per capita consumption of meats, fats and refined carbohydrates is high.

Colorectal cancer is the second leading cause of global cancer morbidity and mortality, and is a prominent disease of the western world. In the United States alone, the American Cancer Society estimates that 112,340 new cases of colon cancer and 41,420 cases of rectal cancer were diagnosed in 2007 (ACS, 2007b). Colorectal cancer is the third most commonly diagnosed cancer and is the second leading cause of cancer deaths in the United States. Established risk factors for colorectal cancer include being over the age of 50, personal history of colorectal cancer, colorectal polyps, inflammatory bowel disease (ulcerative colitis, Crohn disease), and a family history of colorectal cancer (ACS, 2007c; National Cancer Institute, 2007). Other risk factors of colon cancer development include diet, alcohol consumption, and cigarette smoking. Most human colon cancers are considered sporadic in origin, arising from a combination of genetics, environment and lifestyle.

12.2 Features of Colorectal Carcinogenesis

The history of colorectal cancer is well described but the mechanism of colorectal cancer initiation and progression is not well understood. The first step in the development of tumors from normal epithelium is usually the onset of dysplasia. Single dysplastic crypts (unicryptal adenomas) can be seen and are thought to be the first histological manifestation of tumor development. Recently, it has been proposed that aberrant crypt foci (small areas of epithelium with irregular glandular architecture but no evidence of dysplasia) are precursor lesions which give rise to adenomas (Muto et al., 1975). Adenomas can gradually grow in size and change from a tubular to a villous architecture. The cells show first mild, and then moderate to severe dysplasia followed by malignant changes resulting in local invasion with eventual metastasis to distant sites. The multi-step colon cancer model describes an accumulation of genetic events, each conferring a selective growth advantage to an affected colon cell (Fearnhead et al., 2001). Genes which are mutated at different stages of colorectal cancer development include tumor suppressors, proto-oncogenes, DNA repair genes, growth factors and their receptor genes, cell cycle checkpoint genes, and apoptosis-related genes. These mutations ultimately result in uninhibited cell growth, proliferation, and the clonal development of tumors. The cumulative effect of the somatic mutations in these genes is the cause of sporadic colon cancer. A mathematical extrapolation suggests that most cancers require six to ten such clonal events to fully mature (Fearon and Vogelstein, 1990; Beroud and Soussi, 1996). Mutations of proto-oncogene *K-ras* are also detected in up to 50% of sporadic colorectal cancers and in large polyps. Activation of the *K-ras* gene leads to the constitutive activity of the protein, which results in a continuous growth, inhibition of apoptosis, and or differentiation of cells that can be the basis of carcinogenesis (Forrester et al., 1987). Other oncogenes implicated in sporadic colon cancer include *c-myc* and *c-erbB*2 (Hamilton, 1993; Kapitanovic et al., 1997).

In familial adenomatous polyposis (FAP), a germ-line mutation in the *APC* gene is one of the earliest events. If the germ-line mutation in the *APC* gene occurs between codons 1,194 and 1,392, then there is a strong selection of allelic loss of *APC* for a second-hit resulting in the development of a colorectal adenoma. According to Knudson's (1971) two-hit hypothesis, colorectal tumors from FAP patients harbor additional somatic mutations or loss of heterozygosity at the APC locus in addition to the germ-line mutation (Lamlum et al., 1999). If the germ-line mutation is outside of this region, then there is a second hit in the mutation cluster region (MCR) resulting in tumorigenesis (Rowan et al., 2000). Untill now, most of the biological functions of APC have been implicated in cancer cells, thus, exploring the role of truncated APC in various biochemical pathways. However, the function of the wild-type protein in the cells under normal condition or after challenge with environmental mutagens, such as those present in the cigarette smoke, is not yet fully understood.

Mutations in the anti-apoptotic oncogene, *Bcl*-2 lead to the formation of early adenoma. Unlike other oncogenes, this protein blocks cell death and promotes cell survival (McDonnell et al., 1989). The protein does so by physically interacting with mitochondrial membrane (Hockenbery et al., 1990) and prevents the release of cytochrome c from mitochondria. Hypomethylation of genes also leads to the formation of early adenoma (Counts and Goodman, 1995). The K-*ras* gene is mutated in 30–50% of adenomas and carcinoma (Bos et al., 1987). Activation of the K-*ras* oncogene induces progression from early to intermediate adenoma (Bos, 1988), which were among the first to be linked to the pathogenesis of colon cancer (Vogelstein et al., 1988). The loss of APC function usually proceeds with the activation of the K-*ras* oncogene. It has been also observed that APC and K-*ras* mutations are synergestic in promoting β-catenin nuclear translocation, thus enhancing transcriptional expression of Wnt-signaling target genes (Janssen et al., 2006). Genetic instability is also believed to have a role in the transition from adenoma to carcinoma (Shibata et al., 1994). Deletions or mutations in putative tumor suppressor, *deleted in colon cancer* (*DCC*), have a role in the progression to late adenoma (Hedrick et al. 1994). Studies have shown that loss of *DCC* expression is a hallmark of colorectal tumors and not normal colon tissue (Fearon et al., 1990; Schmitt et al., 1998). The transition from adenoma to carcinoma involves mutations in the tumor suppressor gene, *p*53 (Fearon, 1993) and loss of expression of $p27^{Kip}$. The tumor suppressor *p*53 plays a role in sensing the DNA damage, DNA repair, apoptosis, and transcriptional activation of genes (Lane, 1992). P53 is commonly deleted in colorectal carcinomas (Baker et al., 1989). Mutations are rare in the cyclin-dependent kinase inhibitor gene $p27^{Kip}$ and its role in cell growth has been implicated in colorectal carcinogenesis. Loss of its expression plays a role in the prognosis of colorectal cancer and may confer metastatic potential to tumors (Thomas et al., 1998). Mutations in this multi-step process can occur in a somewhat preferential order. There is evidence, however, that the progression of colorectal carcinogenesis may be a heterogeneous process dependent on the cell's intercellular and environmental factors (Fearon and Vogelstein, 1990; Shibata et al., 1994).

12.3 Genes and Individual Susceptibility to Colorectal Cancer

It is important to note that colorectal cancer susceptibility can vary from individual to individual. Individual genetic variations may influence one's susceptibility to environmental carcinogens by altering rates of activation and detoxification of carcinogens (Gertig and Hunter, 1998). The human body has two major enzyme systems that metabolize carcinogens. Phase-I enzymes interact directly with carcinogens and produce metabolites that are often more reactive than the original exposure. Phase-II enzymes detoxify the active metabolites by breaking down or excretion. The genes encoding these enzymes are polymorphic and have common variant forms. Polymorphisms result from genetic mutations that have been passed through generations Polymorphisms have been studied in several metabolic genes (reviewed by Gertig and Hunter, 1998; Mucci et al., 2001). They include MTHFR,

N-acetyltransferase 1 and 2, glutathoine S-transferases, and the cytochrome P450 enzyme, CYP1A1 (Gertig and Hunter, 1998). Identifying individuals who are at increased risk, due to altered metabolism of potential carcinogens, may result in preventive strategies (Gertig and Hunter, 1998).

12.4 Environmental Factors Affecting DNA Repair and Colorectal Cancer Susceptibility

Inherent DNA repair mechanisms are vital in maintaining genomic integrity and preventing microsatellite and chromosomal instability. Indeed, loss of any one of these repair mechanisms leads to instability of the genome. Specifically, the loss of mismatch repair genes leads to microsatellite instability (MIN) and contributes to the development of colorectal cancer. This was first found as a hereditary condition known as hereditary nonpolyposis colorectal cancer (HNPCC) where mutations found to be in the MSH2, MSH6, MLH1, and PMS2 mismatch repair genes dramatically increased the risk of colorectal cancer development (Schafmayer et al., 2007). Recently, another inherited mutation in a DNA repair gene was found to contribute to colorectal cancer. Germ-line mutations in the MutYH gene have been shown to cause a predisposition to MutYH associated polyposis (MAP) which is characterized by colorectal adenomas and carcinomas. It is an autosomal recessive disorder. MutYH is involved in BER as a DNA glycosylase responsible for the removal of adenines that have been misincorporated as a result of 8-oxo-7,8-dihydro-2-deoxyguanosine. It is the most stable product that results from oxidative damage (Al Tassan et al., 2002; Jones et al., 2002; Sampson et al., 2005). As demonstrated by these inherited syndromes, mutations in DNA repair proteins can have a significant effect on carcinogenesis.

Interestingly, upon analysis of sporadic colorectal tumors it was found that these tumors also possessed mutations in mismatch repair (MMR) genes indicating that mutations in these genes could also arise from gene–environment interactions (Schafmayer et al., 2007). Such findings have prompted studies on the development of sporadic colorectal cancer and the effect of single nucleotide polymorphisms present in DNA repair proteins throughout the population. It is thought that the polymorphisms present in these genes may modulate individual repair capacity in response to DNA damage (Naccarati et al., 2007). Moreover, studies have shown that DNA repair capability declines with age indicating that the elderly population may be more susceptible to environmental mutagen-induced DNA damage and thus cancer development (Perera, 1997). A risk factor for colorectal cancer is being over the age of 50 (American Cancer Society, 2007c). Based on the above information, a relationship between susceptibility to colorectal cancer and aging was established which showed that a decreased DNA repair capacity with age may contribute to the development of colorectal cancer in an aging population.

DNA is constantly bombarded by DNA-damaging agents present in the exogenous and endogenous environment (Nohmi and Masumura, 2005). External exposures arise from sunlight, alkylating agents, dietary constituents, alcohol, tobacco smoke, and other pollutants. Endogenous exposures arise from internal stress such as free radicals produced from oxygen metabolism (Paz-Elizur et al., 2005). Both types of exposures can produce harmful lesions such as oxidation, methylation, adduct formation, strand break, and deamination of DNA (Nohmi and Masumura, 2005). Oxidation results from an interaction of free radicals with nucleotides. This modifies the chemical structure of DNA bases and forms DNA lesions. Methylation results from the addition of methyl groups to certain positions of nucleotides, and deamination of DNA occurs when an amino group of a base spontaneously converts to a keto group. The most common deamination is the generation of uracil by spontaneous deamination of cytosine (Spry et al., 2007). These lesions can interfere with many essential processes in the cell, including transcription. Furthermore, these lesions may trigger cell death or carcinogenesis if the mutations are in critical regions of DNA (Paz-Elizur et al., 2005). Fortunately, these events are usually prevented through DNA repair mechanisms which can remove or bypass the damaged site and restore the original sequence of the DNA to maintain the genomic integrity. The cell possesses five major repair mechanisms to deal with genotoxic insults to DNA. These are direct reversal, mismatch repair (MMR), nucleotide excision repair (NER), base excision repair (BER), homologous recombination (HR) and non-homologous end-joining (NHEJ).

12.5 Dietary Components

Diet is associated with 50–80% of all colorectal cancer cases (Willet, 1995). Many studies have identified nutrients and components in foods that play a role in the development or prevention of colorectal cancer. These studies include animal, epidemiological, case-control and cohort studies (Heavey et al., 2004). Epidemiological studies have consistently shown evidence that meat intake is positively related to the risk of colorectal cancer (Heavey et al., 2004). The most convincing reports are case-control studies (Norat and Riboli, 2001). However, other studies have not always shown consistent results. A review of 32 case-control studies and 13 cohort studies concluded that meat consumption was associated with a modest increase in colorectal cancer risk. Red and processed meats showed more consistency than white meats. Many other studies have found similar results (reviewed by Gertig and Hunter, 1998; Ishibe and Freedman, 2001; Ahmed, 2004; Heavey et al., 2004).

Dietary components contain food mutagens that can cause alterations and damage to DNA. Animal studies have provided conflicting results pertaining to the role of meat consumption on colorectal cancer risk (Parnaud and Corpet, 1997). Beef tallow promotes cancer in Fischer F344 rats (Mori et al., 2001), but not in Sprague-Dawley rats (Lipkin et al., 1999). Azoxymethane (AOM) is a metabolite of 1, 2-dimethylhydrazine (DMH), which is used to induce colorectal cancer in rats. It has been observed that red meat is less protective against AOM-induced aberrant crypt foci (ACF) in Wistar-strain rats than whey protein (Belobrajdic et al., 2003).

It has also been suggested that myoglobin in red meat promotes AOM-induced ACF (Pierre et al., 2003).

A number of mechanisms have been proposed by which meat consumption increases colorectal cancer risk. A primary mechanism is production of carcinogenic N-nitroso compounds (NOC) by bacteria in the gut (Hughes et al., 2001). Meat enhances the excretion of NOC in the feces of mice (Mirvish et al., 2003) and volunteers (Hughes et al., 2001). Smoking, grilling, or frying meat produces heterocyclic amines (HCAs) and polycyclic aromatic hydrocarbons (PAHs) that can be broken into free radicals in the gut (Flammang et al., 1992; Sinha et al., 1995; Wurzelmann et al., 1996; Lund et al., 1999). These agents cause colorectal cancer in mouse and rat models (Ito et al., 1991; Ohgaki et al., 1991). However, according to several studies, HCAs may not be a major determinant of colon cancer in human studies. Chicken is an important source of HCAs, but is not considered a risk factor (Sinha et al., 1995). Additionally, the carcinogenic doses given to rodents are 100–1,000 times higher than the equivalent human exposure (Stavric, 1994). Therefore, the colorectal cancer risk in humans is probably associated with cooking methods (Sugimura, 1997), and is not directly to HCA intake (Sinha, 2002).

Food mutagens can induce DNA damage in the cell. The main types of DNA damage caused by food mutagens include nucleotide alterations and gross chromosomal aberrations (Harris, 1991; Strickland and Groopman, 1995). More importantly, the effects of food mutagens on caretaker genes, including DNA repair genes, can become modified based upon inter-individual variation in the form of single nucleotide polymorphisms (Goldman and Shields, 2003). Thus, some individuals will have reduced repair capacity for certain types of DNA damage. PAHs, N-nitrosamines, and HCAs are among the extensively studied food mutagens.

PAHs are formed as a result of the incomplete combustion of organic matter. Studies of PAHs have been mostly limited to exposure as a result of cigarette smoking. It is estimated that exposure to PAH from cigarette smoking is 2–5 μg per pack per day in a regular smoker. Interestingly, it is also estimated that the human diet supplies approximately 3 μg of PAHs per day (Lioy and Greenberg, 1990; Waldman et al., 1991). However, very few studies have focused on dietary intake of PAHs and cancer risk. The data on charcoal-broiled meat intake results showed that there is a higher association with PAH and DNA adducts in the blood than cigarette smoke (Rothman et al., 1990; 2000). The animal studies have shown that diets with PAHs induce foregut tumors on a consistent basis (Benjamin et al., 1991; Culp et al., 1998; Singh et al., 1998). Additionally, evidence also exists for the association of dietary PAH exposure with colorectal cancer (Probst-Hensch et al., 1997; Giovannucci et al., 1994a; Giovannucci, 2001). DNA adducts caused by PAHs have been shown to be repaired by NER (Siede et al., 2006). Depending on the efficiency of the NER system of the individual, consistent exposure to the potent mutagens and carcinogens may lead to the development of colorectal carcinogenesis.

N-Nitrosamines are primarily found in cured meats and fish products (Goldman and Shields, 2003). N-Nitrosamines can also form in the body during ingestion of nitrite or nitrogen oxides and a secondary amine. They are considered carcinogenic as well as mutagenic. Dietary consumption of N-Nitrosamines has been linked to gastrointestinal cancers. The main N-nitrosamine that is formed as a consequence of dietary exposure is N-nitrosodimethylamine. Upon metabolic activation, it causes formation of O^6-methylguanine (O^6-MeG) adducts. Persistence of these adducts has been associated with the induction of colorectal tumors in rats. Therefore, these adducts are pro-carcinogenic. They are usually repaired by O^6-alkylguanine DNA-alkyltransferase (MGMT). It has been found that MGMT activity varies vastly within the colon tumors tend to form in regions of low MGMT activity. Additionally, low MGMT activity in normal mucosa has been associated with the occurrence of GC→AT transition mutations in K-*ras*. This information supports the notion that GC→AT transition mutations in the K-*ras* oncogene can be a result of the persistence of O^6-MeG lesions in the areas of the colon with lower MGMT levels. This also indicates that individual variability of MGMT activity may play a role in the susceptibility of the colon to exposure from endogenous and exogenous alkylating agents (Povey et al., 2002).

Heterocyclic amines are also formed during high temperature cooking of meats such as broiling. Heterocyclic amines result from pyrolysis of proteins, amino acids, or creatine and have been found to be carcinogens and mutagens in animal studies. It is speculated that the formation of the nitrenium ion is the likely culprit which binds to DNA bases (Goldman and Shields, 2003). A model has been proposed relating a heterocyclic amine, 2-amino-1-methyl-6-phenylimidazo[4,5-b]pyrimidine (PhIP), DNA repair, and chromosomal instability. In this model, HCT-116 colon cancer cells were treated with cytotoxic levels of PhIP, which is known to form bulky DNA-adducts formation. Clones that survived this treatment were resistant to the mutagens and were analyzed for chromosomal aberrations. Surprisingly, a striking level of chromosomal instability (CIN) was found in every clone.

12.6 Alcohol

An association between high alcohol consumption and elevated colorectal cancer risk has been demonstrated in many prospective and case-control epidemiological studies (reviewed by Giovannucci, 2003). The relationship of alcohol consumption to colorectal cancer risk remains controversial. However, most studies indicate that alcohol consumption increases the risk of colorectal cancer (Kune and Viterra, 1992). Additionally epidemiological studies have shown a positive association of alcohol consumption and colorectal cancer risk (Gertig and Hunter, 1998).

The mechanism of how alcohol contributes to colorectal cancer risk has yet to be elucidated. Contrary to other dietary factors, alcohol consumption has been shown to contribute to microsatellite instability (MIN) (Slattery et al., 2001). Alcohol has also been shown to inhibit DNA repair. Additionally, acetaldehyde, which is a metabolite of alcohol and cause hangovers, forms DNA adducts (Heavey et al. 2004). It is hypothesized that alcohol may influence histological changes and proliferation of mucosal cells (Kune and Viterra, 1992). Excessive alcohol consumption is commonly associated with a diet deficient in other nutrients that are thought to have a protective effect against colorectal cancer (Heavey et al. 2004). One such nutrient is folate. Consistently higher risk of colorectal adenoma and cancer are observed among frequent alcohol drinkers (Nigro et al., 1979). This may be related to alcohol's antagonistic effect on folate metabolism (Hardman and Cameron, 1995). The relationship between alcohol intake and the folate metabolizing enzyme, methylenetetrahydrofolate reductase (MTHFR) (Burkitt, 1969; Trock et al., 1990; Jacobs et al., 2001; Mason and Choi, 2005) supports the hypothesis that the consequence of alcohol consumption on colorectal cancer risk may be through its influence on folate metabolism (Heavey et al. 2004).

12.7 Cigarette Smoking

Many epidemiological studies suggested an association of cigarette smoking and colorectal cancer risk (IARC, 2004; Giovannucci, 1994a, b). However, other studies were unable to find any association with the cigarette smoking and colorectal cancer risk (Hammond and Horn, 1958; Hammond, 1966; Kahn, 1966; Weir and Dunn, 1970; Doll and Peto, 1976; Doll et al., 1980; Rogot and Murray, 1980). One possible explanation for this discrepancy is that carcinogens in cigarette smoke causes genetic damage in normal colorectal mucosa, but many years are required for carcinogenic events to initiate carcinogenesis (Giovannucci et al., 1994a, b). Early studies may not have considered a sufficient time lag between smoking exposure and risk development. In some cases decades may be needed to fully complete the carcinogenesis pathway (Giovannucci and Martinez, 1996). Even though smoking increases the risk of developing adenomatous polyps, the link between smoking and colorectal cancer is still not clear. Giovannucci extensively reviewed the epidemiology studies conducted until March 2001 (Giovannucci, 2001). He concluded that 21 of 22 studies found that long-term, heavy cigarette smokers have a twofold to threefold increased risk of colorectal cancer. The risk of large precursor adenomas were elevated in smokers in 12 out of 12 studies (Giovannucci, 2001). The combined findings of various studies from the United States and other countries strongly suggest that cigarette smoking is a risk factor for colorectal cancer, especially for those with long smoking histories. Cigarette smoke contains many of the food mutagens mentioned above. Specifically, it contains PAHs, N-nitrosamines, and HCAs (Hoffmann et al., 2001; Nishikawa et al., 2004). The effects of these carcinogens on DNA are similar to other carcinogens in food.

Environmental pollutants and components of cigarette smoke may contribute to oxidative damage of the DNA. Metabolism of some of these carcinogens and/or mutagens may lead to oxidation adducts with DNA and the generation of free radicals. Oxidative damage to DNA has been shown to commonly form 8-oxo-deoxyguanosine (8-oxodG) lesions on DNA. This lesion is known to lead G→T and A→C transversions (Sanders et al., 2004; Hwang and Bowen, 2007), which are repaired through the BER pathway with the damage specific 8-oxodG-DNA glycosylase. Intriguingly, a study on the environment of the colon has shown that the colon environment contains higher basal levels of reactive oxygen species and oxidative damage compared to the small intestine. The study also found that the colon contained higher levels of antioxidant enzymes to compensate for this. It was proposed that the colon is more prone to tumor formation than the small intestine as a result of these increased levels of reactive oxygen species. Therefore, it is concluded that the environment of the colon is pro-oxidant. Furthermore, the study maintained that the DNA repair enzymes involved in the repair of oxidative damage may only be able to make a small contribution, since the amount of DNA damage seen in the colon is thought to exceed the capacity of these enzymes. Once again, individual variability of these repair enzymes may help predispose the colon to mutations resulting from oxidative damage. Additionally, the pro-oxidant environment of the colon may also play a role in the initiation of colorectal carcinogenesis (Sanders et al., 2004).

12.8 Adenomatous Polyposis Coli (APC) in Base Excision Repair and Colorectal Carcinogenesis

Structure and function of APC protein: The gene encoding human APC is localized on chromosome 5q21-q22 and consists of 16 transcribed exons present on a 98-kb genomic fragment (Bodmer et al., 1987; Nishisho et al., 1991; Kinzler et al., 1991; Groden et al., 1991). The size of exons 1–14 range from 85 to 398-bp, while the last exon, exon 15, is remarkably long (6574-bp). Exon 15 comprises more than 75% of the coding sequence of *APC* and is the target for both germ-line and somatic mutations (Groden et al., 1991). With an 8538-nucleotide mRNA, *APC* encodes for a predicted 312-kDa protein consisting of 2,843-amino acids. APC is constitutively expressed within the normal colonic epithelium. It is localized in both the cytoplasm and the nucleus. Due to alternative splicing, post-translational modification and degradation, many forms of APC exists (Horii et al., 1993). The function of these variants is still unknown. The vast majority of germ-line mutations of *APC* are nonsense or frame-shift mutations that result in truncated protein product with abnormal functions. Inactivation of APC function seems to be responsible for both tumor initiation and promotion in the large bowel (Bodmer et al., 1987; Nishisho et al., 1991; Kinzler et al., 1991). About 60% of the *APC* mutations in colorectal tumors are clustered in the central mutation cluster region (MCR, amino acids 1284–1580; Fig. 12.1) (Miyoshi et al., 1992). Colorectal tumors from FAP proteins carry additional somatic mutations or loss of heterozygosity (LOH) in the *APC* gene locus in addition to the original mutation (Nakamura, 1993) (Table 12.1).

Somatic mutations are found in the majority of colorectal adenomas and carcinomas, including adenomas less than 5 mm in size (Powell et al., 1992; Homfray et al., 1998). Somatic mutations result in the loss of both wild-type alleles of the *APC* gene in the majority of sporadic colorectal cancers (Hamada and Bienz, 2002). Most somatic mutations clustered between codons 1,286 and 1,513 are located in the central MCR region of the *APC* gene, in which mutations at codons 1,309 and 1,450 are

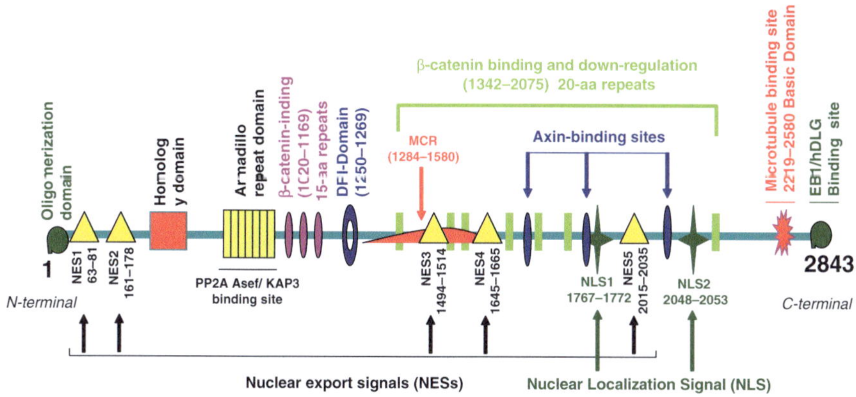

Fig. 12.1 Schematic representation of the Adenomatous polyposis coli protein (APC). APC protein composed of 2843-amino acid displays various regions localized between N-terminal and C-terminal regions. An oligomerization and EB1-binding domains are located near the N-terminus and C-terminus of the protein, respectively. There are two β-catenin-binding domains located at residues 1020–1169 and 1342–2075. The first 15-amino acids repeat located at residues 1,020–1,169 can bind β-catenin, but its functional significance is still obscure, while the 20-amino acids repeat located at residues 1,342–2,075 can bind β-catenin with very high affinity upon phosphorylation. The DRI-domain is upstream of the MCR (located at amino acid 1284–1580) which is involved in the regulation of BER pathway. Most of the mutations in APC occur in the MCR region. As a result of mutation in the MCR, the truncated APC protein is expressed. APC protein also has five NES and two NLS motifs, which could be playing roles in its nuclear export and import, respectively. Asef, APC-stimulated guanine nucleotide exchange factor; DRI, DNA repair inhibitory domain; DLG, Drosophila discs large; EB1, end-binding protein 1, KAP3A, kinesin super-family-associated protein 3A; MCR, mutator cluster region; NES, nuclear export signal; NLS, nuclear localization signal; PP2-B56alpha, protein phosphates 2A B56α subunit

the hot spot mutations. Mutations in *APC* within the MCR region result in truncated APC proteins that lack most of the axin-binding sites. The sequences upstream of the MCR might encode APC protein whose function is essential for cellular survival or tumor progression, while sequences downstream of the MCR might encode APC protein for tumor suppressor function of the *APC* gene (Nakamura, 1993; Fearnhead et al., 2001; Narayan and Roy, 2003). DNA repair inhibitory (DRI)-domain (amino acids 1250–1269) of APC, located upstream of the MCR, is responsible for its interaction with DNA repair proteins DNA-polymerase β (Pol-β) and flap endonuclease 1 (Fen-1) and influence their activity (Narayan et al., 2005; Jaiswal et al., 2006; Balusu et al., 2007).

The APC contains three 15-amino acid and seven 20-amino acid repeats in the central third region of the protein. The residues of the 20-amino acid repeats are highly conserved between the repeats. The Arm-repeats are localized between amino acids 453 and 766 and consist of seven copies of the 42-amino acid motif (Peifer et al., 1994; Hatzfeld, 1999). Varying numbers of Arm repeats have been identified in a variety of proteins with disparate activities including nuclear transport, cell adhesion, cell cycle control, and microtubule stability (Hatzfeld, 1999).

Table 12.1 Genetic mutations and colorectal cancer. This table provides the list of various genes, their chromosomal localization and mutational consequence on the colorectal carcinogenesis. These mutations have been observed in tumor suppressor gene, mismatch repair gene and oncogenes. Mutations in these genes will result in the impairment of normal function and leading to colorectal carcinogenesis

Gene	Locus	Type of mutation	Protein Size	Consequence
Tumor Suppressor Genes				
APC	5q21	Germ line mutation	2843 amino acids	Familial adenomatous polyposis
		Somatic mutation	2843 amino acids	Sporadic colon cancer
p53	17p12	Germ line mutation	393 amino acids	Metastasis
DCC	18q21	Germ line mutation	1447 amino acids	Sporadic colon cancer
MCC	5p	Germ line mutation	829 amino acids	Sporadic colon cancer
SMAD2/ SMAD4	18q21	Germ line mutation	467/552 amino acids	Juvenile polyposis
STK15	20q13	Germ line mutation	403 amino acids	Peutz-Jeghers syndrome
Mismatch repair genes				
hMSH2	2p21	Germ line mutation	1037 amino acids	Hereditary nonpolyposis colon cancer
hMLH1	3p21	Germ line mutation	756 amino acids	Hereditary nonpolyposis colon cancer
hPMS1	2q	Germ line mutation	932 amino acids	Hamartmatous polyposis syndrome
hPMS2	7p22	Germ line mutation	862 amino acids	Hereditary nonpolyposis colon cancer
hMSH3	5q11	Somatic mutation	1137 amino acids	Peutz-Jeghers syndrome
hMSH6	2p16	Germ line mutation	1292 amino acids	Hereditary nonpolyposis colon cancer
Oncogenes				
ras	12p12	Germ line mutation	189 amino acids	Sporadic colorectal cancer
src	20q12/13	Germ line mutation	533 amino acids	Malignant progression to colon cancer and metastasis to liver
c-Myc	8q24	Germ line mutation	439 amino acids	Familial adenomatous polyposis
c-erb2a	17q12	Somatic mutation	1255 amino acids	Sporadic colorectal cancer
c-erb2b	17q12	Somatic mutation	1225 amino acids	Sporadic colorectal cancer

This domain has been designated as a protein-protein interaction domain (Fig. 12.1). There are few proteins identified which bind to APC's Arm repeat region. These are B56 regulatory subunit of the protein phosphatase 2A (PP2A), APC-stimulated Rac-specific guanine nucleotide exchange factor (Asef), and kinesin superfamily-associated protein 3A (KAP3A) (Rubinfeld et al., 1993; Hsu et al., 1999; Jimbo et al., 2002; Jaiswal et al., 2005). PP2A is one of the four major serine/threonine protein phosphatases whose regulatory domain interact with the Arm repeats of

APC, while the catalytic subunit of this enzyme can also bind to Axin (Hsu et al., 1999). The co-localization and functional studies suggest that the APC-Asef complex may regulate the actin/cytoskeletal network, cell morphology, cell migration, and neuronal function.

Both three 15-amino acid repeats and seven 20-amino acid repeats of APC are involved in the binding of β-catenin (Rubinfeld et al., 1993; Su et al., 1993; Rubinfeld et al., 1996); however, the binding of free cytoplasmic β-catenin to the 20-amino acid repeat (consensus TPxxxFSxxxSxSxL) is modulated by phosphorylation through the serine-threonine kinase glycogen synthase kinase-3β (GSK3β) (Rubinfeld et al., 1996). Axin and conductin were originally identified as inhibitors of the Wnt-signaling pathway (Zeng et al., 1997). They form a tetrameric destruction complex together with APC, β-catenin, and GSK3β. This complex promotes the phosphorylation of β-catenin and subsequently mediates its ubiquitination and degradation in the proteasome (Orford et al., 1997; Aberle et al., 1997; Ben-Ze'ev and Geiger, 1998), thereby controlling the Wnt-signaling pathway (Polakis, 1997). The C-terminal region of APC is known as the basic domain region. It contains many arginine, lysine, and proline residues localized between amino acids 2,200 and 2,400. The basic domain of APC contains microtubule binding site (Smith et al. 1994). The C-terminal region of APC may play a role in cell cycle progression or growth control through binding to at least three different proteins, namely EB1 (end-binding protein 1), hDLG (human homologue of Drosophila disc large tumor suppressor gene), and protein tyrosine phosphatase (PTP)-BL (Polakis, 1997; Erdmann et al., 2000; Su et al., 1995; Matsumine et al., 1996). Although little is known about the function of the APC-EB1 complex in mammalian cells, most of the studies have been carried out in Drosophila and yeast to understand the functional role of the APC-EB1 complex. The yeast homologue of EB1, Bim1p, binds α-tubulin and localizes to the mitotic spindle and to cytoplasmic microtubules (Schwartz et al., 1997; Korinek et al., 2000). The association of EB1 with microtubule cytoskeleton of the mitotic spindle is important for spindle assembly throughout the cell cycle. APC's C-terminal amino acids bind through its S/TxV sequence to the PDZ domain of hDLG (Matsumine et al., 1996) and PTP-BL (Polakis, 1997). The hDLG is a member of the family of membrane-associated guanylate kinases, which localize at the sites of the cell-cell contacts of epithelial cells and in the presynaptic nerve termini of the central nervous system. These proteins are involved in the maintenance of cell polarity, migration, and blocking of cell proliferation.

Nuclear localization of APC has been reported in a few cell types (Neufeld et al., 2000). Since APC is too large a protein to diffuse passively into the nucleus, it is possible that APC is shuttled by an unconventional mechanism or else it is also possible that protein configuration tightly regulates its export and import into the nucleus. From the structural analysis of APC, it is apparent that it contains two potential nuclear localization signals (NLSs) comprising amino acids 1,767–1,772 and 2,048–2,053 (Zhang et al., 2000). Both APC NLSs, which are well conserved among human, rat, mouse, and fly, are necessary for the optimal nuclear import of APC. It has been demonstrated that phosphorylation of the NLS may inhibit nuclear import of wild type APC. This provides a regulatory mechanism for nuclear-cytoplasmic shuttling. Recently, several groups identified the presence of nuclear export signals (NES) at the N-terminus of the APC protein. There are at least five nuclear export signals, of which three NESs are located towards the N-terminal amino acids 63–81, 161–178 and 1,494–1,514 and two towards the C-terminal amino acids 1,645–1,665 and 2,015–2,035 (Henderson, 2000; Henderson and Fagotto, 2002). These NESs are located within the 20-amino acid repeats of β-catenin binding domain of APC (Zhang et al., 2000; Henderson, 2000). Only the first two nuclear export signals are functionally active. The highly conserved NES sequences are used to shuttle nuclear β-catenin to the cytoplasmic destruction complex. The absence of the NES sequences lead to the accumulation of β-catenin in the nucleus, which cause an inadvertent activation of Wnt target genes that may possibly be involved in tumor development. The emerging evidence suggest that endogenous APC and β-catenin can interact within the nucleus, and thus APC may export β-catenin from nucleus to cytoplasm (Henderson, 2000; Neufeld et al., 2000) and terminate Wnt-signaling which may block the expression of cell cycle-related genes. β-catenin can exit in the nucleus independent of the chromosome region maintenance 1 (CRM1) mediated mechanism. Although the exact function of nuclear APC is unknown, we recently found that nuclear APC participates in DNA repair pathways (Fig. 12.2) (Narayan et al., 2005; Jaiswal et al., 2006; Balusu et al., 2007).

APC gene expression by mutagens: It has been found that *APC* mRNA and protein levels are up-regulated in response to DNA damage. This was first discovered in a study by Narayan and Jaiswal (1997), in which the colon cancer cell line HCT-116, was treated with several DNA-damaging agents including dimethylhydrazine (DMH), N-methyl-N'-nitro-N-nitrosoguanidine (MNNG), and UV light. An increase in *APC* mRNA expression was seen after treatment with these agents. Furthermore, it was shown that the increased nuclear transcription of the *APC* gene in response to DNA-damaging agents required an increased level of p53. This finding indicated a direct link between APC and p53 in response to alkylation-induced DNA damage and suggested a novel role for p53 in a stress response pathway involving APC (Narayan and Jaiswal, 1997; Jaiswal and Narayan, 2001b). The *APC* gene can also be transcriptionally regulated by upstream stimulating factors 1 and 2 (USF-1 and USF-2) (Jaiswal and Narayan, 2001a). Cigarette smoke condensate (CSC), B[*a*]P, and dimethylbenzanthracine (DMBA) are also known to induce transcriptional activity of the *APC* gene (Jaiswal et al., 2006; Kundu et al. 2007b).

Role of APC in base excision repair: The increase in *APC* gene expression upon exposure of colon cells to DNA damaging agents suggested the possibility of an interaction between APC and DNA repair machinery. Based on these findings, the role of APC was later identified in base excision repair (BER). It has been demonstrated that APC interacts with Pol-β and Fen-1 and blocks both single-nucleotide (SN)- and long-patch (LP)-BER pathways (Narayan et al., 2005; Jaiswal et al., 2006). It is widely accepted that APC acts as a tumor suppressor. Generally, after DNA damage occurs, tumor suppressor genes stimulate DNA repair machinery to protect the integrity of the genome. In contrast, APC has been shown to block

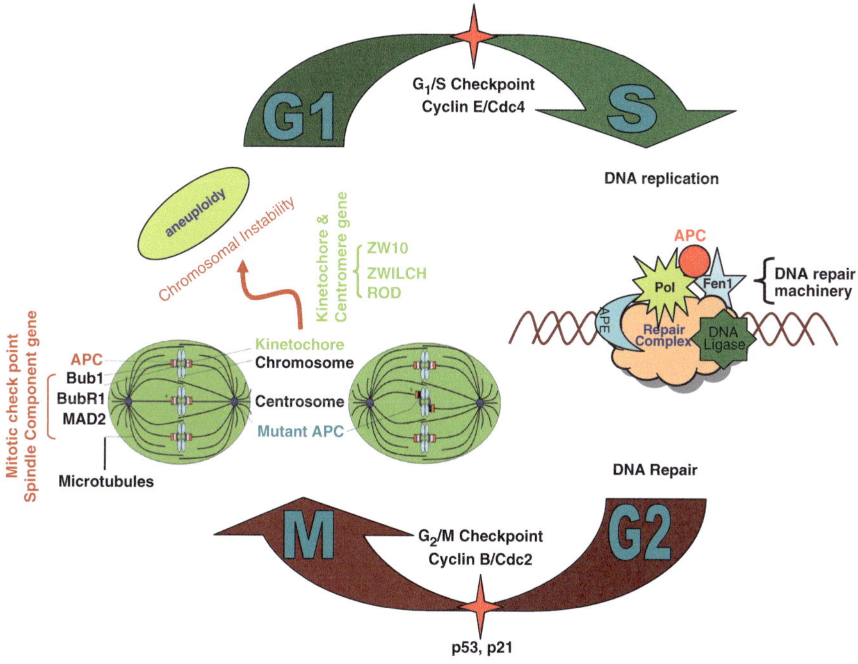

Fig. 12.2 Involvement of APC in various biological functions. APC is the key molecule regulating various physiological functions either directly or through its interaction with other partners such as β-catenin. The role of APC has been implicated in a broad spectrum of functions ranging from cell adhesion, cell migration, regulation of Wnt/β-catenin signaling pathway (transcriptional regulation of target genes), cell cycle control, apoptosis, inappropriate chromosomal segregation at mitosis results in chromosomal instability and recently suspected role in BER pathway

BER. This role could conceivably serve as a tumor suppressor function if, due to the accumulation of DNA damage, it causes the cell to undergo apoptosis. Indeed, studies involving human colon cancer cells and mouse embryonic fibroblast cells treated with methyl methanesulfonate (MMS) have shown that the levels of *APC* are enhanced and the blockage of BER resulted in increased sensitivity to MMS and increased apoptosis of cells harboring damaged DNA (Narayan et al., 2005; Kundu et al., 2007a). Furthermore, an MMS toxicity assay was conducted using colon cancer cells with wild-type levels of APC or colon cancer cells with knocked-down APC with pSiRNA-APC (Narayan et al., 2005). Results showed that cells with wild-type APC levels showed reduced colony formation when compared to cells with knocked-down APC levels (Balusu et al., 2007). These results suggest that increased levels of APC after treatment with MMS block BER and decrease cell growth. On the other hand, it has also been shown that CSC treatment induces APC levels in spontaneously immortalized normal breast epithelial cells, blocks BER, and causes transformation of these cells (Fig. 12.2). This indicates a possible role of APC in carcinogenesis (Kundu et al., 2007b). A larger understanding of the mechanisms that determine the carcinogenic and cytotoxic effects of the APC block on BER in normal cells and tumor cells is necessary in order to develop successful therapeutic strategies based on inhibitors of this interaction. At present, the role of APC is determined only in the BER pathway. Its involvement in damages induced by environmental mutagens which are repaired by other DNA repair pathways such as MMR, NER, HR and NHEJ, has not been shown yet.

12.9 Polymorphism in *APC* Gene and Risk of Colorectal Cancer

Many studies have focused on the relationship between the genetic polymorphisms and risk of colorectal cancer. The overall results of these studies are inconclusive. In last several years correlation between site of mutation in the *APC* gene and clinical phenotype has been observed. There is evidence for a genotype-phenotype correlation with respect to colorectal manifestations. Polymorphism in *APC* gene has been studied in detail. These studies indicate that a mutation in hotspot or mutation cluster region (MCR) is linked with the development of colorectal carcinogenesis. There is consistent correlation between site of mutation in the *APC* gene and clinical phenotype (De la Fuente et al., 2007; Toyooka et al., 1995; Locker and Lynch, 2004; Locker et al., 2006; Friedl and Aretz, 2005). Recently the biological significance of nonsense and frame shift mutations in hot spot or mutation cluster region has been correlated with truncated and nonfunctional APC protein. The significance of missense mutations in APC is still unknown. Allelic loss of *APC* results in loss of APC function. However, in colon cancer where *APC* is mutated shows allelic loss plus truncating mutation in the mutation cluster region. The truncating mutation at nucleotide 3,920 was identified by in vitro synthesized protein method and showed substitution of isoleucine to lysine at codon 1,307(I1307K) (Table 12.2). This germ-line mutation causes a structural abnormality which impairs its biological activity. It was further studied by Laken et al. (1997), and found that these mutations are associated with the development or progression of colorectal cancer. Laken et al. (1997) examined 211 colon cancer affected Ashkenazim Jews and found that 10.4% of the patients harbored this mutation. The study concluded that I1307K predisposes population to colorectal cancer. There is an increased risk for colorectal cancer (OR = 1.24). However, it appears that I1307K mutation is exclusively prominent in Ashkenazi Jews. Other non-Jewish populations do not have this association. Frayling et al. (1998), found that G to A (E1317Q) mutation did not predispose to colorectal cancer. This mutation suppresses the APC/β-catenin pathway thereby predisposing to the development of adenomas. This study showed that a mutation at codon 1307 is critical for the development colon cancer (Liberman et al., 2007). Another study by Friedl and Aretz (2005) found that the most abundant 5 base pair deletion at nucleotides 3,927–3,931 at codon 1309 was critical for the development of colon cancer and was detected in almost 4.8% of the populations tested (Table 12.2). These studies clearly demonstrated that certain mutations occurring in the mutation cluster region increased the risk for colon cancer. Further investigation

Table 12.2 Genetic polymorphism in *APC* gene. This table represents polymorphism in *APC* gene. These mutations spans from exon 5 to exon 16. The most common transversion C→T has been observed and results in nonsense mutation at Arg residue leading to truncated protein with impaired biological activity. The most prevalent mutations are deletion mutation in the mutation cluster region (MCR) or hot spot at codon 1061 and 1309

Variant	Codon	Genotype	Exon	Mutation	Clinical significance
637C>637T	213	C→T	5	Nonsense	Attenuated familial adenomatous polyposis
646C>646T	216	C→T	6	Nonsense	Attenuated familial adenomatous polyposis
694C>694T	232	C→T	6	Nonsense	Familial adenomatous polyposis
790C>790T	264	C→T	7	Nonsense	Familial adenomatous polyposis
1450C>1450T	483	C→T	11	Nonsense (Somatic)	Severe Adenoma
1458T>1458C	486	T→C	11	Nonsense	Predicted role in development of colorectal cancer
1495C>1495T	499	C→T	11	Nonsense	
1539C>1539G	513	C→G	16	Nonsense (Somatic)	Moderate Adenoma
1564T>1564G	521	T→G	16	Nonsense (Somatic)	Moderate Adenoma
1660C>1660T	554	C→T	16	Nonsense	Familial adenomatous polyposis
3183–3187	1061	del ACAAA	15E	Deletion	Typical familial adenomatous polyposis
3202–3205	1068	del TCAA	15E	Deletion	Typical familial adenomatous polyposis
3498T>3498G	1166	T→G	15F	Germline	Unknown malignant potential
3507A>3507T	1169	A→T	15F	Missense	No significant contribution for colorectal cancer development
3920T>3920A	1307	T→A	15G	Missense (Germline)	Significant contribution for colorectal cancer development
3927–3931	1309	del AAAGA	15G	Deletion mutation	Severe familial adenomatous polyposis
4479G>4479A	1493	G→A	15	Silent mutation	Predicted role in development of colorectal cancer
5268T>5268G	1756	T→G	15	Silent mutation	Predicted role in development of colorectal cancer

Table 12.2 (continued)

Variant	Codon	Genotype	Exon	Mutation	Clinical significance
5465A>5465T	1822	A→G	15	Substitution mutation	No predicted role in development of colorectal cancer
Asn1026Ser	1026	A→G	15	Missense	Unknown malignant potential
Val1125Ala	1125	Val→Ala	16	Missense substitution	No significant contribution for colorectal cancer development
Ser1126Arg	1126	Ser→Arg	16	Missense substitution	No significant contribution for colorectal cancer development
Ile1307Lys	1307	Ile→Lys	16	(Germline) Missense	Significant contribution for colorectal cancer development
Glu1317Gln	1317	Glu→Gln	16	(Germline)	controversial role for contribution to colorectal cancer
Ile1458Thr	1458	Ile→Thr	15	Substitution	No significant contribution for colorectal cancer development
Asp1822Val	1822	Asp→Val	15	Substitution	No significant contribution for colorectal cancer development
Gly2502Ser	2502	Gly→Ser	15B	Missense	No significant contribution for colorectal cancer development

revealed new mutations in *APC* gene which were identified in a small study of 30 Chilean patients. Mutations present in exon 15 between codon 1310–2011 have been associated with an increased risk of desmoid tumors. Various mutations found in the *APC* gene are compiled in Table 12.2. Understanding the role of genetic polymorphisms and host susceptibility would provide a better understanding and prospective for screening and management of the disease.

12.10 Conclusion

Although some animal and epidemiological studies show inconsistent results, it is generally understood that high consumption of red meats, alcohol, and heavy smoking contribute to colorectal carcinogenesis. Fruits, vegetables, and macronutrients offer a protective role against colorectal cancer and nutrients such as calcium, vitamin D, and folate also have roles in colorectal cancer prevention. The World Cancer Research Fund reported that diets high in vegetables decrease the risk of colorectal cancer. Diets high in fiber probably reduce risk, but diets high in meat and alcohol probably increase risk to colorectal cancer (World Cancer Research Fund, 1997). The report by the U.S. National Academy of Science on "Diet and Health" implicated that meat, fat, and other energy-producing macronutrients play a role in colorectal carcinogenesis (U.S. National Academy of Sciences, 1989). Studies indicate that diets high in calcium, fruits, and vegetables may curb the carcinogenic effects of high saturated fat and red meat consumption (Bieskalski, 2002; Pierre et al., 2003). The recommended diet consists of reduced intake of fat, broiled foods, and energy-rich foods, while increasing fiber, vegetables, fruits, and minimally processed starchy preparations. This highlights the importance of a balanced diet in the prevention of colorectal cancers.

Gertig and Hunter offered a model of gene–environment interactions in colorectal cancer (Gertig and Hunter, 1998). Ishibe and Freedman, (2001) have also contributed to this model of possible links between environmental, susceptibility factors, and somatic alterations in colorectal carcinogenesis. Tobacco smoke acts on the transition between normal and proliferative epithelium. Alcohol consumption, folate deficiency, and less fiber intake can affect the transition of proliferative epithelium to early adenoma. Consumption of red meat and deficiency of folate and calcium are important for the transition from early to intermediate adenoma. Finally, vegetables and fiber play protective roles in the last transition from late adenoma to carcinoma (Gertig and Hunter, 1998; Ishibe and Freedman, 2001). Emerging evidence also suggests the roles for APC in various biological processes such as blockage of DNA repair, chromosomal instability, cell migration and adhesion (a key step in polyp formation) and apoptosis, which needs to be reconciled in terms of colorectal carcinogenesis. The role of APC in DNA repair is a new finding, which needs further evaluation. Whether all the above functions or one of them of APC are necessary to cause colon cancer development needs to be established, so that a potential target for the intervention of this deadly disease can be sought.

Acknowledgments The work from our laboratory cited in this review was financially supported to Satya Narayan by NIH-grants (R01-CA097031 and R01-CA100247) and Flight Attendant Medical Research Institute, Miami, FL. We thank to Mary Wall for proofreading of the manuscript.

References

Aberle, H., Bauer, A., Stappert, J., Kispert, A., and Kemler, R. 1997. β-Catenin is a target for the ubiquitin-proteasome pathway. EMBO J. 16: 3797–3804.

Ahmed, F. E. 2004. Effects of life style, and other environmental/chemopreventative factors on colorectal cancer development and assessment of the risks. J. Environ. Sci. Health C 22: 91–147.

Alexandrov, K., Rojas, M., Kadlubaer, F. F., Lang, N. P., and Bartsch, H. 1996. Evidence of *anti*-benzo[*a*]pyrene diolepoxide-DNA adduct formation in human colon mucosa. Carcinogenesis 17: 2081–2083.

Al Tassan, N., Chmiel, N. H., Maynard, J., Fleming, N., Livingston, A. L., Williams, G. T., Hodges, A. K., Davies, D. R., David, S. S., Sampson, J. R., and Cheadle, J. P. 2002. Inherited variation of Mut Y associated with somatic G:C->T:A mutations in colorectal tumors. Nat. Genet. 30: 227–232.

American Cancer Society. 2007a. Cigarette smoking. prevention & early detection. http://www.cancer.org/docroot/PED/content/

American Cancer Society. 2007b. What are the key statistics for colorectal cancer? http://www.cancer.org/docroot/CRI/content/

American Cancer Society. 2007c. What are the risk factors for colorectal cancer? http://www.cancer.org/docroot/CRI/content/

Baker, S. J., Fearon, E. R., Nigro, J. M., Hamilton, S. R., Preisinger, A. C., Jessup, J. M., van Tuinen, P., Ledbetter, D. H., Barker, D. F., Nakamura, Y., White, R., and Vogelstein, B. 1989. Chromosome 17 deletions and p53 gene mutations in colorectal carcinomas. Science 244: 217–221.

Balusu, R., Jaiswal, A. S., Armas, M. L., Kundu, C. N., Bloom, L. B., and Narayan, S. Structure/function Analysis of the Interaction of Adenomatous Polyposis Coli (APC) with DNA Polymerase β and its Implications for Base Excision Repair. Biochemistry 2007 Nov 14; 2007 Nov 14; [Epub ahead of print] PMID: 17999539.

Belobrajdic, D. P., McIntosh, G. H., and Owens, J. A. 2003. Whey proteins protect more than red meat against azoxymethane-induced ACF in Wistar rats. Cancer Lett. 198: 45–51.

Benjamin, H., Storkson, J., Nagahara, A., and Pariza, M. W. 1991. Inhibition of benzo(a)pyrene-induced mouse forestomach neoplasia by dietary soy sauce. Cancer Res. 51: 2940–2942.

Ben-Ze'ev, A., and Geiger, B. 1998. Differential molecular interactions of beta-catenin and plakoglobin in adhesion, signaling and cancer. Curr. Opin. Cell Biol. 10: 629–639.

Beroud, C., and Soussi, T. 1996. APC gene: database of germline and somatic mutations in human tumors and cell lines. Nucleic Acids Res. 24: 121–124.

Bieskalski, H. K. 2002. Meat and cancer: meat as a component of a healthy diet. Eur. J. Clin. Nutr. 56(suppl): S2–S11.

Bodmer, W. F., Bailey, C. J., Bodmer, J., Bussey, H. J., Ellis, A., Gorman, P., Lucibello, F. C., Murday, V. A., Rider, S. H., Scambler, P., Sheer, D., Solomon, E., and Spurr, N. K. 1987. Localization of the gene for familial adenomatous polyposis on chromosome 5. Nature 328: 614–616.

Bos, J. L. 1988. The *ras* gene family and human carcinogenesis. Mutat. Res. 195: 255–271.

Bos, J. L., Fearon, E. R., Hamilton, S. R., Verlaan-de Vries, M., van Boom, J. H., van der Eb, A. J., and Vogelstein, B. 1987. Prevalence of *ras* mutations in human colorectal cancers. Nature 327: 293–297.

Burkitt, D. P. 1969. Related disease, related cause? Lancet 2: 1229–1231.

Counts, J., and Goodman, J. 1995. Alternation in DNA methylation may play a variety of roles in carcinogenesis. Cell 83: 13–15.

Culp, S. J., Gaylor, D. W., Sheldon, W. G., Goldstein, L. S., and Beland, F. A. 1998. A comparison of the tumors induced by coal tar and benzo[*a*]pyrene in 2 year bioassay. Carcinogenesis 19: 117–124.

De la Fuente, M. K., Alvarez, K. P., Letelier, A. J., Bellolio, F., Acuña, M. L., León, F. S., Pinto, E., Carvallo, P., and López-Köstner, F. 2007. Mutational screening of the APC gene in Chilean families with familial adenomatous polyposis: nine novel truncating mutations. Dis. Colon Rectum. 50: 2142–2148.

Doll, R., Gray, R., Hafner, B., and Peto, R. 1980. Mortality in relation to smoking: 22 years' observations on female British doctors. Br. Med. J. 280: 967–971.

Doll, R., and Peto, R. 1976. Mortality in relation to smoking: 20 years'observations on male British doctors. Br. Med. J. 2: 1525–1536.

Erdmann, K. S., Kuhlmann, J., Lessmann, V., Herrmann, L., Eulenburg, V., Muller, O., and Heumann, R. 2000. The Adenomatous polyposis coli-protein (APC) interacts with the protein tyrosine phosphatase PTP-BL via an alternatively spliced PDZ domain. Oncogene 19: 3894–3901.

Fearnhead, N. S., Britton, M. P., and Bodmer, W. F. 2001. The ABC of APC. Hum. Mol. Genet. 10: 721–733.
Fearon, E. R. 1993. Molecular genetics studies of the adenoma-carcinoma sequence. Adv. Intern. Med. 39: 123–147.
Fearon, E. R., Cho, K. R., Nigro, J. M., Kern, S. E., Simons, J. W., Ruppert, J. M., Hamilton, S. R., Preisinger, A. C., Thomas, G., Kinzler, K. W., and Vogelstein, B. 1990. Identification of a chromosome 18q gene that is altered in colorectal cancer. Science 247: 49–56.
Fearon, E. R., and Vogelstein, B. 1990. A genetic model for colorectal tumorigenesis. Cell 61: 759–767.
Flammang, T. J., Couch, L. H., and Levy, G. N. 1992. DNA-adduct levels in congenic rapid and slow acetylator mouse strains following chronic administration of 4-aminobiphenyl. Carcinogenesis 13: 1887–1891.
Forrester, K., Almoguera, C., Han, K., Grizzle, W. E., and Perucho, M. 1987. Detection of high incidence of K-*ras* oncogenes during human colon tumorigenesis. Nature 327: 298–303.
Frayling, I. M., Beck, N. E., Ilyas, M., Dove-Edwin, I., Goodman, P., Pack, K., Bell, J. A., Williams, C. B., Hodgson, S. V., Thomas, H. J., Talbot, I. C., Bodmer, W. F., and Tomlinson, I. P. 1998. The APC variants I1307K and E1317Q are associated with colorectal tumors, but not always with a family history. Proc. Natl. Acad. Sci. U.S.A. 95: 10722–10727.
Friedl, W., and Aretz, S. 2005. Familial adenomatous polyposis: Expression from a study of 1164 unrelated german polyposis patients. Hered. Cancer Clin. Pract. 3: 95–114.
Gertig, D. M., and Hunter, D. J. 1998. Genes and environment in the etiology of colorectal cancer. Semin. Cancer Biol. 8: 285–298.
Giovannucci, E. 2001. An updated review of epidemiological evidence that cigarette smoking increased risk of colorectal cancer. Cancer Epidemiol. Biomarkers Prev. 10: 725–731.
Giovannucci, E. 2003. Diet, body weight, and colorectal cancer: a summary of the epidemiologic evidence. J. Womens Health (Larchmt) 12: 173–182.
Giovannucci, E., and Martinez, M. E. 1996. Tobacco, colorectal cancer, and adenomas: a review of the evidence. J. Natl. Cancer Inst. 88: 1717–1730.
Giovannucci, E., Rimm, E. B., Stampfer, M. J., Colditz, G. A., Ascherio, A., Kearney, J., and Willett, W. C. 1994a. A prospective study of cigarette smoking and risk of colorectal adenoma and colorectal cancer in U.S. women. J. Natl. Cancer Inst. 86: 183–191.
Giovannucci, E., Rimm, E. B., Stampfer, M. J., Colditz, G. A., Ascherio, A., and Willet, W. C. 1994b. Intake of fat, meat, and fiber in relatioln to risk of colon cancer in men. Cancer Res. 54: 2390–2397.
Goldman, R., and Shields, P. G. 2003. Food mutagens. J. Nutr. 133: 965S–973S.
Groden, J., Thliveris, A., Samowitz, W., Carlson, M., Gelbert, L., Albertsen, H., Joslyn, G., Stevens, J., Spirio, L., Robertson, M., Sargeant, L., Krapcho, K., Wolff, E., Burt, R., Hughes, J. P., Warrington, J., McPherson, J., Wasmuth, J., Paslier, D. L., Abderrahim, H., Cohen, D., Leppert, M., and White, R. 1991. Identification and characterization of the familial adenomatous polyposis coli gene. Cell 66: 589–600.
Hamada, F., and Bienz, M. 2002. A Drosophila APC tumour suppressor homologue functions in cellular adhesion. Nat. Cell Biol. 4: 208–213.
Hamilton, S. R. 1993. The molecular genetics of colorectal neoplasia. Gastroenterology 105: 3–7.
Hammond, E. C. 1966. Smoking in relation to the death rates of one million men and women. Natl. Cancer Inst. Monogr. 19: 127–204.
Hammond, E. C., and Horn, D. 1958. Smoking and death rates: report on forty-four months of follow-up of 187,783 men. II. Death rate by cause. J. Am. Med. Assoc. 166: 1294–1308.
Hardman, E. E., and Cameron, I. L. 1995. Site-specific reduction of colon cancer incidence, without a concomitant reduction in cryptal cell proliferation in 1,2-dimethylhydrazine-treated rats by diets containing 10% pectin with 5% or 20% corn oil. Carcinogenesis 16: 1425–1431.
Harris, C. C. 1991. Chemical and physical carcinogenesis: advances and perspectives for the 1990s. Cancer Res. 51: 5023S–5044S.

Hatzfeld, M. 1999. The armadillo family of structural proteins. Int. Rev. Cytol. 186: 179–224.
Heavey, P. M., McKenna, D., and Rowland, I. R. 2004. Colorectal cancer and the relationship between genes and the environment. Nutr. Cancer 48: 124–141.
Hedrick, L., Cho, K. R., Fearon, E. R., Wu, T. C., Kinzler, K. W., and Vogelstein, B. 1994. The DCC gene product in cellular differentiation and colorectal tumorigenesis. Genes Dev. 8: 1174–1183.
Henderson, B. R. 2000. Nuclear-cytoplasmic shuttling of APC regulates β-catenin subcellular localization and turnover. Nat. Cell Biol. 2: 653–660.
Henderson, B. R., and Fagotto, F. 2002. The ins and outs of APC and beta-catenin nuclear transport. EMBO Rep. 3: 834–839.
Hockenbery, D., Nuñez, G., Milliman, C., Schreiber, R. D. ,and, and Korsmeyer, S. J. 1990. Bcl-2 is an inner mitochondrial membrane protein that blocks programmed cell death. Nature 348: 334–336.
Hoffman, D., and Hoffman, I. 1997. The changing cigarette, 1950–1995. J. Toxicol. Environ. Health 50: 307–364.
Hoffmann, D., Hoffmann, I., and El-Bayoumy, K. 2001. The less harmful cigarette: a controversial issue. A tribute to Ernst L. Wynder. Chem. Res. Toxicol. 14: 768–790.
Homfray, T. F., Cottrell, S. E., Ilyas, M., Rowan, A., Talbot, I. C., Bodmer, W. F., and Tomlinson, I. P. 1998. Defects in mismatch repair occur after APC mutations in the pathogenesis of sporadic colorectal tumours. Hum. Mutat. 11: 114–120.
Horii, A., Nakatsuru, S., Ichii, S., Nagase, H., and Nakamura, Y. 1993. Multiple forms of the APC gene transcripts and their tissue-specific expression. Hum. Mol. Genet. 2: 283–286.
Hsu, W., Zeng, L., and Costantini, F. 1999. Identification of a domain of Axin that binds to the serine/threonine protein phosphatase 2A and a self-binding domain. J. Biol. Chem. 274: 3439–3445.
Hughes, R., Cross, A. J., Polluck, J. R., and Bingham, S. 2001. Dose-dependent effect of dietary meat on endogenous colonic N-nitrosation. Carcinogenesis 22: 199–202.
Hwang, E., and Bowen, P. E. 2007. DNA damage, a biomarker of carcinogenesis: its measurement and modulation by diet and environment. Crit. Rev. Food Sci. Nutr. 47: 27–50.
International Agency for Research on Cancer. 1986. Tobacco Smoking. IARC Monogr. Eval. Carcinog. Risk Chem. Hum. 38: 1–397.
International Agency for Research on Cancer. 2004. Tobacco Smoke. IARC Monogr. Eval. Carcinog. Risk Chem. Hum. 83: 1005–1187.
Ishibe, N., and Freedman, A. N. 2001. Understanding the interaction between environmental exposures and molecular events in colorectal carcinogenesis. Environ. Carcinogenesis 19: 524–539.
Ito, N., Hasegawa, R., Sano, M., Tamano, S., Esumi, H., Takayama, S., and Sugimura, T. 1991. A new colon and mammary carcinogen in cooked food, 2-amino-1-methyl-6-phenylimidazo[4,5-b]pyridine (PhIP). Carcinogenesis 12: 1503–1506.
Jacobs, E. J., Connell, C. J., Patel, A. V., Chao, A., Rodriguez, C., Seymour, J., McCullough, M. L., Calle, E. E., and Thun, M. J. 2001. Vitamin C and vitamin E supplement use and colorectal cancer mortality in large American Cancer Society cohort. Cancer Epidemiol. Biomarkers Prev. 10: 17–23.
Jaiswal, A. S., Balusu, R., Armas, M. L., Kundu, C. N., and Narayan, S. 2006. Mechanism of adenomatous polyposis coli (APC)-mediated blockage of long-patch base excision repair. Biochemistry 45: 15903–15914.
Jaiswal, A. S., Balusu, R., and Narayan, S. 2005. Involvement of adenomatous polyposis coli in colorectal tumorigenesis. Front. Biosci. 10: 1118–1134.
Jaiswal, A. S., and Narayan, S. 2001a. Upstream stimulating factor-1 (USF1) and USF2 bind to and activate the promoter of *adenomatous polyposis coli* (*APC*) tumor suppressor gene. J. Cell Biochem. 81: 262–277.
Jaiswal, A. S., and Narayan, S. 2001b. p53-dependent transcriptional regulation of the APC promoter in colon cancer cells treated with DNA alkylating agents. J. Biol. Chem. 276: 18193–18199.

Janssen, K. P., Alberici, P., Fsihi, H., Gaspar, C., Breukel, C., Franken, P., Rosty, C., Abal, M., El Marjou, F., Smits, R., Louvard, D., Fodde, R., and Robine, S. 2006. APC and oncogenic KRAS are synergistic in enhancing Wnt signaling in intestinal tumor formation and progression. Gastroenterology 131: 1096–1109.

Jimbo, T., Kawasaki, Y., Koyama, R., Sato, R., Takada, S., Haraguchi, K., and Akiyama, T. 2002. Identification of a link between the tumour suppressor APC and the kinesin superfamily. Nat. Cell Biol. 4: 323–327.

Jones, S., Emmerson, P., Maynard, J., Best, J. M., Jordan, S., Williams, G. T., Sampson, J. R., and Cheadle, J. P. 2002. Biallelic germline mutations in MYH predispose to multiple colorectal adenoma and somatic G:C→ T:A mutations. Hum. Mol. Genet. 11: 2961–2967.

Kahn, H. A. 1966. The Dorn study of smoking and mortality among U.S. veterans: report on eight and one-half years of observation. Natl. Cancer Inst. Monogr. 19: 1–125.

Kapitanovic, S., Radosevic, S., Kapitanovic, M., Andelinovic, S., Ferencic, Z., Tavassoli, M., Primorac, D., Sonicki, Z., Spaventi, S., Pavelic, K., and Spaventi, R. 1997. The expression of p185 (HER-2/neu) correlates with the stage of disease and survival in colorectal cancer. Gastroenterology 112: 1103–1113.

Kinzler, K. W., Nilbert, M. C., Su, L., Vogelstein, B., Bryan, T. M., Levy, D. B., Smith, K. J., Preisinger, A. C., Hedge, P., McKechnie, D., Finniear, R., Markham, A., Groffen, J., Boguski, M. S., Altschul, S. F., Horii, A., Ando, H., Miyoshi, Y., Miki, Y., Nishisho, I., and Nakamura, Y. 1991. Identification of FAP locus genes from chromosome 5q21. Science 253: 661–664.

Knudson, A. G., Jr. 1971. Mutation and cancer: statistical study of retinoblastoma. Proc. Natl. Acad. Sci. U.S.A. 68: 820–823.

Korinek, W. S., Copeland, M. S., Chaudhuri, A., and Chant, J. 2000. Molecular linkage underlying microtubule orientation toward cortical sites in yeast. Science 287: 2257–2259.

Kundu, C. N., Balusu, R., Jaiswal, A. S., Gariola, C. G., and Narayan, S. 2007b. Cigarette Smoke condensate-induced level of adenomatous polyposis coli blocks long-patch base excision repair in breast epithelial cells. Oncogene 26: 1428–1438.

Kundu, C. N., Balusu, R., Jaiswal, A. S., and Narayan, S. 2007a. Adenomatous polyposis coli-mediated hypersensitivity of mouse embryonic fibroblast cell lines to methylmethane sulfonate treatment: implication of base excision repair pathways. Carcinogenesis 28: 2089–2095.

Kune, G. A., Kune, S., Vitetta, L., and Watson, L. F. 1992. Smoking and colorectal cancer risk: data from the Melbourne Colorectal Cancer Study and brief review of literature. Int. J. Cancer 50: 369–372.

Kune, G. A., and Viterra, L. 1992. Alcohol consumption and the etiology of colorectal cancer: a review of the scientific evidence from 1957–1991. Nutr. Cancer 18: 97–111.

Laken, S. J., Petersen, G. M., Gruber, S. B., Oddoux, C., Ostrer, H., Giardiello, F. M., Hamilton, S. R., Hampel, H., Markowitz, A., Klimstra, D., Jhanwar, S., Winawer, S., Offit, K., Luce, M. C., Kinzler, K. W., and Vogelstein, B. 1997. Familial colorectal cancer in Ashkenazim due to a hypermutable tract in APC. Nat. Genet. 17: 79–83.

Lamlum, H., Ilyas, M., Rowan, A., Clark, S., Johnson, V., Bell, J., Frayling, I., Efstathiou, J., Pack, K., Payne, S., Roylance, R., Gorman, P., Sheer, D., Neale, K., Phillips, R., Talbot, I., Bodmer, W. F., and Tomlinson, I. 1999. The type of somatic mutation at APC in familial adenomatous polyposis is determined by the site of the germline mutation: a new facet to Knudson's 'two-hit' hypothesis. Nat. Med. 5: 1071–1075.

Lane, D. P. 1992. p53, guardian of the genome. Nature 358: 15–16.

Liberman, E., Kraus, S., Sagiv, E., Dulkart, O., Kazanov, D., and Arber, N. 2007. The APC E1317Q and I1307K polymorphisms in non-colorectal cancers. Biomed. Pharmacother. 61: 566–569.

Lioy, P. J., and Greenberg, A. 1990. Factors associated with human exposures to polycyclic aromatic hydrocarbons. Toxicol. Ind. Health 6: 209–223.

Lipkin, M., Reddy, B., Newmark, H., and Lamprecht, S. A. 1999. Dietary factors in human colorectal cancer. Annu. Rev. Nutr. 19: 545–586.

Locker, G. Y., Kaul, K., Weinberg, D. S., Gatalica, Z., Gong, G., Peterman, A., Lynch, J., Klatzco, L., Olopade, O. I., Bomzer, C. A., Newlin, A., Keenan, E., Tajuddin, M., Knezetic, J., Coronel,

S., and Lynch, H. T. 2006. The I1307K APC polymorphism in Ashkenazi Jews with colorectal cancer: clinical and pathologic features. Cancer Genet. Cytogenet. 169: 33–38.
Locker, G. Y., and Lynch, H. T. 2004. Genetic factors and colorectal cancer in Ashkenazi Jews. Fam Cancer. 3: 215–221.
Lund, E. K., Wharf, S. G., Fairweather-Tait, S. J., and Johnson, I. T. 1999. Oral ferrous sulfate supplements increase the free radical-generating capacity of feces from healthy volunteers. Am. J. Clin. Nutr. 69: 250–255.
Manabe, S., Tohyama, K., Wada, O., and Aramaki, T. 1991. Detection of a carcinogen, 2-amino-1-methyl-6-phenylimidazo[4,5-b]pyridine(PhIP) in cigarette smoke condensate. Carcinogenesis 12: 1945–1947.
Mason, J. B., and Choi, S. W. 2005. Effects of alcohol on folate metabolism: implications for carcinogenesis. Alcohol 35: 235–241.
Matsumine, A., Ogai, A., Senda, T., Okumura, N., Satoh, K., Baeg, G. H., Kawahara, T., Kobayashi, S., Okada, M., Toyoshima, K., and Akiyama, T. 1996. Binding of APC to the human homolog of the Drosophila discs large tumor suppressor protein. Science 272: 1020–1023.
McDonnell, T. J., Deane, N., Platt, F. M., Nunez, G., Jaeger, U., McKearn, J. P., and Korsmeyer, S. J. 1989. bcl-2-immunoglobulin transgenic mice demonstrate extended B cell survival and follicular lymphoproliferation. Cell 57: 79–88.
Mirvish, S. S., Haorah, J., Zhou, L., Hartman, M., Morris, C. R., and Clapper, M. L. 2003. N-nitrosocompounds in the gastrointestinal tract of rats and in the feces of mice with induced colitis or fed hot dogs or beef. Carcinogenesis 24: 595–603.
Miyoshi, Y., Nagase, H., Ando, H., Ichii, S., Nakatsura, S., Aoki, T., Miki, Y., Mori, T., and Nakamura, Y. 1992. Somatic mutations of the APC gene in colorectal tumors: Mutation cluster region in the APC gene. Hum. Mol. Genet. 1: 229–233.
Mori, T., Imaida, K., Tamon, S., Sano, M., Takahashi, S., Asamoto, M., Takeshita, M., Ueda, H., and Shirai, T. 2001. Beef tallow, but not perilla or corn oil, promotion of rate prostate via intestinal carcinogenesis by 3, 2/-diethyl-4-aminobiphenyl. Jpn. J. Cancer Res. 92: 1026–1033.
Mucci, L. A., Wedren, S., Tamami, R. M., Trichopoulos, D., and Adami, H. O. 2001. The role of gene-environment interactions in the etiology of human cancer: examples from cancer of the large bowel, lung and breast. J. Intern. Med. 249: 477–493.
Muto, T., Bussey, H. J., and Morson, B. C. 1975. The evolution of cancer of the colon and rectum. Cancer 36: 2251–2270.
Naccarati, A., Pardini, P., Hemminki, K., and Pavel, V. 2007. Sporadic colorectal cancer and individual susceptibility: A review of the association studies investigating the role of DNA repair genetic polymorphisms. Mutat. Res. 635: 118–145.
Nakamura, Y. 1993. The role of the adenomatous polyposis coli (APC) gene in human cancers. Adv. Cancer Res. 62: 65–87.
Narayan, S., and Jaiswal, A. S. 1997. Activation of Adenomatous Polyposis Coli (APC) Gene Expression by the DNA-alkylating agent *N*-Methyl-*N'*-nitro-*N*-nitrosoguanidine requires p53. J. Biol. Chem. 272: 30619–30622.
Narayan, S., Jaiswal, A. S., and Balusu, R. 2005. Tumor suppressor APC blocks DNA polymerase β-dependent strand displacement synthesis during long patch but not short patch base excision repair and increases sensitivity to methylmethane sulfonate. J. Biol. Chem. 280: 6942–6949.
Narayan, S., and Roy, D. 2003. Role of APC and DNA mismatch repair genes in the development of colorectal cancers. Mol. Cancer. 2: 41–56.
National Cancer Institute. 2007. What you need to know about colon and rectal cancer: Risk Factors. http://www.cancer.gov/cancertopics/wyntk/colon-and-rectal/page4
Neufeld, K. L., Nix, D. A., Bogerd, H., Kang, Y., Beckerle, M. C., Cullen, B. R., and White, R. L. 2000. Adenomatous polyposis coli protein contains two nuclear export signals and shuttles between the nucleus and cytoplasm. Proc. Natl. Acad. Sci. U.S.A. 97: 12085–12090.
Nigro, N. D., Bull, A. W., Klopfer, B. A., Pak, M. S., and Campbell, R. L. 1979. Effect of dietary fiber on azoxymethane-induced intestinal carcinogenesis in rats. J. Natl. Cancer Inst. 62: 1097–1102.

Nishikawa, A., Mori, Y., Lee, I. S., Tanaka, T., and Hirose, M. 2004. Cigarette smoking metabolic activation and carcinogenesis. Curr.Drug Metabol. 5: 363–373.

Nishisho, I., Nakamura, Y., Miyoshi, Y., Miki, H., Ando, A., Horii, K., Koyama, J., Utsunomiya, S., Baba, S., and Hedge, P. 1991. Mutations of chromosome 5q21 genes in FAP and colorectal cancer patients. Science 253: 665–669.

Nohmi, T., and Masumura, K. 2005. Molecular nature of intrachromosomal deletions and base substitutions induced by environmental mutagens. Environ. Mol. Mutag. 45: 150–161.

Norat, T., and Riboli, E. 2001. Meat consumption and colorectal cancer: a review of epidemiologic evidence. Nutr. Rev. 59: 37–47.

Ohgaki, H., Takahama, J. R., and Sugimura, T. 1991. Carcinogenicities of heterocyclic amines in cooked food. Mutat. Res. 259: 399–410.

Orford, K., Crockett, C., Jensen, J. P., Weissman, A. M., and Byers, S. W. 1997. Serine phosphorylation-regulated ubiquitination and degradation of beta-catenin. J. Biol. Chem. 272: 24735–24738.

Parnaud, G., and Corpet, D. E. 1997. Colorectal cancer: controversial role of meat consumption. Bull. Cancer 84: 899–911.

Paz-Elizur, T., Brenner, D. E., and Livneh, Z. 2005. Interrogating DNA repair in cancer risk assessment. Cancer Epidemiol. Biomarkers Prev. 14: 1585–1587.

Peifer, M. S., Berg, S., and Reynolds, A. B. 1994. A repeating amino acid motif shared by proteins with diverse cellular roles. Cell 76: 789–791.

Perera, F. P. 1997. Environment and cancer: who are susceptible? Science 278: 1068–1073.

Pierre, F., Tache, S., Petit, C. R., Meer, R. V., and Corpet, D. E. 2003. Meat and cancer: hemoglobin and haemin in a low-calcium diet promote colorectal carcinogenesis at the aberrant crypt stated in rats. Carcinogenesis 24: 1683–1690.

Polakis, P. 1997. The adenomatous polyposis coli (APC) tumor suppressor. Biochim. Biophys. Acta 1332: F127–F147.

Povey, A. C., Badawi, A. F., Cooper, D. P., Hall, N., Harrison, K. L., Jackson, P. E., Lees, N. P., O'Connor, P. J., and Margison, G. P. 2002. DNA alkylation and repair in the large bowel: Animal and human studies. J. Nutr. 132: 3518S–3521S.

Powell, S. M., Zilz, N., Beazer-Barclay, Y., Bryan, T. M., Hamilton, S. R., Thibodeau, S. N., Vogelstein, B., and Kinzler, K. W. 1992. APC mutations occur early during colorectal tumorigenesis. Nature 359: 235–237.

Probst-Hensch, N. M., Sinha, R., Longnecker, M. P., Wittle, J. S., Ingles, S. A., Frankl, H. D., Lee, E. R., and Haile, R. W. 1997. Meat preparation and colorectal adenomas in a large sigmoidscopy-based case-control study in California (United States). Cancer Caused Control 8: 175–183.

Rogot, E., and Murray, J. L. 1980. Smoking and causes of death among U.S. veterans: 16 years of observation. Public Health Rep. 95: 213–222.

Rothman, N., Correa-Villasenor, A., Ford, D. P., Poirier, M. C., Haas, R., Hansen, J. A., Rowan, A. J., Lamlum, H., Ilyas, M., Wheeler, J., Straub, J., Papadopoulou, A., Bicknell, D., Bodmer, W. F., and Tomlinson, I. P. 2000. APC mutations in sporadic colorectal tumors: A mutational "hotspot" and interdependence of the "two hits". Proc. Natl. Acad. Sci. U.S.A. 97: 3352–3357.

Rothman, N., Poirier, M. C., Baser, M. E., Hansen, J. A., Gentile, C., Bowman, E. D., and Strickland, P. T. 1990. Formation of polycyclic hydrocarbon-DNA adducts in peripheral white blood cells during consumption of charcoal-broiled beef. Carcinogenesis 11: 1241–1243.

Rowan, A. J., Lamlum, H., Ilyas, M., Wheeler, J., Straub, J., Papadopoulou, A., Bicknell, D., Bodmer, W. F., and Tomlinson, I. P. 2000. APC mutations in sporadic colorectal tumors: A mutational "hotspot" and interdependence of the "two hits". Proc. Natl. Acad. Sci. U.S.A. 97: 3352–3357.

Rubinfeld, B., Albert, I., Porfiri, E., Fiol, C., Munemitsu, S., and Polakis, P. 1996. Binding of GSK3 to the APC-beta-catenin complex and regulation of complex assembly. Science 272: 1023–1026.

Rubinfeld, B., Souza, B., Albert, I., Muller, O., Chamberlain, S. C., Masiarz, F., Munemitsu, S., and Polakis, P. 1993. Association of the APC gene product with catenin. Science 262: 1731–1734.

Sampson, J. R., Jones, S., Dolwani, S., and Cheadle, J. P. 2005. Mut YH (MYH) and colorectal cancer. Biochem. Soc. Trans. 33: 679–683.

Sanders, L. M., Henderson, C. E., Mee, Y. H., Barhoumi, R., Burghardt, R. C., Carroll, R. J., Turner, N. D., Chapkin, R. S., and Lupton, J. R. 2004. Pro-oxidant environment of the colon compared to the small intestine may contribute to greater cancer susceptibility. Cancer Lett. 208: 155–161.

Schafmayer, C., Buch, S., Egberts, J. H., Franke, A., Brosch, M., El Sharawy, A., Conring, M., Koschnick, M., Schwiedernoch, S., Katalinic, A., Kremer, B., Fölsch, U. R., Krawczak, M., Fändrich, F., Schreiber, S., Tepel, J., and Hampe, J. 2007. Genetic investigation of DNA-repair pathway genes PMS2, MLH1, MSH2, MSH6, MUTYH, OGG1 and MTH1 in sporadic colon cancer. Int. J. Cancer 121: 555–558.

Schmitt, C. A., Thaler, K. R., Wittig, B. M., Kaulen, H., Meyer-zum-Büschenfelde, K. H., and Dippold, W. G. 1998. Detection of the DCC gene product in normal and malignant colorectal tissues and its relation to a codon 201 mutation. Br. J. Cancer 77: 588–594.

Schwartz, K., Richards, K., and Botstein, D. 1997. BIM1 encodes a microtubule-binding protein in yeast. Mol. Biol. Cell 8: 2677–2691.

Shibata, D., Peinado, M. A., Ionov, Y., Malkhosyan, S., and Perucho, M. 1994. Genomic instability in repeated sequences is an early somatic event in colorectal tumorigenesis that persists after transformation. Nat. Genet. 6: 273–281.

Siede, W., Kow, Y., and Doetsch, P. W. 2006. DNA damage recognition. New York, NY: CRC Press, pp. 263–267.

Singh, S. V., Benson, P. J., Hu, X., Pal, A., Dunsford, H. A., and Rodriguez, L. V. 1998. Gender-related differences in susceptibility of A/J mouse to benzo[a]pyrene-induced pulmonary and forestomach tumorigenesis. Cancer Lett. 128: 197–204.

Sinha, R. 2002. An epidemiologic approach to studying heterocyclic amines. Mutat. Res. 506/507: 197–204.

Sinha, R., Rothman, N., Brown, E. D., Salmon, C. P., Knize, M. G., Swanson, C. A., Rossi, S. C., Mark, S. D., Levander, O. A., and Felton, J. S. 1995. High concentrations of the carcinogen 2-amino-1 methyl-6-phenylimidazo-[4.5-b]pyridine (PhIP) occur in chicken but are dependent on the cooking method. Cancer Res. 55: 4516–4519.

Slattery, M. L., Anderson, K., Curtin, K., Ma, K. N., Schaffer, D., and Samowitz, W. 2001. Dietary intake and microsatellite instability in colon tumors. Int. J. Cancer 93: 601–607.

Slattery, M. L., Curtin, K., Anderson, K., Ma, K. N., Ballard, L., Edwards, S., Schaffer, D., Potter, J., Leppert, M., and Samowitz, W. S. 2000. Associations between cigarette smoking, lifestyle factors, and microsatellite instability in colon tumors. J. Natl. Cancer Inst. 92: 1831–1836.

Smith, K. J., Levy, D. B., Maupin, P., Pollard, T. D., Vogelstein, B., and Kinzler, K. W. 1994. Wild-type but not mutant APC associates with the microtubule cytoskeleton. Cancer Res. 54: 3672–3675.

Spry, M., Scott, T., Pierce, H., and D'Orazio, J. A. 2007. DNA repair pathways and hereditary cancer susceptibility syndromes. Front. Biosci. 12: 4191–4207.

Stavric, B. 1994. Biological significance of trace levels of mutagenic heterocyclic aromatic amines in human diet: a critical review. Food Chem. Toxicol. 32: 977–994.

Strickland, P. T., and Groopman, J. D. 1995. Biomarkers for assessing environmental exposure to carcinogens in the diet. Am. J. Clin. Nutr. 61: 710S–720S.

Su, L. K., Burrell, M., Hill, D. E., Gyuris, J., Brent, R., Wiltshire, R., Trent, J., Vogelstein, B., and Kinzler, K. W. 1995. APC binds to the novel protein EB1. Cancer Res. 55: 2972–2977.

Su, L. K., Vogelstein, B., and Kinzler, K. W. 1993. Association of the APC tumor suppressor protein with catenins. Science 262: 1734–1737.

Sugimura, T. 1997. Overview of carcinogenic heterocyclic amines. Mutat. Res. 376: 211–219.

Thomas, G. V., Szigeti, K., Murphy, M., Draetta, G., Pagano, M., and Loda, M. 1998. Down-regulation of p27 is associated with development of colorectal adenocarcinoma metastases. Am. J. Pathol. 153: 681–687.

Toyooka, M., Konishi, M., Kikuchi-Yanoshita, R., Iwama, T., and Miyaki, M. 1995. Somatic mutations of the adenomatous polyposis coli gene in gastroduodenal tumors from patients with familial adenomatous polyposis. Cancer Res. 55: 3165–3170.

Trock, B., Lanza, E., and Greenwald, P. 1990. Dietary fiber, vegetables, and colon cancer: critical review and meta-analysis of the epidemiologic evidence. J. Natl. Cancer Inst. 82: 650–661.

U.S. National Academy of Sciences. 1989. Diet and health. Washington, DC: National Academy Press.

Vogelstein, B., Fearson, E. R., Hamilton, S. R., Kern, S. E., Preisinger, A. C., Leppert, M., Nakamura, Y., White, R., Smits, A. M., and Bos, J. L. 1988. Genetic alterations during colorectal tumor development. N. Engl. J. Med. 319: 525–532.

Waldman, J. M., Lioy, P. J., Greenberg, A., and Butler, J. P. 1991. Analysis of human exposure to benzo(a)pyrene via inhalation and food ingestion in the Total Human Exposure Study (THEES). J. Expo. Anal. Environ. Epidemiol. 1: 193–225.

Weir, J. M., and Dunn, J. E., Jr. 1970. Smoking and mortality: a prospective study. Cancer 25: 105–112.

Willet, W. C. 1995. Diet, nutrition, and avoidable cancer. Environ. Health Perspect. 103: 165–170.

World Cancer Research Fund. 1997. Food, nutrition, and the prevention of cancer: a global perspective. Washington, DC: American Institute of Cancer Research, pp. 244–321.

Wurzelmann, J. I., Silver, A., Schreinemachers, D. M., Sandler, R. S., and Everson, R. B. 1996. Iron intake and risk of colon cancer. Cancer Epidemiol. Biomarkers Prev. 5: 503–507.

Yamaski, E., and Ames, B. N. 1977. Concentration of mutagens from urine by absorption with the nonpolar resin XAD-2: cigarette smokers have mutagenic urine. Proc. Natl. Acad. Sci. U.S.A. 74: 3555–3559.

Zeng, L., Fagotto, F., Zhang, T., Hsu, W., Vasicek, T. J., Perry, W. L., Lee, J. J., Tilghman, S. M., Gumbiner, B. M., and Constantini, F. 1997. The mouse fused locus encodes Axin, an inhibitor of the Wnt signaling pathway that regulates embryonic axis formation. Cell 90: 181–192.

Zhang, F., White, R. L., and Neufeld, K. L. 2000. Phosphorylation near nuclear localization signal regulates nuclear import of adenomatous polyposis coli protein. Proc. Natl. Acad. Sci. U.S.A. 97: 12577–12582.

Chapter 13
Gene–Environmental Interactions and Susceptibility to Liver Cancer

John B. Colerangle

Abstract Human liver cancer, specifically hepatocellular carcinoma (HCC), is the fifth most common malignancy worldwide and remains a major cause of cancer death. HCC accounts for over half a million deaths per year. Despite many efforts to understand the pathogenesis of HCC, little is known about its etiology. Hepatitis B and C, and aflatoxin B are the only established cause, and the proportion of cases of liver cancer attributed to Hepatitis B and C and aflatoxin B is about 75–80%. A family history of liver cancer accounts for only 3% of the cases of this disease. The remaining portions of cases are due to yet unrecognized factors. Alcohol is an important risk factor for the development of HCC since hepatic cirrhosis caused by chronic alcohol abuse has long been recognized as a major risk factor for the development of HCC. The pathogenesis of HCC is quite diverse and influenced by a variety of environmental and genetic factors of the host. The link between environmental factors, genetics, and the development of cancer has advanced our understanding of the factors that influence cancer risk. Understanding the relative roles of the environmental factors and genes in cancer etiology may clearly elucidate how each of these factors can disparately affect the health of individual members of a community. Although environmental, occupational, and recreational exposures to carcinogens contribute to cancer risk in humans, variation in incidence and progression of cancer in a population is due to genetic polymorphisms in the population. Functional polymorphisms that influence an individual's susceptibility to liver cancer include gene products involved in activation and detoxification of carcinogens and DNA repair. Gene polymorphisms that play key roles in apoptosis may also provide insight to individual susceptibility to liver cancer. Thus genetic polymorphisms may explain why individuals with shared environmental exposures do not always share cancer morbidity and mortality.

J.B. Colerangle (✉)
Sanofi-Aventis Pharmaceuticals, Regulatory Pharmacology and Toxicology – US, Bridgewater, NJ 08807, USA
e-mail: john.colerangle@sanofi-aventis.com

D. Roy, M.T. Dorak (eds.), *Environmental Factors, Genes, and the Development of Human Cancers*, DOI 10.1007/978-1-4419-6752-7_13,

Keywords Hepatocellular carcinoma (HCC) · Hepatitis B and C · Aflatoxin B · Alcohol · Functional polymorphisms in genes involved in activation and detoxification of carcinogens and DNA repair · Influence an individual's susceptibility to liver cancer

13.1 Gene–Environmental Interactions and Susceptibility to Liver Cancer

Human liver cancer, specifically hepatocellular carcinoma (HCC), is the fifth most common malignancy worldwide and remains a major cause of cancer death. HCC accounts for over half a million deaths per year (Perkin et al., 2001). Despite many efforts to understand the pathogenesis of HCC, little is known about its etiology. Hepatitis B and C, and aflatoxin B are the only established cause, and the proportion of cases of liver cancer attributed to Hepatitis B and C and aflatoxin B is about 75–80% (Kirk et al., 2006). A family history of liver cancer accounts for only 3% of the cases of this disease (Fernandez et al., 1994). The remaining portions of cases are due to yet unrecognized factors. The pathogenesis of HCC is quite diverse and influenced by a variety of environmental and genetic factors of the host. The link between environmental factors, genetics, and the development of cancer has advanced our understanding of the factors that influence cancer risk. Traditional methods for answering questions about the relationship between genes, the environment, and cancer etiology have relied on analyses of cancer incidence in twin pairs and in families (Wilson et al., 2002). Understanding the relative roles of the environmental factors and genes in cancer etiology may clearly elucidate how each of these factors can disparately affect the health of individual members of a community. Although environmental, occupational, and recreational exposures to carcinogens contribute to cancer risk in humans, variation in incidence and progression of cancer in a population is due to genetic polymorphisms in the population. Functional polymorphisms that influence an individual's susceptibility to liver cancer include gene products involved in activation and detoxification of carcinogens and DNA repair. Gene polymorphisms that play key roles in apoptosis may also provide insight to individual susceptibility to liver cancer. Thus genetic polymorphisms may explain why individuals with shared environmental exposures do not always share cancer morbidity and mortality. This chapter will discuss how interactions of various environmental factors with the genetic make-up of the host influence the individual's cancer risk.

13.1.1 Biological Agents in the Environment and Their Interactions with Genes That Predispose to Liver Cancer (Hepatocellular Carcinoma)

Hepatitis B and hepatitis C virus: HBV is a non-cytopathic, partially double stranded hepatotrophic DNA virus. Chronic infection with hepatitis B virus (HBV)

and hepatitis C virus (HCV) are the most significant risk factors for developing HCC in humans (ACS, 2001). HCC is the most common primary liver cancer accounting for 75% of all cases. Rarer forms of the malignant liver cancer include cholangiocarcinomas, angiosarcomas, and hepatoblastomas in children. Although HCC is about ten times more common in East and Southeast Asia and Africa, incidence is rapidly increasing in the United States (ACS, 2001). Rates of HCC in the United States have increased by 70% over the past 20 years (Yu et al., 2000) and similar trends have been observed in Canada and Western Europe. The higher rates observed in recent years has been attributed to the increase in HCV infection (El-Serag, 2001; El-Serag and Mason, 2000). Approximately 80% of HCC cases worldwide are attributed to HBV infection (Yu et al., 2000). However, HBV accounts for only 25% of cases in the United States and infection with HCV plays a much larger role in the incidence of this cancer.

HBV has recently been shown to promote HCC in HBV carriers through several mechanisms. For example, a single case of HBV DNA integration into a retinoic acid receptor gene (Brand et al., 1988) and a cycline A gene (Wang et al., 1990) has been reported, presumably illustrating a "cis-acting" promoter insertion mechanism. Elmore et al. (1997) reported that the HBV oncoprotein, HBx, binds to the C terminus of p53 and inhibit several critical p53-mediated cellular processes, including DNA sequence-specific binding, transcriptional transactivation, and apoptosis. The p53 tumor suppressor protein is involved in several cellular processes that are critical for maintaining the genomic integrity of cells (Levine et al., 1991; Greenblatt et al., 1994). Elmore et al. (1997) have demonstrated that complexing of the distal C-terminus domain of the HBx with p53 in the cytoplasm independent of its transactivation activity, partially prevents its nuclear entry and ability to induce apoptosis. These effects of HBx are thought to contribute to the pathogenesis of HCC. Several studies have demonstrated that the transcriptional transactivation property of HBx contributes to hepatocarcinogenesis (Robinson, 1994; Caselmann, 1995). Although HBx is capable of binding single-stranded DNA (Qadri et al., 1996), it transcriptionally transactivates through protein-protein interactions with cellular transcriptional factors or effectors of signal transduction pathways (Maguire et al., 1991; Lucito and Schneider, 1992; Natoli et al., 1994). HBx which is required for viral infection has been implicated in virus-mediated hepatocarcinogenesis (Benn and Schneider, 1994). Biochemical evidence suggests that HBx activates Ras and rapidly induces a cytoplasmic signaling cascade linking Ras, Raf, and mitogen-activated protein kinase (MAP kinase), leading to transcriptional transactivation (Benn and Schneider, 1994). Ras, a low molecular weight guanosine triphosphate (GTP)-binding protein play key roles in the regulation of cell proliferation by initiating a cascade of threonine and serine phosphorylation events through Raf and MAP kinases (Benn and Schneider, 1994; Lange-Carter et al., 1993; Moodie et al., 1993).

Benn and Schneider, 1995 reported that HBx plays a key role in viral hepatocarcinogenesis by activating the Ras-Raf-MAP kinase signaling cascade, through which it activates transcriptional factors AP-1 and NF-kB, and stimulates cell DNA synthesis. HBx also stimulates cell cycle progression, shortening of the emergence of cells from G_0 and entry into S phase by at least 12 h, and accelerating transit through checkpoint controls at G_0/G_1 and G_2/M. The HBx protein also regulates gene transcription, causing cell proliferation and inducing apoptosis (Shintani et al., 1999).

Hino et al. (1991) reported that chromosomal translocation, deletion, and inversion/duplication directly linked to HBV DNA integration occur frequently in host DNA of human hepatocellular carcinomas. Accumulation of mutations, which may occur during continuous cycles of cell division, may eventually transform some hepatocytes through a multistage process involving, among other things, the permanent loss of activity of genes that suppress cellular proliferation (Wang and Rogler 1988; Buetow et al., 1989; Tsuda et al., 1990; Slagel et al., 1991; Fujimori et al., 1991; Urano et al., 1991) [for example: tumor suppressor genes (Knudson, 1986)]. In addition to these mechanisms, it has been proposed that HBV integration functions as a random mutagen, promoting chromosomal defects in hepatocytes. Experimental evidence in support of this proposal has showed that HBV DNA integration at the sites of chromosomal translocation, cause large deletions, and inversion/duplication in host DNA of HCC (Hino et al., 1986, 1989; Henderson et al., 1988; Rogler et al., 1985; Nagaya et al., 1987; Tokino et al., 1987). These examples have led to the notion that in some instances HBV DNA integration may enhance chromosomal instability.

It thus appears that HBV in addition to other mechanisms induce HCC by a combination of mechanisms, the latter two being: (i) cell killing and stimulation of mitosis that can accumulate the necessary number of events required for cell transformation and (ii) increase of chromosomal instability by the insertion of HBV DNAs into host DNA, mediated by proteins that can stimulate recombination during chronic hepatitis. Based on these data, Hino et al. (1991) hypothesized that integrated HBV DNA might be stable in host DNA without a putative recombinogenic region of HBV DNA or recombinogenic cellular protein(s)-for example, in the healthy HBV carrier state. This mechanism seems to explain why among HBV carriers, HCCs usually develop only in patients with chronic hepatitis and/or cirrhosis.

HCV is a non-cytopathic virus whose positive-stranded RNA genome encodes non-structural proteins (NS2, NS3, NS4A, NS5A and NS5B), which associates with the endoplasmic reticulum (ER) membrane to form the viral replicase and viral envelope proteins (E1 and E2) (Piao et al., 2004). HCV has been reported to possess three biological characteristics distinct from HBV that are relevant for hepatocarcinogenesis (Farazi and DePinho, 2006). First, HCV has a higher likelihood (60–80%) of causing chronic infection relative to 10% for HBV (Piao et al., 2004). Secondly, HCV has a greater propensity to promote liver cirrhosis compared to HBV (Piao et al., 2004). Piao et al. (2004) reported that 5–10% of HCV-infected patients develop cirrhosis after 10 years of infection, a frequency that is 10–20-fold higher than in HBV-infected patients. Third, HCV cannot integrate into host genomes since it is an RNA virus with a DNA intermediate form (Piao et al., 2004).

HCC development requires the interaction of both viral and host factors. One mechanism of HCV-induced hepatocarcinogenesis indicates that continuous cycles of hepatocyte death caused by the immune response to the virus and subsequent

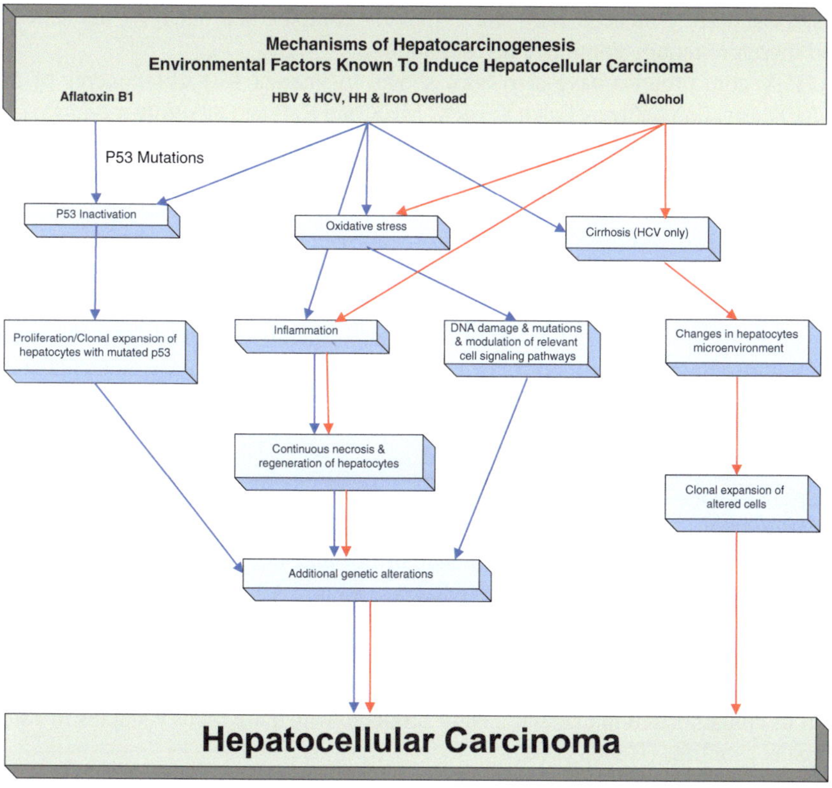

Fig. 13.1 Mechanisms of hepatocarcinogenesis – environmental factors known to induce hepatocellular carcinoma

regeneration provides a means for accumulation and propagation of mutations (Fig. 13.1). It is thought that immune responses to viral infection promote hepatocarcinogenesis in a manner similar to transgenic skin-tumor model in which deficiencies in pro-inflammatory T-cells have been shown to correlate with decreased tumor incidence and progression (Yu et al., 2005). On the contrary, the relevance of the immune-mediated mechanism becomes obscured considering the weak immunological response in chronically HCV-infected livers (Block et al., 2003). This notion is supported by the suggestion that HCV RNA and/or core proteins impair dendritic cell functions that are necessary for T-cell activation (Pachiadakis et al., 2005). In addition, the HCV core proteins and the NS5A non-structural proteins have been implicated in the evasion from immune-mediated cell killing by interacting with various factors involved in this process (for example, tumor necrosis factor-α (TNF-α) receptor, inteferon-α (IFN-α)) (Park et al., 2003; Melen et al., 2004). Other HCV proteins use their protease function to cleave and activate components that are integral for signaling the immune response (Foy et al., 2005; Li et al., 2005). Overall, the pathogenetic interactions between the immune system and HCV-induced HCC are extremely complex and not fully understood, and therefore require continued investigation.

HCV core proteins have also been shown to interact with components of the MAPK signaling pathway (such as ERK, MEK and Raf) and therefore modulate cell proliferation (Hwang et al., 2003; Okabe et al., 2000). NS5A has also been shown to interact with and inactivate p53 by sequestration to the perinuclear membrane, thereby affecting the p53-regulated pathways that control cell-cycle progression, cellular survival, response to hypoxic and genotypic stresses, and tumour angiogenesis (Majumder et al., 2001). The carcinogenic potential of HCV core proteins is also demonstrated by the induction of reactive oxygen species, the development hepatic steatosis, and the development of HCC in transgenic mice that harbor the entire HCV core gene under the control of HBV transcriptional regulatory elements. This raises the possibility that HCV-induced HCC involves an oxidative-stress-mediated mechanism (Kusano et al., 2002) (Fig. 13.1). In addition, core-E1-E2 transgenic mice develop HCCs whose robust tumor growth seems to be due to the inhibition of apoptosis by the E1/E2 HCV proteins (Kitay-Cohen et al., 2001).

Aflatoxins: Aflatoxins are a group of mycotoxins produced mainly by two Aspergillus species which are abundant in hot and humid climates. Aspergillus flavus which produces B aflatoxins (Aflatoxin B_1 and Aflatoxin B_2) are ubiquitous. A. parasiticus which produces both B and G aflatoxins (Aflatoxin G_1 and Aflatoxin G_2), has more limited distribution (IARC, 2002). Human exposure to aflatoxins occurs mainly at levels of nanograms to micrograms per day through consumption of contaminated maize and peanut products which are dietary staples in some tropical countries (IARC, 2002).

Aflatoxin B_1 (AFB_1) is an extremely potent hepatocarcinogen in various species including humans. Epidemiological data have demonstrated a direct relationship between AFB_1 intake and the incidence of primary liver cancer in certain geographical areas (Sengstag, 1997). AFB_1 has been classified by the International Agency for Research on Cancer (IARC) as a Class 1 carcinogen (IARC, 1993).

AFB_1 is metabolized by the cytochrome P450 mono-oxygenase system (CYP1A2, 3A4, 3A5, 3A7) in human and rodent liver to the AFB_1-8,9-exo-epoxide, which binds to DNA mainly at guanine residues, forming the trans-8,9-dihydro-(N^7-guanyl)-9-hydroxy-AFB_1 adduct (Eaton and Gallagher, 1994; IARC, 1993; Chou and Chen, 1997) (Fig. 13.2). This adduct may subsequently hydrolyze to form the stable formamidopyrimidine product. If not excised by the DNA repair machinery, the premutagenic DNA lesions may be fixed as mutations that are predominantly G→T transversions (Sengstag, 1997). G→T transversions occur predominantly at a specific hot-spot, the third base of codon 249, giving rise to a substitute of serine for arginine in the p53 protein (Sengstag, 1997). AFB_1 also induces mitotic recombination which result in chromosomal translocation and gene conversion events. Mitotic recombination is one possible mechanism for loss of heterozygosity (LOH), a phenomenon often observed in cancer cells. LOH is a genetic alteration by which a heterozygous mutation (which may have previously occurred in a tumor suppressor gene (TSG)), is rendered hemizygous or homozygous. This allows the expression of a recessive phenotype that would otherwise be masked by the wild-type

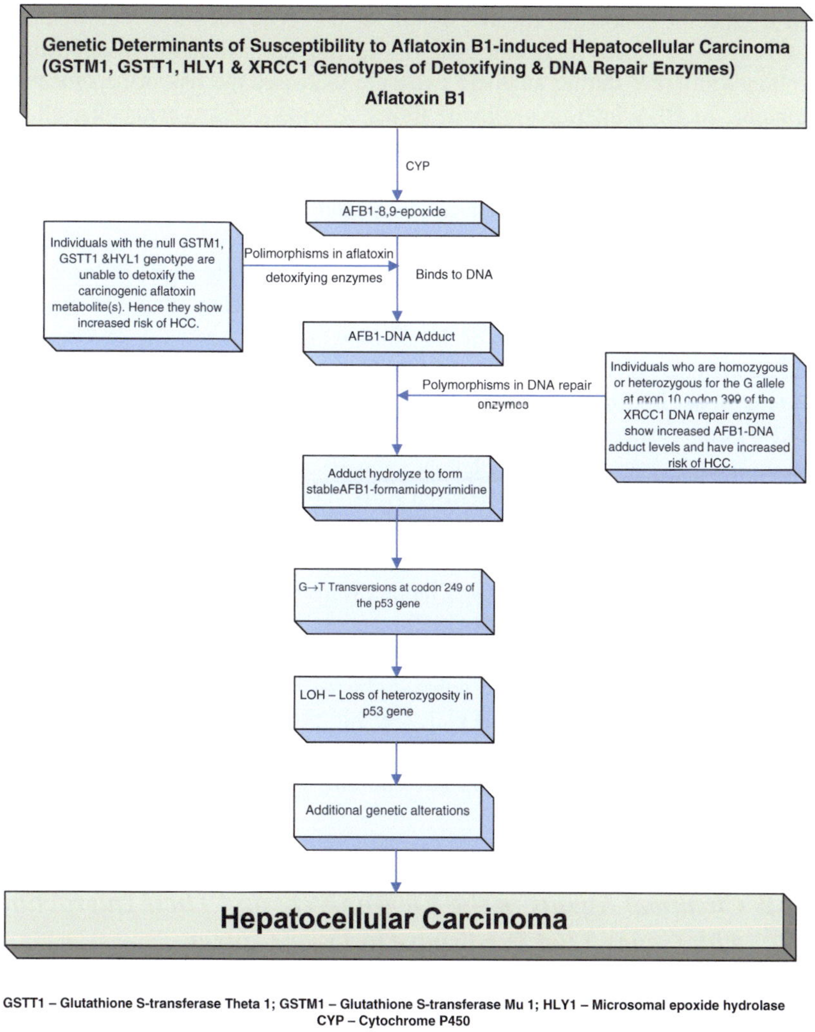

Fig. 13.2 Genetic determinants of susceptibility to aflatoxin B1-induced hepatocellular carcinoma

allele. Besides mutations in the TSGs, loss or silencing of the functional TSG allele appears to be a common mechanism for inactivation. LOH may occur as a result of a large deletion, chromosomal nondisjunction, or through activities related to mitotic recombination (gene conversion and crossing over). Since AFB_1 is highly prone to mitotic recombination events by one of these mechanisms, it contributes to the expression of heterozygous mutations thereby catalyzing an important step of hepatocarcinogenesis (Sengstag, 1997).

Studies of genetic alterations in human hepatocellular cancers (HCCs) from patients living in an AFB_1 contaminated area in China revealed not only an increase in AFB_1-specific codon 249 transversion in the p53 gene but also a high frequency of LOH in the p53 locus (Scorsone et al., 1992). Studies have shown that concurrent infection with HBV during aflatoxin exposure increases the risk of hepatocellular carcinoma. As HBV interferes with the ability of hepatocytes to metabolize aflatoxins, an aflatoxin B_1-DNA conjugate exists for a longer period of time in the liver, increasing the chance of damage to tumor suppressor genes such as p53. This effect is synergistic with the resulting damage far greater than just the sum of aflatoxin or HBV (Williams et al., 2004).

Host genetic differences seem to determine susceptibility to AFB_1-induced HCC. In Gambia, West Africa, HBV infection is high with heavy aflatoxin exposure. However, only a small proportion of the exposed Gambians actually develop HCC. Multivariate analysis of the Gambian Liver Cancer Study (GLCS) showed a modest increase in HCC risk associated with one of the primary enzymes responsible for AFB_1 detoxification (Kirk et al., 2005, 2006). Individuals who were homozygous or heterozygous for the G allele at exon 10 codon 399 of the XRCC1 DNA repair enzyme, associated with increased AFB_1-DNA adduct levels also displayed an increased risk of HCC (Lunn et al., 1999; Kirk et al., 2005) (Fig. 13.2).

A trend of increased HCC risk was observed with XRCC1-399G polymorphism in a study from Taiwan. Strong associations were observed among subjects with both XRCC1 variants and the null GSTT1 genotype (Yu et al., 2003). Kirk et al. (2006) also identified a greater than additive effect on HCC risk with the DNA repair variant in combination with polymorphisms in several aflatoxin detoxifying enzymes including GSTM1 and HYL1. Genetic polymorphisms of AFB_1 metabolizing/detoxifying enzymes (the null GSTM1, GSTT1, HYL1) and DNA repair enzymes (e.g. XRCC1) determine the susceptibility of individuals to HCC following exposure to aflatoxin (Fig. 13.2).

13.1.2 Chemical Agents in the Environment and Their Interactions with Genes That Predispose to Liver Cancer

Vinyl chloride: Vinyl chloride, a gas used in the plastic industry to produce polyvinyl chloride (PVC) and its copolymers has been shown to be a human carcinogen, inducing angiosarcoma of the liver, a very rare type of tumor. The strongest evidence that vinyl chloride causes liver cancer in humans is based on numerous epidemiological studies and case reports that show its association with angiosarcoma of the liver.

The general population is exposed to vinyl chloride through inhalation of contaminated air, ingestion of contaminated water and foods, or dermal contact with consumer products. However, exposure levels are very low for the majority of the population (ASTDR, 1997; HSDB, 2003; Kielhorn et al., 2000). Occupational exposure to vinyl chloride generally occurs after production, when the finished monomer is piped to storage or transportation, or during maintenance. The potential for exposure is high during the process of polymerization to form PVC resins and other materials because vinyl chloride monomers may escape into the air (NCI, 1978).

Vinyl chloride is rapidly absorbed following respiratory exposure and is primarily metabolized in the liver by the cytochrome P450 2E1 system to form chloroethylene oxide, which can undergo spontaneous rearrangement to form chloroacetaldehyde (ASTDR, 1993; Smith et al., 1998) (Fig. 13.3). These metabolites react with DNA bases to form adducts that are known to be mutagenic. The adducts include 7-(2′-oxoethyl) guanine, 1,N^6-thanoadenine, 3,N^4-ehthenocytosinc, and N^2-3-ethenoguanine (ASTDR, 1993; Smith et al., 1998) (Fig. 13.3). The

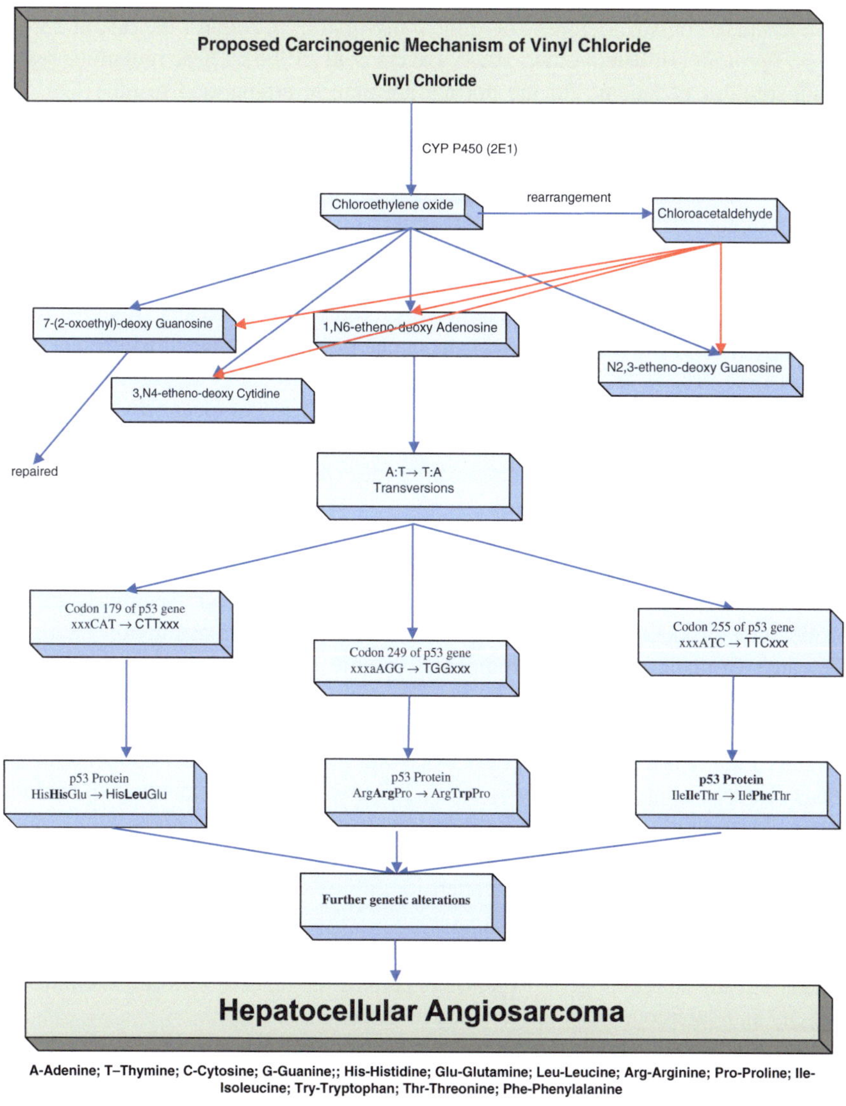

Fig. 13.3 Proposed carcinogenic mechanism of vinyl chloride

oxoethyl adduct is the major liver DNA adduct formed, representing 98% of all adducts but it is least persistent, with a half-life of approximately 62 h (Barbain and Bartsch, 1986). On the contrary, the less common etheno-adducts are highly persistent, with half-lives of more than 30 days, which suggests that they are poorly recognized by the liver DNA repair system, and the ethenoadenine adduct is apparently not repaired at all (Swenberg et al., 1992). The ethenoadenine adducts account for the occurrence of adenine→thymine transversions observed in the p53 tumor suppressor gene in vinyl chloride-associated angiosarcomas of the liver (Fig. 13.3). P53 gene mutations in tumors or cell lines from vinly chloride exposed workers were found to contain adenine→thymine transversions at codon 179, 249, or 255 of the p53 protein (Hollstein et al., 1994; Trivers et al., 1995). These mutations result in substitution of leucine for the normal arginine at amino acid residue 179, the substitution of tryptophan for the normal arginine at amino acid residue 249, or the substitution of phenylalanine for the normal leucine at amino acid residue 255 in the coded p53 protein product (Hollstein et al., 1994; Trivers et al., 1995) (Fig. 13.3). DeVivo et al. (1994), reported a dose-response relationship between vinyl chloride exposure and the serum expression of mutant ras oncogene-encoded p21 protein, presumably produced by guanine→adenine transitions in codon 13 of the K-ras gene caused by the N^2-3-ethenoguanine vinyl chloride-DNA adduct. Together these data suggest that mutation of the p21 oncogene protein and mutant p53 tumor suppressor gene protein are important steps in the development of angiosarcoma of the liver in vinyl chloride-exposed individuals. While it is not clear why some individuals develop angiosarcoma of the liver following exposure to vinly chloride and others do not, it is possible that genetic differences in the efficiency of the liver DNA repair system may play a major role.

Arsenic: Epidemiologic and toxicological studies link human arsenic exposure to various diseases and cancer, including liver diseases and hepatocellular carcinoma. Arsenic, a metalloid, occurs naturally in the soil, water, and air. Arsenicals are by-products of production of various metals, as well as coal consumption (National Research Council, 1999). Environmental arsenic exposure has become a major human health concern due to its carcinogenic potential in multiple organs (National Research Council, 1999; Goering et al., 1999). Arsenic-induced liver toxicity in humans either from the long-term use of Fowler's solution for the treatment of psoriasis (Nevens et al., 1990; Morris et al., 1974, or through contaminated drinking water (Mazumder et al., 1998), food and air (Liu et al., 1992; Zhou, 1993; Zhou et al., 1994), typically manifests as degenerative lesions with jaundice, which often progress to non-cirrhotic portal hypertension, fibrosis, cirrhosis and liver neoplasia, including HCC (National Research Council, 1999). While liver toxicity and HCC are major health concerns in Guizhou province, China, an area of endemic arsenic poisoning, the aberrant gene expression pattern associated with arsenic-induced toxicity and carcinogenicity are not known (Lu et al., 2001).

Lu et al. (2001) reported that in liver biopsy samples obtained from patients in the Guizhou province who had a history of exposure to environmental arsenic for between 6 and 10 years showed an increase in E2F5 (a gene encoding for cell proliferation), and down-regulation of the endothelial plasminogen activator inhibitor 1 (PAI-1). A cDNA microarray performed on these arsenic exposed human liver biopsy samples showed up-regulation of genes encoding for cell proliferation (E2F3, E2F5, and E2F dimerization-partner 2). Black and Azizkhan-Clifford (1999), Muller and Helin (2000) have reported that the E2F family of transcription factors play an important role in cell cycle regulation, oncogenesis and differentiation. The transcription factor E2F plays an important role in the G_1 to S-phase transition of the cell cycle, and is dependent on its association with cyclin A/CDK2, as well as induction of cyclin E, cyclin G_1, and p19ink4 (Kato, 1999; Arata et al., 2000). However, E2F-mediated S-phase transition is not dependent on CDKN1A and CDK4 (Arata et al., 2000). Lu et al. (2001) demonstrated that cyclin A, cyclin E, cyclin G_1, and p19ink4 were all up-regulated in arsenic-exposed human livers, consistent with the hypothesis of cell cycle dysregulation. Chronic exposure of cells to arsenite has been shown to up-regulate E2F1 and the c-myc oncogene resulting in enhanced cell proliferation (Trouba et al., 2000). Similarly, Chen et al. (2000) reported dramatic up-regulation of c-myc, proliferating cell nuclear antigene (PCNA), and cyclin D1 accompanied by marked increase in cell proliferation in chronic arsenite-transforming rat liver TRL1215 cells. In contrast to the marked induction of cyclin D1 (CDKN1A) in chronic arsenite-transformed cells, CDKN1A and cell cyclin dependent kinase 4 (CDK4) were down-regulated in arsenic-exposed human livers (Lu et al., 2001). Johnson and Walker (1999) suggested that overexpression of cyclin D1 and CDK4 may be associated with overt carcinogenic events, as would occur in arsenic-induced malignant cellular transformation (Chen et al., 2001; Zhao et al., 1997).

Huang et al. (1999) have reported alterations in apoptosis-related genes in arsenic-exposed human livers. The expression of apoptosis-related genes during chronic arsenic exposure is quite different from induction of pro-apoptotic genes and initiation of apoptosis following acute arsenic exposure. The expression of caspase 3 and caspase 8, which are dramatically up-regulated during acute arsenic exposure (Akao 2000) remains unchanged in chronic arsenic-exposed human livers. Moreover caspase 4 and caspase 6 expression were down-regulated while caspase 9 and caspase 10 were up-regulated in human liver from arsenic-exposed populations. Several tumor necrosis-associated components, such as TNF (tumor necrosis factor) converting enzyme, and TNF receptor 1 (TNFR1) were also observed to be down-regulated. While TNF-related Fas ligand (FasL) and TNF1-associated death domain protein, TRADD, were down-regulated, the TNF-related apoptosis-inducing ligand, TRAIL, was not.

Arsenic has been shown to produce DNA damage, DNA protein crosslinks, micronuclei (Schaumloffel and Gebel, 1998), DNA strand breaks (Liu and Jan, 2000; Lynn et al., 1998), or alterations in DNA repair enzymes (Hartwig, 1998). Superoxide scavengers such as Cu, Zn-SOD have been reported to suppress arsenic-induced liver damage (Hartwig, 1998; Liu and Jan, 2000; Lynn et al., 1998). Lu et al. (2001) reported up-regulation of the Cu, Zn-SOD gene in livers of arsenic-exposed patients. Lang et al. (1998) have reported up-regulation of nucleotide excision repair genes such as ERCC2, ERCC5, and RAD23A suggestive of activation of the DNA repair machinery in response to arsenic-induced DNA damage. Up-regulation of human topoisomerase II (TOP2A), a key nuclear enzyme involved in DNA replication was observed in arsenic exposed human livers (Lang et al., 1998). Podust and Fanning (1997) reported that replication factor C38 (RFC38) and 40 (RFC40) were up-regulated in arsenic-exposed human livers. RFC is a complex of 5 subunits of an essential protein involved in both DNA replication and repair. Due to the close association of RFC and PCNA functioning in DNA replication, Podust and Fanning (1997) suggested that the up-regulation of RFCs and PCNA induce hyperproliferation and DNA replication in response to arsenic-induced DNA damage. Alterations in cellular regulators and growth factors such as cytokeratin-8 and cytokeratin-18 have been reported by Ramirez et al. (2000). Aberrant expression of cytokeratins in liver disease and HCC has also been reported by Omary and Ku (1997). While the exact role for the aberrant expression of these cytokeratins is not clear, Omary and Ku (1997) suggested that they could be related to liver degenerative lesions and fibrosis.

Endothelin-2 and endothelin-3 were reported to be up-regulated in arsenic-exposed human livers (Lu et al., 2001). Endothelins are potent vasoconstrictors which play a role in increasing intrahepatic vascular resistance thus contributing to portal hypertension in cirrhosis (Petrowsky et al., 1999). Indeed, higher expression of endothelin-1 and endothelin-3 was found to be associated with cirrhosis and liver fibrolamellar carcinoma in Canadian and Chinese populations (Cai et al., 1999). Lu et al. (2001) reported a dramatic down-regulation of endothelial type-1 plasminogen-activator inhibitor (PAI-1) in arsenic-exposed human livers which could have implications in arsenic toxicity and carcinogenesis. PAI-1 is a serine protease inhibitor which inactivates urokinase-type plasminogen activator (UPA) and regulates degradation of the cellular matrix. In addition, the hepatocyte growth factor (HGF), interleukin-6 receptor, and interleukin-1β were all up-regulated in human arsenic-exposed livers, consistent with possible increased cell proliferation. Overall, chronic human exposure to arsenic causes alterations in expression of genes encoding for cell cycle regulation and proliferation, the apoptosis-related genes, the DNA damage-related genes, and genes encoding for cellular regulators and growth factors. While specific alterations in genes associated with increased susceptibility to HCC has not been clearly identified, genetic polymorphism of these arsenic-induced genes may determine which individuals develop HCC and those who do not following arsenic exposure.

Oral Contraceptives and Androgenic Steroids: The liver is morphologically and functionally modulated by sex hormones. Evidence from epidemiological studies has suggested an association between HCC and the use of oral contraceptives (OCs). Long-term use of OCs and anabolic androgenic steroids (AAS) can induce both benign (hemangioma, adenoma, and focal nodular hyperplasia (FNH)) and malignant (HCC) hepatocellular tumors. Long-term use of anabolic steroids may slightly increase the risk of HCC. However, a definite relationship has not been established (ACS, 2001; London and McGlynn, 1996). Hepatic adenomas (HAs) are rare, benign neoplasm usually occurring in young women, the development and the complications of which have been related to the strength of OCs and the duration of their use (Giannitrapani et al., 2006).

Incidence of hepatic adenoma (HA) has fallen since the introduction of pills containing smaller amounts of estrogens. FNH is a benign lesion, most commonly seen in young women, which is thought to represent a local hyperplastic response of hepatocytes to a vascular abnormality. Because of the female predominance and the young age at onset, a role of female hormones has been suggested (Giannitrapani et al., 2006). Furthermore, a large proportion of women with FNH (50–75%) are OC users. Liver hemangiomas are the most common benign liver tumors and are seen more commonly in young adult females. The female predilection and clinical observations of liver hemangioma growth under conditions of estrogenic exposure suggest a possible role for estrogen in the pathogenesis of liver hemangiomas.

Many of the epidemiological studies associating OC use to HCC involved types of OCs that are not currently used. While OCs containing mestranol has been associated with increased HCC risk, it is not known if the newer oral contraceptives which contain different types and doses of estrogen and different combinations of estrogen with other hormones, significantly increase the risk of HCC (ACS, 2001). It has been speculated that long-term anabolic steroid use may slightly increase the risk of HCC, however, a definitive relationship has not been established (ACS, 2001).

OCs that contain the estrogens 17β-estradiol (E_2) and estrone (E_1) are thought to be the etiological agents responsible for HCC. Estradiol and estrone are metabolized via two major pathways: a pathway that generates catechol estrogens (CE), the 2-hydroxy estradiol and 4-hydroxy estradiol and via 16α-hydroxylation (Fig. 13.4). These two CE are mainly inactivated by O-methylation catalyzed by catechol-O-methyltransferases. While other possible conjugations of CE, such as glucuronidation and sulfation may also play a role, if production of these conjugates is inadequate, CE may be oxidized to semiquinones (CE-SQ) and quinones (CE-Q). CE-Q may conjugate with glutathione, catalyzed by S-transferase, or be reduced to CE by quinone reductase. If these two inactivating processes are inadequate, CE-2,3-Q react with DNA to form stable adducts that remain in DNA unless repaired (Dwivedy et al., 1992; Stack et al., 1996; Cavalieri et al., 1997). CE-3,4-Q, if not inactivated, react with DNA to form depurinating adducts, more specifically two rotational conformers bound to the N-7 of guanine (Gua) (Stack et al., 1996); these adducts are lost from DNA by cleavage of the glycosidic bond, leaving apurinic sites.

The primary metabolic conversion of the estrogenic hormones estrone or estradiol in liver of most mammalian species is by 2-hydroxylation (Slaunwhite et al., 1973; Martucci and Fishman, 1993). However, an elevated formation of 4-hydroxyestrogen metabolites by specific estrogen-4-hydroxylases has been detected in hamster kidney (Weisz et al., 1992), mouse uterus (Paria et al., 1990), and rat pituitary (Bui and Weisz, 1989) – all organs in which estrogens are known to induce tumors (Newbold et al., 1990, Walker and Kurth, 1993, Kirkman, 1959). The elevated formation of 4-hydroxyestrogens in rodent organs in which estrogens induce tumors is significant because catecholestrogens, including 4-hydroxyestrogens, may undergo metabolic redox cycling between hydroquinone and quinone forms. The catecholestrogen quinone intermediates may form covalent DNA adducts (Dwivedy et al., 1992; Ashburn et al., 1993; Roy and Liehr,

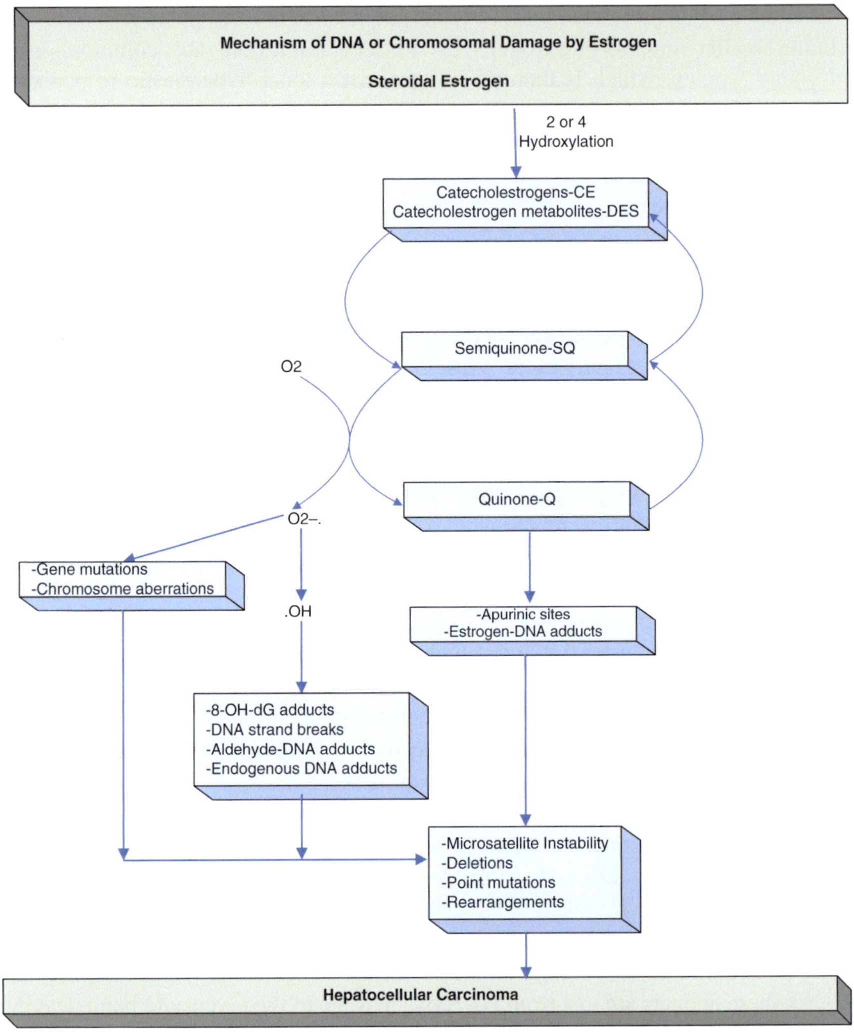

Steroidal estrogens undergo cytochrome P450-mediated hydroxylation to form catecholestrogens (CE). These catecholestrogen metabolites (DES) undergo metabolic redox cycling, which consists of oxidation to quinone (Q) and reduction of the quinone back to the CE/DES catalyzed by Cyp. P450 reductase or other reductases. The SQ formed may react with molecular oxygen to generate superoxide anion, which may be further reduced to hydroxy radical. Several types of DNA and/or chromosomal damage may occur by either estrogen quinones binding covalently to DNA or by free radical action. These DNA and chromosomal damages may lead to various types of gene mutations and finally cause hepatocellular carcinoma.

Fig. 13.4 Mechanism of DNA or chromosomal damage by estrogen

1988) (Fig. 13.4). Moreover, metabolic redox cycling generates free radicals that are capable of direct or indirect covalent modification of DNA (Liehr et al., 1986; Roy and Liehr, 1988). In support of this hypothesis, hydroxy radical damage such as 8-hydroxyguanine bases of DNA or DNA single strand breaks have been detected in the kidney of hamsters treated with estradiol (Han and Liehr, 1994, b, 1995). In addition, intranuclear, site-specific redox cycling involving catecholestrogen metabolites and copper ions may induce DNA damage by reactive oxygen, which is not mediated by metabolizing enzymes (Li et al., 1994).

The involvement of estrogens in carcinogenic processes within estrogen-responsive tissues has been recognized for a number of years. Classically, mitogenicity associated with estrogen receptor-mediated cellular events was believed to be the mechanism by which estrogens contributed to carcinogenesis. Recently, the possibility that estrogens might contribute directly to mutagenesis resulting from DNA damage has been demonstrated. That damage is apparently a result of the formation of catechol estrogens that can be further oxidized to semiquinones and quinones. Those molecules represent reactive oxygen species and electrophilic molecules that can form depurinating DNA adducts, thus having the potential to result in permanent nucleotide mutation. Conjugation of parent estrogens to sulfate and glucuronide moieties or catechol estrogens to methyl, sulfate, and glucuronide conjugates; and of catechol estrogen quinones to glutathione conjugates all represent cellular detoxification reactions that may protect the cell from estrogen induced mitogenicity and mutagenesis. The conjugation pathways of both estrogens and CEs display large inter-individual variations due to common genetic polymorphisms. Therefore, it is possible that common, inherited variations in enzymatic pathways for estrogen bioactivation or inactivation of either the parent compound or metabolites might represent individual risk factors for the occurrence of liver cancer (Raftogianis et al., 2000). Hence genetic polymorphisms of the estrogen bioactivation or inactivation enzymes are the determinants of individual susceptibility to estrogen induced HCC in humans.

While exposure to estrogen has been implicated in the induction of HCC in humans, estrogen is also known to offer protection against HCC especially in women. Men have been reported to have increased (3–5 times) HCC risk relative to women. This disparity by sex has been attributed to the ability of estrogen to inhibit secretion of interleukin-6 (IL-6) from Kupffer cells exposed to necrotic hepatocytes. By suppressing this inflammatory response pathway, estrogen may help prevent further liver injury and excessive cell proliferation that can lead to HCC (Naugler et al., 2007).

It should be noted that while the mechanism(s) of estrogen induced hepatocarcinogenesis has not been clearly elucidated in humans, in vivo studies in rodents suggest that oral contraceptive use may induce hepatocarcinogenesis in a manner similar to those observed in rodents.

Alcohol: Alcohol is an important risk factor for the development of HCC. Hepatic cirrhosis caused by chronic alcohol abuse has long been recognized as a major risk factor for the development of HCC. Chronic alcohol intake has been implicated in causing the production of pro-inflammatory cytokines through monocyte activation (McClain et al., 2002) and provoking increased concentrations of circulating bacterial endotoxin, activating Küpffer cells which release many chemokines and cytokines (including TNFα, interleukin-1β (IL1 β), IL6 and prostaglandin E_2) with adverse effects on hepatocyte survival. With chronic alcohol exposure, hepatocytes show increased sensitivity to the cytotoxic effects of TNFα (Farazi and DePinho, 2006), which sets the stage for chronic hepatocyte destruction–regeneration, stellate cell activation, cirrhosis and ultimately HCC (Fig. 13.5).

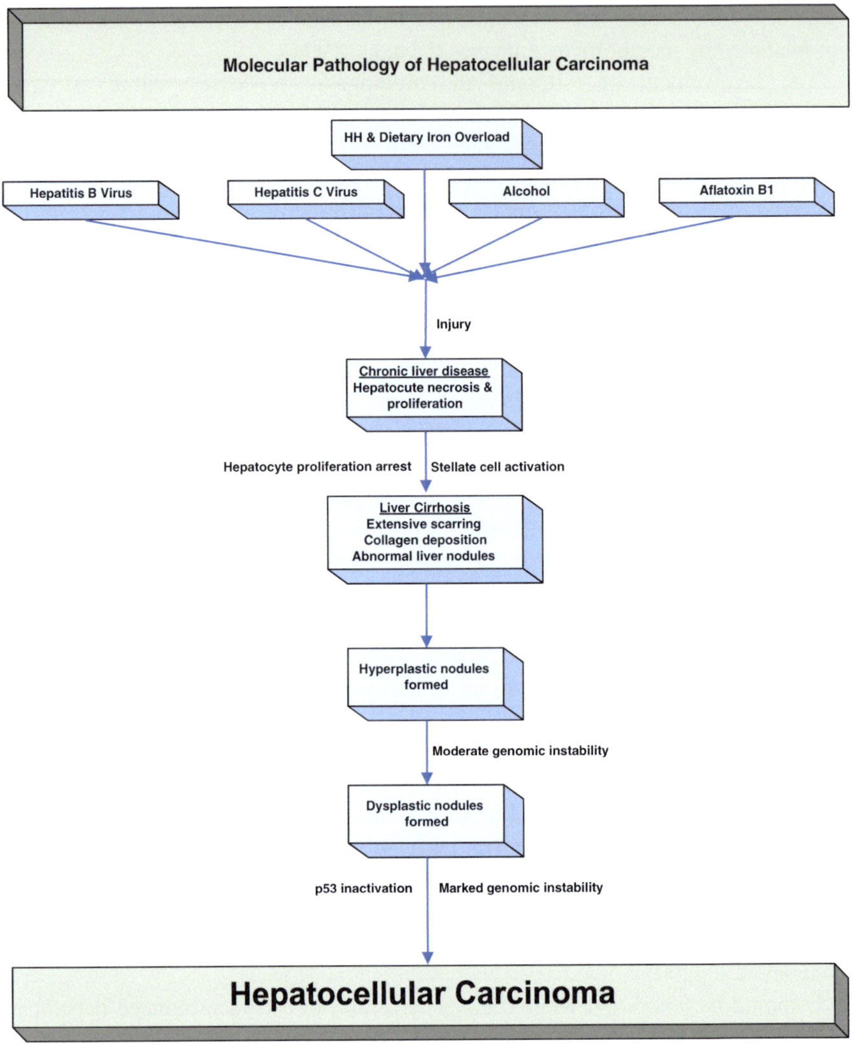

Fig. 13.5 Molecular pathology of hepatocellular carcinoma

Hepatic cirrhosis is a progressive disease that causes inflammation and scar tissue to form on the liver, which can often lead to liver cancer. It has been estimated that 60–80% of HCC cases are associated with cirrhosis. However, it is not clear if cirrhosis itself causes HCC or if the underlying causes of cirrhosis contribute to the development of the disease (Garr et al., 1997). Most cases of liver cirrhosis in the United States are due to chronic alcohol abuse, but HBV and HCV are also major causes of cirrhosis (ACS, 2001). Alcohol also damages the liver through oxidative-stress mechanisms. Alcohol induced hepatitis shows increased isoprostane, a marker of lipid peroxidation (McClain et al., 2002). Oxidative stress contributes to hepatocarcinogenesis in several ways. First, oxidative stress promotes the development of fibrosis and cirrhosis, which are key features of a permissive HCC microenvironment. The pro-carcinogenic effect of the cirrhotic microenvironment has been shown in the mouse, where PDGF transgenic mice develop fibrosis that progresses to HCC (Campbell et al., 2005). Oxidative stress might also cause accumulation of oncogenic mutations. For example, increased oxidative stress associated with hereditary haemochromatosis, an inherited metabolic disorder which causes excess iron accumulation in the liver can lead to cirrhosis (ACS, 2001). The oxidative stress together with cirrhosis and p53 mutations in hepatocytes eventually results in the development of HCC (Marrogi et al., 2001). In addition, other studies have also demonstrated that people with hemochromatosis have an increased risk of developing liver cancer (Francanzani et al., 2001). Despite the fact that chronic alcohol abuse causes cirrhosis and cirrhosis is a major risk factor for liver cancer development, it is not certain whether alcohol is a true carcinogen or if it acts as a cofactor in the presence of coexistent infection with HBV or HCV.

Hereditary Hemochromatosis (HH), Dietary Iron Overload and HCC: Recently an additional environmental hepatocarcinogen has been identified in sub-Saharan Africa namely iron overload. Dietary iron overload occurs with a prevalence of about 10% in some rural areas of sub-Saharan Africa (Gordeuk et al., 1986). It results from the consumption of large volumes over time of iron-rich traditional alcoholic beverages that are home-brewed in cast iron pots or drums. Similar to the iron storage disease, HH, the iron accumulates in its main storage organ, the liver (Bothwell and Bradlow, 1960).

HCC has long been known to occur in patients with HH, and is the most frequent cause of premature death (Niederau et al., 1985; Hsing et al., 1995; Adams, 1998). The mortality rate of HCC from this condition is estimated to be 8% (Kowdley, 2004). Cirrhosis is present in almost all patients who develop HCC. The prevalence of HCC in patients with cirrhosis is higher (18.5%) relative to that of HH patients (10.7%) without cirrhosis (Adams, 1998). Due to the close association between the presence of cirrhosis and the supervention of HCC, a general view has been held that chronic hepatic necroinflammatory disease rather than hepatic iron overload per se was responsible for the malignant transformation. This view is supported by the observation that long-term survival in HH patients in whom cirrhosis was prevented by repeated phlebotomy was comparable to that of the general population (Niederau et al., 1985; Adams et al., 1991). Moreover the risk of HCC development in HH patients with cirrhosis remained even after they had been de-ironed (Bomford and Williams, 1967). Kew and Popper (1984) stated that cirrhosis, whatever its cause is known to contribute to HCC. Comparison between incidence of HCC in HH and in other causes of cirrhosis showed the risk to be similar (Purtilo and Gottlieb, 1973; MacSween and Scott, 1973). This observation supported the belief that cirrhosis played a pivotal role in hepatocarcinogenesis in patients with HH.

Although HCC does occur, but rarely, in HH patients without cirrhosis (Blumberg et al., 1988; Deugnier and Turlin, 1998), this suggests that hepatic iron storage per se might be directly hepatocarcinogenic in addition to its indirect effect via the supervention of cirrhosis. A recent comparison between the incidence of cirrhosis in HH patients and that in other diseases revealed a higher risk of HCC development in the HH patients (Francanzani et al., 2001), suggestive of an added direct hepatocarcinogenic effect of hepatic iron accumulation. This view was also supported by reports of HCC in patients with dietary iron overload (Gordeuk et al., 1996; Moyo et al., 1996; Mandishoma et al., 1998) and of the development of iron-free preneoplastic nodules and HCC in the absence of fibrosis and cirrhosis in an animal model of dietary iron overload (Asare et al., 2006a, b).

Recent case-control studies have documented a causal association between African dietary iron overload and HCC (Gordeuk et al., 1996; Moyo et al., 1996; Mandishoma et al., 1998). In a re-analysis of the pathological material that formed the basis of Strachan's thesis, Gordeuk et al. (1996) calculated a relative risk of HCC development of 23.5 (95% CI: 2.1 and 225) in those subjects with the highest levels of hepatic iron accumulation, after allowing for the confounding effect of cirrhosis. Shortly thereafter, Moyo et al. (1998) reported a relative risk of HCC of 3.1 (95% CI: 1.05 and 9.4) in Zimbabwean Blacks with dietary iron overload, after adjusting for the confounding effects of cirrhosis. Mandishoma et al. (1998) reported a relative risk of HCC of 10.6 (95%CI: 1.5 and 76.8) and a population attributable risk of 29 in rural South African Blacks, after adjusting for the confounding effects of these other risk factors as well as the lesser risk factor in this population, chronic hepatitis C virus infection.

The mechanisms by which free or non-transferrin-bound iron induces malignant transformation have not been fully characterized. The ability of iron to function as an electron donor (Fe^{2+}) and an electron acceptor (Fe^{3+}) in most biochemical reactions also renders iron potentially toxic. Under aerobic conditions which favor the Fenton and Haber-Weiss reactions, catalytic amounts of free iron are sufficient to generate noxious hydroxyl radicals (•OH), collectively known as "reactive oxygen species" (ROS), from superoxide ($^{-}$•O2) and hydrogen peroxide. Iron accumulation thus disrupts the redox balance of the cell and generates chronic oxidative stress, which damages DNA, lipids, and protein in hepatocytes leading to both necrosis and apoptosis (Asare et al., 2006b; Meneghini, 1997; Jungst et al., 2004; Loeb et al., 1988). The resulting chronic necroinflammatory hepatic disease in turn generates further ROS and additional oxidative damage which ultimately result in cirrhosis, a preneoplastic condition (Jungst et al., 2004). Increased lipid peroxidation (LPO) has been shown to contribute to hepatocarcinogenesis in iron overload (Esterbauer et al., 1991; Esterbauer, 1993; Cheeseman, 1993; Cadenzas, 1989). Oxidative stress leads to LPO of unsaturated fatty acids in membranes of cells and organelles. This results in breaks in fatty acid chains with the insertion of hydrophobic groups and cis–trans isomerization. Cytotoxic by-products such as malondialdehyde (MDA), thiobarbituric reactive substances, and 4-hydroxy-20-nonenal (4-HNE) are produced (Esterbauer, 1993; Cadenzas, 1989; Benhar et al., 2002). LPO may also occur through autooxidation of unsaturated lipids by free radicals, the lipoxygenase pathway, or the oxidation of unsaturated lipids by non-heme iron enzymes, catalyzing dioxygenation of polyunsaturated fatty acids. In addition to participating in the initiation and propagation steps of LPO, iron is thought to be involved in β-cleavage of lipid hydroperoxides, producing biogenic aldehydes that interact with DNA to form exocyclic products. The cytotoxic and reactive aldehydic by-products of LPO impair cellular function and protein synthesis (Esterbauer, 1993; Cadenzas, 1989; Benhar et al., 2002). Furthermore, LPO products such as 4-HNE, MDA and acrolein are capable of diffusing from their production sites to more distant sites within the cell to interact with DNA, protein or protein nucleophiles. Both MDA and 4-HNE are cytotoxic as well as genotoxic (Esterbauer, 1993; Cadenzas, 1989; Benhar et al., 2002) and are implicated in carcinogenesis. 4-HNE, for example, can be further metabolized into an epoxide that can interact with DNA to form exocyclic entheno-guanine, -adenine, and -cytosine adducts. The amount of 4-HNEdG adducts significantly increases in the liver of rodents and exocyclic guanine products have been shown to be increased in rodent models of hepatocarcinogenesis (Hagen et al., 1994; Dabbagh et al., 1994).

Deoxyguanosine residues in DNA are also hydroxylated at the C8 position by •OH or singlet oxygen to form 8-hydroxy-20-deoxyguanosine (8OHdG) (Cheng et al., 1992; Ichiba et al., 2003; Kuchino et al., 1989), the major promutagenic adduct produced by ROS and which leads to G:C to T:A transversions (Cheng et al., 1992; Kuchino et al., 1989). 8OHdG also correlates with the rate of DNA unwinding and strand breaks in tissue (Cheng et al., 1992) and has been identified as a biomarker in HCC. An association between DNA unwinding and the risk of HCC formation in HH has been described (Cheng et al., 1992; Kuchino et al., 1989). It is believed that iron-induced chronic oxidative stress eventually leads to mutations in tumor suppressor genes and critical DNA repair genes. This view is supported by the increased LPO and frequency of mutations in the tumor suppressor p53 gene identified in non-tumorous liver samples from patients with HH and Wilson's disease (Vautier et al., 1999; Hussain et al., 2000) (Figs. 13.6 and 13.7).

Increased production of nitric oxide by nitric oxide synthase 2 has been demonstrated in patients with HCC complicating HH (Vadrot et al., 2006; Kim et al., 2000). Possible mechanisms of action include LPO and impaired DNA repair, all of which are important steps in hepatocarcinogenesis (Fig. 13.6).

Tobacco: The results of some epidemiological studies, notably in Japan, have claimed an association of cigarette smoking and primary liver cancer. However, the evidence is not consistent, and residual effects of HBV and HCV cannot be ruled out from the majority of these epidemiologic studies. Nevertheless, recent studies from Taiwan and China have also reported an association of cigarette smoking with liver cancer in the absence of HBV or HCV infection (Wang et al., 2003; Chen et al., 2003). Although results are not totally consistent, some case-control and cohort studies in diverse populations have implicated cigarette smoking as a causal risk factor for HCC (Yuan et al., 2004; Trichopoulos et al., 1987; Chiba et al., 1996; Hsing et al., 1990; Wang et al., 2003; Chen et al., 2003). A case-control that measured DNA adducts of 4-aminobiphenyl, a hepatic carcinogen in animals and a constituent of cigarette smoke, in liver tissues of study subjects showed a statistically significant increase in risk for HCC with increasing levels of adducts (Wang et al., 1998). Because cigarette smoking is a major source of exposure to 4-aminobiphenyl in humans (Yu and Yuan, 2004) this molecular epidemiologic study has strengthened the notion that tobacco smoke is a hepatic carcinogen in humans.

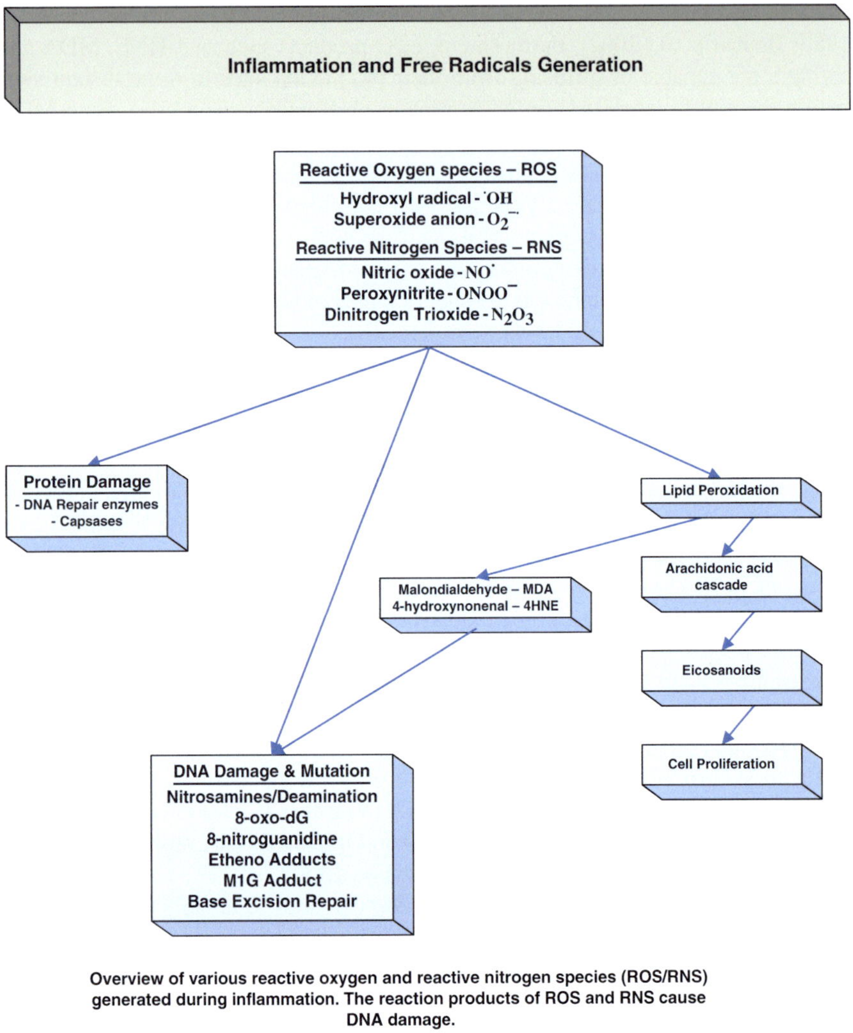

Fig. 13.6 Overview of various reactive oxygen and reactive nitrogen species generated during inflammation

13.1.3 Family History and the Risk of Liver Cancer

A case control study that investigated the relationship between family history and hepatocellular carcinoma and primary liver cancer in first-degree relatives in Italy found significant associations between family history of hepatocellular carcinoma and primary liver cancer [relative risk (RR) = 2.4; 95% confidence interval (CI), 1.3 to 4.4]. The elevated risk of liver cancer associated with family history was not modified by adjustment for tobacco, alcohol, and personal history of cirrhosis and

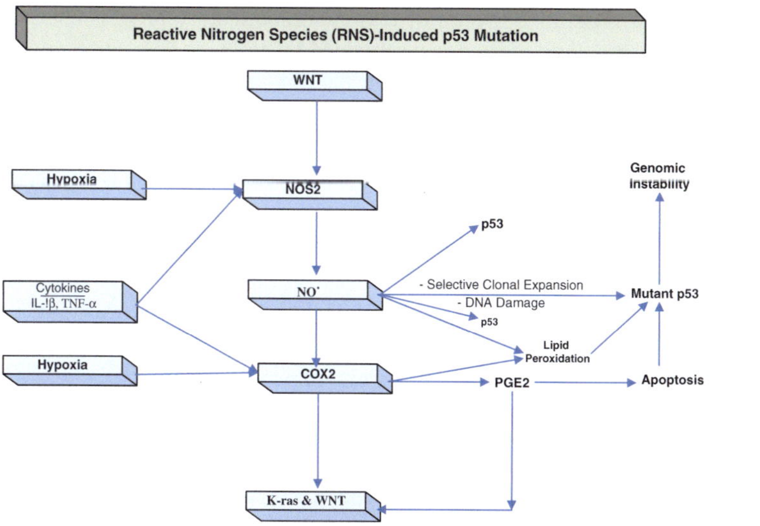

Scheme of the interactive pathways in RNS-induced p53 mutation. NOS2 and COX2 are positively regulated by hypoxia, proinflammatory cytokines, and the WNT signal transduction pathway. NOS2 generates a high concentration of NO that can both damage DNA to induce mutations in cancer-related genes, for example, p53, and induce p53-dependent cell cycle arrest and apoptosis, so that cells containing mutated p53 attain selective clonal growth and survival advantages. NOS2 can physically bind COX2 and activate it by nitrosylation. COX2 can increase lipidperoxidation to generate unsaturated aldehydes that can induce p53 mutations, and increase PGE2 concentrations. PGE2 can attenuate p53-mediated apoptosis and activate the WNT pathway, resulting in increased b-catenin that with TCF-4, transcriptionally activates NOS2 and COX2. High amounts of p53 can participate in negative feedback loops in the regulation of NOS2 and COX2. Lesser amounts of p53 can enhance COX2 accumulation.

Fig. 13.7 Scheme of interactive pathways in reactive nitrogen species-induced TP53 mutation

hepatitis (RR = 2.9; 95% CI, 1.5 to 5.3). The relative risk suggests the existence of a genetic component in the familial aggregation of liver cancer. In terms of population attributable risk, approximately 3% of the newly diagnosed liver cancers could be attributed to this familial component (Fernandez et al., 1994).

13.1.4 Summary of the Diverse Molecular Mechanisms of Hepatocarcinogenesis

The diverse molecular mechanisms of hepatocarcinogenesis share some common pathogenic pathways. A consistent event observed in HBV-, HCV- and aflatoxin-B_1-induced HCC is p53 mutation or inactivation. In addition, inflammation, continuous cycles of necrosis and regeneration and oxidative stress are characteristic of HCV-, HBV- and alcohol-induced hepatocarcinogenesis indicating that these processes contribute to the development of HCC. The molecular mechanisms of hepatocarcinogenesis are illustrated in Fig. 13.1.

Hepatic injury induced by any of the several environmental factors/etiological agents (HBV, HCV, aflatoxin B1, alcohol) leads to necrosis followed by hepatocyte proliferation/hyperplasia. A continuous cycle of this necrotic-regenerative process promotes the development of chronic liver disease which culminates in hepatic cirrhosis. Cirrhosis is the result of chronic inflammatory process characterized by abnormal liver nodule formation surrounded by collagen deposition and scarring of the liver. Additional cellular insults to the abnormal liver nodule lead to the formation of hyperplastic nodules followed by dysplastic nodules and finally HCC. Telomerase reactivation associated with carcinogenesis in general has been associated with hepatocarcinogenesis as well. Hepatocarcinogenesis is also characterized by mutation or inactivation of p53 and genomic instability, as shown in Fig. 13.5.

Chronic inflammation and infection are often associated with increased cancer risk, however, exceptions such as rheumatoid arthritis and human papillomavirus infection (Hussain et al., 2003) exist. Infection with HBV, HCV, and chronic alcohol consumption cause inflammation with the release of chemokines, cytokines and free radicals resulting in DNA damage, cell proliferation, fibrosis and angiogenesis. The p53 pathway plays a key role during inflammatory stress (Staib et al., 2005). Free radicals such as reactive nitrogen species (RNS) and reactive oxygen species (ROS) generated during inflammation directly damage DNA and proteins. They also cause indirect damage to these macromolecules via lipid peroxidation (Fig. 13.6). The p53 pathway responds to lower levels of DNA damage by cell cycle checkpoint arrest, facilitating DNA repair as an adapter in the formation of DNA repair protein complexes and transcriptional transactivation of DNA repair genes (Sengupta and Harris, 2005). Response to extensive DNA damage is mediated through cell death. P53 contributes to these processes by switching from increased expression of anti- to pro-oxidant genes. P53 can transcriptionally repress pro-oxidant/nitrosative genes such as nitric oxide synthase (NOS), and transactivate anto-oxidant genes expressing glutathione peroxidase, aldehyde dehydrogenase and Mn-superoxide dismutase, sestrins and TIGAR (TP53-induced glycolysis and apoptosis) (Fig. 13.7).

Hussain et al. (2007) proposed a model of interactive pathways of nitrosative-stress-induced TP53 mutation. Nitric oxide (NO•), an important bioregulatory signaling molecule play a significant role in carcinogenesis (Nathan and Xie, 1994; Bredt and Snyder, 1994). NO• is catalyzed by the NOS family of enzymes (NOS1, NOS2, NOS3). The isoforms NOS1 and NOS3 are constitutively expressed whereas NOS2 requires induction. Bacterial endotoxin, proinflammatory cytokines or hypoxia induce NOS2 gene expression (Lombard and Guarente, 2000) in many cell types including hepatocytes (Lombard and Guarente, 2000) as well as a variety of human tumors (Ambs et al., 1997). The upregulation of certain proinflammatory cytokines such as tumor necrosis factor-α (TNF-α) and interferon-γ (IFN-γ) have been repeatedly demonstrated during chronic viral hepatitis (Mihm et al., 1996; Gonzalez-Amaro et al., 1994). These proinflammatory cytokines TNF-α, IFN-γ and IL-1 induce NOS2 gene expression which leads to increased NO• concentration in human hepatocytes (Laskin et al., 1998). In addition, NOS2 is also induced directly by HBV and HCV. This is supported by a consistent upregulation of hepatic NOS2 observed in patients with HBV or HCV infection (Kane et al., 1997).

It has been shown that NO•-related DNA damage leads to p53 accumulation and p53-mediated apoptosis (Hussain et al., 2007; Forrester et al., 1996) (Fig. 13.7). Reports have been published indicating that p53 is a transcriptional transrepressor of NOS2 expression in vivo and attenuates excessive NO• production in a regulatory negative feedback loop (Forrester et al., 1996; Ambs et al., 1998b; Hussain et al., 2001). NO• also activates the arachidonic acid pathway by enhancing the enzymatic activity of cyclooxygenase 2 (COX2) (Fig. 13.7). The mechanism of COX2 activation is by NOS2 binding and nitrosylation of COX2 (Kim et al., 2005). Increased COX2 activity then causes the release of prostaglandin E2 (PGE2). PGE2 suppresses the apoptotic pathway and activates the WNT pathway (Castellone et al., 2005; Buchanan and DuBois, 2006). The WNT signal transduction and COX2 pathways play key roles hepatocarcinogenesis (Thorgeirsson and Grisham, 2002). The WNT pathway can also transcriptionally activate both NOS2 and COX2 by T-cell factor (TCF)4-b-catenin binding to positive response elements in their promoters (Araki et al., 2003; Du et al., 2006). Therefore, the NOS2 and COX2 are concomitantly activated by pro-inflammatory cytokines, hypoxia and the WNT pathway. The WNT pathway is frequently activated in HCC associated with high AFB1 exposure (Devereux et al., 2001). COX2 activity is amplified by nitrosylation following its physical interaction with NOS2. NO• can both damage DNA to induce the anticarcinogenic p53 stress response pathway and mutate cancer-related genes including p53. PGE2 attenuates apoptosis (Gupta and DuBois, 2001), which may allow survival of hepatocytes with DNA damage and increase the probability of somatic mutations. As NO•-induced apoptosis can be p53 dependent, cells with mutant p53 have a clonal expansion advantage. Consistent with this model, a significant association as well as a dose-response relationship between p53 mutations (G:C to A:T transition at cytosine guanine dinucleotide (CpG) sites) and an increased NOS2 activity in patients with colon cancer has been observed (Ambs et al., 1999). Furthermore a positive association of NOS2 expression and a comparable p53 mutational spectrum in lung cancer has been demonstrated (Fujimoto et al., 1998; Ambs et al., 1998a). This p53 mutation spectrum is consistent with increased rates of N_2O_3-induced deamination of 5-methylation at CpG sites. In summary, oxidative/nitrosative stress, mediated by free radicals, which is also induced by the cytokine profile of various inflammatory hepatic disorders like HBV and HCV infection, or hemochromatosis, can act as an endogenous carcinogen to induce p53 mutations and provide a microenvironment allowing a clonal growth advantage for cells with p53 mutations.

13.1.5 Biomarkers of Susceptibility to Liver Cancer

Molecular epidemiologic research continues to provide compelling new evidence that environmental factors are the major contributors to human cancer and that their risks are strongly influenced by genetic and acquired susceptibility. At present, many biomarkers exist that are useful in assessing exposure, dose and potential risk for a population. However, these biomarkers are not sufficiently characterized with regards to their ability to predict disease for use in screening, diagnosis, or quantitate individual risk (Perera, 1996). Biomarkers of susceptibility are lacking for most

Table 13.1 The interaction of environmental agents with genetic polymorphisms that predispose to liver cancer. Prevalence among controls and HCC cases and estimate of HCC risk

Agent	Genes	Genotype	# of Cases	# of Controls	OR (95% CI) for HCC Risk	References
Vinyl chloride	P53 gene K-ras gene	–	8	3667	4.5 (1.5–13.3)	Du and Wang (1998) DeVivo et al. (1994)
Oral contraceptives	No specific genes have been identified	–	148	1086	0.75 (0.54–1.03)	MILTS (1997)
Hepatitis B	No specific genes have been identified	–	216	408	16.7 (9.7–28.7)	Kirk et al. (2004)
Hepatitis C	No specific genes have been identified	–	216	408	16.7 (6.9–40.1)	Kirk et al. (2004)
Aflatoxin B1	*GSTM1*	Present	105	218	1	Kirk et al. (2005)
		Null	44	76	2.45 (1.21–4.95)	
	GSTT1	Present	79	162	1	
		Null	70	132	1.11 (0.61–2.05)	
	*HLY1*2*	YY	104	215	1	
		YH	36	66	1.28 (0.62–2.67)	
		HH	9	13	2.83 (0.77–10.4)	
	XRRC1-399G	AA	120	248	1	
		AG	26	43	3.18 (1.35–7.50)	
		GG	3	3	0.48 (0.04–5.50)	
Tobacco	No specific genes have been identified	–	105	37	6.5 (1.6–26.5)	Wang et al. (1998)

environmental factors that contribute to HCC. Therefore, only the currently known biomarkers of susceptibility for some of the environmental agents are discussed in this chapter.

Multivariate analysis of the Gambian Liver Cancer Study (GLCS) showed a modest increase in HCC risk associated with one of the primary enzymes responsible for AFB_1 detoxification (Kirk et al., 2005, 2006). Individuals who were homozygous or heterozygous for the G allele in the 399 locus of the XRCC1

DNA repair enzyme, associated with increased AFB_1-DNA adduct levels also displayed an increase risk of HCC (Lunn et al., 1999; Kirk et al., 2005). A trend of increased HCC risk was observed with XRCC1-399G polymorphism in a study from Taiwan. Strong associations were observed among subjects with both XRCC1 variants and the null GSTT1 (Glutathione S-transferase Theta 1) genotype (Yu et al., 2003). Kirk et al. (2005) also identified a greater than additive effect on HCC risk with the DNA repair variant in combination with polymorphisms in several aflatoxin detoxifying enzymes including GSTM1 (Glutathione S-transferase Mu 1) and HYL1 (Microsomal epoxide hydrolase 1). Genetic polymorphisms of AFB_1 metabolizing/detoxifying enzymes [the null GSTM1, GSTT1, HYL1 and DNA repair enzymes (e.g. XRCC1)] determine the susceptibility of individuals to HCC following exposure to aflatoxin (Table 13.1).

The most widely used biomarker to demonstrate susceptibility to HCC following infection with HBV has been the α-fetoprotein (AFP). AFP L3 (fucosylated AFP), a slightly different version of AFP, is the only biomarker currently approved by the FDA to predict susceptibility to liver cancer (Benowitz, 2007). Scientists have found that levels of fucosylated proteins were higher in HBV patients who had HCC relative to controls or HBV-infected patients who did not have liver cancer (Cottingham, 2009). Thus AFP L3 is the biomarker of susceptibility to HCC following infection with the HBV.

References

Adams, P. C. 1998. Hepatocellular carcinoma in hereditary hemochromatosis. Can. J. Gastroenterol. 129:946–995.

Adams, P. C., Speechley, M., Kertesz, A. E. 1991. Long-term survival analysis in hereditary hemochromatosis. Gastroenterology 101:368–372.

Akao, T. 2000. Competition in the metabolism of glycyrrhizin with glycyrrhetic acid monoglucuronide by mixed Eubacterium sp. GLH and Ruminococcus sp. PO1-3. Biol. Pharm. Bull. 23:149–154.

Ambs, S., Bennett, W. P., Merriam, W. G., Ogunfusika, M. O., Oser, S. M., Harrington, A. M., Shields, P. G., Felley-Bosco, E., Hussain, S. P., Harris, C. C. 1999. Relationship between p53 mutations and inducible nitric oxide synthase expression in human colorectal cancer. J. Natl. Cancer Inst. 91:86–88.

Ambs, S., Bennett, W. P., Merriam, W. G., Ogunfusika, M. O., Oser, S. M., Khan, A. et al. 1998a. Vascular endothelial growth factor and nitric oxide synthase expression in human lung cancer and the relation to p53. Br. J. Cancer 78:233–239.

Ambs, S., Bennett, W. P., Merriam, W. G., Ogunfusika, M. O., Oser, S. M., Khan, M. A., Ambs, S., Hussain, S. P., Harris, C. C. 1997. Interactive effects of nitric oxide and the p53 tumor suppressor gene in carcinogenesis and tumor progression. FASEB J. 11:443–448.

Ambs, S., Ogunfusika, M. O., Merriam, W. G., Bennett, W. P., Billiar, T. R., Harris, C. C. 1998b. Upregulation of NOS2 expression in cancer-prone p53 knockout mice. Proc. Natl. Acad. Sci. U.S.A. 95:8823–8828.

American Cancer Society (ACS). 2001. Cancer facts and figures. Liver cancer. American Cancer Society, Atlanta, GA.

Araki, Y., Okamura, S., Hussain, S. P., Nagashima, M., He, P., Shiseki, M., Miura, K., Harris, C. C. 2003. Regulation of cyclooxygenase-2 expression by the wnt and ras pathways. Cancer Res. 63:728–734.

Arata, Y., Fujita, M., Ohtani, K., Kijima, S., Kato, J. Y. 2000. Cdk2-dependent and -independent pathways in E2F-mediated S-phase induction. J. Biol. Chem. 275:6337–6345.

Asare, G. A., Mossanda, K. S., Kew, M. C., Paterson, A. C., Kahler-Venter, C. P., Siziba, K. 2006a. Hepatocellular carcinoma caused by iron overload: a possible mechanism of direct hepatocarcinogenicity. Toxicology 219:41–52.

Asare, G. A., Paterson, A. C., Kew, M. C., Khan, S., Mossanda, K. S. 2006b. Iron-free neoplastic nodules and hepatocellular carcinoma without cirrhosis in Wistar rats fed a diet high in iron. J. Pathol. 208:82–90.

Ashburn, S. P., Han, X., Liehr, J. G. 1993. Microsomal hydroxylation of 2- and 4-fluoroestradiol to catechol metabolites and their conversion to methyl ethers: catechol estrogens as possible mediators of hormonal carcinogenesis. Mol. Pharmacol. 43:534–541.

ASTDR. 1993. U. S. Public Health Service. Toxicological profile for vinyl chloride (update). Atlanta, GA. U. S. Public Health Service. (DHHS Publication No. TP–92/20).

ASTDR. 1997. Toxicological profile of vinyl chloride. Update (Final Report). NTIS Accession No. P898101132. Atlanta, GA, pp. 274.

Barbain, A., Bartsch, M. 1986. Mutagenic and promutagenic properties of DNA adducts formed by vinyl chloride metabolites. In The role of cyclic nucleic acid adducts in carcinogenesis and mutagenesis, vol. 70. Singer, B. and Bartsch, H. eds. International Agency for Research on Cancer, Lyons, pp. 345–358.

Benhar, M., Engelberg, D., Levitzki, A. 2002. Reactive oxygen stress, stress activated kinases and stress signalling in cancer. EMBO Rep. 3:420–425.

Benn, J., Schneider, R. J. 1994. Hepatitis B virus HBx protein activates Ras-GTP complex formation and establishes a Ras, Raf, MAP kinase signaling cascade. Proc. Natl. Acad. Sci. U.S.A. 91:10350–10354.

Benn, J., Schneider, R. J. 1995. Hepatitis B virus HBx protein deregulates cell cycle checkpoint controls. Proc. Natl. Acad. Sci. U.S.A. 92(24):11215–11219.

Benowitz, S. 2007. Liver Cancer Biomarkers Struggling to Succeed. JNCI News 99(8):590–591.

Black, A. R., Azizkhan-Clifford, J. 1999. Regulation of E2F: A family of transcription factors involved in proliferation control. Gene 237:281–302.

Block, T. M., Mehta, A. S., Fimmel, C. J., Jordan, R. 2003. Molecular viral oncology of hepatocellular carcinoma. Oncogene 22:5093–5107.

Blumberg, R. S., Chopra, S., Ibrahim, R., Crawford, J., Farraye, Y., Zeldis, J., Berman, M. 1988. Primary hepatocellular carcinoma in idiopathic hemochromatosis: occurrence in non-cirrhotic patients. Gastroenterology 95:1399–1402.

Bomford, A., Williams, R. 1967. Long-term results of venesection therapy in idiopathic hemochromatosis. Quart. J. Med. 45:611–623.

Bothwell, T. H., Bradlow, B. A. 1960. Siderosis in the Bantu: a combined histopathological and chemical study. Arch. Path. 70:279–292.

Brand, N., Petkovich, M., Krust, A., Chambon, P., de Thé, H., Marchio, A., Tiollais, P., Dejean, A. 1988. Identification of a second human retinoic acid receptor. Nature 332: 850–853.

Bredt, D. S., Snyder, S. H. 1994. Nitric oxide: a physiologic messenger molecule. Annu. Rev. Biochem. 63:175–195.

Buchanan, F. G., DuBois, R. N. 2006. Connecting COX-2 and Wnt in cancer. Cancer Cell 9: 6–8.

Buetow, K. H., Murray, J. C., Israel, J. L., London, W. T., Smith, M., Kew, M., Blanquet, V., Brechot, C., Redeker, A., Gonvindarajah, S. 1989. Loss of heterozygosity suggests tumor suppressor gene responsible for primary hepatocellular carcinoma. Proc. Natl. Acad. Sci. U.S.A. 86:8852–8856.

Bui, Q. D., Weisz, J. 1989. Monooxygenase mediating catecholestrogen formation by rat anterior pituitary is an estrogen-4-hydroxylase. Endocrinology 124:1085–1087.

Cadenzas, E. 1989. Biochemistry of oxygen toxicity. Annu. Rev. Biochem. 58:79–110.

Cai, L., Wang, G. J., Mukherjee, K., Xu, Z. L., Khalil, M., Cherian, M. G., Chakrabarti, S. 1999. Endothelins and their receptors in cirrhotic and neoplastic livers of Canadian and Chinese populations. Anticancer Res. 19:2243–2247.

Campbell, J. S., Hughes, S. D., Gilbertson, D. G., Palmer, T. E., Holdren, M. S., Haran, A. C., Odell, M. M., Bauer, R. L., Ren, H. P., Haugen, H. S., Yeh, M. M., Fausto, N. 2005. Platelet-derived growth factor C induces liver fibrosis, steatosis, and hepatocellular carcinoma. Proc. Natl. Acad. Sci. U.S.A. 102:3389–3394.

Caselmann, W. H. 1995. Transactivation of cellular gene expression by hepatitis B viral proteins: a possible molecular mechanism of hepatocarcinogenesis. J. Hepatol. 22:34–37.

Castellone, M. D., Teramoto, H., Williams, B. O., Druey, K. M., Gutkind, J. S. 2005. Prostaglandin E2 promotes colon cancer cell growth through a Gs-axin-beta-catenin signaling axis. Science. 310:1504–1510.

Cavalieri, E. L., Stack, D. E., Devanesan, P. D., Todorovic, R., Dwivedy, I., Higginbotham, S., Johansson, S. L., Patil, K. D., Gross, M. L., Gooden, J. K., Ramanathan, R., Cerny, R. L., Rogan, E. G. 1997. Molecular origin of cancer: catechol estrogen-3,4-quinones as endogenous tumor initiators. Proc. Natl. Acad. Sci. U.S.A. 94(20):10937–10942.

Cheeseman, K. H. 1993. Lipid peroxidation in cancer. In DNA and free radicals. Halliwell, B., and Arouma, A. I. Eds. Ellis Horwood, London, pp. 109–144.

Chen, Z. M., Liu, B. Q., Boreham, J., Wu, Y. P., Chen, J. S., Peto, R. 2003. Smoking and liver cancer in China: case-control comparison of 36,000 liver cancer deaths vs. 17,000 cirrhosis deaths. Int. J. Cancer 107(1):106–112.

Chen, H., Liu, J., Merrick, A., Waalkes, M. P. 2000. Genetic events associated with arsenite-induced malignant transformation: application of cDNA microarray technology. Mol. Carcinog. 30:75–87.

Chen, H., Liu, J., Merrick, B. A., Waalkes, M. P. 2001. Genetic events associated with arsenic-induced malignant transformation: applications of cDNA microarray technology. Mol. Carcinogen. 30:80–87.

Cheng, K. C., Cahill, D. S., Kasai, H., Nishimura, S., Loeb, L. A. 1992. 8-Hydroxyl guanine, an abundant form of oxidative DNA damage, causes G-T and A-C substitutions. J. Biol. Chem. 267:166–172.

Chiba, T., Matsuzaki, Y., Abei, M., Shoda, J., Tanaka, N., Osuga, T., Aikawa, T. 1996. The role of previous hepatitis B virus infection and heavy smoking in hepatitis C virus-related hepatocellular carcinoma. Am. J. Gastroenterol. 91:1195–1203.

Chou, M. W., Chen, W. 1997. Food Restriction Reduces Aflatoxin B_1 (AFB_1)-DNA Adduct Formation, AFB_1-Glutathione Conjugation, and DNA Damage in AFB_1-Treated Male F344 Rats and $B6C3F_1$ Mice. The Journal of Nutrition. 127(2):210–217.

Cottingham, K. 2009. Candidate biomarkers for liver cancer. J. Proteom. Res. 8(2):428.

Dabbagh, A. J., Mannion, T., Lynch, S. M., Frei, B. 1994. The effect of iron overload on rat plasma and liver oxidant status in vivo. Biochem. J. 300:799–803.

DeVivo, I., Marion, M. J., Smith, S. J., Carney, W. P., Brandt-Rauf, P. W. 1994. Mutant c-Ki-ras p21 protein in chemical carcinogenes is in humans exposed to vinyl chloride. Cancer Causes Control 5:273–278.

Deugnier, Y., Turlin, B. 1998. Iron and neoplasia. J. Hepatol. 28:21–25.

Devereux, T. R., Stern, M. C., Flake, G. P., Yu, M. C., Zhang, Z. Q., London, S. J., Taylor, J. A. 2001. CTNNB1 mutations and betacatenin protein accumulation in human hepatocellular carcinomas associated with high exposure to aflatoxin B1. Mol. Carcinog. 31:68–73.

Du, Q., Park, K. S., Guo, Z., He, P., Nagashima, M., Shao, L., Sahai, R., Geller, D. A., Hussain, S. P. 2006. Regulation of human nitric oxide synthase 2 expression by Wnt beta-catenin signaling. Cancer Res. 66:7024–7031.

Du, C. L., Wang, J. D. 1998. Increased morbidity odds ratio of primary liver cancer and cirrhosis of the liver among vinyl chloride monomer workers. Occup. Environ. Med. 55:528–532.

Dwivedy, I., Devanesan, P., Cremonesi, P., Rogan, E., Cavalieri, E. S. 1992. ynthesis and characterization of estrogen 2,3- and 3,4-quinones. Comparison of DNA adducts formed by the

quinones versus horseradish peroxidase-activated catechol estrogens. Chem. Res. Toxicol. 5: 828–833.
Eaton, D. L., Gallagher, E. P. 1994. Mechanisms of aflatoxin carcinogenesis. Annu. Rev. Pharmacol. Toxicol. 34:135–172.
El-Serag, H. B. 2001. Epidemiology of hepatocellular carcinoma. Clin. Liver Dis. 5(1):87–107.
El-Serag, H. B., Mason, A. C. 2000. Risk factors for the rising rates of primary liver cancer in the United States. Arch. Intern. Med. 160:3227–3230.
Elmore, L., Hancock, A., Chang, S. F., Wang, X., Chang, S., Callahan, C., Geller, D., Will, H., Harris, C. C. 1997. Hepatitis B virus X protein and p53 tumor suppressor interactions in the modulation of apoptosis. Proc. Natl. Acad. Sci. U.S.A. 94:14707–14712.
Esterbauer, H. 1993. Cytotoxicity and genotoxicity of lipid-oxidation products. Am. J. Clin. Nutr. 57(Suppl.):779–860.
Esterbauer, H., Schaur, R. J., Zollner, H. 1991. Chemistry and biochemistry of 4-hydroxynonenal, malondialdehyde and related aldehydes. Free Radic. Biol. Med. 11(1):81–128.
Farazi, P. A., DePinho, R. A. 2006. Hepatocellular carcinoma pathogenesis: from genes to environment. Nat. Rev. Cancer 6:674–687; Source of Figures 4 and 5.
Fernandez, E., La Vecchia, C., D'Avanzo, B., Negri, E., Franceschi, S. 1994. Family history and the risk of liver, gallbladder, and pancreatic cancer. Cancer Epidemiol. Biomarkers Prev. 3(3): 209–212.
Forrester, K., Ambs, S., Lupold, S. E., Kapust, R. B., Spillare, E. A., Weinberg, W. C., Felley-Bosco, E., Wang, X. W., Geller, D. A., Tzeng, E., Billiar, T. R., Harris, C. C. 1996. Nitric oxide-induced p53 accumulation and regulation of inducible nitric oxide synthase (NOS2) expression by wild-type p53. Proc. Natl. Acad. Sci. U.S.A. 93:2442–2447.
Foy, E., Li, K., Sumpter, R., Loo, Y. M., Johnson, C. L., Wang, C., Fish, P. M., Yoneyama, M., Fujita, T., Lemon, S. M., Gale, M. 2005. Control of antiviral defenses through hepatitis C virus disruption of retinoic acid-inducible gene-I signaling. Proc. Natl. Acad. Sci. U.S.A. 102: 2986–2991.
Francanzani, A. L., Conte, D., Fraquelli, M., Taioli, E., Mattioli, M., Losco, A., Fargioni, S. 2001. Increased cancer risk in a cohort of 230 patients with hereditary hemochromatosis in comparison to matched control patients with non-iron-related chronic liver disease. Hepatology 33:647–665.
Fujimori, M., Tokino, T., Hino, O., Kitagawa, T., Imamura, T., Okamoto, E., Mitsunobu, M., Ishikawa, T., Nakagawa, H., Harada, H., Yagura, M., Matsubara, K., Nakamura, Y. 1991. Allelotype study of primary hepatocellular carcinoma. Cancer Res. 51:89–93.
Fujimoto, H., Sasaki, J., Matsumoto, M., Suga, M., Ando, Y., Iggo, R., Tada, M., Saya, H., Ando, M. 1998. Significant correlation of nitric oxide synthase activity and p53 gene mutation in stage I lung adenocarcinoma. Jpn. J. Cancer Res. 89:696–702.
Garr, B. I., Flickinger, J. C., Lotze, M. T. 1997. Cancer of the liver. In Principles and practice of oncology, 5th Edition. Devita, T., Hellman, S., and Rosenberg, S. eds. Lippincott-Raven Publishers, Philadelphia, PA, pp. 1271–1297.
Giannitrapani, L., Soresi, M., La Spada, E., Cervello, M., D'alessandro, N., Montalto, G. 2006. Sex hormones and risk of liver tumor. Ann. N. Y. Acad. Sci. 1089(1):228–236.
Goering, P. L., Aposhian, H. V., Mass, M. J., Cebrian, M., Beck, B. D., Waalkes, M. P. 1999. The enigma of arsenic carcinogenesis: role of metabolism. Toxicol. Sci. 49:5–14.
Gonzalez-Amaro, R., Garcia-Monzon, C., Garcia-Buey, L., Moreno-Otero, R., Alonso, J. L., Yague, E., Pivel, J. P., Lopez-Cabrera, M., Fernandez-Ruiz, E., Sanchez-Madrid, F. 1994. Induction of tumor necrosis factor alpha production by human hepatocytes in chronic viral hepatitis. J. Exp. Med. 179:841–848.
Gordeuk, V. R., Boyd, R. D., Brittenham, G. H. 1986. Dietary iron overload persists in sub-Saharan Africa. Lancet 1:1310–1313.
Gordeuk, V. R., McLaren, C. E., MacPhail, A. P., Deichsel, D., Bothwell, T. H. 1996. Associations of iron overload in Africa and hepatocellular carcinoma and tuberculosis. Blood 87: 3476–3479.

Greenblatt, M. S., Bennett, W. P., Hollstein, M., Harris, C. C. 1994. Mutations in the p53 tumor suppressor gene: clues to cancer etiology and molecular pathogenesis. Cancer Res. 54: 4855–4878.

Gupta, R. A., DuBois, R. N. 2001. Colorectal cancer prevention and treatment by inhibition of cyclooxygenase-2. Nat. Rev. Cancer 1:11–21.

HSDB. 2003. Hazardous Substances Database. Vinyl chloride. National Library of Medicine. Last updated: 8/29/03.

Hagen, T. M., Huang, S., Curnutte, J., Fowler, P., Martinez, V., Wehr, C. M., Ames, B. N., Chisari, F. V. 1994. Extensive oxidative DNA damage in hepatocytes of transgenic mice with chronic active hepatitis destined to develop hepatocellular carcinoma. Proc. Natl. Acad. Sci. U.S.A. 91:12808–12812.

Han, X., Liehr, J. G. 1994. 8-Hydroxylation of guanine bases in kidney and liver DNA of hamsters treated with estradiol: role of free radicals in estrogen-induced carcinogenesis. Cancer Res. 54:5155–5157.

Han, X., Liehr, J. G. 1994. DNA single strand breaks in kidneys of Syrian hamsters treated with steroidal estrogens. Hormone-induced free radical damage preceding renal malignancy. Carcinogenesis 15:997–1000.

Han, X., Liehr, J. G. 1995. Microsome-mediated 8-hydroxylation of guanine bases of DNA by steroid estrogens: correlation of DNA damage by free radicals with metabolic activation to quinones. Carcinogenesis 16:2571–2574.

Hartwig, A. 1998. Carcinogenicity of metal compounds: possible role of DNA repair inhibition. Toxicol. Lett. 102–103:235–239.

Henderson, A. S., Ripley, S., Hino, O., Rogler, C. E. 1988. Identification of a chromosomal aberration associated with a hepatitis B DNA integration site in human cells. Cancer Genet. Cytogenet. 30:269–275.

Hino, O., Ohtake, K., Rogler, C. E. 1989. Features of two hepatitis B virus (HBV) DNA integrations suggest mechanisms of HBV integration. J. Virol. 63:2638–2643.

Hino, O., Shows, T. B., Rogler, C. E. 1986. Hepatitis B virus integration site in hepatocellular carcinoma at chromosome 17:18 translocation. Proc. Natl. Acad. Sci. U.S.A. 83(21): 8338–8342.

Hino, O., Tabatat, S., Hottat, Y. 1991. Evidence for increased in vitro recombination with insertion of human hepatitis B virus DNA. Proc. Natl. Acad. Sci. U.S.A. 88:9248–9252.

Hollstein, M., Marion, M. -J., Lehman, T., Welsh, J., Harris, C. C., Martel-Planche, G., Kuster, I., Montesano, R. 1994. *p*53 mutations at A: T base pairs in angiosarcomas of vinyl-chloride-exposed factory workers. Carcinogenesis 15:1–3.

Hsing, A. W., McLaughlin, J. K., Hrubec, Z., Blot, W. J., Fraumeni, J. F., Jr. 1990. Cigarette smoking and liver cancer among US veterans. Cancer Causes Control 1:217–221.

Hsing, A. W., McLaughlin, J. K., Olsen, S. H., Mellemkjar, L., Waholder, S., Fraumeni, J. F. 1995. Cancer risk following primary hemochromatosis: a population-based cohort study in Denmark. Int. J. Cancer 60:60–162.

Huang, X. J., Wiernik, P. H., Klein, R. S., Gallagher, R. E. 1999. Arsenic trioxide induces apoptosis of myeloid leukemia cells by activation of caspases. Med. Oncol. 16:58–64.

Hussain, S. P., Hofseth, L. J., Harris, C. C. 2001. Tumor suppressor genes: at the crossroads of molecular carcinogenesis, molecular epidemiology and human risk assessment. Lung Cancer 34(2):S7–S15.

Hussain, S. P., Hofseth, L. J., Harris, C. C. 2003. Radical causes of cancer. Nat. Rev. Cancer 3:276–285.

Hussain, S. P., Raja, K., Amstad, P. A., Sawyer, M., Trudel, T. J., Wogan, G. N., Hofseth, L. J., Shields, P. G., Billiar, T. R., Trautwein, C., Hohler, T., Galle, P. R., Phillips, D. H., Markin, R., Marrogi, A. J., Harris, C. C. 2000. Increased p53 mutation load in non-tumorous human liver of Wilson disease and haemochromatosis: oxyradical overload disease. Proc. Natl. Acad. Sci. U.S.A. 97:12770–12775.

Hussain, S. P., Schwank, J., Staib, F., Wang, X. W., Harris, C. C. 2007. TP53 mutations and hepatocellular carcinoma: insights into the etiology and pathogenesis of liver cancer. Oncogene 26:2166–2176.

Hwang, H. J., Kim, G. J., Lee, G. B., Oh, J. T., Chun, Y. H., Park, S. H. 2003. A comprehensive karyotypic analysis on Korean hepatocellular carcinoma cell lines by cross-species color banding and comparative genomic hybridization. Cancer Genet. Cytogenet. 141: 128–137.

Ichiba, M., Maeta, Y., Mukoyama, T., Saeki, T., Yasui, S., Kanbe, T., Okano, J. I., Tanabe, Y., Hirooka, Y., Yamada, S., Kurimasa, A., Murawaki, Y., Shiota, G. 2003. Expression of 8-hydroxy-20-deoxyguanosine in chronic liver disease and hepatocellular carcinoma. Liver Int. 23(5):338–345.

International Agency for Research on Cancer. 2002. Aflatoxins. IARC Monogr. Eval. Carcinog. Risks Hum. 82:171–300.

International Agency for Research on Cancer. IARC. 1993. Some naturally occurring substances: food items and constituents. IARC Monogr. Eval. Carcinog. Risks Hum. 56:245–395.

Johnson, D. G., Walker, C. L. 1999. Cyclins and cell cycle checkpoints. Annu. Rev. Pharmacol. Toxicol. 39:295–312.

Jungst, C., Cheng, B., Gehrke, R., Schmitz, V., Nischalke, H. D., Ramakers, J., Schramel, P., Schirmacher, P., Sauerbruch, T., Caselmann, W. H. 2004. Oxidative damage is increased in human liver tissue adjacent to hepatocellular carcinoma. Hepatology 39: 1663–1672.

Kane, J. M., III, Shears, L. L., Hierholzer, C., Ambs, S., Billiar, T. R., Posner, M. C. 1997. Chronic hepatitis C virus infection in humans: induction of hepatic nitric oxide synthase and proposed mechanisms for carcinogenesis. J. Surg. Res. 69:321–324.

Kato, J. 1999. Induction of S-phase by G1 regulatory factors. Front Biosci. 4:787–792.

Kew, M. C., Popper, H. 1984. The relationship between hepatocellular carcinoma and cirrhosis. Semin. Liver Dis. 4:136–146.

Kielhorn, J., Melber, C., Wahnschaffe, U., Aitio, A., Mangelsdorf, I. 2000. Vinyl chloride: still a cause for concern. Environ. Health Perspect. 108(7):579–588.

Kim, Y. M., Chung, H. T., Simmons, R. L., Billiar, T. R. 2000. Cellular non-heme iron content is a determinant of nitric oxide-mediated apoptosis, necrosis, and caspase inhibition. J. Biol. Chem. 275:10954–10961.

Kim, S. F., Huri, D. A., Snyder, S. H. 2005. Inducible nitric oxide synthase binds, S-nitrosylates, and activates cyclooxygenase-2. Science 310:1966–1970.

Kirk, G. D., Bah, E., Montesano, R. 2006. Molecular epidemiology of human liver cancer: insights into etiology, pathogenesis and prevention from The Gambia, West Africa. Carcinogenesis 27(10):2070–2082.

Kirk, G. D. ,, Lesi, O. A., Mendy, M., Akano, A. O., Sam, O., Goedert, J. J., Hainaut, P., Hall, A. J., Whittle, H., Montesano, R. 2004. The Gambia liver cancer study: infection with hepatitis B and C and the risk of hepatocellular carcinoma in West Africa. Hepatology 39(1): 211–219.

Kirk, G. D., Turner, P. C., Gong, Y. et al. 2005. Hepatocellular carcinoma and polymorphisms in carcinogen-metabolizing and DNA repair enzymes in a population with aflatoxin exposure and hepatitis B virus endemicity. Cancer Epidemiol. Biomarkers Prev. 14: 373–379.

Kirkman, H. 1959. Estrogen-induced tumors of the kidney in the Syrian hamster. III: growth characteristics in the Syrian hamster. Natl. Cancer Inst. Monogr. 1:1–57.

Kitay-Cohen, Y., Amiel, A., Ashur, Y., Fejgin, M. D., Herishanu, Y., Afanasyev, F., Bomstein, Y., Lishner, M. 2001. Analysis of chromosomal aberrations in large hepatocellular carcinomas by comparative genomic hybridization. Cancer Genet. Cytogenet. 131:60–64.

Knudson, A. G. 1986. Genetics of human cancer. Annu. Rev. Genet. 20:231–251.

Kowdley, K. V. 2004. Iron, hemochromatosis, and hepatocellular carcinoma. Gastroenterology 127:S79–S86.

Kuchino, Y., Mori, F., Kasai, H., Inoue, H., Iwai, S., Miura, K. 1989. Misreading of DNA templates containing 8-hydroxydeoxguanosine at the modified base and at adjacent residues. Nature 327(6117):77–79.

Kusano, N., Okita, K., Shirahashi, H., Harada, T., Shiraishi, K., Oga, A., Kawauchi, S., Furuya, T., Sasaki, K. 2002. Chromosomal imbalances detected by comparative genomic hybridization are associated with outcome of patients with hepatocellular carcinoma. Cancer 94: 746–751.

Lang, A. J., Mirski, S. E., Cummings, H. J., Yu, Q., Gerlach, J. H., Cole, S. P. 1998. Structural organization of the human TOP2A and TOP2B genes. Gene 221:255–266.

Lange-Carter, C. A., Pleiman, C. M., Gardner, A. M., Blumer, K. J., Johnson, G. L. 1993. A divergence in the MAP kinase regulatory network defined by MEK kinase and Raf. Science 260:315–319.

Laskin, D. L., Heck, D. E., Laskin, J.MD. 1998. Role of inflammatory cytokines and nitric oxide in hepatic and pulmonary toxicity. Toxicol. Lett. 102–103:289–293.

Levine, A. J., Momand, J., Findlay, C. A. 1991. The p53 tumor suppressor gene. Nature 351: 453–456.

Li, K., Foy, E., Ferreon, J., Nakamura, M., Ferreon, A. C., Ikeda, M., Ray, S. C., Gale, M., Lemon, S. M. 2005. Immune evasion by hepatitis C virus NS3/4A protease-mediated cleavage of the Toll-like receptor 3 adaptor protein TRIF. Proc. Natl. Acad. Sci. U.S.A. 102: 2992–2997.

Li, Y., Trush, M. A., Yager, J. D. 1994. DNA damage caused by reactive oxygen species orginating from a copper-dependent oxidation of the 2-hydroxycatechol of estradiol. Carcinogenesis 15:1421–1427.

Liehr, J. G., Ulubelen, A. A., Strobel, H. W. 1986. Cytochrome P-450-mediated redox cycling of estrogens. J. Biol. Chem. 261:16865–16870.

Liu, F., Jan, K. Y. 2000. DNA damage in arsenite- and cadmium-treated bovine aortic endothelial cells. Free Radic. Biol. Med. 28:55–63.

Liu, D. N., Lu, X. Z., Li, B. L., Zhou, D. X., Li, F. X., Zheng, D. H., Wang, K. H. 1992. Clinical analysis of 535 cases of chronic arsenic poisoning from coal burning. Chin. J. Med. 31: 560–562.

Loeb, L. A., James, E. A., Waltersdorph, A. M., Klebanofrf, S. J. 1988. Mutagenesis by the autoxidation of iron with isolated DNA. Proc. Natl. Acad. Sci. U.S.A. 85:3918–3932.

Lombard, D. B., Guarente, L. 2000. Nijmegen breakage syndrome disease protein and MRE11 at PML nuclear bodies and meiotic telomeres. Cancer Res. 60:2331–2334.

London, W. T., McGlynn, K. A. 1996. Liver cancer. In Cancer epidemiology and prevention, 2nd Edition. Schottenfeld, D., Fraumeni, J. F. eds. Oxford University Press, New York, NY.

Lu, T., Liu, J., LeCluyse, E. L., Zhou, Y. -S., Cheng, M. -L., Waalkes, M. P. 2001. Application of cDNA microarray to the study of arsenic-induced liver diseases in the population of Guizhou, China. Toxicol. Sci. 59:185–192.

Lucito, R., Schneider, R. J. 1992. Hepatitis B virus X protein activates transcription factor NF-kappa B without a requirement for protein kinase C. J. Virol. 66:983–991.

Lunn, R. M., Langlois, R. G., Hsieh, L. L., Thompson, C. L., Bell, D. A. 1999. XRCC1 polymorphisms: effects on aflatoxin B1-DNA adducts and glycophorin A variant frequency. Cancer Res. 59:2557–2561.

Lynn, S., Shiung, J. N., Gurr, J. -R., Jan, K. Y. 1998. Arsenite stimulates poly(ADP-ribosylation) by generation of nitric oxide. Free Radic. Biol. Med. 24:442–449.

MacSween, R. N., Scott, A. R. 1973. Hepatic fibrosis: a clinico-pathological review of 520 cases. J. Clin. Pathol. 26:9369–9942.

Maguire, H. F., Hoeffler, J. P., Siddiqui, A. 1991. HBV X protein alters the DNA binding specificity of CREB and ATF-2 by protein-protein interactions. Science 252:842–844.

Majumder, M., Ghosh, A. K., Steele, R., Ray, R., Ray, R. B. 2001. Hepatitis C virus NS5A physically associates with p53 and regulates p21/waf1 gene expression in a p53-dependent manner. J. Virol. 75:1401–1407.

Mandishoma, E., MacPhail, A. P., Gordeuk, V. R., Kedda, M. A., Paterson, A. C., Rouault, T. A., Kew, M. C. et al. 1998. Dietary iron overload as a risk factor for hepatocellular carcinoma in Black Africans. Hepatology 27:1563–1566.

Marrogi, A. J., Khan, M. A., van Gijssel, H. E., Welsh, J. A., Rahim, H., Demetris, A. J., Kowdley, K. V., Hussain, S. P., Nair, J., Bartsch, H., Okby, N., Poirier, M. C., Ishak, K. G., Harris, C. C. 2001. Oxidative stress and p53 mutations in the carcinogenesis of iron overload-associated hepatocellular carcinoma. J. Natl. Cancer Inst. 93:1652–1655.

Martucci, C. P., Fishman, J. 1993. P450 enzymes of estrogen metabolism. Pharmacol. Ther. 57:237–257.

Mazumder, D. N., Das Gupta, J., Santra, A., Pal, A., Ghose, A., Sarkar, S. 1998. Chronic arsenic toxicity in West Bengal—the worst calamity in the world. J. Indian Med. Assoc. 96:4–7.

McClain, C. J., Hill, D. B., Song, Z., Deaciuc, I., Barve, S. 2002. Monocyte activation in alcoholic liver disease. Alcohol 27:53–61.

Melen, K., Fagerlund, R., Nyqvist, M., Keskinen, P., Julkunen, I. 2004. Expression of hepatitis C virus core protein inhibits interferon-induced nuclear import of STATs. J. Med. Virol. 73: 536–547.

Meneghini, R. 1997. I ron homeostasis, oxidative stress, and DNA damage. Free Radic. Biol. Med. 23:783–792.

Mihm, S., Hutschenreiter, A., Fayyazi, A., Pingel, S., Ramadori, G. 1996. High inflammatory activity is associated with an increased amount of IFN-gamma transcripts in peripheral blood cells of patients with chronic hepatitis C virus infection. Med. Microbiol. Immunol. (Berlin) 185:95–102.

Moodie, S. A., Willumsen, M. B., Weber, M. J., Wolfman, A. 1993. Complexes of Ras-GTP with Raf-1 and Mitogen-Activated Protein Kinase Kinase. Science 260:1658–1661.

Morris, J. S., Schmid, M., Newman, S., Scheuer, P. J., Sherlock, S. 1974. Arsenic and noncirrhotic portal hypertension. Gastroenterology 66:86–94.

Moyo, V. M., Makinuke, R., Gangaudzo, I. T., Gordeuk, V. R., McLaren, V. R. 1996. Associations of iron overload in Africa and hepatocellular carcinoma and tuberculosis. Blood 87: 3470–3476.

Muller, H., Helin, K. 2000. The E2F transcription factors: key regulators of cell proliferation. Biochim. Biophys. Acta 1470:M1–M12.

Nagaya, T., Nakamura, T., Tokino, T., Tsurimoto, T., Imai, M., Mayumi, T., Kamino, K., Yamamura, K., Matsubara, K. 1987. The mode of hepatitis B virus DNA integration in chromosomes of human hepatocellular carcinoma. Genes Dev. 1:773–782.

Nathan, C., Xie, Q. W. 1994. Nitric oxide synthases: roles, tolls, and controls. Cell 78: 915–918.

National Cancer Institute (NCI). 1978. Vinyl chloride: an information resource. DHEW (NIH) Publication No. 79–1599, Bethesda, MD.

National Research Council (NRC). 1999. Arsenic in drinking water. National Academy Press, Washington, D.C.

Natoli, G., Avantaggiati, M. L., Chirillo, P., Costanzo, A., Artini, M., Balsano, C., Levrero, M. 1994. Induction of the DNA-binding activity of c-jun/c-fos heterodimers by the hepatitis B virus transactivator pX. Mol. Cell Biol. 14:989–998.

Naugler, W. E., Sakurai, T., Kim, S., Maeda, S., Kim, K. H., Elsharkawy, A. M., Karin, M. 2007. Gender disparity in liver cancer due to sex differences in MyD88-dependent IL-6 production. Science. 317(5834):121–124.

Nevens, F., Fevery, J., Van Steenbergan, W., Sciot, R., Desmet, V., De Groot, J. 1990. Arsenic and non-cirrhotic portal hypertension. A report of eight cases. J. Hepatol 11:80–85.

Newbold, R. R., Bullock, B. C., McLachlan, J. A. 1990. Uterine adenocarcinoma in mice following developmental treatment with estrogen. Cancer Res. 50:7677–7681.

Niederau, C., Fischer, R., Sonnenberg, A., Stremmel, W., Trampisch, H. J., Strohmeyer, G. 1985. Survival and causes of death in cirrhotic and noncirrhotic patients with primary hemochromatosis. N. Engl. J. Med. 313:1256–1262.

Okabe, H., Ikai, I., Matsuo, K., Satoh, S., Momoi, H., Kamikawa, T., Katsura, N., Nishitai, R., Takeyama, O., Fukumoto, M., Yamaoka, Y. 2000. Comprehensive allelotype study of hepatocellular carcinoma: potential differences in pathways to hepatocellular carcinoma between hepatitis B virus-positive and-negative tumors. Hepatology 31:1073–1079.

Omary, M. B., Ku, N. O. 1997. Intermediate filament proteins of the liver: emerging disease association and functions. Hepatology 25:1043–1048.

Pachiadakis, I., Pollara, G., Chain, B. M., Naoumov, N. V. 2005. Is hepatitis C virus infection of dendritic cells a mechanism facilitating viral persistence? Lancet Infect. Dis. 5:296–304.

Paria, B. C., Chakraborty, C., Dey, S. K. 1990. Catecholestrogen formation in mouse uterus and its role in implantion. Mol. Cell. Endocrinol 69:25–31.

Park, K. J., Choi, S. H., Choi, D. H., Park, J. M., Yie, S. W., Lee, S. Y., Hwang, S. B. 2003. Hepatitis C virus NS5A protein modulates c-Jun N-terminal kinase through interaction with tumor necrosis factor receptor-associated factor 2. J. Biol. Chem. 278:30711–30718.

Perera, F. P. 1996. Molecular epodemiology: insight into cancer susceptibility, risk assessment, and prevention. J. Natl. Cancer Inst. 88:496–509.

Perkin, D. M., Bray, F. I., Devasa, S. S. 2001. Cancer burden in the year 2000. The global picture. Eur. J. Cancer 37(8):54–66.

Petrowsky, H., Schmandra, T., Lorey, T., Hanisch, E., Herrmann, G. 1999. Endothelin-induced contraction of the portal vein in cirrhosis. Eur. Surg. Res. 31:289–296.

Piao, Y. F., He, M., Shi, Y., Tang, T. Y. 2004. Relationship between microvessel density and telomerase activity in hepatocellular carcinoma. World J. Gastroenterol. 10:2147–2149.

Podust, V. N., Fanning, E. 1997. Assembly of functional replication factor C expressed using recombinant baculoviruses. J. Biol. Chem. 272:6303–6310.

Purtilo, D. T., Gottlieb, L. S. 1973. Cirrhosis and hepatoma occurring at Boston City Hospital (1917–1968). Cancer 32:458–462.

Qadri, I., Conaway, J. W., Conaway, R. C., Schaack, J., Siddiqui, A. 1996. Hepatitis B virus transactivator protein, HBx, associates with the components of TFIIH and stimulates the DNA helicase activity of TFIIH. Proc. Natl. Acad. Sci. U.S.A. 93:10578–10583.

Raftogianis, R., Creveling, C., Weinshilboum, R., Weisz, J. 2000. Estrogen metabolism by conjugation. J. Natl. Cancer Inst. Monogr. 2000(27):113–124.

Ramirez, P., Del Razo, L. M., Gutierrez-Ruiz, M. C., Gonsebatt, M. E. 2000. Arsenite induces DNA–protein crosslinks and cytokeratin expression in the WRL-68 human hepatic cell line. Carcinogenesis 21:701–706.

Robinson, W. S. 1994. Molecular events in the pathogenesis of hepadnavirus-associated hepatocellular carcinoma. Annu. Rev. Med. 45:297–323.

Rogler, C. E., Sherman, M., Su, C. Y., Shafritz, D. A., Summers, J., Shows, T. B., Henderson, A., Kew, M. 1985. Deletion in chromosome 11p associated with a hepatitis B integration site in hepatocellular carcinoma. Science 230:319–322.

Roy, D., Liehr, J. G. 1988. Temporary decrease in renal quinone reductase activity induced by chronic administration of estradiol to male Syrian hamsters. J. Biol. Chem. 263: 3646–3651.

Schaumloffel, N., Gebel, T. 1998. Heterogeneity of the DNA damage provoked by antimony and arsenic. Mutagenesis 13:281–286.

Scorsone, K. A., Zhou, Y. Z., Butel, J. S., Slagle, B. L. 1992. p53 mutations cluster at codon 249 in hepatitis B virus-positive hepatocellular carcinomas from China. Cancer Res. 52(6): 1635–1638.

Sengstag, C. 1997. The molecular mechanism of aflatoxin B1-induced liver cancer: is mitotic recombination involved? Mol. Carcinog. 19:147–152.

Sengupta, S., Harris, C. C. 2005. p53: traffic cop at the crossroads of DNA repair and recombination. Nat. Rev. Cell Mol. Biol. 6:44–55.

Shintani, Y., Hiroshi, Y., Kyoji, M., Hajime, F., Takeya, T., Yumi, K., Satoshi, K., Izumu, S., Kazuhiko, K. 1999. Induction of apoptosis after switch-on of the hepatitis B virus X gene mediated by the Cre/loxP recombination system. J. Gen. Virol. 80:3257–3265.

Slagel, B. L., Zhou, Y. -Z., Butel, J. S. 1991. Hepatitis B virus integration event in human chromosome 17p near the p53 gene identifies the region of the chromosome commonly deleted in virus-positive hepatocellular carcinomas. Cancer Res. 51:49–54.

Slaunwhite, W. R., Kirdani, R. Y., Sandberg, A. A. 1973. Metabolic aspects of estrogens in man. In Handbook of physiology, Section 7: endocrinology, Vol II, Part 1. Greep, R. O., Astwood, E. B., Geiger, S. R. eds. American Physiological Society, Washington, DC, pp. 485–523.

Smith, S. J., Li, Y., Whitley, R., Marion, M. J., Partilo, S., Carney, W. P., Brant-Rauf, P. W. 1998. Molecular epidemiology of p53 protein mutations in workers exposed to vinyl chloride. Am. J. Epidemiol. 147(3):302–308.

Stack, D., Byun, J., Gross, M. L., Rogan, E. G., Cavalieri, E. 1996. Molecular characteristics of catechol estrogen quinones in reactions with deoxyribonucleosides. Chem. Res. Toxicol. 9:851–859.

Staib, F., Robles, A. I., Varticovski, L., Wang, X. W., Zeeberg, B. R., Sirotin, M., Zhurkin, V. B., Hofseth, L. J., Hussain, S. P., Weinstein, J. N., Galle, P. R., Harris, C. C. 2005. The p53 tumor suppressor network is a key responder to microenvironmental components of chronic inflammatory stress. Cancer Res. 65:10255–10264.

Swenberg, J. A., Fedtke, N., Ciroussel, F., Barbin, A., Bartsch, H. 1992. Etheno adducts formed in DNA of vinyl chloride-exposed rats are highly persistent in liver. Carcinogenesis 13: 727–729.

The Collaborative Multicentre International Liver Tumor Study (MILTS) 1997. Oral contraceptives and liver cancer. results of the MILTS study. Contraception 56:275–284.

Thorgeirsson, S. S., Grisham, J. W. 2002. Molecular pathogenesis of human hepatocellular carcinoma. Nat. Genet. 31:339–346.

Tokino, T., Fukushige, S., Nakamura, T., Nagaya, T., Murotsu, T., Shiga, J., Aoki, N., Matsubara, K. 1987. Chromosomal translocation and inverted duplication associated with integrated hepatitis B virus in hepatocellular carcinomas. J. Virol. 61:3848–3854.

Trichopoulos, D., Day, N. E., Kaklamani, E., Tzonou, A., Munoz, N., Zavitsanos, X., Koumantaki, Y., Trichopoulou, A. 1987. Hepatitis B virus, tobacco smoking and ethanol consumption in the etiology of hepatocellular carcinoma. Int. J. Cancer 39:45–49.

Trivers, G. E., Cawley, H. L., DeBenedetti, V. M., Hollstein, M., Marion, M. J., Bennett, W. P., Hoover, M. L., Prives, C. C., Tamburro, C. C., Harris, C. C. 1995. Anti-p53 antibodies in sera of workers occupationally exposed to vinyl chloride. J. Natl. Cancer. Inst. 87: 1400–1407.

Trouba, K. J., Wauson, E. M., Vorce, R. L. 2000. Sodium arseniteinduced dysregulation of proteins involved in proliferative signaling. Toxicol. Appl. Pharmacol. 164:161–170.

Tsuda, H., Zhang, W., Shimosato, Y., Yokota, J., Terada, M., Sugimura, T., Miyamura, T., Hirohashi, S. 1990. Allele loss on chromosome 16 associated with progression of human hepatocellular carcinoma. Proc. Natl. Acad. Sci. U.S.A. 87:6791–6794.

Urano, Y., Watanabe, K., Lin, C. C., Hino, O., Tamaoki, T. 1991. Interstitial chromosomal deletion within 4q11-q13 in a human hepatoma cell line. Cancer Res. 51:1460–1464.

Vadrot, N., Legrand, A., Nello, E., Bringuier, A. F., Guillot, R., Feldman, G. 2006. Inducible nitric oxide synthase could be responsible for resistance or sensitivity to IFN-gamma-induced apoptosis in several human hepatoma cell lines. J. Interferon Cytokine Res. 26: 901–913.

Vautier, G., Bomford, A. B., Portmann, B. ,C., Metivier, E., Williams, R. 1999. P53 mutations in British patients with hepatocellular carcinoma: clustering in genetic hemochromatosis. Gastroenterology 117:154–160.

Walker, B. E., Kurth, L. A. 1993. Pituitary tumors in mice exposed prenatally to diethylstilbestrol. Cancer Res. 53:1546–1549.

Wang, L. Y., Chen, C. J., Zhang, Y. J., Tsai, W. Y., Lee, P. H., Feitelson, M. A., Lee, C. S., Santella, R. M. 1998. 4-Aminobiphenyl DNA damage in liver tissue of hepatocellular carcinoma patients and controls. Am. J. Epidemiol. 147:315–323.

Wang, J., Chenivese, X., Henglein, B., Brechot, C. 1990. Hepatitis B virus integration in a cyclin A gene in a hepatocellular carcinoma. Nature 343:555–557.
Wang, H. P., Rogler, C. E. 1988. Deletions in human chromosome arms 11p and 13q in primary hepatocellular carcinomas. Cytogenet. Cell Genet. 48:72–78.
Wang, L. Y., You, S. L., Lu, S. N., Ho, C. H., Wu, M. H., Sun, C. A., Yang, H. I., Chien-Jen, C. 2003. Risk of hepatocellular carcinoma and habits of alcohol drinking, betel quid chewing and cigarette smoking: a cohort of 2416 HBsAg-seropositive and 9421 HBsAg seronegative male residents in Taiwan. Cancer Causes Control 14(3):241–250.
Weisz, J., Bui, Q. D., Roy, D., Liehr, J. G. 1992. Elevated 4-hydroxylation of estradiol by hamster kidney microsomes: potential pathway of metabolic activation estrogens. Endocrinology 131:655–661.
Williams, J., Phillips, T. D., Jolly, P. E., Stiles, J. K., Jolly, C. M., Aggarwal, D. 2004. Human aflatoxicosis in developing countries: a review of toxicology, exposure, potential health consequences, and interventions. Am. J. Clin. Nutr. 80:1106–1122.
Wilson, S., Jones, L., Coussens, C., and Hanna, K. eds. 2002. Cancer and the environment: gene–environment interactions. The National Academy Press, Washington, DC.
Yu, M. W., Yang, S. Y., Pan, I. J., Lin, C. L., Liu, C. J., Liaw, Y. F., Lin, S. M., Chen, P. J., Lee, S. D., Chen, C. J. 2003. Polymorphisms in XRCC1 and glutathione S-transferase genes and hepatitis B-related hepatocellular carcinoma. J. Natl. Cancer Inst. 95:1485–1488.
Yu, M. C., Yuan, J. M. 2004. Environmental factors and risk for hepatocellular carcinoma. Gastroentorology 127:S72–S78.
Yu, M. C., Yuan, J. M., Govindarajan, S., Ross, R. K. 2000. Epidemiology of hepatocellular carcinoma. Can. J. Gastroenterol. 14(8):703–709.
Yu, C. T., Hsu, J. M., Lee, G. Y. C., Tsou, A. P., Chou, C. K., Huang, F. C. Y. 2005. Phosphorylation and stabilization of HURP by Aurora-A: implication of HURP as a transforming target of Aurora-A. Mol. Cell Biol. 25:5789–5800.
Yuan, J. M., Govindarajan, S., Arakawa, K., Yu, M. C. 2004. Synergism of alcohol, diabetes and viral hepatitis on risk of hepatocellular carcinoma in US blacks and whites. Cancer 101: 1009–1017.
Zhao, C. Q., Young, M. R., Diwan, B. A., Coogan, T. P., Waalkes, M. P. 1997. Association of arsenic-induced malignant transformation with DNA hypomethylation and aberrant gene expression. Proc. Natl. Acad. Sci. U.S.A. 94:10907–10912.
Zhou, Y. S., Zhou, D. X., Zhu, S. L., Jin, D. X., Peng, J. H., Huang, S. Q. 1994. Investigation of arsenic content in food dried by normal coal and high arsenic-containing coal. Chin. Public Health 10:77–79.

Chapter 14
Genetic Epidemiology of Mismatch Repair Deficiency in Ovarian Cancer

Tuya Pal, Jenny Permuth Wey, and Thomas A. Sellers

Abstract This chapter reviews the molecular and histopathologic characteristics of ovarian cancers due to genetic defects in the MMR pathway, highlighting the clinical significance of these findings, including implications for diagnosis, prognosis and treatment as well as interactions between DNA mismatch repair (MMR) pathway and environmental risk factors for ovarian cancer. At least ten per cent of cases of ovarian cancer are due to mutations in BRCA1 and BRCA2 and an additional percentage are due to mutations in other genes, including the mismatch repair genes, MSH2, MLH1 and MSH6. Since the mismatch repair pathway may be impaired in up to one-fifth of ovarian tumors, categorization of ovarian cancers into subtypes based on mismatch repair deficiency is likely to permit more accurate assessment of potential etiologic associations. Furthermore, specific chemotherapeutic regimens may exist specifically for ovarian cancers with microsatellite instability, to improve treatment efficacy and reduce toxicity of drugs which may provide no added benefit. Hence clarification of epigenetic—environment interactions in a large-scale study of ovarian cancers may stimulate the development of novel chemotherapy agents.

Keywords Environmental risk factors · Genetic defects in DNA mismatch repair (MMR) pathway · Ovarian cancers

14.1 Introduction

Ovarian cancer ranks fifth in both cancer incidence and cancer mortality in U.S. women (American Cancer Society I, 2007). An estimated 22,430 women in the United States will be diagnosed and 15,280 deaths will be attributed to this disease during the year 2007 (American Cancer Society I, 2007). Ovarian cancer has the

T. Pal (✉)
Department of Cancer Epidemiology and Genetics, Moffitt Cancer Center, Tampa, FL, USA
e-mail: tuya.pal@moffitt.org

D. Roy, M.T. Dorak (eds.), *Environmental Factors, Genes, and the Development of Human Cancers*, DOI 10.1007/978-1-4419-6752-7_14,

highest mortality rate among gynecologic cancers, with more than two-thirds of patients presenting with late stage metastatic disease at initial diagnosis and a 5-year survival rate of only 20–30% (American Cancer Society I, 2004; Mok et al., 2001; Schwartz and Taylor, 1995; Taylor and Schwartz, 1994; Schink, 1999). Conversely, at early stages, the long-term survival rate approaches 90% (Greenlee et al., 2001).

Overall, an estimated 5–12% of invasive ovarian cancers are considered to be due to hereditary susceptibility (Taylor and Schwartz, 1994; Whittemore, 1994). Based on epidemiologic studies, hereditary breast ovarian cancer syndrome (HBOC), due to gene mutations in *BRCA*1 and *BRCA*2, accounts for 65–75% of all cases of hereditary ovarian cancer (Bewtra et al., 1992; Narod et al., 1994b). Hereditary non-polyposis colorectal cancer (HNPCC) is the third major cause of hereditary ovarian cancer, and is believed to account for an estimated 10–15% of all inherited cases (Bewtra et al., 1992). HNPCC is due to germline mutations in the genes involved in DNA mismatch repair (MMR) pathway, one of the best defined molecular pathways involved in both inherited (Akiyama et al., 1997a; Bronner et al., 1994; Leach et al., 1993; Miyaki et al., 1997; Nicolaides et al., 1994; Papadopoulos et al., 1994) and sporadic cancer (Geisler et al., 2003; Gras et al., 2001; Strathdee et al., 2001) pathogenesis.

One of the consequences of deficient MMR is microsatellite instability (MSI) in tumors (Peltomaki et al., 1993; Woerner et al., 2006). MSI is a hallmark feature of HNPCC-associated tumors. While MSI is a useful molecular marker in colorectal cancer, having etiologic, prognostic and therapeutic significance (Lawes et al., 2003; Jo and Carethers, 2006), its utility in ovarian cancer has not been well studied. The purpose of his chapter is to review the molecular and histopathologic characteristics of ovarian cancers due to genetic defects in the MMR pathway, highlighting the clinical significance of these findings, including implications for diagnosis, prognosis and treatment as well as interactions between MMR pathway and environmental risk factors for ovarian cancer.

14.2 Molecular Basis of Mismatch Repair Defects

To date, seven mismatch repair (MMR) genes, *MLH*1 (Bronner et al., 1994; Papadopoulos et al., 1994), *MSH*2 (Leach et al., 1993), *MSH*6 (Akiyama et al., 1997a; Miyaki et al., 1997), *PMS*1 (Nicolaides et al., 1994), *PMS*2 (Nicolaides et al., 1994), *MSH*3 (Akiyama et al., 1997b), and *MLH*3 (Lipkin et al., 2000) have been shown to be involved in human MMR function. Two of these, MLH1 and *MSH*2, are the most common susceptibility genes for HNPCC, accounting for 80–90% of observed mutations (Bronner et al., 1994; Leach et al., 1993; Papadopoulos et al., 1994; Fishel et al., 1993; Liu et al., 1996; Papadopoulos and Lindblom, 1997; Peltomaki and Vasen, 1997), followed by *MSH*6, which is primarily seen in HNPCC families which do not meet clinical diagnostic criteria (Akiyama et al., 1997a; Miyaki et al., 1997; Trojan et al., 2000; Wagner et al., 2001; Wijnen et al., 1999; Wu et al., 1999; Kolodner et al., 1999; Plaschke et al., 2000; Huang et al., 2001). Additionally, recent evidence has suggested an increased role of *PMS*2 (Nicolaides et al., 1994; Hamilton et al., 1995; de Jong et al., 2004; Halvarsson et al., 2006; Clendenning et al., 2006; Hendriks et al., 2006; Worthley et al., 2005) in HNPCC, with a potentially milder phenotype compared with families with pathogenic *MLH*1 and *MSH*2 mutations. The remaining 3 genes are seldom (*PMS*1) (Nicolaides et al., 1994), or not at all (*MSH*3 (Akiyama et al., 1997b; Hienonen et al., 2003; Liu et al., 2003; Wu et al., 2001; Yamamoto et al., 1999), *MLH*3 (Lipkin et al., 2000; Hienonen et al., 2003; Lipkin et al., 2001; Akiyama et al., 2001; Loukola et al., 2000)) reported to be mutated in the germline.

The intact MMR system has been extensively reviewed (Rhyu, 1996; Jascur and Boland, 2006). Briefly, this system coordinately works in sequential steps to repair DNA mismatch mutations. The steps consist of the recognition of the mismatch/insertion/deletion, protein complex formation, excision of the DNA strand containing the errors, and synthesis of a new, correct strand. Of the seven proteins known to be involved in MMR in humans, the heterodimer between *MSH*2 and *MSH*6 is the one able to recognize the mismatch. A second heterodimer between *MSH*2 and *MSH*3 can also start the process, although it preferentially recognizes insertion/deletion rather than mismatches in DNA (Jiricny, 2000; Jiricny and Nystrom-Lahti, 2000). As a result, defects in *MSH*6 are associated with variable degrees of MSI, as the *MSH*2-*MSH*3 complex can compensate for this activity. The formation of the *MSH*2-*MSH*6 heterodimer leads to a conformational change, allowing it to then accommodate a second heterodimer that contains *MLH*1 and *PMS*2. This protein complex forms a structure that enables repair of the lesion by a process involving exonucleases, DNA polymerase and DNA ligases. It should be noted that *PMS*1 and *MLH*3 can form a heterodimer with *MLH*1 and therefore substitute for *PMS*2. Thus decreased protein expression of *MSH*2 and *MSH*6 is often seen together (de Leeuw et al., 2000) (Fig. 14.1).

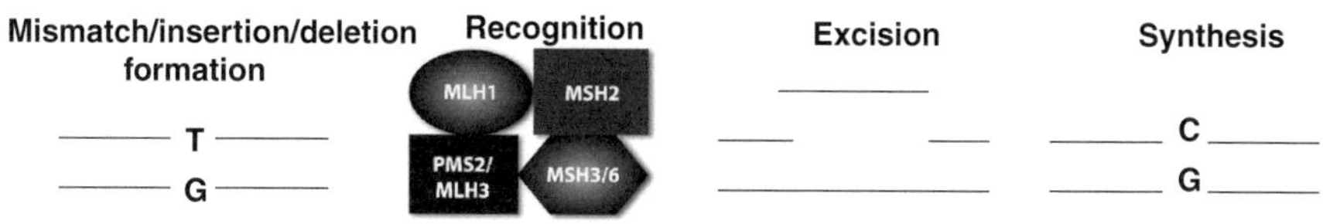

Fig. 14.1 Schematic representation of the human mismatch repair system (adapted from Fig. 1 from Polato and Broggini, 2003, reproduced with permission)

Impaired MMR gene function leads to microsatellite instability (MSI), a hallmark feature of tumors associated with HNPCC (Peltomaki et al., 1993; Boland et al., 1998). Microsatellites are short, polymorphic sequences of DNA between 1 and 5 base pairs which are repeated 15–30 times and distributed across the genome (Thibodeau et al., 1993). Inactivation of the mismatch repair system leads to the accumulation of mutations, particularly in these highly repeated sequences (microsatellites), leading to MSI (Umar et al., 1994; Perucho, 1996; Parsons et al., 1993) (Fig. 14.2).

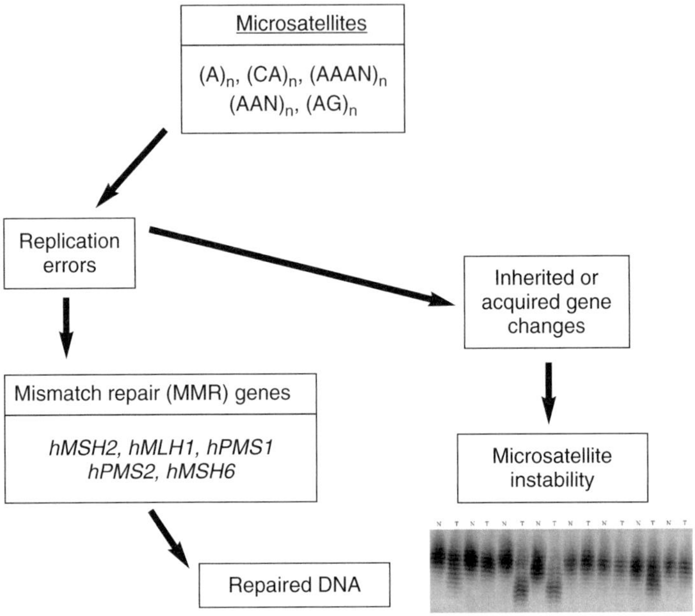

Fig. 14.2 Schematic representation of microsatellite instability. Sample gel from MSI analysis performed for the BAT-26 microsatellite marker. N is for normal DNA control; T is Tumor DNA. Note lanes 2, 6, 8, and 14 have MSI (schematic adapted from Fig. 5 from Prat et al., 2005, reproduced with permission)

Initial studies that sought to estimate the frequency of MSI in ovarian cancer used varying definitions, making it difficult to compare results across studies. In 1997, the National Cancer Institute (NCI) developed uniform criteria to classify MSI (Boland et al., 1998). Five specific markers for microsatellite analysis in colorectal cancer were recommended including two mononucleotide repeats (Bat25 and Bat26) and three dinucleotide repeats (D2S123, D5S346 and D17S250). Tumors were classified as having high level MSI (MSI-H) if two or more of the five markers exhibited variations in microsatellite sequence length, low level MSI (MSI-L) if only one marker showed instability, and stable (MSS) if no marker showed instability.

14.3 Clinical Characteristics of Mismatch Repair Defects

HNPCC was first described by Warthin in 1913, based on his observations and review of pathology records in cancer-rich families. One of these families, family G, became the prototype of cancer families (Warthin, 1913; Lynch and Krush, 1971; Douglas et al., 2005). It took over half a century before Lynch and co-workers collected data that accurately led to the description of these cancer-prone families, whom they initially referred to as being affected by the "cancer family syndrome" (Lynch et al., 1966). In 1991, the International Collaborative Group on Hereditary Non-Polyposis Colorectal Cancer developed the initial criteria, called the "Amsterdam Criteria", to provide a basis for uniformity of diagnosis in multi-center studies (Vasen et al., 1991, 1999). These criteria were too stringent to identify all HNPCC families (Wijnen et al., 1999), thus have been broadened over time to include factors such as extracolonic cancers and small family size [Modified Amsterdam Criteria (Umar et al., 2004) and Amsterdam II Criteria (Vasen et al., 1999)] and tumor characteristics [Bethesda Guidelines (Rodriguez-Bigas et al., 1997) and Revised Bethesda Guidelines (Umar et al., 2004)] in order to identify families in which further analysis for HNPCC is indicated.

HNPCC is characterized by autosomal dominant inheritance of susceptibility to predominantly right-sided colonic cancer, endometrial cancer, ovarian cancer and other extracolonic cancers (including cancer of the renal pelvis, ureter, small bowel, and pancreas), multiple primary cancers, and a young age of onset of cancer (Vasen, 2005). The estimated population incidence is between 1:2,000 and 1:660 (de la Chapelle, 2005). It has previously been suggested that population incidences may vary (Lynch and de la Chapelle, 1999), in part due to the presence or absence of founder mutations that may show considerable enrichment in some populations, including the Finns (Nystrom-Lahti et al., 1995, 1996), Danes (Jager et al., 1997) and Newfoundlanders (Froggatt et al., 1999).

The lifetime risk for ovarian carcinoma in females with HNPCC is estimated to be up to 12%, and the reported relative risk of ovarian cancer has ranged from 3.6 to 13, based on families ascertained from high risk clinics with known or suspected HNPCC (Table 14.1) (Watson and Lynch, 2001; Vasen et al., 1996; Aarnio et al., 1995; Watson and Lynch, 1993; Brown et al., 2001; Aarnio et al., 1999). In these studies, the majority of individuals with known HNPCC had a germline mutation in *MLH*1 or *MSH*2. HNPCC-associated ovarian tumors often develop at a younger

Table 14.1 Ovarian cancer risk in HNPCC

References	Ascertainment source	Location	Sample size	Relative risk	Cumulative inclidence
Watson et al. (1993)	1300 high-risk members from 23 HNPCC kindreds	Nebraska	13	3.5	~
Aarnio et al. (1995)	293 putative HNPCC gene carriers from 40 families	Finland	14	~	9%
Vasen et al. (1996)	382 relatives from 19 families with HNPCC mutations	Netherlands	2	8	~
Aarnio et al. (1999)	1763 high-risk members from 50 HNPCC families	Finland	13	13	12%
Brown et al. (2001)	120 HNPCC families	Australia	24	5 (by age 40)	~

age, with mean ages at diagnosis ranging from 41 to 49 years, compared to sporadic cases with mean ages at diagnosis ranging from 60 to 65 years (Watson and Lynch, 2001; Crijnen et al., 2005; Malander et al., 2006).

Although ovarian cancer risk in *MSH*6 carriers has not been specifically studied in an unselected series of HNPCC families, ovarian cancer is in the *MSH*6 tumor spectrum as evidenced by several case reports where ovarian cancer has been seen in MSH6 family pedigrees (Miyaki et al., 1997; Wagner et al., 2001; Wu et al., 1999; Kolodner et al., 1999; Berends et al., 2002; Suchy et al., 2002). Cederquist et al. (2005) reported a particularly high frequency of ovarian cancers in female members of HNPCC families with mutations in *MSH*6, with a lifetime risk of 33% in the 2 large Swedish pedigrees studied.

As discussed above, the majority of germline MMR mutations are highly penetrant and lead to loss of protein function, genetic instability, and subsequent cancer development. Several investigations have explored whether common polymorphisms in the MMR genes may be associated with varying cancer risks. Colorectal cancer (CRC) susceptibility has been associated with the rare *MLH*1 D132H variant in a study conducted in Israel (Lipkin et al., 2004). However, this finding was not replicated in a study of German patients by Schafmayer et al. (2007). Furthermore, the study by Schafmayer et al. (2007) also considered the MMR genes *PMS*2, *MLH*1, *MSH*2 *and MSH*6, and there was no evidence for an association between CRC and variants in any of these genes. More recently, Song Song et al. (2006) used 44 tagging SNPs (single nucleotide polymorphisms) to investigate common variants in the 7 MMR genes (*MLH*1, *MLH*3, *MSH*2, *MSH*3, *MSH*6, *PMS*1 and *PMS*2) in 1,531 invasive ovarian cancer cases and 2,570 controls from 3 separate studies. Results indicated that common variants in these genes are unlikely to contribute significantly to ovarian cancer susceptibility.

Taken together, the evidence to date suggests that females with germline deleterious mutations in the MMR genes have an elevated risk for ovarian cancer. However, the magnitude of this risk is not well known, and studies to date are severely limited by sample size and varied ascertainment strategies. Larger-scale studies involving known HNPCC cases are needed to explore this issue further, including whether common polymorphisms in these genes may be associated with ovarian cancer risk or MSI in the tumors.

14.4 MSI Status and Ovarian Cancer

The reported prevalence of MSI-H status (as defined by instability in 2 or more markers studied) in ovarian tumors has ranged from 0 to 50% (Table 14.2). This wide variation reflects differences in several factors, including study design, sample size, tumor histotype studied, number and type of microsatellite markers used, and criteria used to define microsatellite instability phenotype. It is noteworthy that many of these studies were completed prior to the development in 1997 of standardized criteria for determining microsatellite instability (Boland et al., 1998). Specifically, several studies have investigated MSI in specific histologic subtypes

Table 14.2 Frequency of ovarian cancers with MSI-H phenotype

References	Sample description	No. of Markers	Sample size	No. of MSI-H (%)
Studies in unselected ovarian cancers				
Allen et al. (2000)	Unselected OC	4	26	1 (4)
Alvi et al. (2001)	Unselected OC	5	43	3 (7)
Buller et al. (2001)	Unselected OC	6	116	24 (20)
Codegoni et al. (1999)	Unselected OC	8	31	8 (26)
Dellas et al. (2004)	Unselected OC	5	66	20 (30)
Fujita et al. (1995)	Unselected OC	4	47	8 (17)
Geisler et al. (2003)	Unselected OC	6	107	21 (20)
Gras et al. (2001)	Unselected OC	5	42	2 (5)
Han et al. (1993)	Unselected OC	4	19	1 (5)
Iwabuchi et al. (1995)	Unselected OC	66	95	6 (6)
King et al. (1995)	Unselected OC	2	41	7 (17)
Kobayashi et al. (1995)	Unselected OC	5	68	2 (3)
Krajinovic et al. (1998)	Unselected OC	8	12	2 (17)
Osborne et al. (1994)	Unselected OC	9	25	2 (8)
Shih et al. (1998)	Unselected OC	69	31	0 (0)
Sood et al. (1996)	Unselected OC	10	68	25 (37)
Sood et al. (2001)	Unselected OC	14	109	13 (12)
Tangir et al. (1996)	Unselected OC	13	31	0 (0)
Studies of specific subgroups of ovarian cancers				
Arzimanoglou et al. (1996)	Familial and sporadic OC	3	90	11 (12)
Chairavalli et al. (2001)	Familial and sporadic OC	3	17	4 (24)
Ichikawa et al. (1999)	HNPCC-associated OC	17	4	4 (100)
Shannon et al. (2003)	52 synchronous OC and EC	5	52	1 (2)
Studies of specific histologic subtypes of ovarian cancer				
Liu et al. (2004)	Endometrioid OC	4	74	15 (20)
Moreno-Bueno et al. (2001)	Endometrioid OC	2	26	5 (19)
Shenson et al. (1995)	Endometrioid OC	28	17	2 (12)
Ohwada et al. (2000)	32 Serous and 29 mucinous OC	5	61	15 (25)
Haas et al. (1999)	Serous OC	6	14	0 (0)
Singer et al. (2004)	53 Serous and 22 non serous OC	5	75	6 (8)
Cai et al. (2004)	Clear cell OC	5	42	6 (14)
Ueda et al. (2005)	Clear cell OC	5	24	6 (25)
Studies of non-ovarian tissues				
Hickey et al. (1999)	Peritoneal fluid	6	20	4 (28)
Orth et al. (1994)	OC cell lines	13	10	5 (50)

(i.e., endometrioid (Shenson et al., 1995; Moreno-Bueno et al., 2001; Liu et al., 2004), serous (Haas et al., 1999; Ohwada et al., 2000; Singer et al., 2004), clear cell (Cai et al., 2004; Ueda et al., 2005), mucinous (Ohwada et al., 2000)), subgroups of ovarian cancers (i.e., HNPCC-associated ovarian cancers only (Ichikawa et al., 1999), familial and sporadic ovarian cancers (Arzimanoglou et al., 1996; Chiaravalli et al., 2001), synchronous cancers of the ovary and endometrium (Shannon et al., 2003) and in non-ovarian tissues (i.e., cell lines (Orth et al., 1994) or peritoneal fluid (Hickey et al., 1999)).

Based on studies of unselected ovarian cancer patients, the true range of MSI is likely between 12 and 20% (Geisler et al., 2003; Sood et al., 2001; King et al., 1995; Fujita et al., 1995; Krajinovic et al., 1998; Buller et al., 2001) (Table 14.2). Furthermore, of the 18 studies of unselected ovarian cancer patients cited in Table 14.2, 11 had a sample size of less than 60 and 8 were performed prior to 1997. Of the 7 studies with a sample size >60, 1 was a Japanese study of 68 cases (Kobayashi et al., 1995) and a MSI-H frequency of 3%. This low estimate may reflect ethnic variation in the frequency of alleles that influence MSI. Another US-based study had a sample size of 95 (Iwabuchi et al., 1995), and had a MSI-H frequency of 6%. Since this was published prior to the development of the 5 NCI-standardized markers, this may be an underestimate. The remaining 5 studies (Geisler et al., 2003; Sood et al., 2001; Buller et al., 2001; Sood and Buller, 1996; Dellas et al., 2004) were all US-based, 4 of which were based at the same center (Geisler et al., 2003; Sood et al., 2001; Buller et al., 2001; Sood and Buller, 1996) and had samples sizes between 66 and 116 and MSI frequencies between 12 and 37%. Thus, data from previous US-based studies suggests that the mismatch repair pathways are etiologically relevant in a significant proportion of ovarian tumors.

14.5 MMR Protein Expression in Ovarian Cancers

Germline or somatic mutations in the MMR genes cause MSI in tumors and result in reduced protein expression (Ichikawa et al., 1999; Orth et al., 1994; Han et al., 1993; Dietmaier et al., 1997; Marcus et al., 1999; Ruszkiewicz et al., 2002; Rigau et al., 2003). Immunohistochemistry (IHC) provides a means to measure protein expression in various tumors. Furthermore, large scale-studies have clearly shown that immunohistochemistry of MSI-H tumors is an accurate screening test for the identification of the specific MMR gene involved in HNPCC-associated tumors (de Leeuw et al., 2000; Ichikawa et al., 1999; Chiaravalli et al., 2001; Orth et al., 1994; Han et al., 1993; Dietmaier et al., 1997; Marcus et al., 1999; Thibodeau et al., 1996; Cawkwell et al., 1999).

Few studies have investigated MMR protein expression in ovarian cancer (Table 14.3). Some studies have investigated IHC in a series of ovarian cancers (Geisler et al., 2003; Domanska et al., 2007; Malander et al., 2004; Rosen et al., 2006), while others have investigated IHC only among cases identified as MSI-H (Liu et al., 2004; Singer et al., 2004; Cai et al., 2004; Ueda et al., 2005; Ichikawa et al., 1999; Chiaravalli et al., 2001). To date, a single published study has comprehensively evaluated the relationship between MSI and protein expression in an unselected series of 107 invasive epithelial ovarian cancers by performing both MSI and MMR protein expression analyses (Geisler et al., 2003). In this study, mRNA

Table 14.3 IHC for MMR protein expression in unselected ovarian cancers

References	Location	Study design	Sample size	No. of MMR loss (%)	Proteins investigated	Method	Comments
Geisler et al. (2003)	Holden Comprehensive Cancer Ctr (Iowa)	Hospital-based	107	10 (9.3)	MLH1, MSH2, MSH3, MSH6, PMS1, PMS2	RT-PCR	No tumors without MSI-H had loss of MMR protein expression
Malander et al. (2004, 2006)	Lund University Hospital (Sweden)	Hospital-based	128	3 (2.3)	MLH1, MSH2, MSH6, PMS2	IHC on TMAs	All tumors with loss of MMR protein expression were MSI-H
Rosen et al. (2006)	MD Anderson (Texas)	Hospital-based	322	7 (2.2)	MLH1, MSH2	IHC on TMAs	All tumors with loss of MMR protein expression were MSI-H
Domanska et al. (2007)	Lund University Hospital/Swedish Cancer Registry (Sweden)	Population-based, age <40	98	6 (6.1)	MLH1, MSH2, MSH6, PMS2	IHC on full section	5/6 tumors with loss of MMR protein expression were MSI-H

Abbreviations: RT-PCR: reverse transcription polymerase chain reaction; TMAs: tissue microarrays

expression of 6 MMR genes was examined by RT-PCR. Results showed loss of *MLH*1 expression in 10 of the 21 MSI-H cases. Eight of the 10 tumors lacking *MLH*1 expression also failed to express *MSH*2 and various other MMR proteins. The remaining MSI-H tumors expressed all MMR proteins and upon subsequent protein truncation testing in the snap frozen tumor, none demonstrated a truncating defect in the *MLH*1 or *MSH*2 genes. Tumors without the MSI-H phenotype expressed all MMR proteins.

To date, 3 studies have evaluated loss of protein expression in unselected invasive epithelial ovarian carcinomas (Malander et al., 2006; Domanska et al., 2007; Rosen et al., 2006). Malander et al. (2006) performed IHC for *MLH*1, *MSH*2, *MSH*6 and *PMS*2, and noted loss of expression in 2.3% (3/128) of cases. Loss of expression of *MLH*1/*PMS*2 was seen in 2 of the cases; 1 of which had a normal result as determined by sequencing and multiplex ligation-dependent probe amplification (MLPA), and the other case had a deletion of exons 4–6 in *MLH*1 that was detected by MLPA but not sequencing. The third case had loss of expression of *MSH*6, and was determined by sequencing to have a truncating mutation in the *MSH*6 gene. Rosen et al. (2006) reported a loss of expression of *MLH*1 and *MSH*2 in 2.2% (7/322) of unselected ovarian cancers, including 5 with loss of *MLH*1 expression and 2 with loss of MSH2 expression. The underlying genetic etiology (either somatic or germline) was not investigated in any of these cases. Finally, Domanska et al. (2007) reported a loss of *MLH*1, *MSH*2, *MSH*6 and *PMS*2 in 6.1% of patients age 40 or below at diagnosis, of which 2 had loss of *MLH*1/*PMS*2, 1 had loss of *MSH*2/*MLH*6, and 3 had loss of *MSH*6 only. This study did not systematically study the underlying genetic etiology of the loss of MMR protein expression, although 1 patient with loss of protein expression of *MSH*6 was diagnosed with an *MSH*6 truncating mutation. These 3 studies (Malander et al., 2006; Domanska et al., 2007; Rosen et al., 2006) all performed MSI analyses in tumors lacking MMR expression, and their results suggest that the majority of tumors lacking expression of MMR proteins have an MSI-H phenotype (Table 14.3).

There have been a number of studies of MMR protein expression in specific subgroups of MSI-H ovarian cancers, including studies of specific histopathologic subtypes (Liu et al., 2004; Singer et al., 2004; Cai et al., 2004; Ueda et al., 2005), as well as studies of high-risk (Ichikawa et al., 1999) and mixed sporadic and familial cases (Chiaravalli et al., 2001). Results of these investigations have shown that the majority have loss of MMR protein expression on IHC, regardless of the specific subgroup studied (Table 14.4).

Thus, studies to date have investigated expression of various numbers of proteins in both unselected ovarian cancers as well as specific ovarian cancer subtypes, and the majority of MSI-H tumors have shown loss of *MLH*1 and *MSH*2 expression as expected. Loss of *MSH*6 expression also appears to be important, especially when early onset cases are investigated. Far less is known regarding the relationship between MSI and other MMR proteins, namely *PMS*2. Not surprisingly, in those studies in which MSI analyses were performed after cases were identified as lacking MMR protein expression, the MSI-H phenotype was identified in the majority.

Table 14.4 IHC for MMR protein expression in MSI-H ovarian cancers

References	Location	Study design	Sample size	No. of MSI-H	No. of MMR loss	Proteins investigated[a]
Cai et al. (2004)	MD Anderson (Texas)	Hospital-based, clear cell	42	6	4	MLH1, MSH2
Liu et al. (2004)	MD Anderson (Texas)	Hospital-based, endometrioid	74	15	9	MLH1, MSH2
Singer et al. (2004)	University of Basel (Switerland)	Hospital-based, serous and non-serous	75	6	5	MLH1, MSH2
Ueda et al. (2005)	Kinki University (Osaka, Japan)	Hospital-based, clear cell	24	9[b]	6	MLH1, MSH2, MSH3, MSH6
Chiaravalli et al. (2001)	University of Insubria (Varese, Italy)	Hospital-based, familial and sporadic	17	4	4[c]	MLH1, MSH2
Ichikawa et al. (1999)	Creighton University (Nebraska)	Clinic-based, high risk families	4	4	3	MLH1, MSH2

[a]All proteins were investigated through IHC on full section slides.
[b]6/9 MSI-H and MSI-L cases had loss of expression on IHC (i.e., MSI-H and MSI-L cases were reported together, thus it was not possible to stratify by MSI-H only).
[c]All 4 tumors showed loss of MLH1 expression only.

14.6 Histology of HNPCC-Associated and/or MSI-H Ovarian Tumors

Classification of ovarian tumors by histologic subtype may be important in identifying ovarian tumors more likely to have defects in the MMR pathway. Overall, approximately 55–70% of all epithelial ovarian cancers have a serous histology, followed by the mucinous (3–9%), endometrioid (8–15%), clear cell (7–13%), mixed (4–6%) and undifferentiated subtypes (Quirk and Natarajan, 2005; Seidman et al., 2004). Based on extensive investigations of both HNPCC-associated and sporadic CRC, the MSI-H tumor phenotype is associated with specific histopathologic characteristics (Lynch et al., 1993; Jass, 2000; Forster et al., 1998; Jass et al., 1999; Konishi et al., 1996; Jass et al., 1998; Bubb et al., 1996; Lothe et al., 1993; Mecklin et al., 1986; Myrhoj et al., 1997; Giacchero et al., 1985). Specifically, evidence suggests an overrepresentation of the less common non-serous histologies, such as endometrioid, mucinous, and clear cell subtypes, in studies of ovarian cancers (Table 14.5).

Table 14.5 Histology of ovarian cancer cases with MMR defects

		Histologic subtypes							
References	Sample size	S	Mu	E	C	U	Mi	NE	NS
HNPCC-associated ovarian cancers									
Aarnio et al. (1999)	13	4	2	1	2	4			5/9 (56)
Bewtra et al. (1992)	4	1		1	2				3/4 (75)
Crijnen et al. (2005)	26	12	1	4	1	1		4	12/24 (50)[a]
Ichikawa et al. (1999)	4	2	1	1					2/2 (50)
Stratton et al. (1999)	2	0	1	1					2/2 (100)
Watson et al. (2001)	79	17	7	13	7	26	4	5	36/53 (68)
MSI-H ovarian cancers									
Chiaravalli et al. (2001)	4	0	3	1					3/4 (75)
Dellas et al. (2004)	20	11	3	3	1	2			9/20 (45)
Fujita et al. (1995)	8	2	1	5					6/8 (75)
Geisler et al. (2003)	21	12	2	6	0	1			9/21 (43)
Gras et al. (2001)	2			1	1				2/2 (100)
King et al. (1995)	7	2		2	1		1	1	5/7 (71)
Sood et al. (2001)	13	7							6/13 (46)
Ovarian cancers with loss of MMR protein expression									
Domanska et al. (2007)	6	0	1	3	2				6/6 (100)
Malander et al. (2006)	3		1		1		1		3/3 (100)
Rosen et al. (2006)	7			1	2		3	1	7/7 (100)

[a] Two histologic subtypes were unknown, thus not included in the percentage: an additional tumor included in the percentage was of undifferentiated subtype.
Abbreviations: S, serous; Mu, mucinous; E, endometrioid; C, clear cell; U, unspecified adenocarcinoma; Mi, mixed; NE, non-epithelial; NS, non-serous.

Information regarding the histopathologic subtypes of MMR-associated ovarian cancers is derived from studies that identified cases with defective MMR based on (1) family history and/or germline mutation analysis or (2) MSI-H status and/or IHC analyses. Studies that have investigated MMR-associated ovarian cancers based on family history or germline mutation status have generally suggested an overrepresentation of non-serous histologies (Bewtra et al., 1992; Watson and Lynch, 2001; Aarnio et al., 1999; Crijnen et al., 2005; Ichikawa et al., 1999; Stratton et al., 1999). However, of the 6 published studies that reported histopathologic subtypes, 5 had a sample size of less than 30, and 3 had a sample size less than 5. Watson and Lynch (2001) have performed the largest study to date investigating HNPCC-associated ovarian cancers with a sample size of 79, and although there was a suggestion of overrepresentation of non-serous histologies, 26 of the cases had unspecified adenocarcinoma, severely limiting the interpretation of results.

Similarly, studies of MMR-associated ovarian cancers detected through MSI or IHC, suggest overrepresentation of endometrioid, mucinous, and clear cell histologic subtypes. Specifically, most (Gras et al., 2001; Chiaravalli et al., 2001; King et al., 1995; Fujita et al., 1995), but not all (Sood et al., 2001; Dellas et al., 2004), studies of MSI-H ovarian cancers found an overrepresentation of non-serous histologies. Furthermore, specific investigations of endometrioid (Shenson et al., 1995; Moreno-Bueno et al., 2001; Liu et al., 2004), mucinous (Ohwada et al., 2000) and clear cell (Cai et al., 2004; Ueda et al., 2005) subtypes have generally observed a higher proportion with MSI-H phenotype, in comparison to studies of serous or unselected ovarian cancers (Table 14.1). Although based on small sample sizes, all studies of MMR protein expression in ovarian cancers that have stratified on histopathologic subtypes (Malander et al., 2006; Domanska et al., 2007; Rosen et al., 2006) have reported non-serous histologies in those with loss of expression.

Hemminki et al. reported a strong familial clustering of ovarian and endometrial cancers that appeared to be specific to endometrioid tumors (Hemminki and Granstrom, 2004). The risk of endometrioid ovarian cancer was elevated 3.4-fold among daughters of mothers with endometrial cancer. The etiology of this familial clustering may reflect HNPCC gene mutations.

Taken together, these data suggest an overrepresentation of endometrioid, mucinous and clear cell subtypes in ovarian cancers with defects in the MMR pathway. Additional research is needed to resolve this question, because knowledge of histology may aid in distinguishing between MMR-associated and non-MMR associated ovarian cancer cases.

14.7 *MLH*1 Promoter Hypermethylation and Somatic Mutations Leading to MSI-H Tumors

Mismatch repair dysfunction can arise through epigenetic and genetic mechanisms (Fig. 14.3). An epigenetic mechanism known to cause inactivation of the mismatch repair system is DNA methylation (Jones and Laird, 1999; Veigl et al., 1998; Wajed et al., 2001). DNA methylation occurs on cytosine bases linked to guanine bases, forming CpG dinucleotide pairs known as islands (Wajed et al., 2001). Localized methylation of CpG islands within the promoter of genes involved in the control of cell proliferation results in their inactivation, leading to carcinogenesis (Jones and Laird, 1999).

As described previously, in HNPCC, mismatch repair inactivation is caused by a heterozygous germline mutation in one of the MMR genes, primarily *MLH*1 *and MSH*2. Consistent with Knudson's two "hit" hypothesis (Knudson, 1971), in HNPCC tumors, loss of the remaining wild-type allele has been attributed to deletions and somatic mutations (Hemminki et al., 1994; Tannergard et al., 1997). Recent evidence also suggests that promoter hypermethylation of *MLH*1 may occur as a second "hit" in hereditary cases (Kuismanen et al., 2000; Ollikainen et al., 2007). Consequently, the detection of promoter hypermethylation does not exclude the possibility of HNPCC. In an effort to differentiate between the clinicopathological characteristics of hereditary and sporadic MSI-H ovarian carcinomas, it may be important to investigate the varying patterns of inherited and somatic events that result as a consequence of genetic and epigenetic mechanisms, which will be the focus of the remainder of this section.

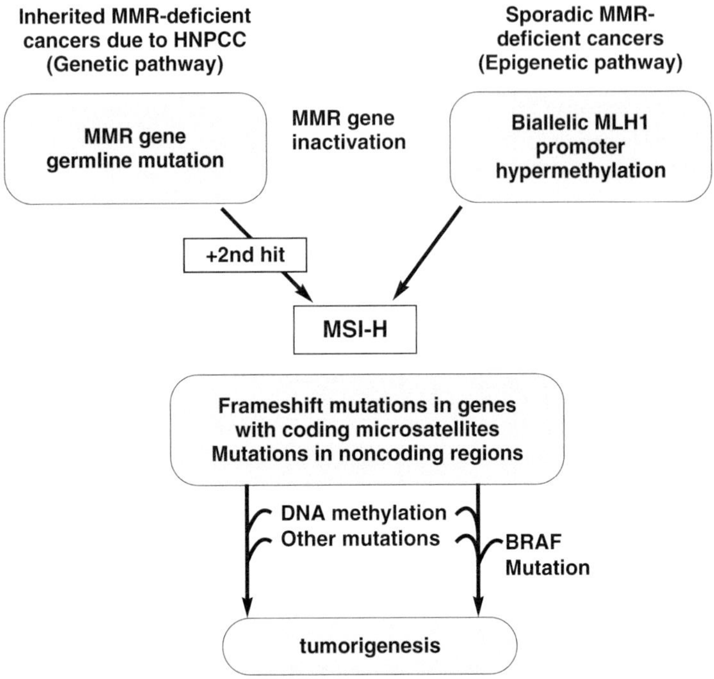

Fig. 14.3 Genetic versus epigenetic pathways leading to MSI-H phenotype and subsequent tumorigenesis. The epigenetic type of MSI-H cancers are frequently accompanied by the BRAF V600E mutation (adapted from Fig. 1 from Imai and Yamamoto, 2007, reproduced with permission)

Promoter hypermethylation of the *MLH*1 gene has been observed in sporadic MSI-H cancers (Ishiguro et al., 2003; Esteller et al., 1999; Brinton et al., 2005; Kane et al., 1997; Fang et al., 2003; Fleisher et al., 2001; Leung et al., 1999; Simpkins et al., 1999; de la Chapelle, 2003),including colorectal, endometrial (Ishiguro et al., 2003; Esteller et al., 1999; Brinton et al., 2005; Kane et al., 1997; Fang et al., 2003; Fleisher et al., 2001; Leung et al., 1999; Simpkins et al., 1999; de la Chapelle, 2003), and ovarian cancer (Geisler et al., 2003; Gras et al., 2001; Strathdee et al., 2001, 1999). Gras et al. (2001) identified *MLH*1 promoter hypermethylation in 50% (3 of 6) of MSI-H cases in their hospital-based series of ovarian cancers. The *MLH*1 promoter was found to be hypermethylated in 3 (10.7%) of a subset of 28 non MSI-H ovarian tumors., suggesting MMR function may be preserved due to less intense hypermethylation. Geisler et al. (2003) reported *MLH*1 promoter hypermethylation in 10 of 21 (47%) MSI-H ovarian tumors. In two additional studies (Strathdee et al., 2001, 1999) of *MLH*1 promoter hypermethylation the MSI status was not reported. Strathdee et al. (1999) identified that 12.5% (3 of 24) of their hospital-based series of ovarian tumors revealed MLH1 promoter hypermethylation. Expression of *MLH*1 was absent in the 3 hypermethylated tumors, while all unmethylated tumors expressed *MLH*1. In a later study, Strathdee et al.

(2001) reported promoter hypermethylation of *MLH*1 in 10% of their hospital-based series of 93 ovarian tumors. Taken together, these studies suggest that MLH1 promoter hypermethylation is observed in a significant proportion of ovarian cancers, especially those which are MSI-H.

To date, the laboratory technique used to detect *MLH*1 promoter hypermethylation in studies of ovarian cancer (Geisler et al., 2003; Gras et al., 2001; Strathdee et al., 2001, 1999) is methylation specific-polymerase chain reaction (MSP), a previously described qualitative technique (Herman et al., 1996). Quantitative PCR methods have recently been used to develop thresholds for methylation determination in CRC tumors, providing cut-off values for *MLH*1 methylation that can discriminate between HNPCC and sporadic MSI-H cases (Bettstetter et al., 2007). Although this method cannot yet exclude the possibility of monoallelic methylation in HNPCC cases (Bettstetter et al., 2007), with improvements, quantitative methods have the potential to provide utility in future diagnostic tests.

Several regions of the *MLH*1 promoter have been evaluated. The distal region of the promoter (known as region A) has traditionally been evaluated because it comprises a dense area of CpG islands (Brinton et al., 2005). However, this region has been demonstrated to have poor correlation with actual *MLH*1 expression (Deng et al., 1999, 2002). On the other hand, methylation status in promoter regions more proximal to the translational start site (called regions C and D) have correlated well with lack of *MLH*1 protein expression (Deng et al., 1999, 2002; Lubomierski et al., 2005). In the study by Geisler et al. (2003), regions A and C of the *MLH*1 promoter were investigated, and coordinated methylation of both regions was observed. Other studies of ovarian tumors (Gras et al., 2001; Strathdee et al., 2001, 1999) have not explicitly reported the region of the promoter studied. These data suggest that MMR protein expression may correlate with methylation in certain regions of the promoter more strongly than others, although further study is needed.

As previously discussed, available evidence infers that MSI-H ovarian tumors can develop as a consequence of both inherited and epigenetic mechanisms. Because the MSI-H phenotype is primarily due to hypermethylation of the *MLH*1 promoter (Veigl et al., 1998; Kane et al., 1997), and not to germline mutations, it has been suggested that it may be cost-effective to define molecular markers (such as promoter hypermethylation and various somatic mutations) that exclude seemingly sporadic cases from further testing of the MMR genes. A specific somatic mutation that has recently been investigated is the *BRAF* proto-oncogene, a kinase encoding gene from the *RAS/RAF/MAPK* pathway (Peyssonnaux and Eychene, 2001). One particular "hotspot" mutation in *BRAF*, known as V600E (previously called V599E), occurs as a result of a single substitution of A to T at nucleotide position 1796, resulting in a valine-to-glutamate substitution at codon 600. This particular mutation has been reported in melanomas (Davies et al., 2002; Kumar et al., 2003), colorectal carcinomas (Fang et al., 2003; Domingo et al., 2004; Rajagopalan et al., 2002), thyroid (Kimura et al., 2003) and ovarian tumors (Gemignani et al., 2003; Ahlgren et al., 2004; Singer et al., 2003; Mayr et al., 2006; Russell and McCluggage, 2004; Sieben et al., 2003). Although other *BRAF* mutations have been reported in non-ovarian tumors (Lubomierski et al., 2005; Davies et al., 2002),only the V600E mutation has been reported in ovarian tissue (Ahlgren et al., 2004; Sieben et al., 2003). Evidence suggests that *BRAF* activation is an early somatic event in the multi-step process of ovarian tumorigenesis, as the mutations occur almost exclusively in serous borderline tumors and low-grade serous carcinomas (Ahlgren et al., 2004; Singer et al., 2003; Mayr et al., 2006; Russell and McCluggage, 2004; Sieben et al., 2003; Ueda et al., 2007). The V600E mutation has not been observed in the germline of ovarian cancer cases and controls (Ueda et al., 2007).

The relationship between the V600E mutation and MMR deficiency has primarily been investigated in colorectal tumors, where it has been found almost exclusively in proximal colon tumors with *MLH*1 promoter hypermethylation (Fang et al., 2003; Domingo et al., 2004). Furthermore, numerous studies have demonstrated that the V600E mutation is not present in MSI-H colorectal tumors of cases known or presumed to harbor a pathogenic mutation in one of the MMR genes (Fang et al., 2003; Bettstetter et al., 2007; Lubomierski et al., 2005; Domingo et al., 2004; Deng et al., 2004; McGivern et al., 2004),providing evidence that the V600E mutation may be of clinical utility in distinguishing between hereditary and sporadic MSI-H tumors.

Limited research has been conducted to investigate the relationship between the V600E mutation and MMR deficiency in ovarian tumors. In a study of 89 invasive and borderline epithelial ovarian tumors of common histological subtypes, 1 tumor of mixed serous/endometrioid histology had a *BRAF* mutation (in the absence of *MLH*1 promoter hypermethylation) (Willner et al., 2007). Additionally, 4 tumors had MLH1 promoter hypermethylation, including 3 endometroid carcinomas and 1 serous carcinoma. Investigation of MMR protein deficiency (through MSI, IHC, or germline mutation testing) was not performed in this study. Further investigations are warranted to determine whether the *BRAF* mutation hotspot is able to help distinguish between sporadic and hereditary MSI-H ovarian cancers.

In summary, there is evidence to suggest that similar to colorectal and endometrial cancers, ovarian cancers are also associated with *MLH*1 promoter hypermethylation in a significant proportion of MSI-H cases. Furthermore, similar to other tumors types, the V600E *BRAF* mutation may provide a reliable, fast, and low cost strategy to simplify genetic testing for HNPCC by excluding ovarian cancer cases that are unlikely to have a hereditary basis (Domingo et al., 2004). It is clear that MSI-H tumors are distinct in terms of their etiology (i.e., genetic and/or epigenetic) and the tumorigenic pathway involved. It is possible that the patterns of genetic and epigenetic events vary depending on germline mutation status and the tissue type involved, possibly explaining the differential tumor susceptibility of different organs in HNPCC (Ollikainen et al., 2007). The use of quantitative PCR methods (Bettstetter et al., 2007) to evaluate *MLH*1 promoter hypermethylation testing of particular promoter regions (Deng et al., 1999, 2002) combined with sequencing of the V600E *BRAF* mutation has the potential to distinguish between hereditary and sporadic MSI-H ovarian cancer cases. The ability to make such distinctions may foster diagnostic, prognostic, and therapeutic utility.

14.8 Epidemiologic Risk Factors and Their Relationship to Microsatellite Instability

There is evidence to suggest an association between specific epidemiologic risk factors and subtypes of colorectal cancer defined by MSI status, however no such studies have yet been reported for ovarian cancer. Interestingly, there are shared epidemiologic risk factors between colorectal and ovarian cancer, possibly related to a hormonal influence on both types of cancers.

Epidemiological risk factors implicated in ovarian carcinogenesis include steroid hormones, primarily estrogens and progesterone. However, it has proved difficult to fully elucidate their mechanisms of action on the tumorigenic process. Epidemiologic studies have suggested an association with certain estrogen-related hormonal risk factors, such as parity and oral contraceptive use, however for other risk factors, the association remains unresolved. There is little consensus regarding the pathogenesis of ovarian cancer, and multiple theories have been postulated, including the theory of incessant ovulation (Fathalla, 1971) and the gonadotropin theory (Cramer and Welch, 1983). Much of the basis of these theories has stemmed from the epidemiology of ovarian cancer. Specifically, endogenous estrogen-related hormonal risk factors such as parity (Casagrande et al., 1979; Kvale et al., 1988)and history of breast-feeding (Gwinn et al., 1990; Rosenblatt and Thomas, 1993)appear to decrease risk, whereas early menarche (Hankinson et al., 1995; Narod et al., 1994a; Whittemore et al., 1992) and late menopause (Booth et al., 1989-Whittemore et al., 1988)appear to slightly increase risk. Similarly, exogenous factors such as use of oral contraceptive pills is protective (Franceschi et al., 1991; Dolcetti et al., 1999; Vessey and Painter, 2006), and the use of hormone replacement therapy possibly increases risk (Beral et al., 2007; Danforth et al., 2007). Obesity has been associated with a slight increase in risk (Olsen et al., 2007), whereas. recreational physical activity may be protective (Olsen et al., 2007). Lifestyle factors such as diet (Schulz et al., 2004) and smoking history (Jordan et al., 2006) may also increase the risk for ovarian cancer.

Although the hormonal basis for ovarian cancer is better established (Hankinson et al., 1995; Whittemore et al., 1992; Ho, 2003; Whiteman et al., 2000; Purdie et al., 1995; Vessey and Painter, 1995; Rodriguez et al., 2001; Farrow et al., 1989), there is also epidemiologic evidence to support a hormonal basis for colorectal cancer, including an increased risk among nulliparous women (Kampman et al., 1997; Marcus et al., 1995), similar to ovarian cancer. In contrast to ovarian cancer, hormone replacement therapy appears to decrease risk (Bray et al., 2005). Obesity (Baker et al., 2007), lack of physical activity (Samad et al., 2005), and cigarette smoking (Giovannucci, 2001) have been shown to increase the risk of colorectal cancer. Due to the lack of information about epidemiologic risk factors in ovarian cancer with mismatch repair deficiency, the remainder of this section will focus on epidemiologic risk factors in colorectal cancers with mismatch repair deficiency, keeping in mind that these factors may also be relevant in ovarian cancer, due to the shared risk factors.

Established and hypothesized risk factors for colorectal cancer, including smoking, reproductive history, hormonal exposure, age, and obesity have been investigated specifically among strata defined by MSI status (Breivik et al., 1997; Slattery et al., 2000). In particular, the hypothesis that estrogens could inhibit the pathway to colon cancer involving mismatch repair deficiency and MSI is based on the observation that the prevalence of MSI in colon tumors is lower among younger than older women (i.e., 5% vs. 42%) (Breivik et al., 1997). Several measures of estrogen exposure were inversely associated with MSI-H tumors, albeit relatively weakly: parity (OR = 0.5; 95% CI = 0.3–0.9), oral contraceptive use (OR = 0.7; 95% CI = 0.4–1.2), and recent use of hormone replacement therapy (OR = 0.8; 95% CI = 0.5–1.4). In a complementary fashion, total ovulatory months increases the risk of an MSI-H tumor. Age was associated with increased risk of MSI-H tumors in women, with statistically significant results ($P<0.01$). The combination of high body mass index and low physical activity level was further associated with increased risk for MSS tumors among women, although results were marginally statistically significant (OR = 1.5;CI = 1.1–2.2). This finding, if verified, could possibly be related to peripheral adipose tissue being a source of estrogens in post-menopausal women. Taken together, these data suggest that estrogen exposure in women protects against MSI-H tumors, whereas lack of estrogen in older women increases the risk of microsatellite instability in tumors.

Slattery et al. (2001) hypothesized that estrogens may specifically prevent MSI-H colon cancers by affecting estrogen responsive DNA mismatch repair genes, *MLH*1 hypermethylation, or DNA methylation processes in general. Presently, there are no data regarding a direct influence of estrogen hormones on methylation. However, existing observational data support further investigation of estrogen hormones as potential modulators of DNA methylation.

The largest study to date to examine associations between multiple environmental exposures and MSI phenotype is a population-based sample of 1,510 colorectal cancer cases and 2,410 controls. The findings revealed that smoking 20 cigarettes per day was associated with MSI-H colon cancers, particularly among women (OR = 2.2; 95% CI = 1.4 to 3.5) (Slattery et al., 2000). Two smaller retrospective studies have also reported positive associations between cigarette smoking and MSI-H tumors. A case-control study of 352 patients showed the risk for MSI-H CRCs was more than sixfold higher among current smokers compared to never smokers ($p < 0.01$) (Yang et al., 2000). A case-control study of 276 patients showed that MSI-H colon cancers were more common among ever smokers than never smokers, although results were not statistically significant (OR = 1.6; 95% CI = 0.7–3.4) (Wu et al., 2001). Conversely, in a population-based case-control study from the Netherlands (n = 425), cigarette smoking was not significantly associated with MSI status (Diergaarde et al., 2003).

Overall, the data suggest that specific epidemiologic risk factors may be important in the development of MSI-H colorectal cancers. Due to the shared epidemiologic risk factors between colorectal cancer and ovarian cancer, these epidemiologic risk factors may also be of etiologic significance in the development of MSI-H ovarian cancers.

14.9 Survival and Treatment Implications Associated with Ovarian Cancers with MMR Deficiency

In addition to providing insight on the pathogenesis of ovarian cancer, the mismatch repair deficiency pathway may also influence treatment and survival. In fact, a number of studies performed in CRC patients suggest that women with HNPCC-associated and/or MSI-H tumors may have improved survival (Thibodeau et al., 1993; Bubb et al., 1996; Lothe et al., 1993; Dolcetti et al., 1999; Kim et al., 1994; Gryfe et al., 2000; Ribic et al., 2003; Halling et al., 1999; Lukish et al., 1998; Wright et al., 2000). It has been suggested that the intrinsic tumor biology leading to the extensive genetic instability associated with microsatellite alterations may ultimately compromise tumor progression (Radman and Wagner, 1993), accounting for improved survival in women with HNPCC associated tumors. To date, a single study has systematically investigated survival in HNPCC-associated ovarian cancers (Crijnen et al., 2005). In this study, survival was investigated in 26 patients identified through the Dutch HNPCC Registry and a population-based control group of 52 cases, matched for age, stage and year of diagnosis. Compared to the control group, ovarian cancer in HNPCC cases was diagnosed at an earlier stage, however the survival rate was not significantly different between cases and controls (64.2 and 58.1%, respectively). Results of this study should be interpreted with caution due to the limited sample size and sampling strategy of the control group.

A survival advantage for ovarian cancers with MMR deficiency is certainly plausible, based on possible overrepresentation of specific histopathologic subtypes and stage at presentation, both of which have the potential to impact survival. As previously reviewed, there has been sufficient data from multiple studies to suggest an overrepresentation of non-serous histologies compared to the more aggressive serous subtype. This may be a contributing factor to any survival advantage of HNPCC-associated and/or MSI-H ovarian tumors.

The distribution of stage at presentation of ovarian tumors with MMR defects has suggested an overrepresentation of early stages at presentation (Hickey et al., 1999; King et al., 1995; Watson et al., 2001). MSI was reported in 50% of ovarian cancer cells obtained from peritoneal fluid in those with stage Ia disease compared to 7% with more advanced disease, suggesting that MSI may be associated with early stage disease (Hickey et al., 1999). In a study of 41 sporadic ovarian cancers, tumors classified as MSI-H were observed in 3/4 (75%) of the patients with stage I tumors versus 4/37 (11%) of the patients with stage II, III and IV tumors ($P = 0.01$) (King et al., 1995). In a series of 80 confirmed or presumed HNPCC-associated ovarian cancers, over 84% of cases were classified as stage I or II, which is significantly different from the 30% of cases diagnosed as stage I or II in the general population (Watson et al., 2001). The overall 5-year survival after diagnosis in this study was ~69% (Watson et al., 2001). Within the stage groups, observed time to death was not significantly different from that expected based on survival in the general population, suggesting that the improved overall survival in HNPCC cases was at least partially due to the favorable stage distribution.

Regarding treatment implications for MMR deficient ovarian tumors, there is in vitro and in vivo data to suggest that MMR deficiency may be a predictor of tumor response to clinical therapy. While studies in primary colorectal cancers initially suggested that MSI may be a favorable indicator for response to chemotherapy (Jo and Carethers, 2006; Ribic et al., 2003; Elsaleh et al., 2001; Hemminki et al., 2000; Elsaleh et al., 2000; Alexander et al., 2001; Watanabe et al., 2001; Chao et al., 2000; Arnold et al., 2003; Warusavitarne and Schnitzler, 2007), more recent studies have shown conflicting results that does not support MMR deficiency as a predictive marker of chemotherapy benefit (Kim et al., 2007; Lamberti et al., 2007).

Platinum-based therapy (such as cisplatin and carboplatin), in combination with taxanes, is the main chemotherapeutic treatment for ovarian cancer (Kaye, 1996). The resistance of mismatch repair deficient cells to platinum-based therapy may be of particular importance in ovarian cancer. There is in vitro evidence to suggest that MMR defects (in tumors with *MLH*1 promoter hypermethylation and/or MSI) are associated with acquired drug resistance to platinum-based agents; in cell lines, drug-induced DNA damage escapes detection and restoration of the MMR activity has been demonstrated to reestablish chemotherapy sensitivity (Strathdee et al., 1999; Massey et al., 2003; Plumb et al., 2000; Anthoney et al., 1996; Aebi et al., 1996; Brown et al., 1997). However, clinical observations from ovarian cancer have shown mixed results for survival and treatment response. Scartozzi et al. (2003) reported that acquired loss of *MLH*1 expression was correlated with improved survival, however others have reported that intrinsic MMR deficiency is not highly predictive of survival (Samimi et al., 2000). Marcelis et al. (2001) described chemotherapy resistance in 2 patients from the same family with inactivating germline mutations in *MSH*2, however others have reported no association between response and MMR status (Samimi et al., 2000; Helleman et al., 2006).

Taken together, the data suggest that despite the fact that acquired loss of expression of *MLH*1 may be associated with improved survival (Scartozzi et al., 2003), in vitro evidence (Strathdee et al., 1999; Massey et al., 2003; Plumb et al., 2000; Anthoney et al., 1996; Aebi et al., 1996; Brown et al., 1997) suggests that MMR-deficient cells may be more resistant to platinum-based treatment, with conflicting results from in vivo studies (Samimi et al., 2000; Marcelis et al., 2001; Helleman et al., 2006). A possible hypothesis to explain this paradoxical finding is that "acquired loss" of *MLH*1 expression due to treatment may lead to poor prognosis because these tumors are intrinsically more aggressive. However, the "initial loss" of *MLH*1 (i.e., leading to MSI-H tumors) may indicate an intrinsically less aggressive tumor, accounting for the survival benefit, despite the tumor possibly being less sensitive to platinum-based chemotherapy.

Although MSI may be a useful genetic marker in prognosis and could be an influential factor in deciding treatment options, its significance in ovarian cancer remains unclear and further evaluation is required. Once the association between drug resistance, treatment response and survival are determined, the basis of the paradoxical finding of improved survival despite drug resistance of MMR-deficient tumors may be dissected out and lead to the development of targeted therapies for MSI-H tumors.

14.10 Conclusion and Future Directions

Of all the common cancers in women, ovarian cancer is the site with the highest hereditary proportion. At least 10% of cases are due to mutations in *BRCA*1 and *BRCA*2 and an additional percentage are due to mutations in other genes, including the mismatch repair genes, *MSH2, MLH*1 and *MSH*6. However, the proportion of hereditary ovarian cancers due to mismatch repair genes remains poorly defined (Watson and Lynch, 1993) and further studies are needed.

Preliminary investigations of the MMR pathway in ovarian tumorigenesis have suggested the possibility of clinical utility for these markers in the diagnosis and treatment of patients with MSI-H ovarian cancer. Since the mismatch repair pathway may be impaired in up to one-fifth of ovarian tumors, categorization of ovarian cancers into subtypes based on mismatch repair deficiency is likely to permit more accurate assessment of potential etiologic associations. Furthermore, specific chemotherapeutic regimens may exist specifically for ovarian cancers with microsatellite instability, to improve treatment efficacy and reduce toxicity of drugs which may provide no added benefit. Hence clarification of epigenetic-environment interactions in a large-scale study of ovarian cancers may stimulate the development of novel chemotherapy agents.

References

Aarnio M, Mecklin JP, Aaltonen LA, Nystrom-Lahti M, Jarvinen HJ. Life-time risk of different cancers in hereditary non-polyposis colorectal cancer (HNPCC) syndrome. *Int J Cancer*. Dec 20 1995;64(6):430–433.

Aarnio M, Sankila R, Pukkala E et al. Cancer risk in mutation carriers of DNA-mismatch-repair genes. *Int J Cancer*. Apr 12 1999;81(2):214–218.

Aebi S, Kurdi-Haidar B, Gordon R et al. Loss of DNA mismatch repair in acquired resistance to cisplatin. *Cancer Res*. Jul 1 1996;56(13):3087–3090.

Ahlgren M, Melbye M, Wohlfahrt J, Sorensen TI. Growth patterns and the risk of breast cancer in women. *N Engl J Med*. Oct 14 2004;351(16):1619–1626.

Akiyama Y, Nagasaki H, Nakajima T, Sakai H, Nomizu T, Yuasa Y. Infrequent frameshift mutations in the simple repeat sequences of hMLH3 in hereditary nonpolyposis colorectal cancers. *Jpn J Clin Oncol*. Feb 2001;31(2):61–64.

Akiyama Y, Sato H, Yamada T et al. Germ-line mutation of the hMSH6/GTBP gene in an atypical hereditary nonpolyposis colorectal cancer kindred. *Cancer Res*. Sep 15 1997a;57(18): 3920–3923.

Akiyama Y, Tsubouchi N, Yuasa Y. Frequent somatic mutations of hMSH3 with reference to microsatellite instability in hereditary nonpolyposis colorectal cancers. *Biochem Biophys Res Commun*. Jul 18 1997b;236(2):248–252.

Alexander J, Watanabe T, Wu TT, Rashid A, Li S, Hamilton SR. Histopathological identification of colon cancer with microsatellite instability. *Am J Pathol*. Feb 2001;158(2): 527–535.

American Cancer Society I. Cancer Facts & Figures 2004. [Internet] http://www.cancer.org/docroots/STT/stt_0.asp. Accessed 2004, 2004.

American Cancer Society I. Cancer Facts & Figures 2007. [Internet] http://www.cancer.org/docroots/STT/stt_0.asp. Accessed 2007, 2007.

Anthoney DA, McIlwrath AJ, Gallagher WM, Edlin AR, Brown R. Microsatellite instability, apoptosis, and loss of p53 function in drug-resistant tumor cells. *Cancer Res.* Mar 15 1996;56(6):1374–1381.

Arnold CN, Goel A, Boland CR. Role of hMLH1 promoter hypermethylation in drug resistance to 5-fluorouracil in colorectal cancer cell lines. *Int J Cancer.* Aug 10 2003;106(1):66–73.

Arzimanoglou II, Lallas T, Osborne M, Barber H, Gilbert F. Microsatellite instability differences between familial and sporadic ovarian cancers. *Carcinogenesis.* Sep 1996;17(9):1799–1804.

Baker JA, Boakye K, McCann SE et al. Consumption of black tea or coffee and risk of ovarian cancer. *Int J Gynecol Cancer.* Jan-Feb 2007;17(1):50–54.

Beral V, Bull D, Green J, Reeves G. Ovarian cancer and hormone replacement therapy in the Million Women Study. *Lancet.* May 19 2007;369(9574):1703–1710.

Berends MJ, Wu Y, Sijmons RH et al. Molecular and clinical characteristics of MSH6 variants: an analysis of 25 index carriers of a germline variant. *Am J Hum Genet.* Jan 2002;70(1):26–37.

Bettstetter M, Dechant S, Ruemmele P et al. Distinction of hereditary nonpolyposis colorectal cancer and sporadic microsatellite-unstable colorectal cancer through quantification of MLH1 methylation by real-time PCR. *Clin Cancer Res.* Jun 1 2007;13(11):3221–3228.

Bewtra C, Watson P, Conway T, Read-Hippee C, Lynch HT. Hereditary ovarian cancer: a clinicopathological study. *Int J Gynecol Pathol.* 1992;11:180–187.

Boland CR, Thibodeau SN, Hamilton SR et al. A National Cancer Institute Workshop on Microsatellite Instability for cancer detection and familial predisposition: development of international criteria for the determination of microsatellite instability in colorectal cancer. *Cancer Res.* Nov 15 1998;58(22):5248–5257.

Booth M, Beral V, Smith P. Risk factors for ovarian cancer: a case-control study. *Br J Cancer.* Oct 1989;60(4):592–598.

Bray F, Loos AH, Tognazzo S, La Vecchia C. Ovarian cancer in Europe: Cross-sectional trends in incidence and mortality in 28 countries, 1953–2000. *Int J Cancer.* Mar 1 2005;113(6):977–990.

Breivik J, Lothe RA, Meling GI, Rognum TO, Borresen-Dale AL, Gaudernack G. Different genetic pathways to proximal and distal colorectal cancer influenced by sex-related factors. *Int J Cancer.* Dec 19 1997;74(6):664–669.

Brinton LA, Sakoda LC, Sherman ME et al. Relationship of benign gynecologic diseases to subsequent risk of ovarian and uterine tumors. *Cancer Epidemiol Biomarkers Prev.* Dec 2005;14(12):2929–2935.

Bronner CE, Baker SM, Morrison PT et al. Mutation in the DNA mismatch repair gene homologue hMLH1 is associated with hereditary non-polyposis colon cancer. *Nature.* Mar 17 1994;368(6468):258–261.

Brown R, Hirst GL, Gallagher WM et al. hMLH1 expression and cellular responses of ovarian tumour cells to treatment with cytotoxic anticancer agents. *Oncogene.* Jul 3 1997;15(1): 45–52.

Brown GJ, St John DJ, Macrae FA, Aittomaki K. Cancer risk in young women at risk of hereditary nonpolyposis colorectal cancer: implications for gynecologic surveillance. *Gynecol Oncol.* Mar 2001;80(3):346–349.

Bubb VJ, Curtis LJ, Cunningham C et al. Microsatellite instability and the role of hMSH2 in sporadic colorectalcancer. *Oncogene.* Jun 20 1996;12(12):2641–2649.

Buller RE, Shahin MS, Holmes RW, Hatterman M, Kirby PA, Sood AK. p53 Mutations and microsatellite instability in ovarian cancer: Yin and yang. *Am J Obstet Gynecol.* Apr 2001;184(5):891–902; discussion 902–893.

Cai KQ, Albarracin C, Rosen D et al. Microsatellite instability and alteration of the expression of hMLH1 and hMSH2 in ovarian clear cell carcinoma. *Hum Pathol.* May 2004;35(5): 552–559.

Casagrande JT, Louie EW, Pike MC, Roy S, Ross RK, Henderson BE. "Incessant ovulation" and ovarian cancer. *Lancet*. Jul 28 1979;2(8135):170–173.
Cawkwell L, Gray S, Murgatroyd H et al. Choice of management strategy for colorectal cancer based on a diagnostic immunohistochemical test for defective mismatch repair. *Gut*. Sep 1999;45(3):409–415.
Cederquist K, Emanuelsson M, Wiklund F, Golovleva I, Palmqvist R, Gronberg H. Two Swedish founder MSH6 mutations, one nonsense and one missense, conferring high cumulative risk of Lynch syndrome. *Clin Genet*. Dec 2005;68(6):533–541.
Chao A, Gilliland F, Willman C et al. Patient and tumor characteristics of colon cancers with microsatellite instability: a population-based study. *Cancer Epidemiol Biomarkers Prev*. Jun 2000;9(6):539–544.
Chiaravalli AM, Furlan D, Facco C et al. Immunohistochemical pattern of hMSH2/hMLH1 in familial and sporadic colorectal, gastric, endometrial and ovarian carcinomas with instability in microsatellite sequences. *Virchows Arch*. Jan 2001;438(1):39–48.
Clendenning M, Hampel H, LaJeunesse J et al. Long-range PCR facilitates the identification of PMS2-specific mutations. *Hum Mutat*. May 2006;27(5):490–495.
Cramer DW, Welch WR. Determinants of ovarian cancer risk. II. Inferences regarding pathogenesis. *J Natl Cancer Inst*. Oct 1983;71(4):717–721.
Crijnen TE, Janssen-Heijnen ML, Gelderblom H et al. Survival of patients with ovarian cancer due to a mismatch repair defect. *Fam Cancer*. 2005;4(4):301–305.
Danforth KN, Tworoger SS, Hecht JL, Rosner BA, Colditz GA, Hankinson SE. A prospective study of postmenopausal hormone use and ovarian cancer risk. *Br J Cancer*. Jan 15 2007;96(1): 151–156.
Davies H, Bignell GR, Cox C et al. Mutations of the BRAF gene in human cancer. *Nature*. Jun 27 2002;417(6892):949–954.
de Jong AE, van Puijenbroek M, Hendriks Y et al. Microsatellite instability, immunohistochemistry, and additional PMS2 staining in suspected hereditary nonpolyposis colorectal cancer. *Clin Cancer Res*. Feb 1 2004;10(3):972–980.
de la Chapelle A. Microsatellite instability. *N Engl J Med*. Jul 17 2003;349(3):209–210.
de la Chapelle A. The incidence of Lynch syndrome. *Fam Cancer*. 2005;4(3):233–237.
de Leeuw WJ, Dierssen J, Vasen HF et al. Prediction of a mismatch repair gene defect by microsatellite instability and immunohistochemical analysis in endometrial tumours from HNPCC patients. *J Pathol*. Nov 2000;192(3):328–335.
Dellas A, Puhl A, Schraml P et al. Molecular and clinicopathological analysis of ovarian carcinomas with and without microsatellite instability. *Anticancer Res*. Jan-Feb 2004;24(1):361–369.
Deng G, Bell I, Crawley S et al. BRAF mutation is frequently present in sporadic colorectal cancer with methylated hMLH1, but not in hereditary nonpolyposis colorectal cancer. *Clin Cancer Res*. Jan 1 2004;10(1 Pt 1):191–195.
Deng G, Chen A, Hong J, Chae HS, Kim YS. Methylation of CpG in a small region of the hMLH1 promoter invariably correlates with the absence of gene expression. *Cancer Res*. May 1 1999;59(9):2029–2033.
Deng D, Deng G, Smith MF et al. Simultaneous detection of CpG methylation and single nucleotide polymorphism by denaturing high performance liquid chromatography. *Nucleic Acids Res*. Feb 1 2002;30(3):E13.
Diergaarde B, Vrieling A, van Kraats AA, van Muijen GN, Kok FJ, Kampman E. Cigarette smoking and genetic alterations in sporadic colon carcinomas. *Carcinogenesis*. Mar 2003;24(3): 565–571.
Dietmaier W, Wallinger S, Bocker T, Kullmann F, Fishel R, Ruschoff J. Diagnostic microsatellite instability: definition and correlation with mismatch repair protein expression. *Cancer Res*. Nov 1 1997;57(21):4749–4756.
Dolcetti R, Viel A, Doglioni C et al. High prevalence of activated intraepithelial cytotoxic T lymphocytes and increased neoplastic cell apoptosis in colorectal carcinomas with microsatellite instability. *Am J Pathol*. Jun 1999;154(6):1805–1813.

Domanska K, Malander S, Masback A, Nilbert M. Ovarian cancer at young age: the contribution of mismatch-repair defects in a population-based series of epithelial ovarian cancer before age 40. *Int J Gynecol Cancer*. Jul-Aug 2007;17(4):789–793.

Domingo E, Espin E, Armengol M et al. Activated BRAF targets proximal colon tumors with mismatch repair deficiency and MLH1 inactivation. *Genes Chromosomes Cancer*. Feb 2004;39(2):138–142.

Douglas JA, Gruber SB, Meister KA et al. History and molecular genetics of Lynch syndrome in family G: a century later. *J Am Med Assoc*. Nov 2 2005;294(17):2195–2202.

Elsaleh H, Joseph D, Grieu F, Zeps N, Spry N, Iacopetta B. Association of tumour site and sex with survival benefit from adjuvant chemotherapy in colorectal cancer. *Lancet*. May 20 2000;355(9217):1745–1750.

Elsaleh H, Powell B, McCaul K et al. P53 alteration and microsatellite instability have predictive value for survival benefit from chemotherapy in stage III colorectal carcinoma. *Clin Cancer Res*. May 2001;7(5):1343–1349.

Esteller M, Catasus L, Matias-Guiu X et al. hMLH1 promoter hypermethylation is an early event in human endometrial tumorigenesis. *Am J Pathol*. Nov 1999;155(5):1767–1772.

Fang DC, Wang RQ, Yang SM et al. Mutation and methylation of hMLH1 in gastric carcinomas with microsatellite instability. *World J Gastroenterol*. Apr 2003;9(4):655–659.

Farrow DC, Weiss NS, Lyon JL, Daling JR. Association of obesity and ovarian cancer in a case-control study. *Am J Epidemiol*. Jun 1989;129(6):1300–1304.

Fathalla MF. Incessant ovulation–a factor in ovarian neoplasia? *Lancet*. Jul 17 1971;2(7716):163.

Fishel R, Lescoe MK, Rao MR et al. The human mutator gene homolog MSH2 and its association with hereditary nonpolyposis colon cancer. *Cell*. Dec 3 1993;75(5):1027–1038.

Fleisher AS, Esteller M, Tamura G et al. Hypermethylation of the hMLH1 gene promoter is associated with microsatellite instability in early human gastric neoplasia. *Oncogene*. Jan 18 2001;20(3):329–335.

Forster S, Sattler HP, Hack M et al. Microsatellite instability in sporadic carcinomas of the proximal colon: association with diploid DNA content, negative protein expression of p53, and distinct histomorphologic features. *Surgery*. Jan 1998;123(1):13–18.

Franceschi S, La Vecchia C, Booth M et al. Pooled analysis of 3 European case-control studies of ovarian cancer: II. Age at menarche and at menopause. *Int J Cancer*. Aug 19 1991;49(1):57–60.

Froggatt NJ, Green J, Brassett C et al. A common MSH2 mutation in English and North American HNPCC families: origin, phenotypic expression, and sex specific differences in colorectal cancer. *J Med Genet*. Feb 1999;36(2):97–102.

Fujita M, Enomoto T, Yoshino K et al. Microsatellite instability and alterations in the hMSH2 gene in human ovarian cancer. *Int J Cancer*. 1995;64:361–366.

Geisler JP, Goodheart MJ, Sood AK, Holmes RJ, Hatterman-Zogg MA, Buller RE. Mismatch repair gene expression defects contribute to microsatellite instability in ovarian carcinoma. *Cancer*. Nov 15 2003;98(10):2199–2206.

Gemignani ML, Schlaerth AC, Bogomolniy F et al. Role of KRAS and BRAF gene mutations in mucinous ovarian carcinoma. *Gynecol Oncol*. Aug 2003;90(2):378–381.

Giacchero A, Aste H, Baracchini P et al. Primary signet-ring carcinoma of the large bowel. Report of nine cases. *Cancer*. Dec 1 1985;56(11):2723–2726.

Giovannucci E. An updated review of the epidemiological evidence that cigarette smoking increases risk of colorectal cancer. *Cancer Epidemiol Biomarkers Prev*. Jul 2001;10(7): 725–731.

Gras E, Catasus L, Arguelles R et al. Microsatellite instability, MLH-1 promoter hypermethylation, and frameshift mutations at coding mononucleotide repeat microsatellites in ovarian tumors. *Cancer*. Dec 1 2001;92(11):2829–2836.

Greenlee RT, Hill-Harmon MB, Murray T, Thun M. Cancer statistics, 2001. *CA Cancer J Clin*. Jan–Feb 2001;51(1):15–36.

Gryfe R, Kim H, Hsieh ET et al. Tumor microsatellite instability and clinical outcome in young patients with colorectal cancer. *N Engl J Med*. 2000;342(2):69–77.

Gwinn ML, Lee NC, Rhodes PH, Layde PM, Rubin GL. Pregnancy, breast feeding, and oral contraceptives and the risk of epithelial ovarian cancer. *J Clin Epidemiol*. 1990;43(6):559–568.
Haas CJ, Diebold J, Hirschmann A, Rohrbach H, Schmid S, Lohrs U. Microsatellite analysis in serous tumors of the ovary. *Int J Gynecol Pathol*. Apr 1999;18(2):158–162.
Halling KC, French AJ, McDonnell SK et al. Microsatellite instability and 8p allelic imbalance in stage B2 and C colorectal cancers. *J Natl Cancer Inst*. Aug 4 1999;91(15):1295–1303.
Halvarsson B, Lindblom A, Rambech E, Lagerstedt K, Nilbert M. The added value of PMS2 immunostaining in the diagnosis of hereditary nonpolyposis colorectal cancer. *Fam Cancer*. 2006;5(4):353–358.
Hamilton SR, Liu B, Parsons RE et al. The molecular basis of Turcot's syndrome. *N Engl J Med*. Mar 30 1995;332(13):839–847.
Han HJ, Yanagisawa A, Kato Y, Park JG, Nakamura Y. Genetic instability in pancreatic cancer and poorly differentiated type of gastric cancer. *Cancer Res*. Nov 1 1993;53(21): 5087–5089.
Hankinson SE, Colditz GA, Hunter DJ et al. A prospective study of reproductive factors and risk of epithelial ovarian cancer. *Cancer*. Jul 15 1995;76(2):284–290.
Helleman J, van Staveren IL, Dinjens WN et al. Mismatch repair and treatment resistance in ovarian cancer. *BMC Cancer*. 2006;6:201.
Hemminki K, Granstrom C. Familial clustering of ovarian and endometrial cancers. *Eur J Cancer*. Jan 2004;40(1):90–95.
Hemminki A, Mecklin JP, Jarvinen H, Aaltonen LA, Joensuu H. Microsatellite instability is a favorable prognostic indicator in patients with colorectal cancer receiving chemotherapy. *Gastroenterology*. Oct 2000;119(4):921–928.
Hemminki A, Peltomaki P, Mecklin JP et al. Loss of the wild type MLH1 gene is a feature of hereditary nonpolyposis colorectal cancer. *Nat Genet*. Dec 1994;8(4):405–410.
Hendriks YM, Jagmohan-Changur S, van der Klift HM et al. Heterozygous mutations in PMS2 cause hereditary nonpolyposis colorectal carcinoma (Lynch syndrome). *Gastroenterology*. Feb 2006;130(2):312–322.
Herman JG, Graff JR, Myohanen S, Nelkin BD, Baylin SB. Methylation-specific PCR: a novel PCR assay for methylation status of CpG islands. *Proc Natl Acad Sci USA*. Sep 3 1996;93(18):9821–9826.
Hickey KP, Boyle KP, Jepps HM, Andrew AC, Buxton EJ, Burns PA. Molecular detection of tumour DNA in serum and peritoneal fluid from ovarian cancer patients. *Br J Cancer*. Aug 1999;80(11):1803–1808.
Hienonen T, Laiho P, Salovaara R et al. Little evidence for involvement of MLH3 in colorectal cancer predisposition. *Int J Cancer*. Aug 20 2003;106(2):292–296.
Ho SM. Estrogen, Progesterone and Epithelial Ovarian Cancer. *Reprod Biol Endocrinol*. Oct 7 2003;1(1):73.
Huang J, Kuismanen SA, Liu T et al. MSH6 and MSH3 are rarely involved in genetic predisposition to nonpolypotic colon cancer. *Cancer Res*. Feb 15 2001;61(4):1619–1623.
Ichikawa Y, Lemon SJ, Wang S et al. Microsatellite instability and expression of MLH1 and MSH2 in normal and malignant endometrial and ovarian epithelium in hereditary nonpolyposis colorectal cancer family members. *Cancer Genet Cytogenet*. Jul 1 1999;112(1):2–8.
Imai K, Yamamoto H. Carcinogenesis and microsatellite instability: The interrelationship between genetics and epigenetics. *Carcinogenesis*. 2007 Oct 17;29(4):673–680.
Ishiguro K, Kawakami K, Maeda K, Ishida Y, Omura K, Watanabe G. Microsatellite instability in gastric cancer is closely associated with hMLH1 hypermethylation at the proximal region of the promoter. *Int J Mol Med*. Oct 2003;12(4):603–608.
Iwabuchi H, Sakamoto M, Sakunaga H et al. Genetic analysis of benign, low-grade, and high-grade ovarian tumors. *Cancer Res*. Dec 15 1995;55(24):6172–6180.
Jager AC, Bisgaard ML, Myrhoj T, Bernstein I, Rehfeld JF, Nielsen FC. Reduced frequency of extracolonic cancers in hereditary nonpolyposis colorectal cancer families with monoallelic hMLH1 expression. *Am J Hum Genet*. Jul 1997;61(1):129–138.

Jascur T, Boland CR. Structure and function of the components of the human DNA mismatch repair system. *Int J Cancer*. Nov 1 2006;119(9):2030–2035.

Jass JR. Pathology of hereditary nonpolyposis colorectal cancer. *Ann N Y Acad Sci*. Jun 2000;910:62–73; discussion 73–64.

Jass JR, Biden KG, Cummings MC et al. Characterisation of a subtype of colorectal cancer combining features of the suppressor and mild mutator pathways. *J Clin Pathol*. Jun 1999;52(6):455–460.

Jass JR, Do KA, Simms LA et al. Morphology of sporadic colorectal cancer with DNA replication errors. *Gut*. May 1998;42(5):673–679.

Jiricny J. Mismatch repair: the praying hands of fidelity. *Curr Biol*. Nov 2 2000;10(21): R788–R790.

Jiricny J, Nystrom-Lahti M. Mismatch repair defects in cancer. *Curr Opin Genet Dev*. Apr 2000;10(2):157–161.

Jo WS, Carethers JM. Chemotherapeutic implications in microsatellite unstable colorectal cancer. *Cancer Biomark*. 2006;2(1–2):51–60.

Jones PA, Laird PW. Cancer epigenetics comes of age. *Nat Genet*. Feb 1999;21(2):163–167.

Jordan SJ, Whiteman DC, Purdie DM, Green AC, Webb PM. Does smoking increase risk of ovarian cancer? A systematic review. *Gynecol Oncol*. Dec 2006;103(3):1122–1129.

Kampman E, Potter JD, Slattery ML, Caan BJ, Edwards S. Hormone replacement therapy, reproductive history, and colon cancer: a multicenter, case-control study in the United States. *Cancer Causes Control*. Mar 1997;8(2):146–158.

Kane MF, Loda M, Gaida GM et al. Methylation of the hMLH1 promoter correlates with lack of expression of hMLH1 in sporadic colon tumors and mismatch repair-defective human tumor cell lines. *Cancer Res*. Mar 1 1997;57(5):808–811.

Kaye SB. Ovarian cancer, from the laboratory to the clinic: challenges for the future. *Ann Oncol*. Jan 1996;7(1):9–13.

Kim GP, Colangelo LH, Wieand HS et al. Prognostic and predictive roles of high-degree microsatellite instability in colon cancer: a National Cancer Institute-National Surgical Adjuvant Breast and Bowel Project Collaborative Study. *J Clin Oncol*. Mar 1 2007;25(7): 767–772.

Kim H, Jen J, Vogelstein B, Hamilton SR. Clinical and pathological characteristics of sporadic colorectal carcinomas with DNA replication errors in microsatellite sequences. *Am J Pathol*. Jul 1994;145(1):148–156.

Kimura ET, Nikiforova MN, Zhu Z, Knauf JA, Nikiforov YE, Fagin JA. High prevalence of BRAF mutations in thyroid cancer: genetic evidence for constitutive activation of the RET/PTC-RAS-BRAF signaling pathway in papillary thyroid carcinoma. *Cancer Res*. Apr 1 2003;63(7): 1454–1457.

King BL, Carcangiu ML, Carter D et al. Microsatellite instability in ovarian neoplasms. *Br J Cancer*. 1995;72:376–382.

Knudson AG Jr. Mutation and cancer: statistical study of retinoblastoma. *Proc Natl Acad Sci USA*. Apr 1971;68(4):820–823.

Kobayashi K, Sagae S, Kudo R, Saito H, Koi S, Nakamura Y. Microsatellite instability in endometrial carcinomas. *Genes, Chromosomes and Cancer*. 1995;14:128–132.

Kolodner RD, Tytell JD, Schmeits JL et al. Germ-line msh6 mutations in colorectal cancer families. *Cancer Res*. Oct 15 1999;59(20):5068–5074.

Konishi M, Kikuchi-Yanoshita R, Tanaka K et al. Molecular nature of colon tumors in hereditary nonpolyposis colon cancer, familial polyposis, and sporadic colon cancer. *Gastroenterology*. Aug 1996;111(2):307–317.

Krajinovic M, Richer C, Gorska-Flipot I et al. Genomic loci susceptible to replication errors in cancer cells. *Br J Cancer*. Oct 1998;78(8):981–985.

Kuismanen SA, Holmberg MT, Salovaara R, de la Chapelle A, Peltomaki P. Genetic and epigenetic modification of MLH1 accounts for a major share of microsatellite-unstable colorectal cancers. *Am J Pathol*. May 2000;156(5):1773–1779.

Kumar R, Angelini S, Hemminki K. Activating BRAF and N-Ras mutations in sporadic primary melanomas: an inverse association with allelic loss on chromosome 9. *Oncogene*. Dec 18 2003;22(58):9217–9224.

Kvale G, Heuch I, Nilssen S, Beral V. Reproductive factors and risk of ovarian cancer: a prospective study. *Int J Cancer*. Aug 15 1988;42(2):246–251.

Lamberti C, Lundin S, Bogdanow M et al. Microsatellite instability did not predict individual survival of unselected patients with colorectal cancer. *Int J Colorectal Dis*. Feb 2007;22(2):145–152.

Lawes DA, SenGupta S, Boulos PB. The clinical importance and prognostic implications of microsatellite instability in sporadic cancer. *Eur J Surg Oncol*. Apr 2003;29(3):201–212.

Leach FS, Nicolaides NC, Papadopoulos N et al. Mutations of a mutS homolog in hereditary nonpolyposis colorectal cancer. *Cell*. Dec 17 1993;75(6):1215–1225.

Leung SY, Yuen ST, Chung LP, Chu KM, Chan AS, Ho JC. hMLH1 promoter methylation and lack of hMLH1 expression in sporadic gastric carcinomas with high-frequency microsatellite instability. *Cancer Res*. Jan 1 1999;59(1):159–164.

Lipkin SM, Rozek LS, Rennert G et al. The MLH1 D132H variant is associated with susceptibility to sporadic colorectal cancer. *Nat Genet*. Jul 2004;36(7):694–699.

Lipkin SM, Wang V, Jacoby R et al. MLH3: a DNA mismatch repair gene associated with mammalian microsatellite instability. *Nat Genet*. Jan 2000;24(1):27–35.

Lipkin SM, Wang V, Stoler DL et al. Germline and somatic mutation analyses in the DNA mismatch repair gene MLH3: Evidence for somatic mutation in colorectal cancers. *Hum Mutat*. May 2001;17(5):389–396.

Liu J, Albarracin CT, Chang KH et al. Microsatellite instability and expression of hMLH1 and hMSH2 proteins in ovarian endometrioid cancer. *Mod Pathol*. Jan 2004;17(1):75–80.

Liu B, Parsons R, Papadopoulos N et al. Analysis of mismatch repair genes in hereditary nonpolyposis colorectal cancer patients. *Nat Med*. Feb 1996;2(2):169–174.

Liu HX, Zhou XL, Liu T et al. The role of hMLH3 in familial colorectal cancer. *Cancer Res*. Apr 15 2003;63(8):1894–1899.

Lothe RA, Peltomaki P, Meling GI et al. Genomic instability in colorectal cancer: relationship to clinicopathological variables and family history. *Cancer Res*. 1993;53:5849–5852.

Loukola A, Vilkki S, Singh J, Launonen V, Aaltonen LA. Germline and somatic mutation analysis of MLH3 in MSI-positive colorectal cancer. *Am J Pathol*. Aug 2000;157(2):347–352.

Lubomierski N, Plotz G, Wormek M et al. BRAF mutations in colorectal carcinoma suggest two entities of microsatellite-unstable tumors. *Cancer*. Sep 1 2005;104(5):952–961.

Lukish JR, Muro K, DeNobile J et al. Prognostic significance of DNA replication errors in young patients with colorectal cancer. *Ann Surg*. Jan 1998;227(1):51–56.

Lynch HT, Krush AJ. Cancer family "G" revisited: 1895–1970. *Cancer*. Jun 1971;27(6): 1505–1511.

Lynch HT, Shaw MW, Magnuson CW, Larsen AL, Krush AJ. Hereditary factors in cancer. Study of two large midwestern kindreds. *Arch Intern Med*. Feb 1966;117(2):206–212.

Lynch HT, Smyrk TC, Watson P et al. Genetics, natural history, tumor spectrum, and pathology of hereditary nonpolyposis colorectal cancer: an updated review. *Gastroenterology*. May 1993;104(5):1535–1549.

Lynch HT, de la Chapelle A. Genetic susceptibility to non-polyposis colorectal cancer. *J Med Genet*. Nov 1999;36(11):801–818.

Malander S, Rambech E, Kristoffersson U et al. The contribution of the hereditary nonpolyposis colorectal cancer syndrome to the development of ovarian cancer. *Gynecol Oncol*. May 2006;101(2):238–243.

Malander S, Ridderheim M, Masback A et al. One in 10 ovarian cancer patients carry germ line BRCA1 or BRCA2 mutations: results of a prospective study in Southern Sweden. *Eur J Cancer*. Feb 2004;40(3):422–428.

Marcelis CL, Van Der Putten HW, Tops C, Lutgens LC, Moog U. Chemotherapy resistant ovarian cancer in carriers of an hMSH2 mutation? *Fam Cancer*. 2001;1(2):109–111.

Marcus VA, Madlensky L, Gryfe R et al. Immunohistochemistry for hMLH1 and hMSH2: A practical test for DNA mismatch repair-deficient tumors. *Am J Surg Pathol.* 1999;23(10):1248–1255.
Marcus PM, Newcomb PA, Young T, Storer BE. The association of reproductive and menstrual characteristics and colon and rectal cancer risk in Wisconsin women. *Ann Epidemiol.* Jul 1995;5(4):303–309.
Massey A, Offman J, Macpherson P, Karran P. DNA mismatch repair and acquired cisplatin resistance in E. coli and human ovarian carcinoma cells. *DNA Repair (Amst).* Jan 2 2003;2(1):73–89.
Mayr D, Hirschmann A, Lohrs U, Diebold J. KRAS and BRAF mutations in ovarian tumors: a comprehensive study of invasive carcinomas, borderline tumors and extraovarian implants. *Gynecol Oncol.* Dec 2006;103(3):883–887.
McGivern A, Wynter CV, Whitehall VL et al. Promoter hypermethylation frequency and BRAF mutations distinguish hereditary non-polyposis colon cancer from sporadic MSI-H colon cancer. *Fam Cancer.* 2004;3(2):101–107.
Mecklin JP, Sipponen P, Jarvinen HJ. Histopathology of colorectal carcinomas and adenomas in cancer family syndrome. *Dis Colon Rectum.* Dec 1986;29(12):849–853.
Miyaki M, Konishi M, Tanaka K et al. Germline mutation of MSH6 as the cause of hereditary nonpolyposis colorectal cancer. *Nat Genet.* Nov 1997;17(3):271–272.
Mok SC, Chao J, Skates S et al. Prostasin, a potential serum marker for ovarian cancer: identification through microarray technology. *J Natl Cancer Inst.* Oct 3 2001;93(19):1458–1464.
Moreno-Bueno G, Gamallo C, Perez-Gallego L, de Mora JC, Suarez A, Palacios J. beta-Catenin expression pattern, beta-catenin gene mutations, and microsatellite instability in endometrioid ovarian carcinomas and synchronous endometrial carcinomas. *Diagn Mol Pathol.* Jun 2001;10(2):116–122.
Myrhoj T, Bisgaard ML, Bernstein I, Svendsen LB, Sondergaard JO, Bulow S. Hereditary nonpolyposis colorectal cancer: clinical features and survival. Results from the Danish HNPCC register. *Scand J Gastroenterol.* Jun 1997;32(6):572–576.
Narod SA, Madlensky L, Bradley L et al. Hereditary and familial ovarian cancer in Southern Ontario. *Cancer.* 1994a;74:2341–2346.
Narod SA, Tonin P, Lynch H, Watson P, Feunteun J, Lenoir G. Histology of BRCA-1 associated ovarian tumours. *Lancet.* 1994b;343:236.
Nicolaides NC, Papadopoulos N, Liu B et al. Mutations of two PMS homologues in hereditary nonpolyposis colon cancer. *Nature.* Sep 1 1994;371(6492):75–80.
Nystrom-Lahti M, Kristo P, Nicolaides NC et al. Founding mutations and Alu-mediated recombination in hereditary colon cancer. *Nat Med.* Nov 1995;1(11):1203–1206.
Nystrom-Lahti M, Wu Y, Moisio AL et al. DNA mismatch repair gene mutations in 55 kindreds with verified or putative hereditary non-polyposis colorectal cancer. *Hum Mol Genet.* Jun 1996;5(6):763–769.
Ohwada M, Suzuki M, Saga Y, Sato I. DNA replication errors are frequent in mucinous cystadenocarcinoma of the ovary. *Cancer Genet Cytogenet.* Feb 2000;117(1):61–65.
Ollikainen M, Hannelius U, Lindgren CM, Abdel-Rahman WM, Kere J, Peltomaki P. Mechanisms of inactivation of MLH1 in hereditary nonpolyposis colorectal carcinoma: a novel approach. *Oncogene.* Jul 5 2007;26(31):4541–4549.
Olsen CM, Green AC, Whiteman DC, Sadeghi S, Kolahdooz F, Webb PM. Obesity and the risk of epithelial ovarian cancer: a systematic review and meta-analysis. *Eur J Cancer.* Mar 2007;43(4):690–709.
Orth K, Hung J, Gazdar A, Bowcock A, Mathis JM, Sambrook J. Genetic instability in human ovarian cancer cell lines. *Proc Natl Acad Sci.* 1994;91:9495–9499.
Papadopoulos N, Lindblom A. Molecular basis of HNPCC: mutations of MMR genes. *Hum Mutat.* 1997;10(2):89–99.
Papadopoulos N, Nicolaides NC, Wei YF et al. Mutation of a mutL homolog in hereditary colon cancer. *Science.* Mar 18 1994;263(5153):1625–1629.
Parazzini F, La Vecchia C, Negri E, Gentile A. Menstrual factors and the risk of epithelial ovarian cancer. *J Clin Epidemiol.* 1989;42(5):443–448.

Parsons R, Li GM, Longley MJ et al. Hypermutability and mismatch repair deficiency in RER+ tumor cells. *Cell*. Dec 17 1993;75(6):1227–1236.

Peltomaki P, Lothe RA, Aaltonen LA et al. Microsatellite instability is associated with tumors that characterize the hereditary non-polyposis colorectal carcinoma syndrome. *Cancer Res*. Dec 15 1993;53(24):5853–5855.

Peltomaki P, Vasen HF. Mutations predisposing to hereditary nonpolyposis colorectal cancer: database and results of a collaborative study. The International Collaborative Group on Hereditary Nonpolyposis Colorectal Cancer. *Gastroenterology*. Oct 1997;113(4): 1146–1158.

Perucho M. Cancer of the microsatellite mutator phenotype. *Biol Chem*. Nov 1996;377(11): 675–684.

Peyssonnaux C, Eychene A. The Raf/MEK/ERK pathway: new concepts of activation. *Biol Cell*. Sep 2001;93(1–2):53–62.

Plaschke J, Kruppa C, Tischler R et al. Sequence analysis of the mismatch repair gene hMSH6 in the germline of patients with familial and sporadic colorectal cancer. *Int J Cancer*. Mar 1 2000;85(5):606–613.

Plumb JA, Strathdee G, Sludden J, Kaye SB, Brown R. Reversal of drug resistance in human tumor xenografts by 2′-deoxy-5-azacytidine-induced demethylation of the hMLH1 gene promoter. *Cancer Res*. Nov 1 2000;60(21):6039–6044.

Polato F, Broggini M. Microsatellite instability and genetic alterations in ovarian cancer. *Minerva Ginecol*. 2003;55:129–138.

Prat F, Ribe A, Gallardo A. Hereditary ovarian cancer. *Hum Pathol*. 2005;36:861–870.

Purdie D, Green A, Bain C et al. Reproductive and other factors and risk of epithelial ovarian cancer: an Australian case-control study. Survey of Women's Health Study Group. *Int J Cancer*. Sep 15 1995;62(6):678–684.

Quirk JT, Natarajan N. Ovarian cancer incidence in the United States, 1992–1999. *Gynecol Oncol*. May 2005;97(2):519–523.

Radman M, Wagner R. Missing mismatch repair. *Nature*. 1993;366:722.

Rajagopalan H, Bardelli A, Lengauer C, Kinzler KW, Vogelstein B, Velculescu VE. Tumorigenesis: RAF/RAS oncogenes and mismatch-repair status. *Nature*. Aug 29 2002;418(6901):934.

Rhyu MS. Molecular mechanisms underlying hereditary nonpolyposis colorectal carcinoma. *J Natl Cancer Inst*. Mar 6 1996;88(5):240–251.

Ribic CM, Sargent DJ, Moore MJ et al. Tumor microsatellite-instability status as a predictor of benefit from fluorouracil-based adjuvant chemotherapy for colon cancer. *N Engl J Med*. Jul 17 2003;349(3):247–257.

Rigau V, Sebbagh N, Olschwang S et al. Microsatellite instability in colorectal carcinoma. The comparison of immunohistochemistry and molecular biology suggests a role for hMSH6 [correction of hMLH6] immunostaining. *Arch Pathol Lab Med*. Jun 2003;127(6):694–700.

Rodriguez C, Patel AV, Calle EE, Jacob EJ, Thun MJ. Estrogen replacement therapy and ovarian cancer mortality in a large prospective study of US women. *J Am Med Assoc*. Mar 21 2001;285(11):1460–1465.

Rodriguez-Bigas MA, Boland CR, Hamilton SR et al. A National Cancer Institute Workshop on Hereditary Nonpolyposis Colorectal Cancer Syndrome: meeting highlights and Bethesda guidelines. *J Natl Cancer Inst*. Dec 3 1997;89(23):1758–1762.

Rosen DG, Cai KQ, Luthra R, Liu J. Immunohistochemical staining of hMLH1 and hMSH2 reflects microsatellite instability status in ovarian carcinoma. *Mod Pathol*. Nov 2006;19(11):1414–1420.

Rosenblatt KA, Thomas DB. Lactation and the risk of epithelial ovarian cancer. The WHO Collaborative Study of Neoplasia and Steroid Contraceptives. *Int J Epidemiol*. Apr 1993;22(2):192–197.

Russell SE, McCluggage WG. A multistep model for ovarian tumorigenesis: the value of mutation analysis in the KRAS and BRAF genes. *J Pathol*. Jun 2004;203(2):617–619.

Ruszkiewicz A, Bennett G, Moore J et al. Correlation of mismatch repair genes immunohistochemistry and microsatellite instability status in HNPCC-associated tumours. *Pathology*. Dec 2002;34(6):541–547.
Samad AK, Taylor RS, Marshall T, Chapman MA. A meta-analysis of the association of physical activity with reduced risk of colorectal cancer. *Colorectal Dis*. May 2005;7(3): 204–213.
Samimi G, Fink D, Varki NM et al. Analysis of MLH1 and MSH2 expression in ovarian cancer before and after platinum drug-based chemotherapy. *Clin Cancer Res*. Apr 2000;6(4): 1415–1421.
Scartozzi M, De Nictolis M, Galizia E et al. Loss of hMLH1 expression correlates with improved survival in stage III-IV ovarian cancer patients. *Eur J Cancer*. May 2003;39(8):1144–1149.
Schafmayer C, Buch S, Egberts JH et al. Genetic investigation of DNA-repair pathway genes PMS2, MLH1, MSH2, MSH6, MUTYH, OGG1 and MTH1 in sporadic colon cancer. *Int J Cancer*. Aug 1 2007;121(3):555–558.
Schink JC. Managing the care of patients with advanced ovarian cancer. *Semin Oncol*. 1999;26(1 Suppl 1):59–61.
Schulz M, Lahmann PH, Riboli E, Boeing H. Dietary determinants of epithelial ovarian cancer: a review of the epidemiologic literature. *Nutr Cancer*. 2004;50(2):120–140.
Schwartz PE, Taylor KJ. Is early detection of ovarian cancer possible? *Ann Med*. Oct 1995;27(5):519–528.
Seidman JD, Horkayne-Szakaly I, Haiba M, Boice CR, Kurman RJ, Ronnett BM. The histologic type and stage distribution of ovarian carcinomas of surface epithelial origin. *Int J Gynecol Pathol*. Jan 2004;23(1):41–44.
Shannon C, Kirk J, Barnetson R et al. Incidence of microsatellite instability in synchronous tumors of the ovary and endometrium. *Clin Cancer Res*. Apr 2003;9(4):1387–1392.
Shenson DL, Gallion HH, Powell DE, Pieretti M. Loss of heterozygosity and genomic instability in synchronous endometrioid tumors of the ovary and endometrium. *Cancer*. Aug 15 1995;76(4):650–657.
Sieben NL, Kolkman-Uljee SM, Flanagan AM et al. Molecular genetic evidence for monoclonal origin of bilateral ovarian serous borderline tumors. *Am J Pathol*. Apr 2003;162(4):1095–1101.
Simpkins SB, Bocker T, Swisher EM et al. MLH1 promoter methylation and gene silencing is the primary cause of microsatellite instability in sporadic endometrial cancers. *Hum Mol Genet*. Apr 1999;8(4):661–666.
Singer G, Kallinowski T, Hartmann A et al. Different types of microsatellite instability in ovarian carcinoma. *Int J Cancer*. Nov 20 2004;112(4):643–646.
Singer G, Oldt R 3rd, Cohen Y et al. Mutations in BRAF and KRAS characterize the development of low-grade ovarian serous carcinoma. *J Natl Cancer Inst*. Mar 19 2003;95(6):484–486.
Slattery ML, Curtin K, Anderson K et al. Associations between cigarette smoking, lifestyle factors, and microsatellite instability in colon tumors. *J Natl Cancer Inst*. Nov 15 2000;92(22): 1831–1836.
Slattery ML, Potter JD, Curtin K et al. Estrogens reduce and withdrawal of estrogens increase risk of microsatellite instability-positive colon cancer. *Cancer Res*. Jan 1 2001;61(1):126–130.
Song H, Ramus SJ, Quaye L et al. Common variants in mismatch repair genes and risk of invasive ovarian cancer. *Carcinogenesis*. Nov 2006;27(11):2235–2242.
Sood AK, Buller RE. Genomic instability in ovarian cancer: a reassessment using an arbitrarily primed polymerase chain reaction. *Oncogene*. Dec 5 1996;13(11):2499–2504.
Sood AK, Holmes R, Hendrix MJ, Buller RE. Application of the National Cancer Institute international criteria for determination of microsatellite instability in ovarian cancer. *Cancer Res*. Jun 1 2001;61(11):4371–4374.
Strathdee G, Appleton K, Illand M et al. Primary ovarian carcinomas display multiple methylator phenotypes involving known tumor suppressor genes. *Am J Pathol*. Mar 2001;158(3): 1121–1127.

Strathdee G, MacKean MJ, Illand M, Brown R. A role for methylation of the hMLH1 promoter in loss of hMLH1 expression and drug resistance in ovarian cancer. *Oncogene*. Apr 8 1999;18(14):2335–2341.

Stratton JF, Thompson D, Bobrow L et al. The genetic epidemiology of early-onset epithelial ovarian cancer: a population-based study. *Am J Hum Genet*. Dec 1999;65(6):1725–1732.

Suchy J, Kurzawski G, Jakubowska A, Lubinski J. Ovarian cancer of endometrioid type as part of the MSH6gene mutation phenotype. *J Hum Genet*. 2002;47(10):529–531.

Tannergard P, Liu T, Weger A, Nordenskjold M, Lindblom A. Tumorigenesis in colorectal tumors from patients with hereditary non-polyposis colorectal cancer. *Hum Genet*. Nov 1997;101(1):51–55.

Taylor KJ, Schwartz PE. Screening for early ovarian cancer. *Radiology*. Jul 1994;192(1):1–10.

Thibodeau SN, Bren G, Schaid D. Microsatellite instability in cancer of the proximal colon. *Science*. 1993;260:816–819.

Thibodeau SN, French AJ, Roche PC et al. Altered expression of hMSH2 and hMLH1 in tumors with microsatellite instability and genetic alterations in mismatch repair genes. *Cancer Res*. Nov 1 1996;56(21):4836–4840.

Trojan J, Raedle J, Zeuzem S. [Germline mutations of the MSH6 gene in patients with an atypical hereditary nonpolyposis colorectal carcinoma (HNPCC)]. *Z Gastroenterol*. Jul 2000;38(7):607–609.

Ueda M, Toji E, Noda S. Germ line and somatic mutations of BRAF V599E in ovarian carcinoma. *Int J Gynecol Cancer*. Jul-Aug 2007;17(4):794–797.

Ueda H, Watanabe Y, Nakai H, Hemmi H, Koi M, Hoshiai H. Microsatellite status and immunohistochemical features of ovarian clear-cell carcinoma. *Anticancer Res*. Jul-Aug 2005;25(4):2785–2788.

Umar A, Boyer JC, Thomas DC et al. Defective mismatch repair in extracts of colorectal and endometrial cancer cell lines exhibiting microsatellite instability. *J Biol Chem*. May 20 1994;269(20):14367–14370.

Umar A, Risinger JI, Hawk ET, Barrett JC. Testing guidelines for hereditary non-polyposis colorectal cancer. *Nat Rev Cancer*. Feb 2004;4(2):153–158.

Vasen HF. Clinical description of the Lynch syndrome [hereditary nonpolyposis colorectal cancer (HNPCC)]. *Fam Cancer*. 2005;4(3):219–225.

Vasen HF, Mecklin JP, Khan PM, Lynch HT. The International Collaborative Group on Hereditary Non-Polyposis Colorectal Cancer (ICG-HNPCC). *Dis Colon Rectum*. May 1991;34(5): 424–425.

Vasen HF, Watson P, Mecklin JP, Lynch HT. New clinical criteria for hereditary nonpolyposis colorectal cancer (HNPCC, Lynch syndrome) proposed by the International Collaborative group on HNPCC. *Gastroenterology*. Jun 1999;116(6):1453–1456.

Vasen HF, Wijnen JT, Menko FH et al. Cancer risk in families with hereditary nonpolyposis colorectal cancer diagnosed by mutation analysis. *Gastroenterology*. Apr 1996;110(4):1020–1027.

Veigl ML, Kasturi L, Olechnowicz J et al. Biallelic inactivation of hMLH1 by epigenetic gene silencing, a novel mechanism causing human MSI cancers. *Proc Natl Acad Sci USA*. Jul 21 1998;95(15):8698–8702.

Vessey MP, Painter R. Endometrial and ovarian cancer and oral contraceptives–findings in a large cohort study. *Br J Cancer*. Jun 1995;71(6):1340–1342.

Vessey M, Painter R. Oral contraceptive use and cancer. Findings in a large cohort study, 1968–2004. *Br J Cancer*. Aug 7 2006;95(3):385–389.

Wagner A, Hendriks Y, Meijers-Heijboer EJ et al. Atypical HNPCC owing to MSH6 germline mutations: analysis of a large Dutch pedigree. *J Med Genet*. May 2001;38(5):318–322.

Wajed SA, Laird PW, DeMeester TR. DNA methylation: an alternative pathway to cancer. *Ann Surg*. Jul 2001;234(1):10–20.

Warthin A. Heredity with reference to carcinoma. *Arch Intern Med*. 1913;4:681–696.

Warusavitarne J, Schnitzler M. The role of chemotherapy in microsatellite unstable (MSI-H) colorectal cancer. *Int J Colorectal Dis*. Jul 2007;22(7):739–748.

Watanabe T, Wu TT, Catalano PJ et al. Molecular predictors of survival after adjuvant chemotherapy for colon cancer. *N Engl J Med*. Apr 19 2001;344(16):1196–1206.
Watson P, Butzow R, Lynch HT et al. The clinical features of ovarian cancer in hereditary nonpolyposis colorectal cancer. *Gynecol Oncol*. Aug 2001;82(2):223–228.
Watson P, Lynch HT. Extracolonic cancer in hereditary nonpolyposis colorectal cancer. *Cancer*. 1993;71:677–685.
Watson P, Lynch HT. Cancer risk in mismatch repair gene mutation carriers. *Fam Cancer*. 2001;1(1):57–60.
Whiteman DC, Murphy MF, Cook LS et al. Multiple births and risk of epithelial ovarian cancer. *J Natl Cancer Inst*. Jul 19 2000;92(14):1172–1177.
Whittemore AS. Characteristics relating to ovarian cancer risk: implications for prevention and detection. *Gynecol Oncol*. 1994;55:S15–S19.
Whittemore AS, Harris R, Itnyre J. Characteristics relating to ovarian cancer risk: collaborative analysis of 12 US case-control studies. II. Invasive epithelial ovarian cancers in white women. Collaborative Ovarian Cancer Group. *Am J Epidemiol*. Nov 15 1992;136(10):1184–1203.
Whittemore AS, Wu ML, Paffenbarger RS Jr. et al. Personal and environmental characteristics related to epithelial ovarian cancer. II. Exposures to talcum powder, tobacco, alcohol, and coffee. *Am J Epidemiol*. Dec 1988;128(6):1228–1240.
Wijnen J, de Leeuw W, Vasen H et al. Familial endometrial cancer in female carriers of MSH6 germline mutations. *Nat Genet*. Oct 1999;23(2):142–144.
Willner J, Wurz K, Allison KH et al. Alternate molecular genetic pathways in ovarian carcinomas of common histological types. *Hum Pathol*. Apr 2007;38(4):607–613.
Woerner SM, Kloor M, von Knebel Doeberitz M, Gebert JF. Microsatellite instability in the development of DNA mismatch repair deficient tumors. *Cancer Biomark*. 2006;2(1–2): 69–86.
Worthley DL, Walsh MD, Barker M et al. Familial mutations in PMS2 can cause autosomal dominant hereditary nonpolyposis colorectal cancer. *Gastroenterology*. May 2005;128(5): 1431–1436.
Wright CM, Dent OF, Barker M et al. Prognostic significance of extensive microsatellite instability in sporadic clinicopathological stage C colorectal cancer. *Br J Surg*. Sep 2000;87(9): 1197–1202.
Wu Y, Berends MJ, Mensink RG et al. Association of hereditary nonpolyposis colorectal cancer-related tumors displaying low microsatellite instability with MSH6 germline mutations. *Am J Hum Genet*. Nov 1999;65(5):1291–1298.
Wu AH, Shibata D, Yu MC, Lai MY, Ross RK. Dietary heterocyclic amines and microsatellite instability in colon adenocarcinomas. *Carcinogenesis*. Oct 2001;22(10):1681–1684.
Yamamoto H, Perez-Piteira J, Yoshida T et al. Gastric cancers of the microsatellite mutator phenotype display characteristic genetic and clinical features. *Gastroenterology*. Jun 1999;116(6):1348–1357.
Yang P, Cunningham JM, Halling KC et al. Higher risk of mismatch repair-deficient colorectal cancer in alpha(1)-antitrypsin deficiency carriers and cigarette smokers. *Mol Genet Metab*. Dec 2000;71(4):639–645.

Part III
Case Studies

Chapter 15
Betel Nut and Susceptibility to Cancer

Rajesh N. Sharan and Yashmin Choudhury

Abstract Betel nut is a widely masticated natural product, which is consumed by over 600 million people across the globe. The ancient habit of betel nut chewing, either as dry or raw/wet nut, in association with betel leaf and a host of region specific additives, including chewing tobacco, is believed to be an important etiological factor for human cancer. Alkaloids and their betel nut specific nitrosamine derivatives produced upon metabolic activation interact with DNA and other cellular targets to produce highly variable mutagenic, genotoxic, cytostatic, immunostatic and teratogenic effects. At molecular level the betel nut or its constituents strongly influence gene expression patterns, especially that of tumor suppressor genes. Structural damage to nucleus and mitochondria, etc. are also induced. The review dwells upon these aspects of betel nut induced carcinogenesis to show that genetic susceptibility to cancer through generations progressively increased due to exposure to betel nut.

Keywords Betel nut specific nitrosamine derivatives and alkaloids · Mutagenic and genotoxic effects · Tumor suppressor genes · Susceptibility to oral cancer

15.1 Introduction

Areca nut is the seed of fruit of a tropical palm, *Areca catechu* L (Fig. 15.1a). It forms the most basic ingredient of a variety of widely used social and habitual masticatory products, which are often wrapped in the leaf of another tropical creeper, *Piper betle* L., commonly known as the betel leaf. Hence, the *Areca* nut is more commonly known as betel nut (BN) (Warnakulasuriya, 2002). The earliest use of BN as a masticatory by humans has been mentioned by Theophrastus in scripts dating around 430 BCE (Before Common Era), which described use of *Areca* nut as a

R.N. Sharan (✉)
Radiation and Molecular Biology Unit, Department of Biochemistry, North-Eastern Hill University, Shillong 793 022, India
e-mails: rnsharan@nehu.ac.in; rnsharan@gmail.com

D. Roy, M.T. Dorak (eds.), *Environmental Factors, Genes, and the Development of Human Cancers*, DOI 10.1007/978-1-4419-6752-7_15,

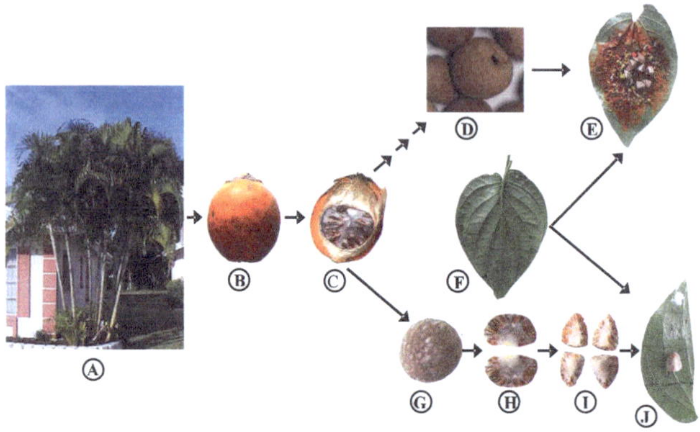

Fig. 15.1 Patterns of betel nut usage: *Areca catechu* L. palm trees in its natural habitat (**a**); a ripe betel fruit (**b**) and its cross section showing the betel nut (BN) encased within its fibrous shell (**c**). After appropriate curing, sun drying and removal of the shell, the dry and very hard variety of BN (**d**) is prepared, which is usually cut into small to very small pieces for mastication along with *Piper betle* leaf (**f**) as a betel quid (BQ) supplemented with a large variety of additives (**e**) (see text for details). BN is also masticated in its raw and wet form (**g**), which is usually cut into 4 pieces (**h** and **i**) and consumed as a simple BQ (**j**) comprising betel leaf (**f**), slacked lime and a piece of wet/raw variety of nut

component of the betel morsel. Chinese texts of 150 BCE, also mention BN as "*pin-lang*". In Persia (modern Iran), it is believed that around 30,000 shops sold BN in the capital town during the reign of Khosrau II, the King of Persia during 590–628 AD. There is also mention of use of BN in one or the other form in different parts of the world including South and South-East Asia, several Pacific islands, many regions of the former Soviet Union, parts of North America and Europe (Sharan, 1996). The use of BN is deeply ingrained in highly variable socio-cultural and religious practices across the globe (Warnakulasuriya, 2002). BN is believed to be used by both men and women across all age groups and social classes though in some societies the latter predominate (Warnakulasuriya, 2002). In old Indian scripts such as *Vagbhata* (fourth century), and *Bhavamista* (thirteenth century), BN has also been described as a "therapeutic agent". BN users report increased well-being and stamina, a soothing effect on the digestion, protection of the mouth and gums, and some euphoria. Its use was recommended in wide ranging human diseases and other disorders, which included vitiligo or leucoderma, leprosy, anemia, digestive disorders and infections, urinary and dental infections, and obesity. It has been suggested that BN chewing may confer protection against dental caries and other infections. In vitro evidence indicates that *Areca* tannins may have anti-microbial activity, which may contribute to the cariostatic properties of BN. Furthermore, betel stain, which coats the teeth of chewers, may act as a protective varnish (Trivedy et al., 2002). BN is also reported to have aphrodisiac property and has been recommended as a general stimulant. In China, it has been used as a vermifuge since the sixth century (Sharan, 1996). The BN is predominantly consumed in its dry form, which is usually a very hard nut (Fig. 15.1d). To make it easy to masticate or chew, the BN is cut into small to very small pieces (Fig. 15.1e). In contrast, people in several parts of the world, including the whole of the north-eastern region of India, masticate the raw and wet form, which is relatively soft (Fig. 15.1 g). Hence, larger pieces of the nut are masticated (Fig. 15.1i). Aged people may masticate even powdered form of raw/wet or dry variety of BN.

Areca nut is normally harvested as unripe (green) or ripe (orange/red) fruit from the *Areca* palm (Fig. 15.1b, c). The *Areca* fruits may be sun dried for several weeks, fibrous shells removed and the hard, dry nuts are ready for use (Fig. 15.1d). Alternatively, the ripe *Areca* fruits are boiled for several hours in an aqueous solution containing the bark of the plant *Eugenia jambolana*, jaggery or brown sugar, and various edible oils, to "cure" it. The cured fruits are sun dried for several weeks, fibrous shell removed and very hard, brown nuts are ready for use (Fig. 15.1d). In contrast, ripe, partly ripe or unripe *Areca* fruits are freshly picked (Fig. 15.1b, c), fibrous shells removed and the relatively soft nuts are ready for masticated (Fig. 15.1 g). Occasionally, the fruits can be cured by burying them into moist pits for 1–2 weeks for fermentation (maturation) before deshelling and use. Such raw and wet variety of BN in the north-eastern part of India is locally called "*kwai*"or "*tambul*" (Fig. 15.1 g–i).

The BN is either consumed alone or with a wide variety of region and socio-culture specific additives as betel quid (BQ). In latter case, dry variety of BN is usually wrapped along with slaked lime (calcium oxide and calcium hydroxide or slacked lime) and catechu (*Acacia catechu*) without or with a host of additives, which may also include a variety of tobacco products, perfumes, stimulants, etc., in a piece of betel leaf (Fig. 15.1e, f). The raw/wet variety of BN is usually masticated with slaked lime wrapped in a betel leaf (Fig. 15.1e, j) and occasionally supplemented with chewing tobacco (IARC, 1985; Sharan, 1996; Warnakulasuriya, 2002). In India, most habitual chewers of BQ add tobacco, while in some countries, such as Papua New Guinea and China, tobacco is not added. Betel leaf is perishable and the preparation of BQ is somewhat complex (Fig. 15.1e). Hence, over the past three decades, commercial BQ substitutes, flavored and sweetened dry mixture of *Areca* nut, catechu and slaked lime with tobacco (*gutkha*) or without tobacco (*pan masala*), have become increasingly popular among habitual BN chewers (Nair et al., 2004).

15.1.1 Constituents of Betel Nut and Its Active Principles

The constituents of BN include carbohydrates, crude fiber, fats, polyphenols, alkaloids, tannins, proteins, ash and water. Trace amounts of fluorine, sapogenein, and free amino acids have also been reported in some forms. The relative amounts of these constituents are highly variable in dry or raw/wet variety of BN. Geographical and climatic conditions of growth of the *Areca* palm tree and the methods of curing BN also contribute to the observed variation in the constituents (Sharan, 1996). Table 15.1 shows the approximate content of different constituents of dry and raw/wet variety of BN. The raw and wet variety of BN is relatively rich in all constituents as compared to the dry variety. Notwithstanding these variations, the active

Table 15.1 Constituent of betel nut (BN): Approximate average percent constituent of dry and raw/wet varieties BN (IARC, 1985, 2004; Sharan, 1996)

Constituent	Dry variety (%)	Raw/wet variety (%)
Alkaloids		
Combined	0.25	0.35–0.49
Arecoline	0.15	0.18–0.24
Arecaidine	0.10	0.10–0.20
Others	Trace	0.14
Polyphenols	15	23
Tannins	18	22
Carbohydrates	25	30
Proteins	7.5	12
Fats	1.2	2.5
Fiber	15	18
Water	Low	High
Ash	Low	High

components of both forms of BN, which produce betel nut associated effects, are primarily the alkaloids, polyphenols, and tannins.

(a) *Alkaloids*: Alkaloids are reduced pyridines. BN contains primarily two alkaloids that are biologically highly relevant. Arecoline (1,2,4,5-tetrahydro-1-methyl-pyridinecarboxylic acid; molecular weight 155. 19 Da) is the most abundant alkaloid of BN followed by arecaidine (1,2,5,6-tetrahydro-1-methyl-3-pyridinecarboxylic acid; molecular weight 141. 17 Da). Other alkaloids such as, guvacine (methyl ester of arecaidine), guvacoline (methyl ester of guvacine) and arecolinidine are also present in small to very small or trace amounts (Table 15.1) (Sharan, 1996).

(b) *Polyphenols and tannins*: The main polyphenols of BN are catechin, flavanoids, flavan-3:4-diols, leucocyanidins and hexahydroxyflavans. When oxidized in the presence of lime, these give the characteristic red color to saliva, teeth and lips of BQ masticator. The predominant tannin of BN is gallotannic acid. In addition, minor amounts of gallic acid, D-catechol and phiobatannin are also present (Sharan, 1996).

(c) *Betel nut specific nitrosamines (BSNA)*: Numerous and highly complex nitrosamine derivatives are produced from different alkaloids of BN essentially by nitrosation of the alkaloid in the mouth and stomach, especially in acidic milieu, and in the presence of nitric oxide generated by bacterial action (Wary and Sharan, 1991; Boucher and Mannan, 2002). Figure 15.2 shows a typical and representative metabolic pathway of arecoline nitrosation and production of different derivatives. The major biologically relevant nitrosamines of arecoline, appropriately grouped as betel nut specific nitrosamines (BSNA), are N-(methylnitrosamino) propionaldehyde (NMPA), N-(methylnitrosamino) propionitrile (NMPN) and N-nitosoguvacoline. Of these, MNPA was reported to be the most potent BSNA on a molar basis effecting both survival and thiol content

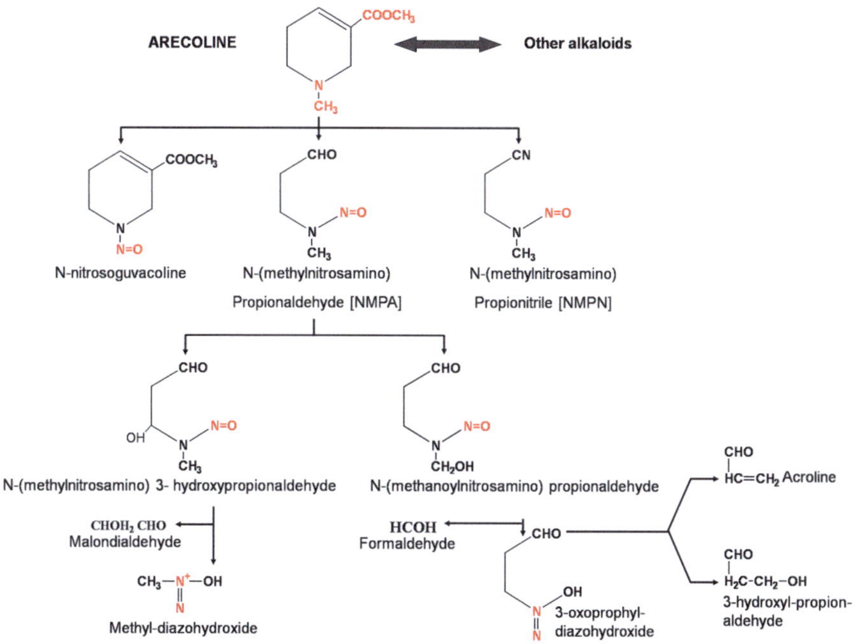

Fig. 15.2 Representative chemical pathway of metabolic activation of arecoline, the major carcinogenic alkaloid of BN. Different nitrosamine and their derivative are produced from the alkaloids, which have been called as betel nut specific nitrosamines (BSNA)

of cultured human buccal epithelial cells and causing significant formation of DNA single strand breaks (Sundqvist et al., 1989). It is proposed that NMPA may further generate N-(methylnitrosamino) 3-hydroxypropionaldehyde and N-(methanoylnitrosamino) propionaldehyde derivatives, each of which can potentially produce several diazohydroxide derivatives (see Fig. 15.2). Presence of most of these derivatives has been demonstrated in the saliva of BQ chewers (IARC, 1985; Nair et al., 1985).

(d) *Reactive oxygen species (ROS)*: Aqueous extracts of *Areca* nut and catechu were found to be capable of generating superoxide anion radicals ($O_2{\bullet}^-$) and hydrogen peroxide (H_2O_2) at pH greater than 9.5 (Nair et al., 1987). While saliva was found to inhibit both $O_2{\bullet}^-$ and H_2O_2 formation from BQ ingredients, ROS are formed in the alkaline chewing mixture within the saliva of a chewer due to the addition of slaked lime (Stich and Anders, 1989).

15.1.2 General Effects of Betel Nut Consumption

BN is masticated or chewed for its psycho-stimulating effects (Norton, 1998). When BN is masticated, it usually produces mild psychoactive and cholinergic effects. Due to this, it is estimated that over 600 million individuals are habitual consumers of BN in one form or the other world-wide (Sharan, 1996). Only three other "addictive" substances—nicotine, ethanol and caffeine, are reported to be more widely used by human beings (Norton, 1998). In north-east India, a raw/wet variety of BN called *kwai* or *tambul*, consumed with betel leaf and slaked lime, causes an immediate thermogenic physiological response lasting 2–3 min with significant perspiration on the forehead and reddening of ear pinnae (Sharan, 1996). There is copious production of blood-red saliva that stains oral structures. After years of chewing, the teeth may become red–brown to nearly black (Sharan, 1996; Boucher and Mannan, 2002). In vitro studies have demonstrated that *Areca* extracts containing arecoline inhibit growth and attachment of and protein synthesis in human cultured periodontal fibroblasts. These findings suggest that *Areca* may be cytotoxic to periodontal fibroblasts and may exacerbate preexisting periodontal disease as well as impair periodontal reattachment (Trivedy et al., 2002). The use of BQ was also found to be associated with the appearance of lichenoid lesions on the buccal mucosa and tongue, and betel chewer's mucosa, characterized by a brownish–red discoloration of the oral mucosa, often accompanied by encrustation of the affected mucosa with quid particles which are not easily removed, and with a tendency for desquamation and peeling (Trivedy et al., 2002).

Acute ill effects are also reported at high rates of usage of BN and include cardiac arrhythmia, exacerbation of asthma, acute psychosis and acute gut upset (Boucher and Mannan, 2002). Significant hyperglycemia was observed in male mice administered with BSNA, NMPN. In fact, a population study revealed increase in waist size and weight, taken as markers for hyperglycemia, in direct relation to *paan*, a type of Indian BQ, usage among Asians. These studies, thus, suggest that BN may be diabetogenic (Boucher and Mannan, 2002). BN chewing was found to be independently associated with increased urinary albumin excretion and albuminuria in Taiwanese male patients of type-2 diabetes (Tseng, 2006). BN alkaloids, especially arecoline, have anti-muscarinic effects on the smooth muscle. They are proposed to bind to GABA receptors in the brain, contributing to their psychoactive effects. BN chewing is thought to reduce the severity of symptoms in schizophrenia with reduction in both positive and negative symptoms. Withdrawal symptoms such as mood swings, anxiety, irritability, reduced concentration, sleep disturbance and craving were found to be associated with trying to quit the habit of BN chewing. These findings are regarded to be consistent with the existence of a dependence syndrome among regular users. In rare cases, *Areca* nut psychosis has been reported to occur in heavy users following abrupt cessation of the habit (IARC, 2004). One study of cases between 1988 and 1998 also reports toxicity of BN manifested in different individuals by tachycardia/palpitations, tachypnea/dyspnea, hypotension, sweating, vomiting, dizziness, chest discomfort, abdominal colic, nausea, numbness, coma, and acute myocardial infarction with its related manifestations (Deng et al., 2001).

15.1.3 Link Between Betel Nut and Carcinogenesis

Today, there is sufficient evidence that *Areca* nut or BN as well as BQ without or with tobacco is carcinogenic to humans (Sharan, 1996; IARC, 1985, 2004). BQ without tobacco causes oral cancer, while BQ with tobacco causes cancers of the oral cavity, pharynx and oesophagus (IARC, 2004). A causal association between tobacco and BQ chewing habits and oral mucosal diseases such as leukoplakia, oral submucous fibrosis (OSF) and oral cancer has been established, and heavy users have a significantly increased mortality rate. Oral cancer is the fifth most common cancer worldwide (Nair et al., 2004). Of the 390,000 oral and oro-pharyngeal cancers estimated to occur annually worldwide, 58% occur in south and south east Asia. In India, there is reported addition of 75,000–80,000 new cases of oral cancer each year and the incidence rates of cancers of the oral cavity in both males and females in all urban cancer registries are among the highest in the world. Time-trend analysis of cancers at all sites for the period 1990–1996 showed a decrease in cancers of the oral cavity in Indian population based registries, but an increase in the incidence of mouth cancer was reported among those aged < 50 years between 1983–1987 and 1995, consistent with the hypothesis of an increase in oral cancer among the young due to increased consumption of the alternative chewing products such as, *gutkha* and *pan masala* (Nair et al., 2004). In Taiwan, data on oral cavity cancer from the period between 1986 and 1997 indicated that those who chew BN belong to a high-risk group (Lin et al., 2005).

15.1.3.1 Induction of Pre-cancerous Lesions by Betel Nut

As an early sign of damage to the oral mucosa, chewers of BN or BQ with or without tobacco often develop clinically visible whitish (leukoplakia) or reddish (erythroplakia) lesions, which may or may not be accompanied by stiffening of the oral mucosa and OSF. These manifestations are well established precancerous lesions and are taken as early and important indicators of oral cancer risk to an individual. Some 2–12% of these lesions have been reported to turn malignant over several years. OSF, which is predominantly caused by the use of *Areca* nut, is a seriously debilitating and progressive disease marked by stiffening of the oral mucosa, development of fibrous bands and loss of elasticity of the mucosa, resulting in a progressive restriction of mouth opening. Flavonoids, catechins and tannins of BN cause collagen fibers to crosslink making them less susceptible to collagenase. This can cause increased fibrosis due to increased collagen production and decreased collagen breakdown. OSF is irreversible and persists even after cessation of the chewing habit, suggesting that components of the *Areca* nut initiate OSF and then affect gene expression in the fibroblasts, which then produce greater amounts of normal collagen (Nair et al., 2004). Considerable amounts of copper have been found in BN products. Copper salts significantly increase the production of collagen by oral fibroblasts in vitro supposedly by upregulation of activity of a copper-dependent enzyme, lysyl oxidase, which catalyses the cross linking of collagens and elastin and is implicated in the pathogenesis of OSF (Nair et al., 2004). In recent years, studies in India, China, south east Asia and South Africa, and on Asian migrants in the UK have shown a clear link between *Areca* nut chewing and OSF (Nair et al., 2004).

15.1.3.2 Betel Nut and Betel Nut Extracts in Carcinogenesis

An increased incidence of local tumors was observed in mice after subcutaneous injection of aqueous extracts of BQ without tobacco. Local tumors were produced in mice and local mesenchymal tumors in rats following subcutaneous injection of aqueous extracts of betel nut (AEBN). In hamsters, administration of *Areca* nut and application of its aqueous or dimethyl sulphoxide extracts to the cheek-pouch mucosa resulted in squamous cell carcinomas (SCC) of the cheek pouch and carcinomas of the fore-stomach (IARC, 1985). While BQ has various components (IARC, 1985; Sharan, 1996; Warnakulasuriya, 2002), a study on Syrian hamsters revealed that BN fiber and cold aqueous extract are the major components of BQ that may promote carcinogenesis in the hamster buccal pouch, leading to tumor formation. AEBN has been shown to induce conformational changes in mouse liver high mobility group (HMG) proteins similar to that induced by a hepatocarcinogen, diethylnitrosamine (DEN), leading to the development of preneoplastic nodules in the liver (Pariat and Sharan, 1998a, b). The post-translational modification of proteins such as, poly-ADP-ribosylation of HMG (Pariat et al., 1999; Pariat and Sharan, 2002) and histone (Saikia et al., 1998, 1999a, b) proteins was also strongly affected by exposure to BN resulting in alterations in chromatin organization.

(a) *Cytotoxicity: Areca* nut extract was found to decrease cell survival, vital dye accumulation and membrane integrity of cultured human buccal epithelial cells in a dose-dependent manner. BN also caused formation of both DNA single strand breaks and DNA protein cross links (Wary and Sharan, 1988; Sundqvist et al., 1989, Wary and Sharan, 1991). Different extracts of BN such as, AEBN, acetic acid extract (AAEBN), HCl extract (HEBN) and ethanol extract (EEBN) as well as arecoline showed different extents of cytostatic and cytotoxic effects on Hep2 cells in vitro, with arecoline, HEBN and EEBN being the most potent (Sharan and Wary, 1992). Cultured normal human oral keratinocytes (NHOK) exposed to ripe BN extract also showed significant decrease in population doubling, increase in senescence, cell cycle arrest at G_1/S phase and decrease in cell proliferation (Lu et al., 2006). Hamsters fed with powdered diet containing BN or BQ showed significant decrease in the survival rate, body weight, and hyperkeratosis and acanthosis of cheek pouch indicating that BN and BQ components may induce alterations in proliferation and differentiation of oral epithelial cells (Chiang et al., 2004).

(b) *Genotoxicity:* BQ and its components were found to be genotoxic. Interestingly, they also stimulated cell proliferation making the observed biological effects very complex. For instance, while the extracts of BN and inflorescence of *Piper betle* (IPB) induced DNA strand break, the extracts of BN, IPB, the BN polyphenol (+/−)catechin and arecoline decreased cell survival and proliferation. On the other hand, another component of BQ, the aqueous extract of lime, was found to increase cell proliferation (Jeng et al., 1994). AEBN was found to reduce glutathione synthetase (GSH) levels, induce chromosomal aberrations (CA) and delay cell kinetics in mouse bone marrow cells with the induction of sister chromatid exchange (SCE) probably involving TP53 dependant changes in cell proliferation (Kumpawat et al., 2003). Ethyl acetate and *n*-butanol extracts of BN as well as betel leaf are reported to induce CA in human lymphocytes and Chinese hamster ovary (CHO) cells (IARC, 1985). All components of BQ have been shown to individually enhance chromatid breaks and exchanges in the range of 12–37% in human cells in vitro. Frequency of SCE was elevated in mouse bone marrow cells when mice were exposed to the AEBN and its tannin (Panigrahi and Rao, 1989). AEBN also induced DNA strand breaks and enhanced cell proliferation in mouse kidney cells in vitro (Wary and Sharan, 1988). A study revealed that OSF was largely associated with BN and the exfoliated oral mucosal cells of such patients had significantly higher numbers of micronucleated cells. The patients also exhibited increased SCE in circulating lymphocytes indicating that the carcinogenic agents in BN produce damage not only in target tissue but also in other host cells such as circulating lymphocytes (Desai et al., 1996).

(c) *Immunotoxicity:* Aqueous extracts of raw *Areca* nut without husk as well as with husk were found to inhibit the phagocytic activity of human neutrophils in a dose dependent manner (Hung et al., 2005). BQ also influenced cytokine production of peripheral blood mononuclear cell. The mononuclear cells of persons suffering from SCC, with a long history of BQ chewing, produced lower levels of TGF-β, TNF-α and IFN-γ in comparison to normal persons (Hsu et al., 2001). This was indicative of compromised immune system under the influence of BQ or BN chewing.

(d) *Mutagenicity:* Aqueous extracts of BQ without tobacco induced mutations in *Salmonella typhimurium* but not in Chinese hamster V79 cells. BQ also did not induce any significant micronuclei in Swiss albino mice (IARC, 1985). AEBN, on the other hand, induced mutations in *Salmonella typhimurium* and in Chinese hamster V79 cells besides inducing gene conversion in *Saccharomyces cerevisiae* as well as CA in CHO cells. It also induced micronuclei in bone marrow cells of Swiss albino mice while BN tannin fraction induced gene conversion in *Saccharomyces cerevisiae* (IARC, 1985). Arecoline, AEBN, AAEBN, HEBN and EEBN induced variable levels of dose dependent unscheduled DNA synthesis (UDS) in Hep2 cells in vitro (Sharan and Wary, 1992; Sharan, 1996). Ames test using *Salmonella typhimurium* strain TA 1535 revealed that arecoline, AEBN and HEBN were weak mutagens while AAEBN and EEBN were strong mutagens suggesting that the mutagenic potential of alkaloids (arecoline) could be significantly enhanced by other constituents of BN (Sharan, 1994; Balachandran and Sharan, 1995; Sharan, 1996). Exposure to BN extracts was found to induce mutations at the *hypoxanthine phosphoribosyltransferase* (*HPRT*) locus in human keratinocytes (HaCaT cells), which also increased frequency of appearance of micronuclei, intracellular levels of reactive oxygen species and 8-hydroxyguanosine in the cells suggesting that stress caused by long-term BN extract exposure enhanced oxidative stress and genetic damage in HaKaT cells (Lai and Lee, 2006). When aqueous extracts of different brands of *pan masala* and scented BN or *supari* were tested for mutagenicity by the

Salmonella typhimurium assay using tester strains TA98 and TA100 their mutagenic effects were found to be similar to that produced by BN extracts (Polasa et al., 1993). A study involving patients of head and neck cancer suggested that BQ chewing may increase mitochondrial DNA (mtDNA) mutation in human oral tissues and that accumulation of mtDNA deletions and subsequent cytoplasmic segregation of these mutations during cell division could be important contributors to the early phase of oral carcinogenesis (Lee et al., 2001).

(e) *Teratogenesis:* Aqueous extracts of dry as well as raw/wet varieties of BN were reported to be fetotoxic in Swiss albino mice leading to death, enhanced resorption and reduced weight of fetuses. Other abnormalities such as hematomas, curved tails, abnormal ribs and delay in skeletal maturity have also been reported (Sinha and Rao, 1985a).

15.1.3.3 Betel Nut Alkaloids in Carcinogenesis

Alkaloids of BN are suspected to be its main carcinogenic constituent (IARC, 1985, 2004; Sharan, 1996; Norton, 1998; Jeng et al., 2001; Trivedy et al., 2002). Early studies found that the application of arecaidine to the oral mucosa of experimental animals failed to have any carcinogenic effects unless it was supplemented with a known promoter such as, croton oil (Trivedy et al., 2002). Arecoline given by gavage produced lung adenocarcinomas, stomach SCC and liver haemangiomas in male mice (IARC, 2004). Cheek-pouch application of arecoline following application of slaked lime produced an esophageal papilloma in female hamsters, while local application of arecaidine to the cheek pouch did not produce tumors in male hamsters (IARC, 2004). To explain the variable observation, it is proposed that the alkaloids first required metabolic activation via nitrosation to develop its carcinogenicity (Wary and Sharan, 1991). In rats, the major metabolic pathway of arecoline activation is via de-esterification and production via conjugated mercapturic acid. In vitro data suggest that arecoline is metabolized by carboxylesterase (EC 3.1.1.1) in mouse liver and kidney. Male Swiss albino mice fed *Areca* nut powder or arecoline showed enhanced levels of the hepatic cytochrome P450 and b_5 and decreased levels of hepatic GSH (IARC, 2004). Exposure of Swiss albino mice to arecoline was found to lower poly-ADP-ribosylation of most cellular and histone proteins and induce relaxation of chromatin, thereby allowing the N-nitrosamines of arecoline easy access to genomic DNA for interaction, while the absence of PADPR induced repair may favor the accumulation of DNA damage (Saikia et al., 1999b).

(a) *Cytotoxicity*: Arecoline was found to inhibit cell attachment, cell spreading and cell migration in a dose dependent manner in cultured human gingival fibroblasts (HGF) (Jeng et al., 1996). In Hep2 cells in vitro, arecoline inhibited both DNA and protein syntheses in a dose dependent manner, which ultimately resulted in cytostatic effect on cell division (Wary and Sharan, 1991). Crude alkaloid extracts of green *Areca* fruit consumed in Taiwan and arecoline were found to be mutagenic in *Salmonella typhimurium* TA100, and

N-Nitrosoguvacoline (NG) was weakly mutagenic in TA98 and TA100, with the formation of NG being favored at neutral pH (Wang and Peng, 1996). Arecoline alone was also only weakly mutagenic (Balachandran and Sharan, 1995). In vitro studies have shown that arecoline and arecaidine may stimulate cultured fibroblasts to proliferate and synthesize collagen, an important step in development of OSF. However, subsequent in vitro studies have failed to show similar effects of arecoline on cultured OSF fibroblast. It has also been shown that arecoline inhibited collagen synthesis and fibroblast proliferation in vitro, indicating the cytotoxic properties of arecoline. The disparity of results from in vitro studies might be indicative of other agents, in addition to arecoline, being important in the pathogenesis of OSF (Trivedy et al., 2002). The cytotoxicity of arecoline on the oral mucosal fibroblast (OMF) or on Hep2 cells was found to be associated with cellular GSH levels and esterase activities on one hand (Jeng et al., 1999), and the agents that facilitate metabolic activation and nitrosation of alkaloids, on the other (Wary and Sharan, 1991). In fact, GSH depletion and reduction of glutathione *S*-transferase activity have been demonstrated in cultured human oral keratinocytes and in fibroblasts treated with arecoline (IARC, 2004). Arecoline was also reported to be cytotoxic to human buccal fibroblasts in a dose dependent manner wherein the cellular glutathione-S-transferase (GST) activity was downregulated in a dose dependent manner without increase in lipid peroxidation. Addition of extracellular nicotine acted synergistically on the arecoline-induced cytotoxicity, indicating that arecoline may render human OMF more vulnerable to other reactive agents in cigarettes via GST reduction. These observations could explain why patients who practice the combined habit of BQ chewing and cigarette smoking are at greater risk of contracting oral cancer (Chang et al., 2001a).

Global gene expression profiling in HGF exposed to arecoline revealed that four genes related to maintenance of genome stability and DNA repair were repressed by arecoline (Chiang et al., 2007). They are *FANCG*, also known as *XRCC9* (tumor suppressor capable of correcting CA), *CHAF*1 and *CHAF*2 (encoding chromatin assembly factor I, CAF1), and *BRCA*1 (breast cancer susceptibility gene implicated in DNA damage response and DNA repair). Among them, at least the *BRCA*1 response was dose dependent. *COX-2/PTGS*2, which are involved in cancer initiation and progression, were over expressed in HGF cells. *HSP*4*A*1 and *DNAAJA*1, which belong to the *HSP*70 family of stress induced proteins, and GDF15/MIC-1 were also upregulated by arecoline in a dose dependent manner (Chiang et al., 2007).

(b) *Genotoxicity*: Arecoline was found to induce mutations in *Salmonella typhimurium* and Chinese hamster V79 cells, and CA in CHO cells. It also induced micronuclei, CA and SCE in bone marrow cells of Swiss albino mice (IARC, 1985; Deb and Chatterjee, 1998). However, upon withdrawal of arecoline exposure regime from Hep2 cells in vitro the inhibited DNA synthetic index fully recovered (Wary and Sharan, 1991) suggesting existence of weak interaction between BN genotoxin and DNA. Arecaidine induced mutations in *Salmonella typhimurium* and Chinese hamster V79 cells. It also induced SCE but not micronuclei in bone marrow cells of Swiss albino mice (IARC, 1985). This arecoline induced DNA damage was found to be influenced by endogenous GSH levels with the frequency of CA and SCE increasing when arecoline was given to mice treated with buthionine sulfoximine (BSO), a GSH depleting agent (Lu et al., 2006).

(c) *Immunotoxicity*: Arecoline was found to cause inhibition of both humoral and cell-mediated immune responses in mice (IARC, 2004). It is reported to interfere with the immune system by targeting the muscarinic acetylcholine receptors of the non-neuronal cholinergic system (Wen et al., 2006). Arecoline was also found to inhibit the phagocytic activity of human neutrophils (Hung et al., 2005).

(d) *Cell-cycle alterations*: Arecoline inhibited growth of human KB epithelial cells in dose- and time dependent manners by causing cell cycle arrest in late-S and G2/M phases due to induction of cyclin Bl, Wee 1, and phosphorylated cdc2 proteins and inhibition of p21 protein expression in KB cancer cells. In primary human gingival keratinocyes (HGK) arecoline effect was mediated differently. In this case, arecoline induced p21 but inhibited cdc2 and cyclin B1 proteins. This clearly suggests that differential regulation of S and/or G2/M cell cycle related proteins in the HGK and KB cells play crucial roles in different stages of BQ mediated carcinogenesis (Lee et al., 2006). Arecoline, which was cytotoxic to HGF cells due to depletion of intracellular thiols and inhibition of mitochondrial activity, induced cell cycle arrest in HGF cells at G2/M phase in a dose dependent manner (Chang et al., 2001b).

(e) *Teratogenicity*: Arecoline has been reported to induce abnormality in the shape of sperm heads and unscheduled DNA synthesis (UDS) in the early spermatid stages of Swiss albino mice (Sinha and Rao, 1985b). It also induced micronuclei formation in fetal mouse blood after transplacental exposure to BN (Sinha and Rao, 1985c). Arecoline caused general developmental retardation of zebra fish embryos predominantly due to a general cytotoxic effect induced by depletion of intracellular thiols (Chang et al., 2001c). Arecoline hydrobromide has been reported to have teratogenic effects on developing chick embryos leading to embryo mortality, retarded development of fetuses and other abnormalities. The abnormalities included reduced body size, scanty feathering, general edema with light body color, shortened lower beak, clubfoot, missing or unossified rib and shortening of long bones (Paul et al., 1999).

15.1.4 Betel Nut and Tumor Suppressor Genes **TP53, BRCA1** *and* **BRCA2**

Tumor suppressor genes are critical in carcinogenesis because loss of their function(s) results in promotion of malignancy (Kinzler and Vogelstein, 1997). Prominent among them is *TP*53 gene encoding a 393-amino acid residue long p53 protein, which is maintained at low cellular level in normal cells due to MDM2 mediated rapid turnover (Lane, 1992; Levine, 1997). Cells exposed to carcinogen or other stresses rapidly accumulate p53 due to its stabilization and/or mutation. Mutated or stabilized p53 induces cell cycle arrest at G1/S or G2 checkpoints. The quiescent cells are now in a position to repair the damage caused by the carcinogen or other stress factors and come out of it. Thus, TP53 functions as a "gatekeeper" tumor suppressor. The breast cancer susceptibility genes *BRCA*1 and *BRCA*2 are other two tumor suppressor genes relevant to human carcinogenesis. Both Brca1 and Brca2 proteins are functionally grouped as "caretakers" as they are involved with repair of DNA breaks, especially the critical double stranded breaks (DBS), via homologous recombination (HR) repair pathway in association with RAD family and other proteins.

Consistent with projected functions of *TP*53, *BRCA*1 and *BRCA*2 tumor suppressor genes, mutation or alteration in expression or both is expected in these tumor suppressor genes/proteins during carcinogenesis. Indeed, *TP*53 gene, one of the most extensively studied tumor suppressor genes, is known to be mutated in a variety of human and experimental animal cancers. Similarly, change in cellular level of p53 protein is also known to occur. Accumulation of p53 protein or its stabilization is an important indicator of the presence of mutant p53 protein (Hollstein et al., 1991, Harris and Hollstein, 1993). However, reports pertaining to *TP*53 mutation status of cancers associated with BN chewing have been widely contradicting. A study of Sri Lankan subjects with histologically confirmed oral squamous cell carcinoma (OSCC) and the habit of BN chewing with tobacco revealed low expression of p53 protein (Ranasinghe et al., 1993). A similar study in BN and tobacco associated OSCC from Southern India showed nuclear TP53 staining and TP53 expression indicating that carcinogens derived from tobacco and BN chewing may induce TP53 mutations (Kuttan et al., 1995). BQ chewers in Taiwan exhibited significantly higher incidence of *TP*53 gene mutations than non-chewers in esophageal squamous cell carcinoma (ESCC). The A:T $\rightarrow$ G:C transition and G:C $\rightarrow$ T:A transversion were the prevalent spectra of *TP*53 gene mutations and alcohol consumption could enhance this peculiar spectrum of *TP*53 mutation in ESCC suggesting that *TP*53 might be an important molecular target of BQ carcinogens in the development of ESCC in Taiwanese (Goan et al., 2005). Another study on patients of OSCC in Taiwan revealed that G:C $\rightarrow$ A:T transitions were the predominant mutations in the *TP*53 gene associated with BQ and tobacco use (Hsieh et al., 2001). Mutations in the *TP*53 gene were also frequent in OSCC specimens from Sri Lanka obtained from BQ chewers. They exhibited point, small deletion and addition type of mutations mainly clustered in exon 5 of the *TP*53 gene. These results indicate that exon 5 of the *TP*53 gene could be one of the specific targets for some BQ ingredients, and BQ chewing may be a critical environmental factor in the development of OSCC (Chiba et al., 1998). A study of potentially malignant oral lesions (leukoplakia) and OSCC associated with BQ consumption in northern India revealed a good correlation between TP53 missense mutations, p53 antibodies and p53 protein accumulation in matched potentially malignant and malignant oral lesions (Ralhan et al., 2001). Alternatively, incidence of *TP*53 mutations was reported to be infrequent or absent in oral premalignant lesions and OSCC in subjects chewing BQ with tobacco (Kannan et al., 1999) and without tobacco (Thomas et al., 1994; IARC, 2004). Mutations in both BRCA genes are known to be prevalent in familial as well as sporadic breast cancers (Rajan et al., 1996, Nadeau et al., 2000). However, not much is known about the status of these two important tumor suppressor proteins in BN associated carcinogenesis in mice or men.

We have made a systematic effort to study the effect of long term and transgenerational exposure of Swiss albino mice to AEBN on expression of TP53, Brca1 and Brca2 proteins as well induction of mutation in exons 5 and 7 of the *TP*53 gene and exon 11 of the *Brca*1 gene. Chronic exposure to AEBN in drinking water led to an upregulation of p53 protein in liver, spleen and peripheral blood lymphocytes (PBL) of exposed parental (P) generation mice from 2 weeks onwards reaching a maximum (2.5 folds of the age-matched control) after 6 weeks of exposure in the liver and spleen and 4 weeks of exposure in PBL (Fig. 15.3, panel A). Subsequently, the level of p53 protein declined gradually reaching control level after 16 weeks of exposure concomitant with the appearance of pre-neoplastic nodules in the liver (Fig. 15.3, panel A). After 24 weeks of exposure p53 protein was below control

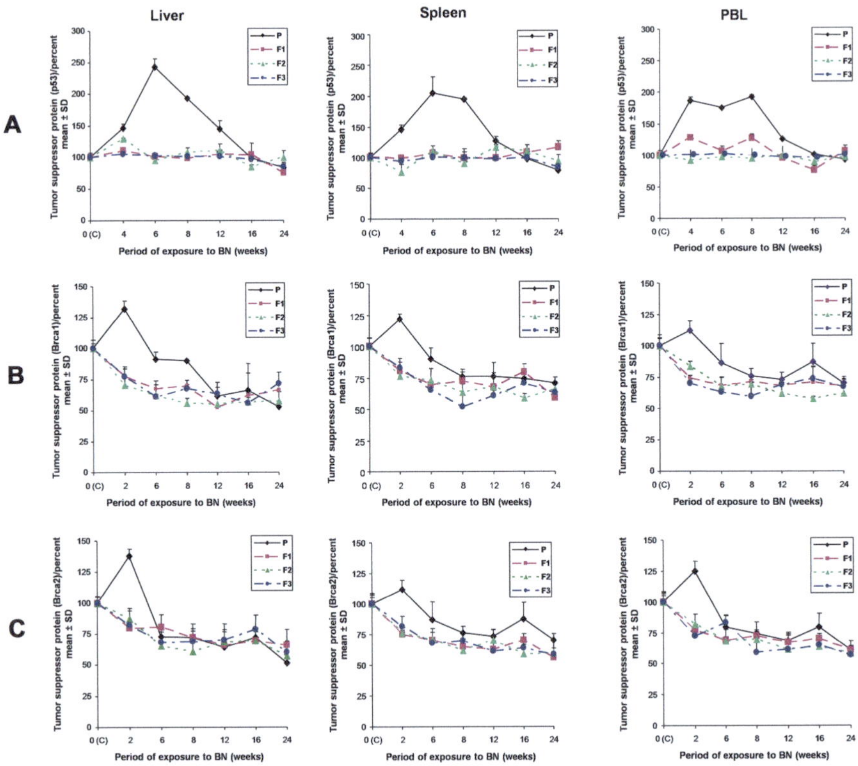

Fig. 15.3 Graphs showing cellular levels of three tumor suppressor proteins, p53 (**a**), Brca1 (**b**) and Brca2 (**c**), in liver, spleen and peripheral blood lymphocytes (PBL) of mice chronically and transgenerationally exposed to aqueous extract of betel nut (AEBN) in drinking water from parental (P) generation to F1 through F3 generations of mice

level, and the pre-neoplastic nodules were well developed. The expression of Brca1 (Fig. 15.3, panel B) and Brca2 (Fig. 15.3, panel C) proteins showed immediate elevation in liver, spleen and PBL after 2 weeks of exposure followed by a decline to 60% of that of age-matched control after 16 weeks of exposure and 50% after 24 weeks of exposure. No mutation in exons 5 and 7 of the *TP53* gene (GenBank accession # EF570972 and EF634061) (Choudhury and Sharan, 2009) and exon 11 of the *Brca1* gene (Choudhury and Sharan, 2010) were detected. Transmission electron microscope (TEM) study of the liver pre-neoplastic nodules after 24 weeks of exposure revealed a large number of binucleated cells with enlarged and abnormally shaped nuclei (Fig. 15.4b) as compared to the controls (Fig. 15.4a). Disruption of nuclear membrane as well as chromatin condensation and marginalization were also observed in a significant number of nuclei (Fig. 15.4c, d). Damage to mitochondria was most noticeable. The size of normal mitochondria (Fig. 15.4e) was significantly reduced (Fig. 15.4f) in all cases showing shrinkage. This was also accompanied with membrane disruptions (Fig. 15.4c, f; arrow head). The rough endoplasmic reticulum membrane organization (Fig. 15.4 h) was also severely damaged (Fig. 15.4i; arrow head).

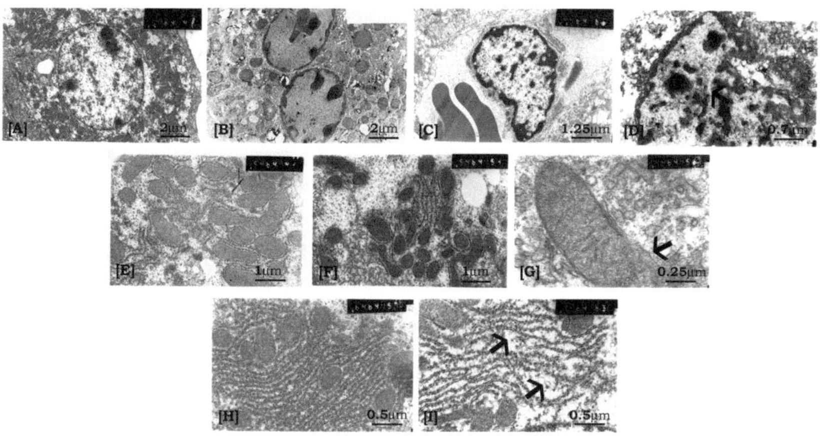

Fig. 15.4 Transmission electron micrographs of normal and transformed liver sections of mice exposed to aqueous extract of betel nut (AEBN) in drinking water. A normal liver cell with regular nucleus (**a**), which upon exposure to AEBN often showed binucleated cells (**b**), deformed nucleus (**c**) and/or nucleus with condensed and marginalized chromatin (**d**). The regular mitochondria of a normal cell (**e**), exhibited shrinkage and reduction in size upon exposure to AEBN (**f**) often accompanied with disrupted mitochondrial membrane (**g**). The normal arrangement of membrane in the endoplasmic reticulum (ER) (**h**) also exhibited pronounced disruptions (**i**)

Extensive damage of the mitochondrial membrane is a pro-apoptotic signal and extensive disruption of the ER could lead to calcium release from the ER lumen, which can potentially trigger ER-stress induced apoptosis. Thus, chronic exposure to AEBN caused serious molecular and metabolic damage to cells characterized by enlarged nuclei, high frequency of abnormally shaped nuclei, chromatin condensation and marginalization, and damaged membrane (Fig. 15.4) along with downregulated p53, Brca1 and Brca2 proteins (Fig. 15.3). After 16 weeks of chronic exposure to AEBN, an inability to upregulate TP53 beyond control level, combined with compromised DNA repair due to downregulation of Brca1 and Brca2, are sufficient to allow progression of hepatocarcinogenesis.

The effect of prenatal and transgenerational chronic exposure to AEBN has been followed up to F3 generation by breeding. In striking contrast to the P generation, the liver, spleen and PBL of AEBN exposed F1, F2 and F3 generation mice exhibited invariant expression of p53 protein in comparison to age matched controls throughout the period of exposure (Fig. 15.3a). Similarly, the expression of Brca1 (Fig. 15.3b) and Brca2 (Fig. 15.3c) proteins progressively declined to approximately 80% that of age matched controls only after 2 weeks of exposure in all the three tissues examined. Thus, while the P generation mice exhibited an induction of the tumor suppressive functions of the p53, Brca1 and Brca2 proteins during the initial periods of AEBN exposure, the transgenerationally exposed mice failed to induce these tumor suppressors (Fig. 15.3). Concomitantly, a significant advancement in the appearance of liver pre-neoplastic nodules was observed with each subsequent generation suggesting progressive enhancement of transmission of carcinogenic risk due to exposure to BN constituents (Table 15.2). Abnormalities, which were not observed in P generation mice, also developed in the transgenerationally exposed mice. Though statistically insignificant up to F3 generation, these abnormalities included enlargement of lymph nodes of the neck, development of protuberant pus-filled sacs, necrosis of the liver and development of solid tumors. No mutations in exons 5 and 7 of the *TP*53 gene were observed in the liver nodules as well as solid tumors of even the transgenerationally exposed mice. Thus, while inactivation of the TP53 gene apparently plays a crucial role in BN associated cancer in mice, the inactivation is not ubiquitously through *TP*53 mutation and other routes of inactivation require to be investigated. One possible alternative mechanism for TP53 inactivation in BN carcinogenesis may be over-expression of MDM2 protein as has been shown in OSCC (Shwe et al., 2001). In contrast BN induced solid tumors in Swiss albino mice carried a G $\rightarrow$ C (codon 156; –TGT– $\rightarrow$ –TCT–) transversion mutation in exon 11 of the *Brca*1 gene (Fig. 15.5). Exon 11 of the *Brca*1 gene encodes the two nuclear localization motifs and a region of the gene believed to be essential for binding of RAD51 (Cressman et al., 1999). Mutation in exon 11 would, therefore, disrupt normal functioning of the *Brca*1 gene leading to DNA repair defects, which could be pivotal for the development of the solid tumors. Thus, AEBN can possibly

Table 15.2 Estimated transgenerational cancer transmission risk in mice from BN (Choudhury and Sharan, 2009)

Chronic AEBN administration in drinking water to mice	Appearance of pre-neoplastic nodules on liver
P generation	16 weeks
F1 generation	8 weeks
F2 generation	6 weeks
F3 generation	4 weeks

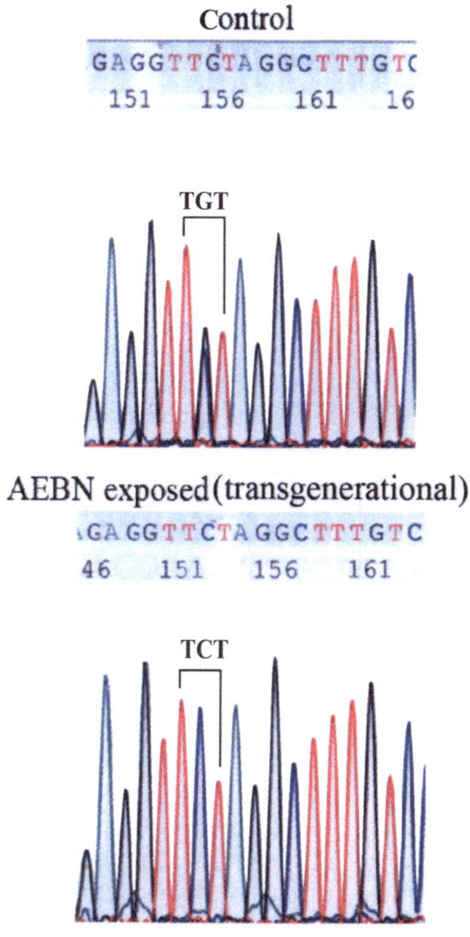

Fig. 15.5 Part of the nucleotide sequence chromatograms of PCR amplicons representing exon 11 of *Brca*1 gene of control (*top*) and F1 generation of AEBN exposed (*bottom*) mice liver. It shows induction of a G → C transversion type point mutation

lead to transgenerational transmission of carcinogenic risk in Swiss Albino mice by compromising the functions of the tumor suppressor genes *TP*53, *BRCA*1 and *BRCA*2 via different mechanisms.

15.1.5 Betel Nut Polyphenol and Tannins in Carcinogenesis

Toxicity studies relating to BN specific polyphenols and tannins are not conclusive with both carcinogenic and anti-carcinogenic effects being reported. It is reported that ROS produced during auto-oxidation of BN polyphenols in the BQ chewer's saliva are crucial in the initiation and promotion of oral cancer (Jeng et al., 2001). Incidences of certain cancers, such as esophageal cancer, have been reported to be related to consumption of tannins-rich foods such as BN suggesting that tannins might be carcinogenic. However, other reports indicated that the carcinogenic activity of tannins might be related to components associated with tannins rather than tannins themselves (Chung et al., 1998).

15.1.6 Betel Nut and Human Genetic Susceptibility to Oral Cancer

Exposure to BN carcinogens, particularly the alkaloids, enhances the risk of cancer in BN or BQ chewers in general. However, correlation between prevalence of cancer in human populations in different parts of the world and habit of BN/BQ mastication is not absolute. This suggests that the genetic makeup of the masticator has its own influence on the ultimate manifestation of BN induced cancer. It is becoming obvious that the interplay between the genetic constitution and the environmental factor(s), determine the final risk of human oral cancer following exposure to BN or BQ alone or in combination with additives, including tobacco. Mere exposure to BN or BQ does not commit the chewer to cancer. For any given level of exposure to BN carcinogen, only a proportion of exposed individuals will develop cancer, indicating the prevalence of inter-individual differences in susceptibility (Spitz and Bondy, 1993). Individual susceptibility to cancer may result from several factors including (a) differences in metabolism, (b) status of DNA repair pathways and related genes, (c) patterns of expression of proto-oncogenes and tumor suppressor genes, and (d) nutritional status of the masticator, etc. Variations in an individual's metabolic phenotype, i.e., phenotypic polymorphism, have also been detected in a variety of enzymes involved in activation and detoxification of chemical carcinogens. It is becoming clearer now that different phenotypic and/or metabolic variations stem from genetic polymorphisms prevalent in different population groups (Bartsch and Hietanen, 1996). A number of genetic polymorphisms have been identified, which seem to be associated with risk of BN induced oral cancer in human sub-populations. Table 15.3 depicts the up to date list of polymorphisms observed in BN exposed human sub-populations with manifestation of oral cancer.

15.1.7 Possible Mechanism of Betel Nut Induced Carcinogenesis

BN is a natural plant product characterized by a very complex and highly variable mixture of different biochemical and nutraceutical constituents (Table 15.1). Some of these are recognized as potent carcinogens (e.g., alkaloids, polyphenols, tannins, etc.). However, many others, especially those present in small to trace amounts, have largely unknown biological functions. As with nutraceuticals, it is anticipated that in a complex cellular environment some of these may function as mediators, some as modulators, affecters, promoters, and/or inhibitors, etc. eliciting a variety of biological effects and responses. The highly variable constituents of BN should also chemically and otherwise interact differently with different biomolecules. The

Table 15.3 Genetic polymorphism and susceptibility to oral cancer in humans

No.	Gene/region	Polymorphism	Effect	Population group	References
1	Matrix metallo-proteinase-9 (MMP9) promoter	1562 C-to-T polymorphism	MMP-9-1562 C>T polymorphism—enhanced OSCC risk in young male BN chewers	Taiwanese	Tu et al. (2007)
2	Matrix metallo-proteinase-3 (MMP3) promoter	Insertion/deletion (-1171 5A→>6A) polymorphisms	5A genotype polymorphism—enhanced risk of OSF but not OSCC among male BN users	Asian	Tu et al. (2006)
3	NFKB1 promoter	Insertion (ins)/deletion (del) polymorphism (-94 ins/del ATTG) in NFKB1 promoter.	NFKB1 ins and HO-1 L allelotypes—significantly enhanced risks for different subsets of OSCC in male BN chewers	Asian	Lin et al. (2006)
4	DNA repair genes *XRCC1* and *XPD*	Polymorphisms Arg194Trp, Arg280His, and Arg399Gln of the XRCC1 gene and Lys751Gln of the XPD gene	Variant allele of XRCC1 399 codon and XPD—enhanced risk of oral cancer among BQ chewers and smokers	South Indian	Ramachandran et al. (2006)
5	Heme oxygenase-1 (*HMOX1*)	Polymorphisms in a (GT)n microsatellite repeat in HMOX1 promoter in short (S), medium (M) and long (L) alleles	Longer (GT)n repeat allele L—higher risk of BN related OSCC; (GT)n repeat allele S—may be protective for OSCC	Asian	Chang et al. (2004)
6	Cytochrome gene *CYP2A6*	*CYP2A6**4C* mutation-gene deletion type of polymorphism	Deficient *CYP2A6* activity due to deletion—reduced risk of oral cancer risk in BQ chewers	Sri Lankan	Topcu et al. (2002)
7	Cytochrome gene *CYP1A1*	*CYP1A1 A/G* genotype (Ile/Val) and *G/G* genotype (Val/Val) in exon 7	*CYP1A1* exon 7 containing *G* allele—enhanced risk for OSCC and oral precancerous lesion (OPL) in BN chewer and smoker	Chinese	Kao et al. (2002)

Table 15.3 (continued)

No.	Gene/region	Polymorphism	Effect	Population group	References
8	Collagen related genes: Collagen 1A1 and 1A2 (COL1A1 and COL1A2), Collagenase-1 (MMP1), transforming growth factor β1 (TGFB1), Lysyl oxidase (LOX), and Cystatin C (CST3)	Polymorphisms of six collagen related genes, COL1A1, COL1A2, MMP1, TGFB1, LOX, and CST3	Multigenic mechanisms involving the collagen related genes enhance susceptibility to OSF among BQ chewers	Taiwanese	Chiu et al. (2002)
9	Tumor necrosis factor-α (TNFA)	Bi-allelic promoter region (-308) polymorphism on the TNFA gene	The high production allele, TNF2—significantly lower among individuals with OSF	Taiwanese	Chiu et al. (2001)
10	Glutathione-S-transferase genes GSTM1 and GSTT1	GSTM1 and GSTT1 null genotypes (GSTM1*2 and GSTT1*2)	Null genotypes of either or both GSTM1 and GSTT1—enhanced risk of development of leukoplakia following exposure to tobacco with or without BQ	South Indian	Nair et al. (1999)
11		Genetic polymorphism of GSTM1 and GSTT1	Homozygous deletion of GSTM1 gene—enhanced risk for oral cancer, which is further compounded by exposure to cigarette smoke, alcohol, and BQ	Thai	Kietthubthew et al. (2001)

situation is further complicated by the fact that a host of region, culture and society specific additives, notably different types of chewing tobacco, are invariably added to BN preparation by a traditional masticator (Fig. 15.1). Therefore, it is only expected that the mechanism of BN induced carcinogenesis would also be highly variable and complex. Nonetheless, certain conclusions can be drawn from the wealth of knowledge available to us (see Fig. 15.6). The overall perception is that alkaloids are the main carcinogenic constituents of BN. Polyphenols and tannins may also contribute positively to carcinogenic potency of the alkaloids. It

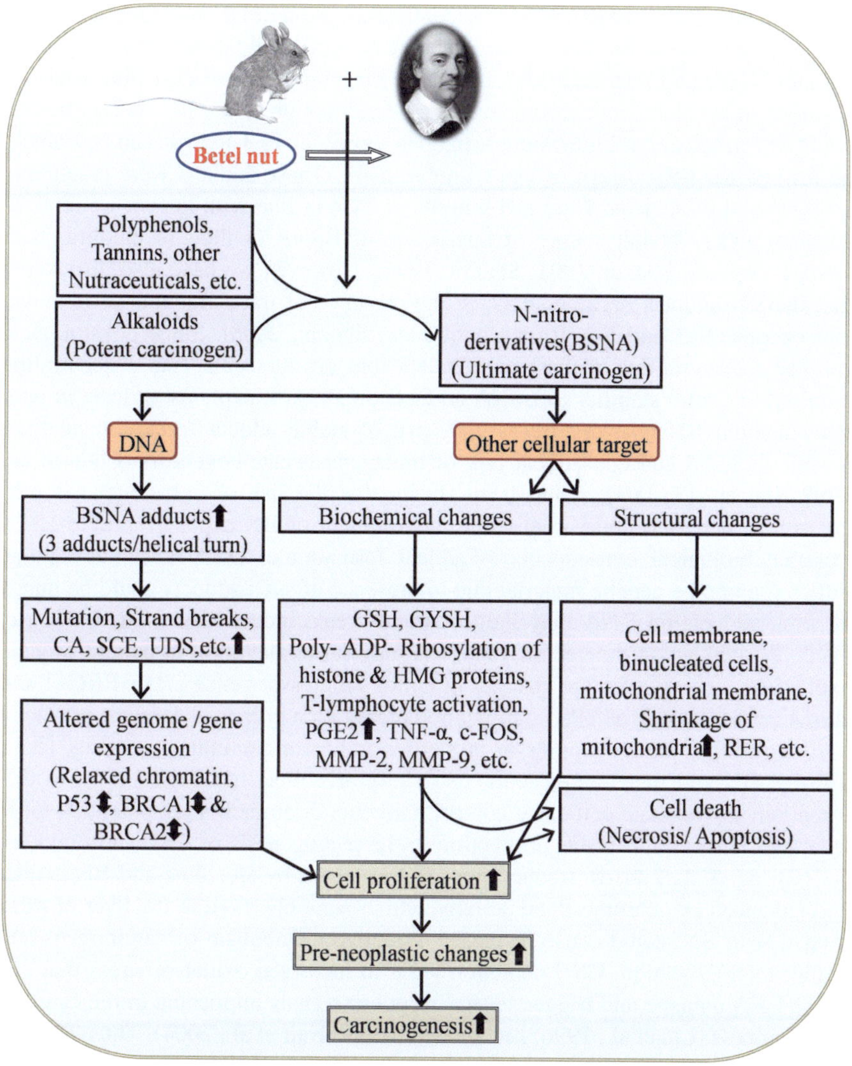

Fig. 15.6 Schematic diagram of major metabolic events and milestones in the pathway of betel nut induced carcinogenesis (see text for details)

is now accepted that alkaloids, the primary suspected carcinogen of BN, should first undergo metabolic activation and nitrosation to produce the ultimate carcinogenic derivatives together called BSNA (Fig. 15.2). This may be achieved by de-esterification using carboxylesterase and may also involve cytochrome P450, b_5 and GSH besides other metabolites. The activated or ultimate carcinogen(s) acquires capability of interaction with target biomolecules. The interaction of BSNA or their activated derivatives with cellular targets forming adducts of different kinds may be the beginning of carcinogenesis (Chen et al., 1999; Liu et al., 2004). Using different physic-chemical methods evidence of existence of BSNA adducts has been amply demonstrated (IARC, 1985). Recently, formation of DNA adducts by AEBN and its consequences has been directly shown on a plasmid DNA construct, pMTa4 (Bhattacharjee and Sharan, 2008). Using the plasmid model in vitro and in vivo it has been shown that under chronic exposure condition up to one BN specific adduct could be formed every 3 nucleotides. In other words, up to 3 adducts can potentially be formed per helical turn of DNA double helix. These adducts were essentially unstable and dissociated from DNA in about 24 h in line with known weak, non-covalent and reversible nature of interaction of BSNA or their metabolites with DNA (Wary and Sharan, 1991; Sharan, 1996). However, we have also discovered that the BN adducts became stable in the presence of trace amounts of monovalent cations, Na^+ and K^+ (Bhattacharjee and Sharan, 2008). Since physiological cellular concentrations of these monovalent ions are more than the concentration required to confer stability to BSNA adducts on DNA, it explains, at least in part, why habitual BN chewers are at high risk of stable adduct formation on their genetic material and consequent risk of mutagenesis/carcinogenesis (Chen et al., 1999; Liu et al., 2004). It has been shown that the risk of carcinogenesis progressively increased under continuing environment of BN exposure (Table 15.2). Possible biological consequence of adduct formation on DNA as well as damage inflicted upon the genetic material due to presence of such adducts could be many. At first, adducts on DNA may induce strand break, induce CA, SCE, UDS, etc. Secondly, damage to the genetic materials may cause alteration in pattern of gene expression. In particular, the changes in tumor suppressor genes *TP*53, *BRCA*1 and *BRCA*2 either by way of TP53 stabilization or mutation in critical domains are likely to diminish their tumor suppressor properties and favor carcinogenesis (Fig. 15.3). Thirdly, BN and their constituents, especially arecoline, has been shown to differentially dysregulate cell cycle control, mitochondrial membrane potential, GSH level and intracellular H_2O_2 production in the pathogenesis of OSF and oral cancer (Chang et al., 2001d). Reduction of GSH content by arecoline and BN extract and enhanced cytochrome P450 activity, which were observed in the liver of mice treated with BN, could cause increased oxidative metabolism of carcinogens and reduced detoxification. GSH depletion leads to increased oxidative stress that can cause DNA damage and trigger several response signals implicated in the carcinogenic process (Liu et al., 1996; Liu and Chi, 1999; Nair et al., 2004). Thus, BN and its constituents potentially interfere with cell signaling pathways. Little is understood about these aspects and more research is needed to unravel the influence of BN exposure on the complex cell signaling pathways. In spite of this, it is known that

BQ chewing contributes to the pathogenesis of cancer and OSF also by impairing T cell activation and by induction of PGE2, TNF-α and IL-6 production, which favors oral mucosal inflammation and growth of OMF and oral epithelial cells (Jeng et al., 2003). Similar end may also be achieved by activation of the MEK1/ERK/c-Fos pathway, which promotes keratinocyte inflammation, cell survival, and affects cell cycle progression (Chang et al. 2004). Alternatively, MMP-2, an enzyme belonging to matrix metalloproteinases (MMP) group of proteins that degrade extracellular matrix proteins and contribute to the tumor invasion and metastasis, was found to be elevated in most oral tumor patients with long term BQ usage while short term BQ usage increased the secretion of MMP-2 by oral epithelial cells and fibroblasts. This is suggestive of BQ consumption promoting oral tumor progression through the induction of MMP-2 secretion (Kato et al., 2005, Liu et al., 2005a). Elevation of MMP-9 was also observed following BQ chewing showing its role in the pathogenesis of oral mucosal lesions (Liu et al., 2005b). Due to this, levels of both MMP-2 and MMP-9 have been suggested as possible markers of human oral cancer (Patel et al., 2007). In all this, it has to be kept in mind that mere exposure to BN does not commit a cell or an organism to carcinogenesis. There are metabolic escape routes available to the exposed cell or organism by way of complete repair of damage and attainment of normalcy or necrotic or apoptotic programmed cell death (Fig. 15.6). Metabolic, cellular and other genetic factors, in complex and largely unclear ways, influence the path of carcinogenesis triggered by exposure to BN.

Acknowledgments RNS acknowledges contributions of all research associates and scholars whose work has been cited in this review. Grants of UGC, CSIR, DST and ICMR, which supported different aspects of research embodied in this chapter, are also acknowledged. Part of the ongoing research is being carried out under a research scheme partly funded by the UPE-NEHU grant. YC was supported by a fellowship (NET-JRF/SRF) from the UGC and is currently working as a Lecturer, Department of Biotechnology, Assam University, Silchar, 788 011, India.

References

Balachandran, B., Sharan, R. N. 1995. Induction of mutations by different extracts of betel nut and radiation: Their implication in carcinogenesis. In Radiation Research 1895–1995, eds. U. Hagen, H. Jung, and C. Streffer, pp 165, vol. 1, Würzburg: Universitätsdruckerei H. Stürtz AG.

Bartsch, H., Hietanen, E. 1996. The role of individual susceptibility in cancer burden related to environmental exposure. Environ Health Perspect 104:569–577.

Bhattacharjee, C., Sharan, R. N. 2008. Aqueous extract of betel nut (AEBN) induced adducts on pMTa4 DNA acquires stability in the presence of Na^+ and K^+ ions. Mol. Med. Rep. 1:435–441.

Boucher, B. J., Mannan, N. 2002. Metabolic effects of the consumption of *Areca catechu*. Addict. Biol. 7:103–110.

Chang, M. C., Ho, Y. S., Lee, P. H., Chan, C. P., Lee, J. J., Hahn, L. J., Wang, Y. J., Jeng, J. H. 2001d. Areca nut extract and arecoline induced the cell cycle arrest but not apoptosis of cultured oral KB epithelial cells: association of glutathione, reactive oxygen species and mitochondrial membrane potential. Carcinogenesis 22:1527–1535.

Chang, Y. C., Hu, C. C., Lii, C. K., Tai, K. W., Yang, S. H., Chou, M. Y. 2001b. Cytotoxicity and arecoline mechanisms in human gingival fibroblasts in vitro. Clin. Oral Investig. 5:51–56.

Chang, Y. C., Hu, C. C., Tseng, T. H., Tai, K. W., Lii, C. K., Chou, M. Y. 2001a. Synergistic effects of nicotine on arecoline-induced cytotoxicity in human buccal mucosal fibroblasts. J. Oral Pathol. Med. 30:458–464.

Chang, B., Liao, M., Kuo, M. Y., Chen, C. 2001c. Developmental toxicity of arecoline, the major alkaloid in betel nuts, in zebrafish embryos. Birth Defects Res. 70:28–36.
Chang, M. C., Wu, H. L., Lee, J. J., Lee, P. H., Chang, H. H., Hahn, L. J., Lin, B. R., Chen, Y. J., Jeng, J. H. 2004. The induction of prostaglandin E2 production, interleukin-6 production, cell cycle arrest, and cytotoxicity in primary oral keratinocytes and KB cancer cells by areca nut ingredients is differentially regulated by MEK/ERK activation. J Biol Chem 279:50676–50683.
Chen, C. L., Chi, C. W., Chang, K. W., Liu, T. Y. 1999. Safrole-like DNA adducts in oral tissue from oral cancer patients with a betel quid chewing history. Carcinogenesis 20:2331–2334.
Chiang, C., Chang, M., Lee, J., Chang, J. Y., Lee, P., Hahn, L., Jeng, J. 2004. Hamsters chewing betel quid or areca nut directly show a decrease in body weight and survival rates with concomitant epithelial hyperplasia of cheek pouch. Oral Oncol. 40:720–727.
Chiang, S., Jiang, S., Wang, Y., Chiang, H., Chen, P., Tu, H., Ho, K., Tsai, Y., Chang, I., Ko, Y. 2007. Characterization of arecoline-induced effects on cytotoxicity in normal human gingival fibroblasts by global gene expression profiling. Toxicol Sci 100:66–74.
Chiba, I., Muthumala, M., Yamazaki, Y., Zaman, A. U., Iizuka, T., Amemiya, A., Shibata, T., Kashiwazaki, H., Sugiura, C., Fukuda, H. 1998. Characteristics of mutations in the *p*53 gene of oral squamous-cell carcinomas associated with betel-quid chewing in Sri Lanka. Int J Cancer 77:839–842.
Chiu, C. J., Chang, C. P., Hahn, L. J., Hsieh, L. L., Chen, C. J. 2002. Interaction of collagen-related genes and susceptibility to betel quid-induced oral submucous fibrosis. Cancer Epidemiol. Biomarkers. Prev. 11:646–653.
Chiu, C. J., Chiang, C. P., Chang, M. L., Chen, H. M., Hahn, L. J., Hsieh, L. L., Kuo, Y. S., Chen, C. J. 2001. Association between genetic polymorphism of tumor necrosis factor-alpha and risk of oral submucous fibrosis, a pre-cancerous condition of oral cancer. J. Dent. Res. 80: 2055–2059.
Choudhury, Y., Sharan, R. N. 2009. Altered p53 response and enhanced transgenerational transmission of carcinogenic risk upon exposure of mice to betel nut. Environ. Toxicol. Pharmacol. 27:127–138.
Choudhury, Y., Sharan, R. N. 2010. Altered BRCA1 and BRCA2 response and mutation of BRCA1 gene m mice exposed chronically and transgenerationally to aqueous extract of betel nut. Environ. Toxicol. Pharmacol. (in communication)
Chung, K. T., Wong, T. Y., Wei, C. I., Huang, Y. W., Lin, Y. 1998. Tannins and human health: a review. Crit. Rev. Food Sci. Nutr. 38:421–464.
Cressman, V. L., Backlund, D. C., Avrutskaya, A., Leadon, S. A., Godfrey, V., Koller, B. H. 1999. Growth retardation, DNA repair defects, and lack of spermatogenesis in BRCA1-deficient mice. Mol Cell Biol 19:7061–7075.
Deb, S., Chatterjee, A. 1998. Influence of buthionine sulfoximine and reduced glutathione on arecoline-induced chromosomal damage and sister chromatid exchange in mouse bone marrow cells in vivo. Mutagenesis 13:243–248.
Deng, J. F., Ger, J., Tsai, W. J., Kao, W. F., Yang, C. C. 2001. Acute toxicities of betel nut: rare but probably overlooked events. J Toxicol Clin Toxicol 39:355–360.
Desai, S. S., Ghaisas, S. D., Jakhi, S. D., Bhide, S. V. 1996. Cytogenetic damage in exfoliated oral mucosal cells and circulating lymphocytes of patients suffering from precancerous oral lesions. Cancer Lett. 109:9–14.
Goan, Y. G., Chang, H. C., Hsu, H. K., Chou, Y. P., Cheng, J. T. 2005. Risk of *p*53 gene mutation in esophageal squamous cell carcinoma and habit of betel quid chewing in Taiwanese. Cancer Sci. 96:758–765.
Harris, C. C., Hollstein, M. 1993. Clinical implications of the p53 tumor-suppressor gene. N Engl J Med 329:1318–1327.
Hollstein, M., Sidransky, D., Vogelstein, B., Harris, C. C. 1991. P53 mutation in human cancer. Science 253:49–53.
Hsieh, L. L., Wang, P. F., Chen, I. H., Liao, C. T., Wang, H. M., Chen, M. C., Chang, J. T., Cheng, A. J. 2001. Characterisics of mutations of the *p*53 gene in oral squamous cell carcinoma associated with betel quid chewing and cigarette smoking in Taiwanese. Carcinogenesis 22:1497–1503.

Hsu, H. J., Chang, K. L., Yang, Y. H., Shieh, T. Y. 2001. The effects of arecoline on the release of cytokines using cultured peripheral blood mononuclear cells from patients with oral mucous diseases. Kaohsiung J Med Sci 17:175–182.

Hung, S., Cheng, Y., Peng, J., Chang, L., Liu, T., Chen, Y. 2005. Inhibitory effects of areca nut extracts on phagocytosis of *Actinobacillus actinomycetemcomitans* ATCC 33384 by neutrophils. J. Periodontol. 76:373–379.

IARC. 1985. International Agency for Research on Cancer (IARC) – Tobacco habits other than smoking: Betel quid and Areca-nut chewing and some related nitrosamines. IARC Monogr Eval Carcinog Risks Hum 37:263, Lyon: IARC.

IARC. 2004. International Agency for Research on Cancer (IARC) – Summaries & Evaluations: Betel-quid and areca-nut chewing. IARC Monogr Eval Carcinog Risk Chem Hum 85:39, Lyon: IARC.

Jeng, J. H., Chang, M. C., Hahn, L. J. 2001. Role of areca nut in betel quid-associated chemical carcinogenesis: current awareness and future perspectives. Oral Oncol. 37:477–492.

Jeng, J. H., Kuo, M. L., Hahn, L. J., Kuo, M. Y. 1994. Genotoxic and non-genotoxic effects of betel quid ingredients on oral mucosal fibroblasts in vitro. J. Dental Res. 73:1043–1049.

Jeng, J. H., Lan, W. H., Hahn, L. J., Hsieh, C. C., Kuo, M. Y. 1996. Inhibition of the migration, attachment, spreading, growth and collagen synthesis of human gingival fibroblasts by arecoline, a major areca alkaloid, in vitro. J. Oral Pathol. Med. 25:371–375.

Jeng, J. H., Tsai, C. L., Hahn, L. J., Yang, P. J., Kuo, Y. S., Kuo, M. Y. 1999. Arecoline cytotoxicity on human oral mucosal fibroblasts related to cellular thiol and esterase activities. Food Chem Toxicol 37:751–756.

Jeng, J. H., Wang, Y. J., Chiang, B. L., Lee, P. H., Chan, C. P., Ho, Y. S., Wang, T. M., Lee, J. J., Hahn, L. J., Chang, M. C. 2003. Roles of keratinocyte inflammation in oral cancer: regulating the prostaglandin E2, interleukin-6 and TNF-α production of oral epithelial cells by areca nut extract and arecoline. Carcinogenesis 24:1301–1315.

Kannan, K., Munirajan, A. K., Krishnamurthy, J. 1999. Low incidence of p53 mutation in betel quid and tobacco chewing-associated oral squamous carcinoma from India. Int J Oncol 15:1133–1136.

Kao, S. Y., Wu, H. C., Lin, S. C., Yap, S. K., Chang, C. S., Wong, Y. K., Chi, L. Y., Liu, T. Y. 2002. Genetic polymorphism of cytochrome P4501A1 and susceptibility to oral squamous cell carcinoma and oral precancer lesions associated with smoking/betel use. J. Oral Pathol. Med. 31:505–511.

Kato, K., Hara, A., Kuno, T., Kitaori, N., Huilan, Z., Mori, H., Toida, M., Shibata, T. 2005. Matrix metalloproteinases 2 and 9 in oral squamous cell carcinomas: manifestation and localization of their activity. J. Cancer Res. Clin. Oncol. 131:340–346.

Kietthubthew, S., Sriplung, H., Au, W. W. 2001. Genetic and environmental interactions on oral cancer in Southern Thailand. Environ Mol Mutagen 37:111–116.

Kinzler, K. W., Vogelstein, B. 1997. Gatekeeprs and caretakers. Nature 386:761–763.

Kumpawat, K., Deb, S., Ray, S., Chatterjee, A. 2003. Genotoxic effect of raw betel-nut extract in relation to endogenous glutathione levels and its mechanism of action in mammalian cells. Mutat Res 538:1–12.

Kuttan, N. A. A., Rosin, M. P., Ambika, K., Priddy, R. W., Bhakthan, N. M. G., Zhang, L. 1995. High prevalence of expression of p53 oncoprotein in oral carcinomas from India associated with betel and tobacco chewing. Eur J Cancer 31:169–173.

Lai, K., Lee, T. 2006. Genetic damage in cultured human keratinocytes stressed by long-term exposure to areca nut extracts. Mutat. Res. Fundam. Mol. Mech. Mutag. 599:66–75.

Lane, D. P. 1992. Cancer: p53 guardian of the genome. Nature 358:15–16.

Lee, P., Chang, M., Chang, W., Wang, T., Wang, Y., Hahn, L., Ho, Y., Lin, C., Jeng, J. 2006. Prolonged exposure to arecoline arrested human KB epithelial cell growth: Regulatory mechanisms of cell cycle and apoptosis. Toxicology 220:81–89.

Lee, H., Yin, P., Yu, T., Chang, Y., Hsu, W., Kao, S., Chi, C., Liu, T., Wei, Y. 2001. Accumulation of mitochondrial DNA deletions in human oral tissues — effects of betel quid chewing and oral cancer. Mutat. Res. Genetic Toxicol. Environ. Mutagen. 493:67–74.

Levine, A. J. 1997. P53, the cellular gatekeeper for growth and division. Cell 88:323–331.

Lin, Y., Jen, Y., Wang, B., Lee, J., Kang, B. 2005. Epidemiology of oral cavity cancer in Taiwan with emphasis on the role of betel nut chewing. *ORL J. Otorhinolaryngol. Relat. Spec.* 67: 230–236.

Lin, S. C., Liu, C. J., Yeh, W. I., Lui, M. T., Chang, K. W., Chang, C. S. 2006. Functional polymorphism in NFKB1 promoter is related to risks of oral squamous cell carcinoma occurring on older male areca (betel) chewers. Cancer Lett. 243:47–54.

Liu, T., Chen, C., Chi, C. 1996. Oxidative damage to DNA induced by areca nut extract. Mutat. Res. Genetic Toxicol. 367:5–31.

Liu, T. Y., Chi, C. W. 1999. Areca nut extracts stimulate DNA strand breaks by generation of nitric oxide. Toxicol Lett 95:112.

Liu, T. Y., Chung, Y. T., Wang, P. F., Chi, C. W., Hsieh, L. L. 2004. Safrole-DNA adducts in human peripheral blood—an association with areca quid chewing and CYP2E1 polymorphisms. Mutat. Res. Genetic Toxicol. Environ. Mutagen. 559:59–66.

Liu, S. Y., Lin, M. H., Yang, S. C., Huang, G. C., Chang, L., Chang, S., Yen, C. Y., Chiang, W. F., Kuo, Y. Y., Chen, L. L., Lee, C. H., Liu, Y. C. 2005a. Increased expression of matrix metalloproteinase-2 in oral cells after short-term stimulation and long-term usage of areca quid. J. Formos. Med. Assoc. 104:390–397.

Liu, S. Y., Lin, M. H., Yang, S. C., Huang, G. C., Chang, L., Chang, S., Yen, C. Y., Chiang, W. F., Lee, C. H., Kuo, Y. Y., Liu, Y. C. 2005b. Areca quid chewing enhances the expression of salivary matrix metalloproteinase-9. J. Formos. Med. Assoc. 104:113–119.

Lu, S., Chang, K., Liu, C., Tseng, Y., Lu, H., Lee, S., Lin, S. 2006. Ripe areca nut extract induces G_1 phase arrests and senescence-associated phenotypes in normal human oral keratinocyte. Carcinogenesis 27:1273–1284.

Nadeau, G., Boufaied, N., Moisan, A., Lemieux, K. M., Cayanan, C., Monteiro, A. N. A., Gaudreau, L. 2000. BRCA1 can stimulate gene transcription by a unique mechanism. EMBO Rep. 3:260–265.

Nair, U., Bartsch, H., Nair, J. 2004. Alert for an epidemic of oral cancer due to use of the betel quid substitutes gutkha and pan masala: a review of agents and causative mechanisms. Mutagenesis 19:251–262.

Nair, U., Floyd, R. A., Nair, J., Bussachini, V., Friesen, M., Bartsch, H. 1987. Formation of reactive oxygen species and of 8-hydroxydeoxyguanosine in DNA in vitro with betel quid ingredients. Chem Biol Interact 63:157–169.

Nair, U. J., Nair, J., Mathew, B., Bartsch, H. 1999. Glutathione S-transferase M1 and T1 null genotypes as risk factors for oral leukoplakia in ethnic Indian betel quid/ tobacco chewers. Carcinogenesis 20:743–748.

Nair, J., Ohshima, H., Friesen, M., Croisy, A., Bhide, S. V., Bartsch, H. 1985. Tobacco-specific and betel nut-specific N-nitroso compounds: occurrence in saliva and urine of betel quid chewers and formation in vitro by nitrosation of betel quid. Carcinogenesis 6:295–303.

Norton, S. A. 1998. Betel: consumption and consequences. J Am Acad Dermatol 38:81–88.

Panigrahi, G. B., Rao, A. R. 1989. Study of the genotoxicity of the total aqueous extract of betel nut and its tannin. Carcinogenesis 7:37–39.

Pariat, T., Balachandran, B., Sharan, R. N. 1999. Effects of carcinogen exposure on poly-ADP-ribosylation of HMG Proteins and on chromatin organization. In Recent Aspects of Cellular and Applied Radiobiology, eds. F. H. A. Schneeweiss and R. N. Sharan, pp 158–161, vol. 30, International co-operation bilateral seminars series, Juelich: Forschungszentrum Juelich GmbH.

Pariat, T., Sharan, R. N. 1998a. Betel nut and diethylnitrosamine induced conformational changes in the liver HMG proteins in vivo. *In* Trends in Radiation and Cancer Biology, ed. R. N. Sharan, pp 162–165, vol. 29, International co-operation bilateral seminars series, Juelich: Forschungszentrum Juelich GmbH.

Pariat, T., Sharan, R. N. 1998b. Qualitative change in mice liver HMG proteins after low dose chronic administration of aqueous extract of betel nut and diethynitrosamine. Hepatol Res 12:177–185.

Pariat, T., Sharan, R. N. 2002. Role of mouse spleen cell HMG proteins and its poly-ADP-ribosylation in betel nut induced carcinogenesis. Indian J Biochem Biophys 39:130–132.
Patel, B. P., Shah, S. V., Shukla, S. N., Shah, P. M., Patel, P. S. 2007. Clinical significance of MMP-2 and MMP-9 in patients with oral cancer. Head Neck 29:564–572.
Paul, K., Moitra, P. K., Mukherjee, I., Maity, C., Ghosal, S. K. 1999. Teratogenicity of arecoline hydrobromide on developing chick embryos: A preliminary report. Bull Environ Contam Toxicol 62:356–362.
Polasa, K., Babu, S., Shenolikar, I. S. 1993. Dose-dependent genotoxic effect of pan masala and areca nut in *Salmonella typhimurium* assay. Food Chem Toxicol 31:439–442.
Rajan, J. V., Wang, M., Marquis, S. T., Chodosh, L. A. 1996. Brca2 is coordinately regulated with Brca1 during proliferation and differentiation in mammary epithelial cells. Proc. Natl. Acad. Sci. (USA) 93:13078–13083.
Ralhan, R., Agarwal, S., Nath, N., Mathur, M., Wasylyk, B., Srivastava, A. 2001. Correlation between p53 gene mutations and circulating antibodies in betel- and tobacco-consuming North Indian population. Oral Oncol. 37:243–250.
Ramachandran, S., Ramadas, K., Hariharan, R., Rejnish, K. R., Radhakrishna, P. M. 2006. Single nucleotide polymorphisms of DNA repair genes XRCC1 and XPD and its molecular mapping in Indian oral cancer. Oral Oncol. 42:350–362.
Ranasinghe, A. W., Warnakulasuriya, K. A. A. S., Johnson, N. W. 1993. Low prevalence of expression of p53 oncoprotein in oral carcinomas from Sri Lanka associated with betel and tobacco chewing. Eur J Cancer 29:147–150.
Saikia, J. R., Schneeweiss, F. H. A., Sharan, R. N. 1998. Effects of chronic low-dose arecoline administration on the macromolecular components of bone marrow and spleen cells of mice. Cancer J. 11:94–98.
Saikia, J. R., Schneeweiss, F. H. A., Sharan, R. N. 1999a. Chronic low dose arecoline exposure affects DNA, RNA and protein contents and cellular poly-ADP-ribosylation in mice in vivo. *In* Recent Aspects of Cellular and Applied Radiobiology, eds. F. H. A. Schneeweiss, and R. N. Sharan, pp 149–152, vol. 30, International co-operation bilateral seminars series, Juelich: Forschungszentrum Juelich GmbH.
Saikia, J. R., Schneeweiss, F. H. A., Sharan, R. N. 1999b. Arecoline-induced changes of poly-ADP-ribosylation of cellular proteins and its influence on chromatin organization. Cancer Lett. 139:59–65.
Sharan, R. N. 1994. Biochemical investigation of carcinogenic potency of betel nut (*Kwai*) of north-east India. In, Oral Oncology, pp. 190–193, vol. III, New Delhi: Mac Millan India Ltd.
Sharan, R. N. 1996. Association of betel nut with carcinogenesis – A review. Cancer J. 9:13–19.
Sharan, R. N., Wary, K. K. 1992. Study of unscheduled DNA synthesis following exposure of human cells to arecoline and extracts of betel nut in vitro. Mutat Res 278:271–276.
Shwe, M., Chiguchi, G., Yamada, S., Nakajima, T., Maung, K. K., Takagi, M., Amagasa, T., Tsuchida, N. 2001. P53 and MDM2 co-expression in tobacco and betel chewing-associated oral squamous cell carcinomas. J. Med. Dent. Sci. 48:113–119.
Sinha, A., Rao, A. R. 1985a. Embryotoxicity of betel nuts in mice. Toxicol. 37:315–326.
Sinha, A., Rao, A. R. 1985b. Induction of shape abnormality and unscheduled DNA synthesis by arecoline in the germ cells of mice. Mutat Res 158:189–192.
Sinha, A., Rao, A. R. 1985c. Transplacental micronucleus inducing ability of arecoline, a betel nut alkaloid in mice. Mutat Res 158:193–194.
Spitz, M. R., Bondy, M. L. 1993. Genetic susceptibility to cancer. Cancer. 72:991–995.
Stich, H. F., Anders, F. 1989. The involvement of reactive oxygen species in oral cancers of betel quid/tobacco chewers. Mutat Res 214:47–61.
Sundqvist, K., Liu, Y., Nair, J., Bartsch, H., Arvidson, K., Grafström, R. C. 1989. Cytotoxic and genotoxic effects of areca nut-related compounds in cultured human buccal epithelial cells. Cancer Res 49:5294–5298.
Thomas, S., Brennan, J., Martel, G. 1994. Mutations in the conserved regions of p53 are infrequent in betel-associated oral cancers from Papua New Guinea. Cancer Res 54:3588–3593.

Topcu, Z., Chiba, I., Fujieda, M., Shibata, T., Ariyoshi, N., Yamazaki, H., Sevgican, F., Muthumala, M., Kobayahi, H., Kamataki, T. 2002. CYP2A6 gene deletion reduces oral cancer risk in betel quid chewers in Sri Lanka. Carcinogenesis 23:595–598.

Trivedy, C. R., Craig, G., Warnakulasuriya, S. 2002. The oral health consequences of chewing areca nut. Addict. Biol. 7:115–125.

Tseng, C. 2006. Betel nut chewing is independently associated with urinary albumin excretion rate in type 2 diabetic patients. Diabetes Care 29:462–463.

Tu, H. F., Liu, C. J., Chang, C. S., Lui, M. T., Kao, S. Y., Chang, C. P., Liu, T. Y. 2006. The functional (-1171 5A→>6A) polymorphisms of matrix metalloproteinase 3 gene as a risk factor for oral submucous fibrosis among male areca users. J. Oral Pathol. Med. 35:99–103.

Tu, H. F., Wu, C. H., Kao, S. Y., Liu, C. J., Liu, T. Y., Lui, M. T. 2007. Functional-1562 C-to-T polymorphism in matrix metalloproteinase-9 (MMP-9) promoter is associated with the risk for oral squamous cell carcinoma in younger male areca users. J. Oral Pathol. Med. 36:409–414.

Wang, C. K., Peng, C. H. 1996. The mutagenicities of alkaloids and *N*-nitrosoguvacoline from betel quid. Mutat Res Environ Mutagen Relat Subj 360:165–171.

Warnakulasuriya, S. 2002. Areca nut use: an independent risk factor for oral cancer. Br. Med. J. 324:799–800.

Wary, K. K., Sharan, R. N. 1988. Aqueous extract of betel-nut of North-East India induces DNA strand breaks and enhances rate of cell proliferation in vitro. J. Cancer Res. Clin. Oncol 114:579–582.

Wary, K. K., Sharan, R. N. 1991. Cytotoxic and cytostatic effects of arecoline and sodium nitrite on human cells in vitro. Int J Cancer 47:396–400.

Wen, X., Zhang, Y., Liu, X., Guo, S., Wang, H. 2006. Immune responses in mice to arecoline mediated by lymphocyte muscarinic acetylcholine receptor. Cell Biol. Int. 30:1048–1053.

Chapter 16
Birth Weight and Cancer Associations

Nadia Barahmani and M. Fatih Okcu

Abstract Birth weight is an established risk factor for development of childhood acute lymphoblastic leukemia (ALL); however, the biological mechanism of this correlation is unknown. Some possible mechanisms of birth weight association in childhood cancer are increased cell proliferation rate; the combination of high IGF and low IGFBP levels; maternal estrogen level; and higher iron (nutrient for cancer cells) levels in heavier babies. Birth weight increases with gestational age; therefore it is important to adjust birth weight for gestational age or use percentile of weight for gestational age or fetal growth rate in birth weight related studies. Further studies are still needed to explore biological reasons of confounder of the association between birth weight and cancer, so ultimately, preventive and therapeutic interventions can be initiated.

Keywords Birth weight · Gestational age or fetal growth rate · IGF · IGFBP · Maternal estrogen · Iron · Childhood cancer

16.1 Importance of Birth Weight

Birth weight is a major predictive factor of perinatal survival and maternal health (Godfrey, 2001; Boulet et al., 2003; Melve and Skjaerven, 2003; Heiskanen et al., 2006). Birth weight is also associated with childhood cancers (Ross, 2006), adult cancers (McCormack et al., 2005; Ahlgren et al., 2007) and adult metabolic disorders (Simmons, 2005). Although the association between birth weight and infant survival is among the strongest seen in epidemiology (babies weighing less than 1,500 g have a mortality risk at least 100–fold higher than babies at the optimum weight), the biologic mechanism of this correlation is unknown. The correlation may

N. Barahmani (✉)
Section of Hematology-Oncology, Department of Pediatrics, Childhood Cancer Epidemiology and Prevention Center, Texas Children's Cancer Centre, Baylor College of Medicine, Houston, TX 77030, USA
e-mail: nxbarahm@txccc.org

D. Roy, M.T. Dorak (eds.), *Environmental Factors, Genes, and the Development of Human Cancers*, DOI 10.1007/978-1-4419-6752-7_16,

be due to an unmeasured confounding factor (Basso et al., 2006). Epidemiological analyses often regard birth weight as on the causal pathway to health outcomes associated with it but the link between birth weight and health outcomes may not be causal (Wilcox, 2001). In any case, biological mechanisms that link birth weight to health outcomes are of great interest, even if they are not causal (Wilcox, 2001). It has been suggested that there may be metabolism or growth genes that determine fetal size and that go on to regulate child development in ways that affect later risk of disease (Wilcox, 2001). Although most of the previous discussions of birth weight and health outcomes concerned the low birth weight and infant mortality link, the doubts about causality of birth weight in any health outcome are equally valid. It is however still important to identify the mechanism of confounder of the association between birth weight and cancer to be able to design preventive and therapeutic interventions.

16.2 Determinants of Birth Weight

Birth weight determination is multifactorial. Known factors include maternal age, multiparity (birth order), preeclampsia during pregnancy, previous stillbirth, maternal diabetes, smoking, iron deficiency; while maternal birth weight and pre-pregnancy body size, previous sibling birth weight, and maternal iron status show some correlation (Peters et al., 1983; Wilcox et al., 1993; Meis et al., 1997; Melve and Skjaerven, 2003; Storms and Van Howe, 2004; Scholl, 2005; Dunger et al., 2007). Birth weight increases with gestational age. In birth weight association studies, it is important to adjust birth weight for gestational age. Alternatively percentile of weight for gestational age or fetal growth rate can be used (Milne et al., 2007; Schuz and Forman, 2007; Laurvick et al., 2008; Milne et al., 2008; 2007; 2009; Sprehe et al., 2009).

Positive associations with high birth weight or macrosomia (>4,500 g) have been found for advanced age, multiparity, a previous macrosomic infant or pregnancy loss, male fetus, postdatism (>42 weeks of gestation), maternal and paternal high birth weight, maternal high height, maternal obesity (BMI >25 before pregnancy), ethnicity, gestational diabetes or hypertension, preeclampsia, increased interpregnancy interval, and non-smoking (Boulet et al., 2003; Heiskanen et al., 2006; Ahlsson et al., 2007). However, most studies suggest that high prepregnancy body mass index, along with weight gain during pregnancy are the most important predictors of having a high-birth weight infant (Yang and Yu, 2000; Surkan et al., 2004; Ricart et al., 2005; Ahlsson et al., 2007). It is thus important to also take into account pre-pregnancy maternal weight and weight gain during pregnancy in genetic association studies of birth weight.

Iron has attracted attention because of the high prevalence of iron deficiency in the developing and even in the developed world (Allen, 2000; Fosset et al., 2004). Iron deficiency is associated with low birth weight (Scholl and Hediger, 1994; Milman, 2006; Palma et al., 2008). Cord blood iron levels modestly correlate with birth weight (Srivastava et al., 2002) (very much like the correlation between IGF1 levels and birth weight, discussed later). There is, however, a gap in knowledge in terms of the effects of iron excess. Iron excess during pregnancy could occur if iron supplementation was applied non-selectively (Haram et al., 2001) or in genetically predisposed women (Datz et al., 1998). Mothers with a reduced store of iron at term can still provide sufficient iron for developing fetus (Wong and Saha, 1990) due to physiological mechanisms that favor iron transport. Iron deficiency, however, still causes low-birth weight and iron supplementation reduces the risk for low-birth weight (Agarwal et al., 1991; Allen, 2000; Mitchell et al., 2004). Iron supplementation in iron-replete women during pregnancy increases average birth weight (Cogswell et al., 2003; Siega-Riz et al., 2006) suggesting that iron transport to fetus continues even when iron levels are optimal. This would be further augmented if the mother is genetically prone to develop iron excess. Correlation of birth weight with maternal (Gambling and McArdle, 2004) and cord blood (Srivastava et al., 2002) iron levels or maternal iron supplementation during pregnancy (Cogswell et al., 2003; Siega-Riz et al., 2006) has been documented. In the study by Cogswell et al. (2003), women who were not iron deficient were given supplemental iron during pregnancy and this was enough to increase the birth weight by 205 g on average (from 3,072 to 3,277 g).

Birth weight is considered to be a cumulative index of prenatal exposures in disease association studies but it has very little predictive value for at least steroid hormone levels during pregnancy (Peck et al., 2003) despite showing a correlation as also observed in another study (Petridou et al., 1990). Its use as a surrogate marker for other exposures may also be doubtful.

Genetic determinants of birth weight have been sought extensively but so far only in candidate gene studies. Linkage studies have identified genomic regions that may harbor genetic variants involved in birth weight determination (Arya et al., 2006; Fradin et al., 2006) and a large number of studies have identified genetic variants that are associated with low or high birth weight. A complete list of those variants is presented in Table 16.1. These variants may also prove useful in the study of the connection between birth weight and cancer susceptibility as discussed in the next section.

Table 16.1 Gene variants associated with birth weight and/or cancer[a]

Gene – GeneID	Variant(s)	dbSNP ID	Minor allele frequency[b]	Marker frequency[b]	References
HFE – 3077	C282Y	rs1800562	0.042	0.085	Dorak et al. (2009)
	H63D	rs1799945	0.129	0.259	
TFRC – 7037	G142S	rs3817672	0.417	0.667	Dorak et al. (2009)
MTHFR – 4524	677C>T (A222V)	rs1801133	0.242	0.417	Relton et al. (2005)
	1298AC (E429A)	rs1801131	0.358	0.583	

Table 16.1 (continued)

Gene – GeneID	Variant(s)	dbSNP ID	Minor allele frequency[b]	Marker frequency[b]	References
HLA-G – 3135	HLA-G*010102 (indel polymorphism)	rs1704 (formerly rs16375)	0.320	0.435 (exp)	Hviid (2004)
	-725C>G	rs1233334	0.167	0.333	
IGF1 – 3479	intron 3, C>G	rs1520220	0.173	0.306	Al-Zahrani et al. (2006); Diorio et al. (2008)
	exon 4 (3′ UTR), G>A	rs6220	0.303	0.500	
IGF1R – 3480	Exon 16, E1043E, G>A	rs2229765	0.400	0.683	Al-Zahrani et al. (2006); Diorio et al. (2008)
IGFBP3 – 3486	5′ UTR, A>C	rs2854744	0.409	0.546	Al-Zahrani et al. (2006); Diorio et al. (2008)
LEP – 3952	G>A	rs7799039	0.491	0.724	Ong et al. (1999); Hoffstedt et al. (2002); Jiang et al. (2004)
INS – 3630	5′ STR	–	–	–	Dunger et al. (1998)
	-23 HphI, A>T	rs689	0.284	0.691	
LRP8 – 7804	Exon 9, C>A (G419G)	rs2297660	0.467	0.717	Wang et al. (2006)
GC – 2638	D432E	rs7041	0.425	0.700	Jiang et al. (2007)
	T436K	rs4588	0.292	0.517	
	3′ UTR	rs17467825	0.292	0.517	
H19 – 283120	C>T	rs2107425	0.297	0.492	Petry et al. (2005)
	C>T	rs217727	0.167	0.298	
EGF – 1950	5′ UTR (61G>A)	rs4444903	0.392	0.617	Dissanayake et al. (2007)
	M798I (c.2566G>A)	rs2237051	0.375	0.600	
TPK1 – 27010	C>T	rs228581	0.342	0.583	Fradin and Bougneres (2007)
	A>G	rs228582	0.467	0.700	
	C>T	rs228584	0.475	0.695	
PPARG – 5468	C>G (P12A)	rs1801282	0.075	0.134	Pihlajamaki et al. (2004), see also Pfab et al. (2006)
UCP2 – 7351	C>T	rs659366	0.333	0.883	Esterbauer et al. (2001)
GCK – 2645	G>A	rs1799884 and other rare ones	0.203	0.322	Hattersley et al. (1998); Weedon et al. (2006); Freathy et al. (2007)
TCF7L2 – 6934	T>C	rs7903146	0.375	0.516	Freathy et al. (2007)

Table 16.1 (continued)

Gene – GeneID	Variant(s)	dbSNP ID	Minor allele frequency[b]	Marker frequency[b]	References
CDKAL1 – 54901	C>A	rs10946398	0.308	0.533	Freathy et al. (2009)
HHEX-IDE – 3087	G>A	rs1111875	0.558	0.683	Freathy et al. (2009)
PON2 – 5445	A148G, C>G	rs12026	0.242	0.433	Busch et al. (1999)

[a]PGM1 (5236) (Gloria-Bottini et al., 2001), ACP1 (52) (Amante et al., 1990; Gloria-Bottini et al., 2008) and ADA (100) (Gloria-Bottini et al., 2008) polymorphisms have only been examined at the protein level and not included in this table. Some of these variants show their associations when present in the mother and some when present in the offspring.
[b]The frequencies are from HapMap or dbSNP and for Europeans (exp = expected frequency based on Hardy-Weinberg equilibrium); marker frequency is the combined heterozygous and homozygous genotypes for the variant (minor allele positivity).

16.3 Birth Weight and Cancer Connection

Although no mechanism is known and causality is not established, associations between higher birth weight and cancer risk have been observed consistently. The associations are stronger for childhood than in adult cancers.

In childhood the most common cancers are leukemias and brain tumors and the most common subtypes of each group are associated with heavy birth weight as recent meta-analyses have confirmed: acute lymphoblastic and myeloblastic leukemias (ALL and AML) (Hjalgrim et al., 2003; Caughey and Michels, 2009) and astrocytoma and medulloblastoma (Harder et al., 2008). Childhood cancer associations have also been observed in population-based prospective cohort studies (Westergaard et al., 1997; Milne et al., 2007). High birth weight has been associated with a 23% increase risk of ALL (95% CI: 1.15–1.32) while it is 35% for overall leukemia (95% CI: 1.24–1.48) (Caughey and Michels, 2009). For ALL patients this relationship is most consistent and strongest in patients diagnosed at an age younger than 5 years (Daling et al., 1984; Robison et al., 1987; Kaye et al., 1991; Ross et al., 1997; Yeazel et al., 1997; Okcu et al., 2002). The relationship between high birth weight and increased cancer risk may be present only in boys but not in girls in leukemia and lymphomas (Dorak et al., 2007; Milne et al., 2008). The risk of AML shows a U-shaped relationship with birth weight, being increased in children of either low or high birth weight (Caughey and Michels, 2009). Non-Hodgkin Lymphoma shows a dose-response association for every 500 g increase in birth weight by increasing the risk by 42% (95% CI: 1.04–1.92) (Petridou et al., 2007). High birth weight is also a risk factor for astrocytoma (OR = 1.38; 95% CI: 1.07–1.79) and medulloblastoma (OR = 1.27; 95% CI: 1.02–1.60), the two most common types of brain tumor in childhood. No association was found for ependymoma and high birth weight (Harder et al., 2008). These observations further suggest that the relationship between birth weight and cancer is complex and perhaps interacting with other determinants of cancer susceptibility.

For adult malignancies, several studies have shown positive associations between high birth weight and specific cancers, most notably with breast (Xue and Michels, 2007; Park et al., 2008; Silva Idos et al., 2008), prostate (Nilsen et al., 2005b; Eriksson et al., 2007), colon cancer (Nilsen et al., 2005a), and general cancer risk (McCormack et al., 2005; Ahlgren et al., 2007).

Not all birth weight associations with cancer are unidirectional. Like AML, testicular cancer shows a U-shaped association; both low and high birth weight increase the risk (Michos et al., 2007) although low birth weight association is more often reported (Ahlgren et al., 2007). An inverse association between high birth weight and lower risk for endometrial cancer has also been reported (McCormack et al., 2005).

Recent studies started to point out that it is the fetal growth rate rather than size at birth that is associated with increased cancer risk (Milne et al., 2007; Schuz and Forman, 2007; Laurvick et al., 2008; Milne et al., 2008; Sprehe et al., 2009). This is an important observation that may help distinguish between the alternative hypotheses for the mechanism of birth weight and cancer connection (discussed below).

16.4 Possible Mechanisms of Birth Weight Association in Childhood Cancer

The mechanisms involved in the associations between birth weight or other parameters of size at birth are unknown. It is expected that the mechanism is complex and involves interactions of various factors. It has been commented that unraveling the mechanism will be difficult to disentangle particularly for adult malignancies, and studies of childhood cancer are more likely to yield results (Ross, 2006). Furthermore, there is evidence that average birth weight has been increasing gradually over the last few decades (Kramer et al., 2002; Surkan et al., 2004) along with an increase in childhood leukemia incidence (Ross, 2006) but it is unlikely that a single mechanism is responsible for this.

To date, four hypotheses have been put forward to explain the mechanism of the birth weight association in cancer:

(1) The simplest speculation is that the heavier the baby at birth, the more cells are at risk for a transformation event (Westergaard et al., 1997). Since birth weight and fetal weight both correlate with bone marrow volume (Hudson, 1965; Wilpshaar et al., 2002) this idea is plausible. High birth weight itself reflects increased cell proliferation rate which is a recognized risk factor for cancer (Albanes and Winick, 1988; Preston-Martin et al., 1990). The reason that boys are naturally heavier than girls at birth (Storms and Van Howe, 2004; Heiskanen et al., 2006) is obviously their increased cell proliferation rate during

fetal development (Mittwoch, 1993; Kochhar et al., 2001). The higher frequency of cancer, including childhood cancer, in males (Ashley, 1969; Pearce and Parker, 2001; Cartwright et al., 2002; Linet et al., 2003) may be the cumulative end-result of higher cell proliferation rate and the subsequent high birth weight.

A correlation between an HLA-G genotype and fetoplacental growth has been reported (Hviid, 2004). HLA-G is the human equivalent of the mouse preimplantation embryo development (*Ped*) gene (Comiskey et al., 2003). The *Ped* gene regulates the cell proliferation rate during embryonic development in mice. Further investigation of this gene in cancer may be informative in elucidating the mechanism of birth weight and cancer link.

(2) Insulin-like growth factors (IGFs; somatomedins) are mitogens that regulate cell proliferation, differentiation and apoptosis (Baker et al., 1993; Yu and Rohan, 2000). Two IGFs are present in humans: IGF1 (somatomedin C), and IGF2 (somatomedin A) (somatomedin B is not an IGF, but vitronectin). Their action is modulated by a network of molecules, including binding proteins (IGFBP1–10), proteases (pregnancy-associated plasma protein A, PAPPA; HtrA serine peptidase 1, HTRA1; Kazal-type serine peptidase inhibitor domain 1, KAZALD1) and receptors (IGF1R/CD221, IGF2R/CD222). IGF1R is a cellular receptor that seems to have a role in transformation, tumorigenicity, and metastasis. It is expressed in leukemia, meningioma, breast, ovarian, endometrial, gastric, pancreatic, colon, lung, prostate and bladder cancer cells (Ouban et al., 2003). IGF-binding proteins (IGFBPs) can inhibit or enhance the actions of IGFs. The combination of high IGF levels and low IGF binding protein levels is associated with cancer risk in many studies. High levels of circulating IGF1 and low levels of IGFBP3 are associated with increased risk of common cancers, including prostate, breast, colorectal and lung cancers (Renehan et al., 2004). High-energy diet may increase IGF1 levels and in animal experiments, IGFs abolish the inhibitory effect of calorie restriction on cancer growth (Yu and Rohan, 2000). IGFs are commonly expressed by tumor cells, and/or the nearby stroma and may act as an autocrine growth factor. IGFs may promote cell cycle progression and inhibition of apoptosis either by directly or indirectly by interacting with other molecules such as the steroid hormones, integrins, ataxin 1, TP53/cyclin-dependent kinase inhibitor 1A (CDKN1A) and vascular endothelial growth factor (Moschos and Mantzoros, 2002). Besides acting synergistically with other mitogenic growth factors and steroids, the IGF axis also antagonizes the effect of antiproliferative molecules on cancer growth. Their effect on breast carcinogenesis may have a synergistic interaction with sex hormones (Yu et al., 2003).

IGF1 and its principal binding protein IGFBP3 are also fetal growth factors and have been implicated in childhood leukemia pathogenesis (Ross et al., 1996; Petridou et al., 2000; Yang and Yu, 2000; Baik et al., 2005; Ross, 2006) (reviewed in Ref. (Tower and Spector, 2007; Callan and Milne, 2009)). IGF1 levels positively correlate with birth weight (Petridou et al., 2000; Yang and Yu, 2000; Boyne et al., 2003; Skalkidou et al., 2003) and may be the link between birth weight and cancer risk. In this connection, no causality is implied but birth weight increase is an epiphenomenon of increased growth factor stimulation (Ross et al., 1996). No genetic data in childhood ALL have been presented in direct support of this relationship but in breast cancer, a genetic association study revealed results expected from correlations with serum IGF1 and IGFBP3 levels. The C allele of IGF1 SNP rs1520220 is associated with higher rates of circulating IGF1 in females (P-trend = 0.003) and higher risk of breast cancer (OR (CC/GG) = 1.41; 95% CI: 1.11–1.79). The A allele of IGFBP3 SNP rs2854744 is associated with higher circulating IGFBP3 rates and a protective factor for breast cancer (OR (AA/CC) = 0.87; 95% CI: 0.77–0.99) (Al-Zahrani et al., 2006). SNPs that correlate with serum IGF1 levels, however, do not show any association with birth weight, childhood growth or glucose metabolism (Vella et al., 2008).

Like the first hypothesis presented above, the IGF axis hypothesis also fits in with the sex effect in childhood cancer. The study of healthy children has shown that girls have a higher level of IGFBP3 which is the protective member of the IGF axis (Petridou et al., 2000). This finding may be interpreted as a possible mechanism for the greater protection of females from cancer in all age groups (Ashley, 1969; Pearce and Parker, 2001; Cartwright et al., 2002; Linet et al., 2003). Although a very attractive hypothesis, the link between the IGF system and birth weight-cancer connection and whether it contributes to the sex effect need more exploration.

(3) Maternal estrogen levels correlate with birth weight (Petridou et al., 1990; Peck et al., 2003) and Shu et al. proposed that in-utero exposure to high endogenous estrogen levels is involved in the etiology of childhood ALL (Shu et al., 2002). This is a plausible hypothesis and requires further exploration. Given the possible interaction between IGF system and estrogens in breast carcinogenesis (Yu et al., 2003), such mechanism is worth exploring in childhood leukemia.

(4) Besides being a nutrient for the fetus, iron is also a nutrient for cancer cells (Trowbridge and Domingo, 1981; Trowbridge and Lopez, 1982; Cazzola et al., 1990; Le and Richardson, 2002). The connection between even moderate elevation of serum iron levels and increased cancer risk is well-established (Stevens et al., 1988; 1994; Wu et al., 2004). Furthermore, the hereditary hemochromatosis gene (HFE) variants C282Y and H63D have shown associations with a variety of cancers (Dorak et al., 2005; Dorak, 2006) but most notably with childhood ALL (Dorak et al., 1999; 2005). These associations appear to be the genetic counterpart of the previous longitudinal studies in large cohorts that linked higher iron levels to increased cancer risk. In their report of the birth weight association in childhood ALL with sex effect, Dorak et al. hypothesized that iron, like the IGF system, may be the link between birth weight and cancer risk (Dorak et al., 2007). In a study of birth weight and childhood ALL in North of England, the results suggested a correlation between birth weight and HFE variants which also conferred increased risk to ALL (Dorak et al., 2009).

16.5 Obesity and Cancer

Recent genome-wide association studies have identified a number of SNP associations with obesity ((Herbert et al., 2006; Dina et al., 2007; Frayling et al., 2007; Meyre et al., 2009; Thorleifsson et al., 2009); reviewed in (Hofker and Wijmenga, 2009)). Obesity risk markers do not overlap with the markers for heavy birth weight. Since obesity increases the risk for several cancers, in particular breast cancer, it is of interest to examine their associations with cancer. For example, the fat mass and obesity associated (FTO) gene variants increase the risk for type-2 diabetes because of their effect on obesity (Frayling et al., 2007). A similar approach can be tried to identify their associations in cancer. One such association seems to be the association of the prolactin gene PRL variants with both obesity (Meyre et al., 2009) and breast cancer (Vaclavicek et al., 2006). Likewise, the GC group-specific component (vitamin D binding protein) rs7041 (D432E) and rs4588 (T436K) polymorphisms correlate with serum 25-hydroxyvitamin D and 1,25–dihydroxyvitamin D concentrations (Engelman et al., 2008; Sinotte et al., 2009) and modify the risk for postmenopausal breast cancer independent from serum vitamin D levels (Abbas et al., 2008). More research is needed to clarify the link, if any, between birth weight and obesity, and whether their connections with cancer are linked or independent.

References

Abbas, S., Linseisen, J., Slanger, T., Kropp, S., Mutschelknauss, E.J., Flesch-Janys, D., Chang-Claude, J., 2008. The Gc2 allele of the vitamin D binding protein is associated with a decreased postmenopausal breast cancer risk, independent of the vitamin D status. Cancer Epidemiol Biomarkers Prev 17, 1339–1343.

Agarwal, K.N., Agarwal, D.K., Mishra, K.P., 1991. Impact of anaemia prophylaxis in pregnancy on maternal haemoglobin, serum ferritin & birth weight. Indian J Med Res 94, 277–280.

Ahlgren, M., Wohlfahrt, J., Olsen, L.W., Sorensen, T.I., Melbye, M., 2007. Birth weight and risk of cancer. Cancer 110, 412–419.

Ahlsson, F., Gustafsson, J., Tuvemo, T., Lundgren, M., 2007. Females born large for gestational age have a doubled risk of giving birth to large for gestational age infants. Acta Paediatr 96, 358–362.

Albanes, D., Winick, M., 1988. Are cell number and cell proliferation risk factors for cancer? J Natl Cancer Inst 80, 772–774.

Allen, L.H., 2000. Anemia and iron deficiency: effects on pregnancy outcome. Am J Clin Nutr 71, 1280S–1284S.

Al-Zahrani, A., Sandhu, M.S., Luben, R.N., Thompson, D., Baynes, C., Pooley, K.A., Luccarini, C., Munday, H., Perkins, B., Smith, P., Pharoah, P.D., Wareham, N.J., Easton, D.F., Ponder, B.A., Dunning, A.M., 2006. IGF1 and IGFBP3 tagging polymorphisms are associated with circulating levels of IGF1, IGFBP3 and risk of breast cancer. Hum Mol Genet 15, 1–10.

Amante, A., Gloria-Bottini, F., Bottini, E., 1990. Intrauterine growth: association with acid phosphatase genetic polymorphism. J Perinat Med 18, 275–282.

Arya, R., Demerath, E., Jenkinson, C.P., Goring, H.H., Puppala, S., Farook, V., Fowler, S., Schneider, J., Granato, R., Resendez, R.G., Dyer, T.D., Cole, S.A., Almasy, L., Comuzzie, A.G., Siervogel, R.M., Bradshaw, B., Defronzo, R.A., Maccluer, J., Stern, M.P., Towne, B., Blangero,

J., Duggirala, R., 2006. A quantitative trait locus (QTL) on chromosome 6q influences birth weight in two independent family studies. Hum Mol Genet 15, 1569–1579.

Ashley, D.J., 1969. A male-female differential in tumour incidence. Br J Cancer 23, 21–25.

Baik, I., Devito, W.J., Ballen, K., Becker, P.S., Okulicz, W., Liu, Q., Delpapa, E., Lagiou, P., Sturgeon, S., Trichopoulos, D., Quesenberry, P.J., Hsieh, C.C., 2005. Association of fetal hormone levels with stem cell potential: evidence for early life roots of human cancer. Cancer Res 65, 358–363.

Baker, J., Liu, J.P., Robertson, E.J., Efstratiadis, A., 1993. Role of insulin-like growth factors in embryonic and postnatal growth. Cell 75, 73–82.

Basso, O., Wilcox, A.J., Weinberg, C.R., 2006. Birth weight and mortality: causality or confounding? Am J Epidemiol 164, 303–311.

Boulet, S.L., Alexander, G.R., Salihu, H.M., Pass, M., 2003. Macrosomic births in the United States: determinants, outcomes, and proposed grades of risk. Am J Obstet Gynecol 188, 1372–1378.

Boyne, M.S., Thame, M., Bennett, F.I., Osmond, C., Miell, J.P., Forrester, T.E., 2003. The relationship among circulating insulin-like growth factor (IGF)-I, IGF-binding proteins-1 and -2, and birth anthropometry: a prospective study. J Clin Endocrinol Metab 88, 1687–1691.

Busch, C.P., Ramdath, D.D., Ramsewak, S., Hegele, R.A., 1999. Association of PON2 variation with birth weight in Trinidadian neonates of South Asian ancestry. Pharmacogenetics 9, 351–356.

Callan, A.C., Milne, E., 2009. Involvement of the IGF system in fetal growth and childhood cancer: an overview of potential mechanisms. Cancer Causes Control 20(10), 1783–1798.

Cartwright, R.A., Gurney, K.A., Moorman, A.V., 2002. Sex ratios and the risks of haematological malignancies. Br J Haematol 118, 1071–1077.

Caughey, R.W., Michels, K.B., 2009. Birth weight and childhood leukemia: A meta-analysis and review of the current evidence. Int J Cancer 124, 2658–2670.

Cazzola, M., Bergamaschi, G., Dezza, L., Arosio, P., 1990. Manipulations of cellular iron metabolism for modulating normal and malignant cell proliferation: achievements and prospects. Blood 75, 1903–1919.

Cogswell, M.E., Parvanta, I., Ickes, L., Yip, R., Brittenham, G.M., 2003. Iron supplementation during pregnancy, anemia, and birth weight: a randomized controlled trial. Am J Clin Nutr 78, 773–781.

Comiskey, M., Goldstein, C.Y., De Fazio, S.R., Mammolenti, M., Newmark, J.A., Warner, C.M., 2003. Evidence that HLA-G is the functional homolog of mouse Qa-2, the Ped gene product. Hum Immunol 64, 999–1004.

Daling, J.R., Starzyk, P., Olshan, A.F., Weiss, N.S., 1984. Birth weight and the incidence of childhood cancer. J Natl Cancer Inst 72, 1039–1041.

Datz, C., Haas, T., Rinner, H., Sandhofer, F., Patsch, W., Paulweber, B., 1998. Heterozygosity for the C282Y mutation in the hemochromatosis gene is associated with increased serum iron, transferrin saturation, and hemoglobin in young women: a protective role against iron deficiency? Clin Chem 44, 2429–2432.

Dina, C., Meyre, D., Gallina, S., Durand, E., Korner, A., Jacobson, P., Carlsson, L.M., Kiess, W., Vatin, V., Lecoeur, C., Delplanque, J., Vaillant, E., Pattou, F., Ruiz, J., Weill, J., Levy-Marchal, C., Horber, F., Potoczna, N., Hercberg, S., Le Stunff, C., Bougneres, P., Kovacs, P., Marre, M., Balkau, B., Cauchi, S., Chevre, J.C., Froguel, P., 2007. Variation in FTO contributes to childhood obesity and severe adult obesity. Nat Genet 39, 724–726.

Diorio, C., Brisson, J., Berube, S., Pollak, M., 2008. Genetic polymorphisms involved in insulin-like growth factor (IGF) pathway in relation to mammographic breast density and IGF levels. Cancer Epidemiol Biomarkers Prev 17, 880–888.

Dissanayake, V.H., Tower, C., Broderick, A., Stocker, L.J., Seneviratne, H.R., Jayasekara, R.W., Kalsheker, N., Broughton Pipkin, F., Morgan, L., 2007. Polymorphism in the epidermal growth factor gene is associated with birthweight in Sinhalese and white Western Europeans. Mol Hum Reprod 13, 425–429.

Dorak, M.T., 2006. HFE H63D variant and leukemia susceptibility. Leuk Lymphoma 47, 2269–2270.

Dorak, M.T., Burnett, A.K., Worwood, M., 2005. HFE gene mutations in susceptibility to childhood leukemia: HuGE review. Genet Med 7, 159–168.

Dorak, M.T., Hammal, D.M., Pearce, M.S., McNally, R.J., Parker, L., 2007. Examination of gender effect in birth weight and miscarriage associations with childhood cancer. Cancer Causes Control 18, 219–228.

Dorak, M.T., Mackay, R.K., Relton, C.L., Worwood, M., Parker, L., Hall, A.G., 2009. Hereditary hemochromatosis gene (HFE) variants are associated with birth weight and childhood leukemia risk. Pediatr Blood Cancer 53, 1242–1248.

Dorak, M.T., Sproul, A.M., Gibson, B.E., Burnett, A.K., Worwood, M., 1999. The C282Y mutation of *HFE* is another male-specific risk factor for childhood ALL. Blood 94, 3957–3958.

Dunger, D.B., Ong, K.K., Huxtable, S.J., Sherriff, A., Woods, K.A., Ahmed, M.L., Golding, J., Pembrey, M.E., Ring, S., Bennett, S.T., Todd, J.A., 1998. Association of the INS VNTR with size at birth. ALSPAC Study Team. Avon Longitudinal Study of Pregnancy and Childhood. Nat Genet 19, 98–100.

Dunger, D.B., Petry, C.J., Ong, K.K., 2007. Genetics of size at birth. Diabetes Care 30 Suppl 2,S150–S155.

Engelman, C.D., Fingerlin, T.E., Langefeld, C.D., Hicks, P.J., Rich, S.S., Wagenknecht, L.E., Bowden, D.W., Norris, J.M., 2008. Genetic and environmental determinants of 25-hydroxyvitamin D and 1,25-dihydroxyvitamin D levels in Hispanic and African Americans. J Clin Endocrinol Metab 93, 3381–3388.

Eriksson, M., Wedel, H., Wallander, M.A., Krakau, I., Hugosson, J., Carlsson, S., Svardsudd, K., 2007. The impact of birth weight on prostate cancer incidence and mortality in a population-based study of men born in 1913 and followed up from 50 to 85 years of age. Prostate 67, 1247–1254.

Esterbauer, H., Schneitler, C., Oberkofler, H., Ebenbichler, C., Paulweber, B., Sandhofer, F., Ladurner, G., Hell, E., Strosberg, A.D., Patsch, J.R., Krempler, F., Patsch, W., 2001. A common polymorphism in the promoter of UCP2 is associated with decreased risk of obesity in middle-aged humans. Nat Genet 28, 178–183.

Fosset, C., McGaw, B.A., Abramovich, D., McArdle, H.J., 2004. Interrelations between ceruloplasmin and Fe status during human pregnancy. Biol Trace Elem Res 98, 1–12.

Fradin, D., Bougneres, P., 2007. Three common intronic variants in the maternal and fetal thiamine pyrophosphokinase gene (TPK1) are associated with birth weight. Ann Hum Genet 71, 578–585.

Fradin, D., Heath, S., Lepercq, J., Lathrop, M., Bougneres, P., 2006. Identification of distinct quantitative trait loci affecting length or weight variability at birth in humans. J Clin Endocrinol Metab 91, 4164–4170.

Frayling, T.M., Timpson, N.J., Weedon, M.N., Zeggini, E., Freathy, R.M., Lindgren, C.M., Perry, J.R., Elliott, K.S., Lango, H., Rayner, N.W., Shields, B., Harries, L.W., Barrett, J.C., Ellard, S., Groves, C.J., Knight, B., Patch, A.M., Ness, A.R., Ebrahim, S., Lawlor, D.A., Ring, S.M., Ben-Shlomo, Y., Jarvelin, M.R., Sovio, U., Bennett, A.J., Melzer, D., Ferrucci, L., Loos, R.J., Barroso, I., Wareham, N.J., Karpe, F., Owen, K.R., Cardon, L.R., Walker, M., Hitman, G.A., Palmer, C.N., Doney, A.S., Morris, A.D., Smith, G.D., Hattersley, A.T., McCarthy, M.I., 2007. A common variant in the FTO gene is associated with body mass index and predisposes to childhood and adult obesity. Science 316, 889–894.

Freathy, R.M., Bennett, A.J., Ring, S.M., Shields, B., Groves, C.J., Timpson, N.J., Weedon, M.N., Zeggini, E., Lindgren, C.M., Lango, H., Perry, J.R., Pouta, A., Ruokonen, A., Hypponen, E., Power, C., Elliott, P., Strachan, D.P., Jarvelin, M.R., Smith, G.D., McCarthy, M.I., Frayling, T.M., Hattersley, A.T., 2009. Type 2 diabetes risk alleles are associated with reduced size at birth. Diabetes 58, 1428–1433.

Freathy, R.M., Weedon, M.N., Bennett, A., Hypponen, E., Relton, C.L., Knight, B., Shields, B., Parnell, K.S., Groves, C.J., Ring, S.M., Pembrey, M.E., Ben-Shlomo, Y., Strachan, D.P., Power,

C., Jarvelin, M.R., McCarthy, M.I., Davey Smith, G., Hattersley, A.T., Frayling, T.M., 2007. Type 2 diabetes TCF7L2 risk genotypes alter birth weight: a study of 24,053 individuals. Am J Hum Genet 80, 1150–1161.

Gambling, L., McArdle, H.J., 2004. Iron, copper and fetal development. Proc Nutr Soc 63, 553–562.

Gloria-Bottini, F., Lucarini, N., La Torre, M., Lucarelli, P., Bottini, E., 2001. Birth weight and parental PGM1 alleles. Am J Hum Biol 13, 417–420.

Gloria-Bottini, F., Pietropolli, A., Coppeta, L., Magrini, A., Bergamaschi, A., Bottini, E., 2008. The genetics of feto-placental development: a study of acid phosphatase locus 1 and adenosine deaminase polymorphisms in a consecutive series of newborn infants. Reprod Biol Endocrinol 6, 38.

Godfrey, K.M., 2001. The 'gold standard' for optimal fetal growth and development. J Pediatr Endocrinol Metab 14 Suppl 6,1507–1513.

Haram, K., Nilsen, S.T., Ulvik, R.J., 2001. Iron supplementation in pregnancy–evidence and controversies. Acta Obstet Gynecol Scand 80, 683–688.

Harder, T., Plagemann, A., Harder, A., 2008. Birth weight and subsequent risk of childhood primary brain tumors: a meta-analysis. Am J Epidemiol 168, 366–373.

Hattersley, A.T., Beards, F., Ballantyne, E., Appleton, M., Harvey, R., Ellard, S., 1998. Mutations in the glucokinase gene of the fetus result in reduced birth weight. Nat Genet 19, 268–270.

Heiskanen, N., Raatikainen, K., Heinonen, S., 2006. Fetal macrosomia–a continuing obstetric challenge. Biol Neonate 90, 98–103.

Herbert, A., Gerry, N.P., McQueen, M.B., Heid, I.M., Pfeufer, A., Illig, T., Wichmann, H.E., Meitinger, T., Hunter, D., Hu, F.B., Colditz, G., Hinney, A., Hebebrand, J., Koberwitz, K., Zhu, X., Cooper, R., Ardlie, K., Lyon, H., Hirschhorn, J.N., Laird, N.M., Lenburg, M.E., Lange, C., Christman, M.F., 2006. A common genetic variant is associated with adult and childhood obesity. Science 312, 279–283.

Hjalgrim, L.L., Westergaard, T., Rostgaard, K., Schmiegelow, K., Melbye, M., Hjalgrim, H., Engels, E.A., 2003. Birth weight as a risk factor for childhood leukemia: a meta-analysis of 18 epidemiologic studies. Am J Epidemiol 158, 724–735.

Hoffstedt, J., Eriksson, P., Mottagui-Tabar, S., Arner, P., 2002. A polymorphism in the leptin promoter region (-2548 G/A) influences gene expression and adipose tissue secretion of leptin. Horm Metab Res 34, 355–359.

Hofker, M., Wijmenga, C., 2009. A supersized list of obesity genes. Nat Genet 41, 139–140.

Hudson, G., 1965. Bone-marrow volume in the human foetus and newborn. Br J Haematol 11, 446–452.

Hviid, T.V., 2004. HLA-G genotype is associated with fetoplacental growth. Hum Immunol 65, 586–593.

Jiang, Y., Wilk, J.B., Borecki, I., Williamson, S., DeStefano, A.L., Xu, G., Liu, J., Ellison, R.C., Province, M., Myers, R.H., 2004. Common variants in the 5′ region of the leptin gene are associated with body mass index in men from the National Heart, Lung, and Blood Institute Family Heart Study. Am J Hum Genet 75, 220–230.

Jiang, H., Xiong, D.H., Guo, Y.F., Shen, H., Xiao, P., Yang, F., Chen, Y., Zhang, F., Recker, R.R., Deng, H.W., 2007. Association analysis of vitamin D-binding protein gene polymorphisms with variations of obesity-related traits in Caucasian nuclear families. Int J Obes (Lond) 31, 1319–1324.

Kaye, S.A., Robison, L.L., Smithson, W.A., Gunderson, P., King, F.L., Neglia, J.P., 1991. Maternal reproductive history and birth characteristics in childhood acute lymphoblastic leukemia. Cancer 68, 1351–1355.

Kochhar, H.P., Peippo, J., King, W.A., 2001. Sex related embryo development. Theriogenology 55, 3–14.

Kramer, M.S., Morin, I., Yang, H., Platt, R.W., Usher, R., McNamara, H., Joseph, K.S., Wen, S.W., 2002. Why are babies getting bigger? Temporal trends in fetal growth and its determinants. J Pediatr 141, 538–542.

Laurvick, C.L., Milne, E., Blair, E., de Klerk, N., Charles, A.K., Bower, C., 2008. Fetal growth and the risk of childhood non-CNS solid tumours in Western Australia. Br J Cancer 99, 179–181.

Le, N.T., Richardson, D.R., 2002. The role of iron in cell cycle progression and the proliferation of neoplastic cells. Biochim Biophys Acta 1603, 31–46.

Linet, M.S., Wacholder, S., Zahm, S.H., 2003. Interpreting epidemiologic research: lessons from studies of childhood cancer. Pediatrics 112, 218–232.

McCormack, V.A., dos Santos Silva, I., Koupil, I., Leon, D.A., Lithell, H.O., 2005. Birth characteristics and adult cancer incidence: Swedish cohort of over 11,000 men and women. Int J Cancer 115, 611–617.

Meis, P.J., Michielutte, R., Peters, T.J., Wells, H.B., Sands, R.E., Coles, E.C., Johns, K.A., 1997. Factors associated with term low birthweight in Cardiff, Wales. Paediatr Perinat Epidemiol 11, 287–297.

Melve, K.K., Skjaerven, R., 2003. Birthweight and perinatal mortality: paradoxes, social class, and sibling dependencies. Int J Epidemiol 32, 625–632.

Meyre, D., Delplanque, J., Chevre, J.C., Lecoeur, C., Lobbens, S., Gallina, S., Durand, E., Vatin, V., Degraeve, F., Proenca, C., Gaget, S., Korner, A., Kovacs, P., Kiess, W., Tichet, J., Marre, M., Hartikainen, A.L., Horber, F., Potoczna, N., Hercberg, S., Levy-Marchal, C., Pattou, F., Heude, B., Tauber, M., McCarthy, M.I., Blakemore, A.I., Montpetit, A., Polychronakos, C., Weill, J., Coin, L.J., Asher, J., Elliott, P., Jarvelin, M.R., Visvikis-Siest, S., Balkau, B., Sladek, R., Balding, D., Walley, A., Dina, C., Froguel, P., 2009. Genome-wide association study for early-onset and morbid adult obesity identifies three new risk loci in European populations. Nat Genet 41, 157–159.

Michos, A., Xue, F., Michels, K.B., 2007. Birth weight and the risk of testicular cancer: a meta-analysis. Int J Cancer 121, 1123–1131.

Milman, N., 2006. Iron prophylaxis in pregnancy–general or individual and in which dose? Ann Hematol 85, 821–828.

Milne, E., Laurvick, C.L., Blair, E., Bower, C., de Klerk, N., 2007. Fetal growth and acute childhood leukemia: looking beyond birth weight. Am J Epidemiol 166, 151–159.

Milne, E., Laurvick, C.L., Blair, E., de Klerk, N., Charles, A.K., Bower, C., 2008. Fetal growth and the risk of childhood CNS tumors and lymphomas in Western Australia. Int J Cancer 123, 436–443.

Milne, E., Royle, J.A., de Klerk, N.H., Blair, E., Bailey, H., Cole, C., Attia, J., Scott, R.J., Armstrong, B.K., 2009. Fetal growth and risk of childhood acute lymphoblastic leukemia: results from an Australian case-control study. Am J Epidemiol 170, 221–228.

Mitchell, E.A., Robinson, E., Clark, P.M., Becroft, D.M., Glavish, N., Pattison, N.S., Pryor, J.E., Thompson, J.M., Wild, C.J., 2004. Maternal nutritional risk factors for small for gestational age babies in a developed country: a case-control study. Arch Dis Child Fetal Neonatal Ed 89, F431–F435.

Mittwoch, U., 1993. Blastocysts prepare for the race to be male. Hum Reprod 8, 1550–1555.

Moschos, S.J., Mantzoros, C.S., 2002. The role of the IGF system in cancer: from basic to clinical studies and clinical applications. Oncology 63, 317–332.

Nilsen, T.I., Romundstad, P.R., Troisi, R., Potischman, N., Vatten, L.J., 2005a. Birth size and colorectal cancer risk: a prospective population based study. Gut 54, 1728–1732.

Nilsen, T.I., Romundstad, P.R., Troisi, R., Vatten, L.J., 2005b. Birth size and subsequent risk for prostate cancer: a prospective population-based study in Norway. Int J Cancer 113, 1002–1004.

Okcu, M.F., Goodman, K.J., Carozza, S.E., Weiss, N.S., Burau, K.D., Bleyer, W.A., Cooper, S.P., 2002. Birth weight, ethnicity, and occurrence of cancer in children: a population-based, incident case-control study in the State of Texas, USA. Cancer Causes Control 13, 595–602.

Ong, K.K., Ahmed, M.L., Sherriff, A., Woods, K.A., Watts, A., Golding, J., Dunger, D.B., 1999. Cord blood leptin is associated with size at birth and predicts infancy weight gain in humans. ALSPAC Study Team. Avon Longitudinal Study of Pregnancy and Childhood. J Clin Endocrinol Metab 84, 1145–1148.

Ouban, A., Muraca, P., Yeatman, T., Coppola, D., 2003. Expression and distribution of insulin-like growth factor-1 receptor in human carcinomas. Hum Pathol 34, 803–808.

Palma, S., Perez-Iglesias, R., Prieto, D., Pardo, R., Llorca, J., Delgado-Rodriguez, M., 2008. Iron but not folic acid supplementation reduces the risk of low birthweight in pregnant women without anaemia: a case-control study. J Epidemiol Community Health 62, 120–124.
Park, S.K., Kang, D., McGlynn, K.A., Garcia-Closas, M., Kim, Y., Yoo, K.Y., Brinton, L.A., 2008. Intrauterine environments and breast cancer risk: meta-analysis and systematic review. Breast Cancer Res 10, R8.
Pearce, M.S., Parker, L., 2001. Childhood cancer registrations in the developing world: still more boys than girls. Int J Cancer 91, 402–406.
Peck, J.D., Hulka, B.S., Savitz, D.A., Baird, D., Poole, C., Richardson, B.E., 2003. Accuracy of fetal growth indicators as surrogate measures of steroid hormone levels during pregnancy. Am J Epidemiol 157, 258–266.
Peters, T.J., Golding, J., Butler, N.R., Fryer, J.G., Lawrence, C.J., Chamberlain, G.V., 1983. Plus ca change: predictors of birthweight in two national studies. Br J Obstet Gynaecol 90, 1040–1045.
Petridou, E.T., Dikalioti, S.K., Skalkidou, A., Andrie, E., Dessypris, N., Trichopoulos, D., 2007. Sun exposure, birth weight, and childhood lymphomas: a case control study in Greece. Cancer Causes Control 18, 1031–1037.
Petridou, E., Panagiotopoulou, K., Katsouyanni, K., Spanos, E., Trichopoulos, D., 1990. Tobacco smoking, pregnancy estrogens, and birth weight. Epidemiology 1, 247–250.
Petridou, E., Skalkidou, A., Dessypris, N., Moustaki, M., Mantzoros, C., Spanos, E., Trichopoulos, D., 2000. Endogenous risk factors for childhood leukemia in relation to the IGF system (Greece). The Childhood Haematologists-Oncologists Group. Cancer Causes Control 11, 765–771.
Petry, C.J., Ong, K.K., Barratt, B.J., Wingate, D., Cordell, H.J., Ring, S.M., Pembrey, M.E., Reik, W., Todd, J.A., Dunger, D.B., 2005. Common polymorphism in H19 associated with birthweight and cord blood IGF-II levels in humans. BMC Genet 6, 22.
Pfab, T., Poralla, C., Richter, C.M., Godes, M., Slowinski, T., Priem, F., Halle, H., Hocher, B., 2006. Fetal and maternal peroxisome proliferator-activated receptor gamma2 Pro12Ala does not influence birth weight. Obesity (Silver Spring) 14, 1880–1885.
Pihlajamaki, J., Vanhala, M., Vanhala, P., Laakso, M., 2004. The Pro12Ala polymorphism of the PPAR gamma 2 gene regulates weight from birth to adulthood. Obes Res 12, 187–190.
Preston-Martin, S., Pike, M.C., Ross, R.K., Jones, P.A., Henderson, B.E., 1990. Increased cell division as a cause of human cancer. Cancer Res 50, 7415–7421.
Relton, C.L., Pearce, M.S., Burn, J., Parker, L., 2005. An investigation of folate-related genetic factors in the determination of birthweight. Paediatr Perinat Epidemiol 19, 360–367.
Renehan, A.G., Zwahlen, M., Minder, C., O'Dwyer, S.T., Shalet, S.M., Egger, M., 2004. Insulin-like growth factor (IGF)-I, IGF binding protein-3, and cancer risk: systematic review and meta-regression analysis. Lancet 363, 1346–1353.
Ricart, W., Lopez, J., Mozas, J., Pericot, A., Sancho, M.A., Gonzalez, N., Balsells, M., Luna, R., Cortazar, A., Navarro, P., Ramirez, O., Flandez, B., Pallardo, L.F., Hernandez-Mijas, A., Ampudia, J., Fernandez-Real, J.M., Corcoy, R., 2005. Body mass index has a greater impact on pregnancy outcomes than gestational hyperglycaemia. Diabetologia 48, 1736–1742.
Robison, L.L., Codd, M., Gunderson, P., Neglia, J.P., Smithson, W.A., King, F.L., 1987. Birth weight as a risk factor for childhood acute lymphoblastic leukemia. Pediatr Hematol Oncol 4, 63–72.
Ross, J.A., 2006. High birthweight and cancer: evidence and implications. Cancer Epidemiol Biomarkers Prev 15, 1–2.
Ross, J.A., Perentesis, J.P., Robison, L.L., Davies, S.M., 1996. Big babies and infant leukemia: a role for insulin-like growth factor-1? Cancer Causes Control 7, 553–559.
Ross, J.A., Potter, J.D., Shu, X.O., Reaman, G.H., Lampkin, B., Robison, L.L., 1997. Evaluating the relationships among maternal reproductive history, birth characteristics, and infant leukemia: a report from the Children's Cancer Group. Ann Epidemiol 7, 172–179.
Scholl, T.O., 2005. Iro n status during pregnancy: setting the stage for mother and infant. Am J Clin Nutr 81, 1218S–1222S.

Scholl, T.O., Hediger, M.L., 1994. Anemia and iron-deficiency anemia: compilation of data on pregnancy outcome. Am J Clin Nutr 59, 492S–500S discussion 500S–501S.

Schuz, J., Forman, M.R., 2007. Birthweight by gestational age and childhood cancer. Cancer Causes Control 18, 655–663.

Shu, X.O., Han, D., Severson, R.K., Chen, Z., Neglia, J.P., Reaman, G.H., Buckley, J.D., Robison, L.L., 2002. Birth characteristics, maternal reproductive history, hormone use during pregnancy, and risk of childhood acute lymphocytic leukemia by immunophenotype (United States). Cancer Causes Control 13, 15–25.

Siega-Riz, A.M., Hartzema, A.G., Turnbull, C., Thorp, J., McDonald, T., Cogswell, M.E., 2006. The effects of prophylactic iron given in prenatal supplements on iron status and birth outcomes: a randomized controlled trial. Am J Obstet Gynecol 194, 512–519.

Silva Idos, S., De Stavola, B., McCormack, V., 2008. Birth size and breast cancer risk: re-analysis of individual participant data from 32 studies. PLoS Med 5, e193.

Simmons, R., 2005. Developmental origins of adult metabolic disease: concepts and controversies. Trends Endocrinol Metab 16, 390–394.

Sinotte, M., Diorio, C., Berube, S., Pollak, M., Brisson, J., 2009. Genetic polymorphisms of the vitamin D binding protein and plasma concentrations of 25-hydroxyvitamin D in premenopausal women. Am J Clin Nutr 89, 634–640.

Skalkidou, A., Petridou, E., Papathoma, E., Salvanos, H., Kedikoglou, S., Chrousos, G., Trichopoulos, D., 2003. Determinants and consequences of major insulin-like growth factor components among full-term healthy neonates. Cancer Epidemiol Biomarkers Prev 12, 860–865.

Sprehe, M.R., Barahmani, N., Cao, Y., Wang, T., Forman, M.R., Bondy, M., Okcu, M.F., 2009. Comparison of birth weight corrected for gestational age and birth weight alone in prediction of development of childhood leukemia and central nervous system tumors. Pediatr Blood Cancer 54 2, 242–249.

Srivastava, S., Mehrotra, P.K., Srivastava, S.P., Siddiqui, M.K., 2002. Some essential elements in maternal and cord blood in relation to birth weight and gestational age of the baby. Biol Trace Elem Res 86, 97–105.

Stevens, R.G., Graubard, B.I., Micozzi, M.S., Neriishi, K., Blumberg, B.S., 1994. Moderate elevation of body iron level and increased risk of cancer occurrence and death. Int J Cancer 56, 364–369.

Stevens, R.G., Jones, D.Y., Micozzi, M.S., Taylor, P.R., 1988. Body iron stores and the risk of cancer. N Engl J Med 319, 1047–1052.

Storms, M.R., Van Howe, R.S., 2004. Birthweight by gestational age and sex at a rural referral center. J Perinatol 24, 236–240.

Surkan, P.J., Hsieh, C.C., Johansson, A.L., Dickman, P.W., Cnattingius, S., 2004. Reasons for increasing trends in large for gestational age births. Obstet Gynecol 104, 720–726.

Thorleifsson, G., Walters, G.B., Gudbjartsson, D.F., Steinthorsdottir, V., Sulem, P., Helgadottir, A., Styrkarsdottir, U., Gretarsdottir, S., Thorlacius, S., Jonsdottir, I., Jonsdottir, T., Olafsdottir, E.J., Olafsdottir, G.H., Jonsson, T., Jonsson, F., Borch-Johnsen, K., Hansen, T., Andersen, G., Jorgensen, T., Lauritzen, T., Aben, K.K., Verbeek, A.L., Roeleveld, N., Kampman, E., Yanek, L.R., Becker, L.C., Tryggvadottir, L., Rafnar, T., Becker, D.M., Gulcher, J., Kiemeney, L.A., Pedersen, O., Kong, A., Thorsteinsdottir, U., Stefansson, K., 2009. Genome-wide association yields new sequence variants at seven loci that associate with measures of obesity. Nat Genet 41, 18–24.

Tower, R.L., Spector, L.G., 2007. The epidemiology of childhood leukemia with a focus on birth weight and diet. Crit Rev Clin Lab Sci 44, 203–242.

Trowbridge, I.S., Domingo, D.L., 1981. Anti-transferrin receptor monoclonal antibody and toxin-antibody conjugates affect growth of human tumour cells. Nature 294, 171–173.

Trowbridge, I.S., Lopez, F., 1982. Monoclonal antibody to transferrin receptor blocks transferrin binding and inhibits human tumor cell growth in vitro. Proc Natl Acad Sci U S A 79, 1175–1179.

Vaclavicek, A., Hemminki, K., Bartram, C.R., Wagner, K., Wappenschmidt, B., Meindl, A., Schmutzler, R.K., Klaes, R., Untch, M., Burwinkel, B., Forsti, A., 2006. Association of prolactin and its receptor gene regions with familial breast cancer. J Clin Endocrinol Metab 91, 1513–1519.

Vella, A., Bouatia-Naji, N., Heude, B., Cooper, J.D., Lowe, C.E., Petry, C., Ring, S.M., Dunger, D.B., Todd, J.A., Ong, K.K., 2008. Association analysis of the IGF1 gene with childhood growth, IGF-1 concentrations and type 1 diabetes. Diabetologia 51, 811–815.

Wang, L., Wang, X., Laird, N., Zuckerman, B., Stubblefield, P., Xu, X., 2006. Polymorphism in maternal LRP8 gene is associated with fetal growth. Am J Hum Genet 78, 770–777.

Weedon, M.N., Clark, V.J., Qian, Y., Ben-Shlomo, Y., Timpson, N., Ebrahim, S., Lawlor, D.A., Pembrey, M.E., Ring, S., Wilkin, T.J., Voss, L.D., Jeffery, A.N., Metcalf, B., Ferrucci, L., Corsi, A.M., Murray, A., Melzer, D., Knight, B., Shields, B., Smith, G.D., Hattersley, A.T., Di Rienzo, A., Frayling, T.M., 2006. A common haplotype of the glucokinase gene alters fasting glucose and birth weight: association in six studies and population-genetics analyses. Am J Hum Genet 79, 991–1001.

Westergaard, T., Andersen, P.K., Pedersen, J.B., Olsen, J.H., Frisch, M., Sorensen, H.T., Wohlfahrt, J., Melbye, M., 1997. Birth characteristics, sibling patterns, and acute leukemia risk in childhood: a population-based cohort study. J Natl Cancer Inst 89, 939–947.

Wilcox, A.J., 2001. On the importance–and the unimportance–of birthweight. Int J Epidemiol 30, 1233–1241.

Wilcox, M., Gardosi, J., Mongelli, M., Ray, C., Johnson, I., 1993. Birth weight from pregnancies dated by ultrasonography in a multicultural British population. BMJ 307, 588–591.

Wilpshaar, J., Joekes, E.C., Lim, F.T., Van Leeuwen, G.A., Van den Boogaard, P.J., Kanhai, H.H., Willemze, R., Falkenburg, J.H., 2002. Magnetic resonance imaging of fetal bone marrow for quantitative definition of the human fetal stem cell compartment. Blood 100, 451–457.

Wong, C.T., Saha, N., 1990. Inter-relationships of storage iron in the mother, the placenta and the newborn. Acta Obstet Gynecol Scand 69, 613–616.

Wu, T., Sempos, C.T., Freudenheim, J.L., Muti, P., Smit, E., 2004. Serum iron, copper and zinc concentrations and risk of cancer mortality in US adults. Ann Epidemiol 14, 195–201.

Xue, F., Michels, K.B., 2007. Intrauterine factors and risk of breast cancer: a systematic review and meta-analysis of current evidence. Lancet Oncol 8, 1088–1100.

Yang, S.W., Yu, J.S., 2000. Relationship of insulin-like growth factor-I, insulin-like growth factor binding protein-3, insulin, growth hormone in cord blood and maternal factors with birth height and birthweight. Pediatr Int 42, 31–36.

Yeazel, M.W., Ross, J.A., Buckley, J.D., Woods, W.G., Ruccione, K., Robison, L.L., 1997. High birth weight and risk of specific childhood cancers: a report from the Children's Cancer Group. J Pediatr 131, 671–677.

Yu, H., Rohan, T., 2000. Role of the insulin-like growth factor family in cancer development and progression. J Natl Cancer Inst 92, 1472–1489.

Yu, H., Shu, X.O., Li, B.D., Dai, Q., Gao, Y.T., Jin, F., Zheng, W., 2003. Joint effect of insulin-like growth factors and sex steroids on breast cancer risk. Cancer Epidemiol Biomarkers Prev 12, 1067–1073.

Chapter 17
Iron Excess and Cancer

Charronne F. Davis and M. Tevfik Dorak

Abstract In the last two decades, strong observational and experimental evidence has been presented for the role of iron excess in cancer development. The hereditary hemochromatosis gene HFE variants that increase body iron levels are associated with increased cancer risk. The first such association was reported by us in childhood acute lymphoblastic leukemia. With the identification of molecular mechanisms of potentiation of carcinogenesis by iron, epidemiologic associations have been gaining more weight. Experimental data also increase the credibility of suggestions that iron excess can both initiate (genotoxic effect) and promote (via its effect on immune function) cancer development. Both environmental and genetic factors may lead to iron excess but the effect is strongest in combination. Iron excess may contribute to cancer development in many different ways, most of which yet unappreciated and most relevant of those possible connections are discussed in this chapter. Since reduction in smoking, alcohol and red meat consumption eliminates excessive exposure to iron, eating fruits and vegetables does not expose the body to too much bioavailable iron and perhaps replaces other iron-rich food stuff and avoidance of excess iron levels reduces infections, iron is indirectly involved in the success of these preventive measures. Perhaps it is time to emphasize lower exposure to environmental iron directly as an important factor to reduce the cancer burden in the industrialized world.

Keywords Iron excess · Gentoxic effects · Gene variants · Development of cancer

17.1 Introduction

Modern life style is often blamed for increasing cancer incidence in developed countries. Since genetic constitution of human populations has not changed in the last few decades, increasing carcinogenic exposures must be responsible for this.

M.T. Dorak (✉)
Department of Environmental and Occupational Health, Robert Stempel College of Public Health & Social Work, Florida International University, Miami, FL 33199-0001, USA
e-mail: mdorak@fiu.edu

D. Roy, M.T. Dorak (eds.), *Environmental Factors, Genes, and the Development of Human Cancers*, DOI 10.1007/978-1-4419-6752-7_17,

There is now almost a consensus that the role of environment in cancer development is greater than heritable component (Lichtenstein et al., 2000; Le Marchand, 2005; Colditz et al., 2006; Hemminki et al., 2006). Modern life style in developed countries is suspected to have some carcinogenetic elements. Large epidemiologic studies have identified "smoking, heavy alcohol use, obesity, a lack of physical activity, having a low fruit and vegetable intake, unsafe sex, urban air pollution, indoor smoke from household use of coal" as potential culprits (Danaei et al., 2005). Of the 7 million deaths from cancer worldwide in 2001, an estimated 2.4 million (35%) were attributable to these potentially modifiable risk factors. In high-income countries, smoking, alcohol use, and being overweight and obesity are the most important causes of cancer (Danaei et al., 2005).

Breast cancer is a particularly striking example of a temporal increase in incidence, which is noted not only in Westernized world but also in Asia (see the Breast Cancer chapter). Incidence and mortality has been increasing for many decades. In Britain, the age-standardized incidence of breast cancer per 100,000 women increased from 74 in 1975 to 123 in 2005. Over the 25 year period (1981–2005) the incidence rate increased by 57% (Cancer Research UK: http://info.cancerresearchuk.org/cancerstats/types/breast/incidence). The strongest evidence for the role played by environment comes from immigrant studies which show that migrants from low-risk Asian societies to the U.S. suffer elevated risk of breast cancer in their own lifetimes (Bray et al., 2004).

Something about the modern Western lifestyle apparently increases the cancer risk. High income is estimated to account for about 19% of breast cancer cases when analyzed by itself (Madigan et al., 1995), which has no biological interpretation and must reflect attributes of lifestyle and/or environment that increase risk (Stevens, 2002). At least half of breast cancer risk in the U.S., and other industrialized societies, is in excess of that found in non-industrialized societies for unknown reasons. Among the candidate factors are smoking, alcohol use, overweight/obesity (Danaei et al., 2005), smaller family size and higher induced abortion rates (Beral et al., 2004), stress (Kiecolt-Glaser et al., 2002; Chida et al., 2008) and disrupted circadian rhythm (Stevens, 2002).

General cancer risk factors smoking and alcohol use both contribute to or are associated with iron excess (Kato et al., 2000), which is know to increase the risk for most cancers (Huang, 2003; Papanikolaou and Pantopoulos, 2005; Toyokuni, 2009), in particular breast cancer (Elliott et al., 1993; Kabat and Rohan, 2007; Huang, 2008), colon cancer (Butterworth, 2006; Shi et al., 2009), esophageal cancer (Hsing et al., 1995; Boult et al., 2008; Zhang et al., 2009) and liver cancer (Deugnier and Turlin, 2001; Kowdley, 2004; Kew, 2008). Furthermore, iron also potentiates the effects of estrogen and radiation (Stevens and Kalkwarf, 1990; Stevens, 2000; Liehr and Jones, 2001; Kabat and Rohan, 2007), mediates oxidative damage (Herbert et al., 1994; Lipinski et al., 2000; De Freitas and Meneghini, 2001; Eaton and Qian, 2002; McCord, 2004; Valko et al., 2005; Tuomainen et al., 2007) and induces inflammation (Dai et al., 2004; Kell, 2009).

17.2 Iron and Its Pro-Carcinogenic Effect

In the last two decades, strong observational and experimental evidence has been presented for the role of iron excess in cancer development (Table 17.1). Even mildly elevated serum iron levels are associated with increased cancer risk in prospective cohort studies (Weinberg, 1984; Stevens et al., 1986; Selby and Friedman, 1988; Stevens et al., 1988; Sussman, 1992; Knekt et al., 1994; Stevens et al., 1994; van Asperen et al., 1995; Wurzelmann et al., 1996; Nelson, 2001; Lee et al., 2004; Mainous et al., 2004; Wu et al., 2004a; Lee et al., 2005; Mainous et al., 2005a; Mainous et al., 2005b; Zhou et al., 2005; Balder et al., 2006) and cancer incidence declines with regular phlebotomy (Merk et al., 1990; Zacharski et al., 2008). Only occasional studies failed to observe the correlation between body iron levels and cancer risk (Kabat et al., 2007). The hereditary hemochromatosis gene *HFE* variants that increase body iron levels are associated with increased cancer risk (Dorak et al., 2005; Dorak, 2006). The first such association was reported in childhood ALL (Dorak et al., 1999; Davis and Dorak, 2010; Dorak et al., 2009). An interaction between *HFE* and transferrin receptor gene (*TFRC*) variants has also been reported in modification of cancer risk (Beckman et al., 1999). Specific cancer types that are associated with either iron excess or iron regulatory gene polymorphisms are listed in Table 17.2. Overall these data overwhelmingly suggest that iron-induced phenomena contribute to carcinogenesis in humans.

Table 17.1 Evidence for and mechanisms of a pro-carcinogenic role of iron excess

– Iron-induced oxidative DNA damage (Herbert et al., 1994; Lipinski et al., 2000; De Freitas and Meneghini, 2001; Eaton and Qian, 2002; McCord, 2004; Valko et al., 2005; Tuomainen et al., 2007)
– Iron-induced abnormalities of immune function (Good et al., 1988; de Sousa, 1989; Brock and Mulero, 2000; Walker and Walker, 2000; Porto and De Sousa, 2007)
– Iron as an essential nutrient for proliferating neoplastic cells (Bergeron, 1986; Cazzola et al., 1990; Sussman, 1992; Kwok and Richardson, 2002; Butterworth, 2006)
– Animal experiments showing pro-carcinogenic effect of iron (Hann et al., 1988; Hann et al., 1991; Toyokuni, 1996; Weinberg, 1996; Toyokuni, 2009)
– Substitution of zinc in zinc finger proteins by iron interfering with gene expression regulation (Conte et al., 1996)
– Transcriptional activation of HAMP by P53 to lower body iron levels (Weizer-Stern et al., 2007)
– Increased hepatic and extra-hepatic cancers in hereditary hemochromatosis patients and their relatives (Ammann et al., 1980; Tiniakos and Williams, 1988; Hsing et al., 1995; Mallory and Kowdley, 2001; Geier et al., 2002; Elmberg et al., 2003)
– Correlation between serum iron levels and cancer risk (Stevens et al., 1986; Selby and Friedman, 1988; Stevens et al., 1988; Sussman, 1992; Knekt et al., 1994; Stevens et al., 1994; van Asperen et al., 1995; Wurzelmann et al., 1996; Nelson, 2001; Lee et al., 2004; Mainous et al., 2004; Wu et al., 2004a; Lee et al., 2005; Mainous et al., 2005a; Mainous et al., 2005b; Zhou et al., 2005; Balder et al., 2006)
– Correlation between regular blood donation and reduced cancer risk (Merk et al., 1990; Edgren et al., 2008)

Table 17.2 Cancers that have been associated with excessive iron intake or iron regulatory gene polymorphisms that increase body iron levels

– Childhood acute lymphoblastic leukemia (Dorak et al., 1999; Davis and Dorak, 2010; Dorak et al., 2009)
– Hepatocellular carcinoma (Deugnier and Turlin, 2001; Kowdley, 2004; Kew, 2008)
– Breast cancer (Elliott et al., 1993; Beckman et al., 1999; Kabat and Rohan, 2007; Huang, 2008)
– Colon cancer (Beckman et al., 1999; Butterworth, 2006; Shi et al., 2009)
– Multiple myeloma (Beckman et al., 1999)
– Myelodysplastic syndrome (Varkonyi et al., 2003; Nearman et al., 2007)
– Brain tumors (Martinez di Montemuros et al., 2001)
– Esophagus cancer (Hsing et al., 1995; Boult et al., 2008; Zhang et al., 2009)

Animal studies have also generated supportive data for the iron and cancer connection. Iron excess induces several cancers in animal models (Toyokuni, 1996, 2009). Increased tumor growth rates are observed in animals fed with iron (Hann et al., 1988; Hann et al., 1991). Furthermore, iron-rich diet synergizes with cancer induction by other agents including estrogen. An elevated dietary iron intake enhances the incidence of carcinogen-induced mammary cancer in rats and estrogen-induced kidney tumors in Syrian hamsters (Liehr and Jones, 2001). Results of in vitro studies on cell lines also suggest a direct involvement of iron in tumor growth (Chen et al., 2007). The pro-carcinogenic activity of iron is due to absolute requirement of any proliferating cell for iron (Bergeron, 1986; Cazzola et al., 1990; Kwok and Richardson, 2002), which is evident by emergence of transferrin receptor on the surface of transformed cells to increase iron uptake (Trowbridge and Omary, 1981; Trowbridge and Lopez, 1982).

In humans, both males and females are at risk for iron-induced cancer susceptibility. Although pre-menopausal women are believed to have lower body iron levels due to regular blood loss, detailed studies showed that genetic effects were more than twice as great in women as the effects of menstrual blood loss or pregnancies on iron stores (Whitfield et al., 2003), a finding which has support from mouse models (Courselaud et al., 2004). In women, additive genetic effects on iron stores are at least as equally strong as in men (Whitfield et al., 2000). In the general female population, serum iron parameters increase after menopause (Zacharski et al., 2000) but women with *HFE* variants show iron excess even during the reproductive period (Datz et al., 1998; Greenwood et al., 2005). Thus, iron excess due to genetic variants is plausible in women during pre- and post-menopausal periods.

Iron is the most abundant redox active metal in human body. Ingested iron is absorbed but excretion is minimal (Dunn et al., 2007). In general, body iron stores show gradual increase with age and this process starts earlier in life in males, with levels reaching toxic levels in a proportion of healthy adults (Milman, 1996; Zacharski et al., 2000; Fleming et al., 2001b; Liu et al., 2003; Milman et al., 2003; Sullivan, 2004; Cade et al., 2005; Mainous et al., 2005a; Kabat and Rohan, 2007; Pedersen and Milman, 2009a). At the molecular level, iron is a genotoxic agent through induction of oxidative stress (Herbert et al., 1994; Lipinski et al., 2000; De Freitas and Meneghini, 2001; McCord, 2004; Valko et al., 2005; Tuomainen et al., 2007). This pro-oxidant effect coupled with effect of iron on cell cycle (Le and Richardson, 2002; Butterworth, 2006; Sanchez et al., 2006; Yu et al., 2007) is the basis of its pro-carcinogenic role. Iron mediates hydrogen peroxide-induced mutagenesis and the formation of several types of DNA lesions in mammalian cells including sister chromatid exchanges (Mello Filho et al., 1984; Larramendy et al., 1987; Martins et al., 1995; Meneghini, 1997). The effect on cell cycle is due to regulation of a number of cell cycle control molecules by iron. These molecules include p53 (TP53), p27 (CDKN1B), cyclin D1 (CCND1), cyclin-dependent kinase 2 (CDK2), BCL2, growth differentiation factor 15 (GDF15) and the metastasis suppressor gene, N-myc downstream regulated gene-1 (NDRG1) (Simonart et al., 2001; Kovacevic and Richardson, 2006; O'Donnell et al., 2006; Yu et al., 2007; Lakhal et al., 2009).

In recent years research identified other molecular interactions involving cellular iron relevant in carcinogenesis. The oncogenic transcription factor c-Myc manipulates intracellular iron levels to promote tumor growth (Wu et al., 1999; Butterworth, 2006). c-Myc activates TFRC transcription through a conserved c-Myc binding site also located within the first intron of the TFRC gene (O'Donnell et al., 2006). Cytokine-activated transcription factor STAT5A/B regulates iron delivery through transcriptional activation of the transferrin receptor gene TFRC (Kerenyi et al., 2008). This finding also implies the involvement of iron in inflammation since STAT5 is a transcription factor for NFKB1. Matrix metalloproteinase-9 (MMP-9), whose overexpression is implicated in the invasion and metastasis of head and neck squamous cell carcinoma (HNSCC) is upregulated in vitro by iron treatment of HNSCC cell lines (Kaomongkolgit et al., 2008). Finally, iron excess may also be involved in epigenetic changes observed in cancer (Butterworth, 2006; Lehmann et al., 2007). Thus, with the identification of molecular mechanisms of potentiation of carcinogenesis by iron, epidemiologic associations have been gaining more weight. Experimental data also increase the credibility of suggestions that iron excess can both initiate (genotoxic effect) and promote (via its effect on immune function) cancer development.

17.3 Environmental Sources of Iron

17.3.1 Red Meat

Iron in red meat may increase oxidative damage and increase the formation of N-nitroso compounds (Sinha et al., 2009), which is implicated in increased colon cancer risk (Wurzelmann et al., 1996; Kato et al., 1999). Iron is therefore relevant in the mechanism of the association between red meat intake and cancer (Lee et al., 2004). The highest amount of bioavailable iron is ingested in red meat (Sinha et al., 2009) and red meat intake correlates with body iron stores (Rossi et al., 2001; Cade et al., 2005; Milward et al., 2008; Pedersen and Milman, 2009a). One study tested the hypothesis that the iron-containing heme protein in red meat may be responsible for its association with colon cancer and this association may be modified by chlorophyll, the pigment in green vegetables (Balder et al., 2006). Chlorophyll inhibits heme metabolism and prevents the heme-induced colonic cytotoxicity and epithelial proliferation (de Vogel et al., 2005). In cohort study a (Balder et al., 2006), an association was present between heme intake and colon cancer among men but subjects with the lowest chlorophyll and the highest heme intake had the highest risk of colon cancer. It is therefore possible that heme-iron plays a role in the association between red meat intake and colon cancer, and this is modifiable by green vegetables. Likewise, heme-iron in red meat also contributes to general increase in body iron content and may increase the risk to other cancers.

17.3.2 Home Brewed Beer in Africa

African iron overload due to consumption of home-brewed beer is associated with high incidence of esophageal cancer in South Africa (Matsha et al., 2006). Iron overload in sub-Saharan Africa results from increased dietary iron derived from traditional home-brewed beer, which contains 258-fold higher iron than the commercial beer (Matsha et al., 2006). Despite the obvious environmental exposure, a genetic component may also contribute to African iron overload (Gordeuk et al., 1992). Regardless of genetic variants, African iron induced by excessive iron intake is associated with liver cancer (Kew and Asare, 2007), as in other iron overload conditions in non-African populations (Bradbear et al., 1985).

17.3.3 Other Food Stuff

As a result of a post-world war II legislation adopted globally, common food stuff is currently iron fortified in almost all countries (except in Scandinavia). Flour and breakfast cereals are the most commonly iron fortified foods. The iron fortification may supply up to 25% of total iron intake for adults (Olsson et al., 1997; Osler et al., 1999; Milman et al., 2003). In a Swedish study which covered the period with and without iron fortification of food, it was concluded that after withdrawal of fortification people with genetic hemochromatosis will accelerate into clinical disease at a slower rate (Olsson et al., 1997). Conversely, this also means that in developed countries, mandatory iron fortification of food may contribute to the development of iron overload in genetically prone individuals although experimental findings do not universally support this conclusion (Hunt and Zeng, 2004). In Denmark where mandatory iron fortification was abolished in 1987, a study documented that during the 10 years covering the last few years of the fortification area and the beginning of the post-fortification era, body iron stores were unchanged in premenopausal women but the prevalence of iron overload in postmenopausal women increased significantly although changes in dietary habits may have contributed to this result (Milman et al., 2003).

The Framingham Heart Study cohort is an iron-replete elderly population with a high prevalence of elevated iron stores in contrast with a low prevalence of iron deficiency, with insignificant effects of chronic disease on these iron status estimates. The likely liability in free-living, elderly white Americans eating a Western diet is, thus, high iron stores not iron deficiency (Fleming et al., 2001b).

Another important source of iron intake is the supplements voluntarily used by individuals. The Framingham study has shown that in the elderly age group the strongest predictor of increased iron stores is supplemental iron intake (Fleming et al., 1998; Fleming et al., 2002). Other studies confirmed the positive correlation between supplemental iron use and serum iron parameters (Kato et al., 2000; Liu et al., 2003; Blanck et al., 2005).

It is noteworthy that increased consumption of red meat and common use of iron-containing supplements together with ongoing iron fortification of common food stuff put the Western populations at higher risk for iron excess, It is estimated that on average, 5–10% of adult population at such countries have excessive levels of iron (Milman, 1996; Zacharski et al., 2000; Fleming et al., 2001b; Liu et al., 2003; Milman et al., 2003; Sullivan, 2004; Cade et al., 2005; Mainous et al., 2005a; Kabat and Rohan, 2007; Pedersen and Milman, 2009a). This figure is usually lower for pre-menopausal women and may be higher in the elderly in both sex reflecting the gradual accumulation of iron with age. In the presence of genetic predisposition, however, even reproductive age women may show biochemical signs of iron excess (Datz et al., 1998).

Dietary vitamin C, alcohol, fruit intake, whole grains, nuts, tea and coffee consumption also have some effect on iron status (Fleming et al., 1998; Temme and Van Hoydonck, 2002; Cade et al., 2005; Pedersen and Milman, 2009a). Whole grains, fruits and nuts contain phytochemicals that are generally associated with protection from cancer (Waladkhani and Clemens, 1998). Their inhibitory role in iron absorption should be included in discussions of the mechanism of this association (Waladkhani and Clemens, 1998).

17.3.4 Soil

The distribution of endemic form of Kaposi sarcoma, a rare skin tumor, corresponds to continental rifts and presence of iron-oxide-rich volcanic clays (Simonart et al., 1998; Simonart, 2006).

17.3.5 Occupational Exposures

There are several occupations in which exposure to iron is possible but there has not been an unambiguous connection with increased cancer risk. Workers in ferriferous industries have an elevated risk of respiratory tract neoplasia. A weak lung cancer excess in many populations exposed to iron oxides has been reported but causality is unclear (Wild et al., 2009). Although iron exposure may be directly involved in increased cancer risk, some investigators have also suggested that inhaled iron compounds may be just carriers of other carcinogens (Weinberg, 1999). Cancer accounted for a higher proportion of deaths among the iron-steel workers than the general male population and risks of stomach cancer appeared to be highest among workers employed in jobs with exposure to iron (Xu et al., 1996). A dramatic case report on the occurrence of Kaposi sarcoma in the palm of a metallurgist (Simonart et al., 2003) further strengthen the proposed connection between iron exposure and Kaposi sarcoma first exemplified in areas where soil is rich in iron (see above).

Knowledge about the sources of iron is helpful to find ways to avoid excessive iron intake. A summary of such measures is given in Table 17.3.

Table 17.3 Measures to avoid excessive iron intake (unless documented iron deficiency exists)

– Regular blood donation (if not possible, medical phlebotomy by regular aspirin intake unless medically contra-indicated)
– Avoidance of excessive red meat intake and alcohol consumption
– Avoidance of iron containing supplements
– Avoidance of vitamin C intake with iron containing food
– Intake of whole grains, milk, eggs and green vegetables
– Substitution of iron-fortified foods

17.4 Genetic Control of Iron Homeostasis

With the discovery of the hereditary hemochromatosis gene *HFE* in 1996 (Feder et al., 1996) the work on genetic regulation of iron homeostasis gained momentum. Besides discovery of a large number of iron regulatory genes, in the last few years, genome-wide screens have been performed to identify yet unknown genes or variants of known genes involved in iron overload and iron-related phenotypes (Acton et al., 2007; Andrews, 2009; Benyamin et al., 2009a; Benyamin et al., 2009b; Chambers et al., 2009; Ganesh et al., 2009; Soranzo et al., 2009; Tanaka et al., 2009). As more genes are identified, interactions among them are also unraveled and genetic or environmental factors influencing expressivity and penetrance of genetic variants are determined (Milet et al., 2007; Deugnier and Mosser, 2008). Animal studies confirm a polygenic control of iron homeostasis and strain differences in iron overload levels in *hfe* disrupted mice (Fleming et al., 2001c; Dupic et al., 2002; Bensaid et al., 2004; Coppin et al., 2007) suggest the importance of *hfe*-modifier loci in iron homeostasis. Indeed, one of the human genome-wide studies showed that only 40% of the genetic variation in serum transferrin levels (which reflects the body iron content) are explained by genetic variants within the *HFE* and transferrin (*TF*) genes (Benyamin et al., 2009b). It is now clear that a large number of genes are involved in regulation of iron homeostasis (Whitfield et al., 2000; McGregor et al., 2004; Pietrangelo, 2004). 23 and 31% of the variance in iron, 66 and 49% of the variance in

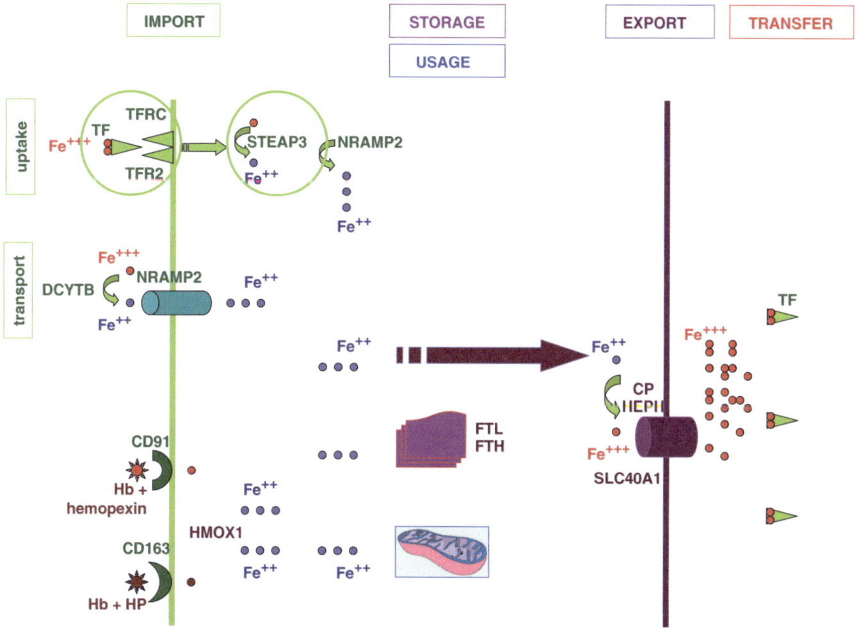

Fig. 17.1 Molecules involved in iron transport across cell membranes. After iron molecule is transported inside the cell by one of the mechanisms shown, it may be used in physiological reactions (as in mitochondria), stored in ferritin molecules or exported outside the cell. Extracellular transfer of iron is achieved by transferrin (TF). Other molecules shown are TFRC (transferrin receptor), TFR2 (transferrin receptor), DCYTB (formally CYBRD1, cytochrome b reductase 1), NRAMP2 (formally SLC11A2, proton-coupled divalent metal ion transporter 2), CD91 (formally LRP1, alpha-2-macroglobulin receptor), CD163 (macrophage-associated antigen), HP (haptoglobin), HMOX1 (heme oxygenase type 1), STEAP3 (STEAP family member 3), FTL (ferritin light chain), FTH (ferritin heavy chain), CP (ceruloplasmin), HEPH (hephaestin), SLC40A1 (ferroportin)

transferrin, 33 and 47% of the variance in transferrin saturation, and 47 and 47% of the variance in ferritin could be explained by additive genetic factors, for men and women, respectively. There are highly significant effects of other as-yet-unidentified genes on iron stores, in addition to *HFE* genotype (Whitfield et al., 2000). In Fig. 17.1, the genes taking part in iron transport are shown. The iron-related genes that modify the penetrance of *HFE* in humans are listed in Table 17.4.

In females, environmental effects, mainly regular blood loss during the premenopausal period, have a stronger influence on iron homeostasis. In a study of more than 2,000 female twin pairs, significant effects of age, menopausal status and magnitude of menstrual blood loss on body iron content as measured by serum ferritin levels were demonstrated, accounting for up to 18% of variance in serum ferritin (Whitfield et al., 2003). Genetic effects were more than twice as great as sex-specific effects. Despite obvious environmental effects on body iron content such as regular blood loss and pregnancy, genetics still play a major role in iron

Table 17.4 Modifiers of body iron stores

(a) Genetics
– *HFE* and modifiers of *HFE* penetrance (Deugnier and Mosser, 2008)
HLA-A3B7 haplotype (Barton et al., 1997)
HLA-A1B8 haplotype (Olsson et al., 2007)
HLA-A1, -A2, -A3 (Cruz et al., 2006)
Ancestral HFE haplotype (Barton et al., 1996; Piperno et al., 1998)
Calreticulin levels (Pinto et al., 2008)
– Other iron regulatory genes:
TF (Benyamin et al., 2009b)
LTF (Ward and Conneely, 2004)
TFRC (Chua et al., 2008)
*TFR*2 (Chua et al., 2008)
HJV (Milet et al., 2007)
HAMP (Jacolot et al., 2004)
*TMPRSS*6 (Benyamin et al., 2009a; Benyamin et al., 2009b; Tanaka et al., 2009)
*SLC*11*A*2 (Courville et al., 2006)
*SLC*40*A*1 (Donovan et al., 2005)
*BMP*2, *BMP*4, *BMP*6 (Milet et al., 2007; Meynard et al., 2009)
(b) Environmental
– Dietary factors: red meat, ascorbic acid, iron supplements, whole grains and nuts, non-citrus fruits, milk, eggs, tea and coffee (Cook et al., 1984; Fleming et al., 1998; Kaltwasser et al., 1998; Temme and Van Hoydonck, 2002; Blanck et al., 2005; Cade et al., 2005; Milward et al., 2008; Pedersen and Milman, 2009a)
– Smoking (Mussalo-Rauhamaa et al., 1986; Weinberg, 1999, 2009) and alcohol consumption (Weinberg, 1996; Rossi et al., 2001; Deugnier and Mosser, 2008; Heath et al., 2008; Milward et al., 2008; Pedersen and Milman, 2009a)
– Regular blood transfusion (as in congenital hemolytic anemias or hemodialysis causing transfusional hemosiderosis)
– Blood loss (Milman, 1996; Heath et al., 2008; Pedersen and Milman, 2009a) including aspirin use (Fleming et al., 2001a; Liu et al., 2003; Mascitelli et al., 2009)
– Cessation of regular blood loss in menopause (Milman, 1996; Zacharski et al., 2000; Liu et al., 2003; Nakano et al., 2003)
– Iron loss through pregnancy (Milman et al., 1992; Milman, 1996)
– Exercise (Lauffer, 1991)
– Obesity (Kohgo et al., 2007; Miraglia Del Giudice et al., 2009; Tussing-Humphreys et al., 2009; Zafon et al., 2009)
– Occupational exposure in ferriferous industries (Weinberg, 1996)

For reviews, see (Weinberg, 1996; Deugnier and Mosser, 2008).

homeostasis in females. Thus, genetics has a measurable effect on iron status alongside environment.

17.5 Population at Risk for Iron Excess

Both environmental and genetic factors may lead to iron excess but the effect is strongest in combination. The most common mutation of the *HFE* gene is C282Y and homozygosity for this mutation is responsible for 90% of hereditary hemochromatosis which is a severe iron overload disease. Conversely, not all C282Y homozygotes develop iron overload (Olynyk et al., 1999; Jackson et al., 2001; Mura et al., 2001). They are however, at even higher risk for iron overload if their iron intake is high (Cade et al., 2005; Deugnier and Mosser, 2008). Other *HFE* genotypes that increase the risk for iron overload are compound heterozygosity for C282Y and H63D (Pedersen and Milman, 2009b), or homozygosity for H63D (Samarasena et al., 2006; Pedersen and Milman, 2009b). Heterozygosity for either mutation only causes increased serum iron levels in a proportion of individuals (biochemically manifesting heterozygotes) without clinical iron overload (Adams, 1994; Bulaj et al., 1996; Datz et al., 1998; Distante et al., 1999; de Valk et al., 2000; Mura et al., 2000; Rossi et al., 2001; Gochee et al., 2002; Raddatz et al., 2003; Pedersen and Milman, 2009b). Even without *HFE* mutations, it is possible to have iron overload. In Denmark, among people with wildtype genotypes in C282Y, 6% have elevated transferrin saturation, 13% have elevated ferritin, and 1% have elevation of both iron status markers (Pedersen and Milman, 2009b). Another Scandinavian study (Bell et al., 2000) as well as clinical observations (Jalihal and Barlow, 1984; Green et al., 1989; Barton et al., 2006) also showed that it is possible to develop iron overload with excessive iron intake only.

The *HFE* mutations C282Y and H63D show different geographic distributions (Rochette et al., 1999; Merryweather-Clarke et al., 2000). While C282Y is only seen in Northwestern European populations (at highest frequencies in Celts and Scandinavians), H63D has a more global distribution. In a study of more than 6,700 middle-aged women in the UK, C282Y homozygosity rate was 0.5 and 13.2% were heterozygote. Compound heterozygosity for C282Y and H63D was observed in 2.5% of the sample (Cade et al., 2005). H63D homozygosity and heterozygosity were observed in 2.5 and 25.8%, respectively. In a representative subsample of these middle-aged women ($n = 2{,}528$), 3% had high serum ferritin values. Since middle-aged women are at lower risk to develop iron excess than older women and men, this is the lowest estimate of iron excess in a Western adult population.

Other studies that investigated iron indexes in otherwise healthy adult populations in Western countries reported that on average 5–10% have biochemical iron excess (Milman, 1996; Distante et al., 1999; Zacharski et al., 2000; Fleming et al., 2001b; Liu et al., 2003; Milman et al., 2003; Sullivan, 2004; Cade et al., 2005; Mainous et al., 2005a; Kabat and Rohan, 2007; Pedersen and Milman, 2009a). Specifically, 7.3% of the US population has a serum transferrin saturation of more than 45% at baseline and thus, are at risk for cancer if they consume high levels of dietary iron (Mainous et al., 2005a). 13% of Framingham study subjects have increased iron levels (Fleming et al., 2001b). In post-menopausal women, 9.8% had an elevated ferritin concentration (Liu et al., 2003).

17.6 Gene and Environment Interactions in Iron Excess and Cancer Connection

Iron deficiency is the most common nutritional deficiency in the world. In an iron-deficient population, excessive iron intake or genetic variation will only bring the individual's iron level to normal values but not to excessive levels. As an iron-related phenotype, iron and birth weight association provides a good example to illustrate this concept. Iron excess is likely to cause excessive birth weight (Dorak et al., 2009) and iron supplementation of iron-replete women during pregnancy increases birth weight of their offspring (Cogswell et al., 2003). However, supplementation in iron deficient women only prevents low-birth weight (Palma et al., 2008) or makes no difference in birth weight (Preziosi et al., 1997). An equivalent situation would be the pro-carcinogenic effect of iron depending on the average iron levels in the population. Environmentally-induced or genetically-determined changes in body iron content and its phenotypic consequences may be different for the same magnitude of change in different populations. This concept is illustrated in Fig. 17.2.

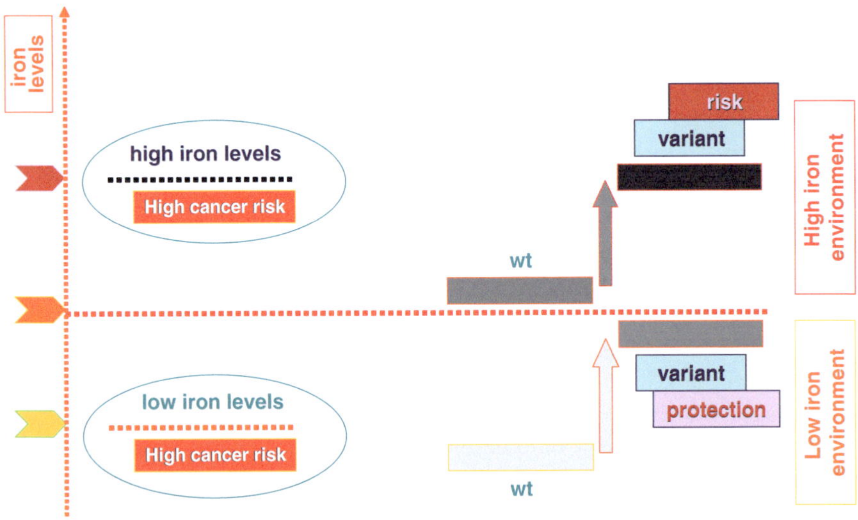

Fig. 17.2 Iron-related gene variants may be markers for protection or risk for cancer depending on the background iron levels in the population. Iron regulatory gene variants will increase the body iron levels to the normal range on average when the population is iron-deficient but the same variants will increase the levels to excessive levels in iron-replete populations. Since both iron deficiency and excess are risk for cancer development, the same variants may act as markers for protection or risk in different populations

While iron intake on its own or genetic variants of iron regulatory genes may not cause a gross change in iron status, the combination may have measurable effects. In a study of 2,531 women in the UK, *HFE* C282Y homozygosity doubled the effect of heme iron intake from meat, fish or poultry on serum ferritin levels (Greenwood et al., 2005) although heterozygosity for C282Y mutation does not show the same effect (Greenwood et al., 2005) nor increases the iron absorption significantly (Roe et al., 2005).

Several studies investigated the gene (*HFE*) and environment (iron intake) interactions in cancer. In a study of variants of genes involved in iron homeostasis or anti-oxidants, the associations with breast cancer risk were stronger in iron supplement users (Hong et al., 2007). Likewise, in colon cancer, the risk conferred by *HFE* mutations increases with increasing age and total iron intake (Shaheen et al., 2003) reflecting the interaction between the genetic variants and total bosy iron stores. A gene and environment interaction is also observed in the association of two iron regulatory gene variants on HIV mortality (McDermid et al., 2009). A combination of antioxidant gene polymorphisms from *NFE2L2* (NRF2), *NQO1*, *NOS3* or *HMOX1* and high iron intake or usage of iron supplements increase the risk (OR > 2.9, $P < 0.05$ for both) for breast cancer (Hong et al., 2007).

Failure to find an association of iron regulatory gene polymorphisms with cancer will not be surprising in a group of iron deficient individuals from developing countries and even gene and environment interaction studies may not be able to unravel a risk association. In Western societies however there is a well-defined proportion of populations who are already at risk (elderly, male, high iron intake -especially with alcohol, iron-containing supplement users) and this subgroup will show the strongest associations with genetic variants.

17.7 Biomarkers for Iron Intake and Body Iron Levels

To date, cohort studies have mostly used biomarkers including serum iron, serum ferritin, transferrin saturation level, total iron-binding capacity (TIBC), and toenail iron levels, as well as dietary iron and supplemental iron intake computed from food-frequency questionnaires. It has been pointed out that these markers may be inadequate (Kabat and Rohan, 2007). Due to the fact that iron stored in iron proteins is tightly bound, serum iron (also known as transferrin iron), serum ferritin, transferrin saturation level, and TIBC do not provide direct markers of bioavailable "free" iron, which is responsible for the adverse effects of iron. This may be one reason for inconsistencies in epidemiologic studies of the association of iron with various cancers.

An increase in serum iron and a decrease in TIBC are early indicators of iron overload, but their sensitivity and specificity are not very high. Iron stored in iron proteins such as transferrin or ferritin is tightly bound and not bioavailable for adverse health effects. Transferrin iron (known as serum iron), transferrin saturation and TIBC represent only 0.1% of total body iron storage (Worwood, 1997). Serum iron has a low reliability coefficient (Ali et al., 2003). With greater variability of serum iron, a single measurement would include a large degree of measurement error and, as a consequence, observed association such as relative risk would be increasingly attenuated. Therefore, the low reliability coefficient of serum iron may contribute to discrepancies of results in studies.

Most commonly used biomarker to assess iron status is serum ferritin levels. In healthy individuals, serum ferritin levels correlate well with total body iron stores as measured by phlebotomy, and with directly measured liver iron but two individuals with the same ferritin level can have very different amounts of iron (Borgna-Pignatti and Castriota-Scanderbeg, 1991). This is because ferritin is also an acute phase reactant which increases in cases of chronic disease, disseminated malignancy, or inflammatory disorders (Hallberg et al., 1997; Hallberg and Hulthen, 2003). In obesity, for example, ferritin is usually found elevated despite actual iron deficiency (Lecube et al., 2008; Zafon et al., 2009). Ferritin concentration can also be influenced by sex, age, infection and frequency of blood donation (Leggett et al., 1990). It has been proposed that the molar ratio of iron to ferritin may provide a better marker of cancer risk than ferritin alone (Huang, 2003). Similarly, serum ferritin-iron measurement is proposed to be a reliable estimate of true ferritin levels not confounded by inflammatory conditions (Herbert et al., 1997).

Non-transferrin bound iron (NTBI), i.e., iron that circulates in plasma unbound to transferrin, is potentially toxic since it is capable of taking part in free radical-mediated reactions that result in irreversible tissue damage. This iron can be measured with a HPLC based assay. At present the most accurate way of estimating the iron burden is by direct measurement of iron concentration in tissues (Brissot et al., 1981; Borgna-Pignatti and Castriota-Scanderbeg, 1991). The liver is the main iron storage site and most accessible but liver biopsy is not acceptable or practical to do routinely for this purpose. A highly correlated non-invasive method may be magnetic resonance imaging of the liver (Kaltwasser et al., 1990) Alternative markers for iron status include reticulocyte hemoglobin content, percentage of hypochromic red cells, and soluble transferrin receptor (Wish, 2006).

Possibly the most significant consequence of iron excess is expansion of the labile iron pool (LIP), the intra-cellular form of NTBI. It is redox-active and it is the iron form that does the harm (Lipinski et al., 2000; Kakhlon and Cabantchik, 2002; Le Lan et al., 2005). Even the trace amounts of free iron can catalyze production of a highly toxic hydroxyl radical via Fenton/Haber-Weiss reaction cycle. LIP and reactive oxygen species (ROS) levels show similar patterns as a result of changes in cellular physiology. To avoid an excess of harmful "free" iron, the LIP is kept at the lowest sufficient level by transcriptional and posttranscriptional control of the expression of principal proteins involved in iron homeostasis (Kruszewski, 2003). It is however detected at high levels in iron overloaded subjects regardless of etiology and in C282Y homozygous subjects (Le Lan et al., 2005). Unfortunately, there is no easy way to measure the levels of LIP routinely. Thus, development of a method to measure the LIP that can be used widely will greatly help to better assess the contribution of iron excess to cancer development.

17.8 Possible Contribution of Iron to Epidemiologic Associations with Cancer

Iron excess may contribute to cancer development in many different ways, most of which is yet unappreciated (Table 17.5). Most relevant of those possible connections are discussed below.

Table 17.5 Possible contribution of iron to epidemiologic associations with cancer

(a) Increased cancer risk
– Modern life style
– Sex (males) and age (increased age) factors
– Smoking, alcohol and asbestos
– Inflammation
– Chronic viral hepatitis
– Suboptimal cancer immune surveillance
– Multivitamin supplements
– Birth weight association in childhood cancer
– Radiation
(b) Decreased cancer risk
– Mediterranean diet and red wine consumption
– Aspirin use and cancer
– Protective effect of pregnancy and maternal effect in breast cancer
– Blood donors and reduced cancer risk
– Exercise

Smoking and alcohol: In high-income countries, smoking, alcohol use, and overweight and obesity were the most important causes of cancer (Danaei et al., 2005) and there is now evidence that smoking and alcohol consumption correlates with iron indexes (Kato et al., 2000; Rossi et al., 2001; Cade et al., 2005; Heath et al., 2008; Milward et al., 2008; Pedersen and Milman, 2009a). Iron is a main component of tobacco smoke (Weinberg, 2009), alcohol increases iron absorption and a strong co-factor in iron excess of genetic or environmental origin (Rossi et al., 2001; Deugnier and Mosser, 2008; Milward et al., 2008; Pedersen and Milman, 2009a). Chronic and excessive alcohol consumption result in iron excess by decreasing hepcidin transcription via its effect on transcriptional factor C/EBPa (Bridle et al., 2006; Harrison-Findik, 2007; Harrison-Findik et al., 2007), induction of reactive oxygen species production (Harrison-Findik et al., 2006) and causing damage on the liver (Bridle et al., 2006). Tobacco smoking increases the risk for a number of cancers and mechanism of this carcinogenetic effect has been well studied (Wu et al., 2004b). Iron excess may well be another factor contributing to the carcinogenic effect of tobacco smoke (Weinberg, 2009). It has been estimated that a one pack a day smoker inhales around 1 μg of iron in a day (Thompson et al., 1991). This aspect of alcohol and smoking needs better recognition in future studies.

Increasing cancer incidence with increasing age: Age is a strong modifier of serum iron parameters (Milman, 1996; Kabat and Rohan, 2007; Pedersen and Milman, 2009a). In post-adolescent men, there is a gradual increase in serum ferritin levels until 30 years of age. Subsequently, serum ferritin remains relatively constant until old age. After menopause, serum ferritin gradually rises and approaches male levels (Milman, 1996). Other studies confirmed the lower serum iron parameters in premenopausal women which increase to male levels in postmenopausal period (Zacharski et al., 2000; Nakano et al., 2003). Although, immune senescence, slow growth of many tumors, decreased DNA repair capacity are better known factors that contribute to increased incidence of cancer in the elderly (Ershler, 1993; Feng et al., 2007), increases in body iron stores may also contribute to this observation.

Higher cancer incidence in men: Being male is itself a risk factor for many cancers (Cartwright et al., 2002). As has been discussed above, males have higher body iron content throughout their lives and this may be one of the reasons why they have higher susceptibility to cancer.

Inflammation and cancer: Chronic inflammation and cancer development are closely linked (Hussain et al., 2003; Kell, 2009). The mechanism includes the production of ROS and subsequent genotoxic damage. ROS production increase by inflammation is augmented by iron (Toyokuni, 2002). For example, release of the pro-inflammatory cytokine interleukin-6 (IL-6) is increased from a mouse epidermal cell line by iron in a dose-dependent manner (Dai et al., 2004). Body iron contributes to excess oxidative stress even at non-iron overload concentrations (Tuomainen et al., 2007). Thus, iron excess also facilitates inflammation-induced neoplastic transformation.

Immune surveillance and cancer: Immune surveillance has an important role in keeping cancer development under control (Dunn et al., 2004; Kinlen, 2004) (see the Genetic Immunology chapter). Immunosuppressive phenomena, best exemplified by congenital immune deficiencies, HIV infection and post-transplant immunosuppression, increase cancer risk (Schwartz, 2001; Kinlen, 2004). Imune senescence accompanying ageing is though to be one of the reasons for higher cancer incidence in the elderly (Ershler, 1993). Any other factor that has an adverse effect on the immune function may contribute to an increase in cancer risk.

The deleterious effects of iron overload on the immune system have been recognized for a long time (Good et al., 1988; de Sousa, 1989; Brock and Mulero, 2000; Walker and Walker, 2000; Porto and De Sousa, 2007) and has been suggested as a contributory factor to cancer susceptibility (Kabat and Rohan, 2007). With increasing popularity of cancer immune surveillance concept, this aspect of iron excess needs better recognition for its involvement in cancer susceptibility.

Red wine and chronic diseases: Strict adherence to a Mediterranean-style diet is associated with reduced risk for mortality and chronic disease (Sofi et al., 2008) including cancer (de Lorgeril et al., 1998). A Mediterranean-style diet includes high intake of vegetables, fruits, legumes, cereals and fish, with moderate consumption of *red wine with meals*. Besides other beneficial effects in moderation, red wine also inhibits iron absorption.

Mediterranean diet and cancer: Chlorophyll in green plants has cancer preventive effects (Waladkhani and Clemens, 1998) and one of them is to antagonize the harmful effect of heme-iron on carcinogenesis (de Vogel et al., 2005; Balder et al., 2006). Furthermore, elements of the "Mediterranean" diet that are usually considered to be beneficial due to their antioxidant capabilities but many of the polyphenolic compounds so implicated may also act to chelate iron as well (Kell, 2009). Thus, iron may also participate in this common observation that Mediterranean diet has components protective from cancer.

Multivitamin supplementation: It has been unambiguously established that multivitamin supplement usage—unless medically indicated—has no beneficial effect for cancer occurrence (Greenwald et al., 2007). In fact, some deleterious effect has been reported, for example, in prostate cancer (Lawson et al., 2007). The Women's Health Initiative (WIN) study provided convincing evidence that multivitamin use has little or no influence on the risk of common cancers (Neuhouser et al., 2009).

Iron deficiency is the most common nutritional deficiency all around the world. In USA, 25% of 20–30 year old women consume iron less than 50% of recommended amount (Ames and Wakimoto, 2002). However, it is also clear that a proportion has iron excess. For example, 7.3% of US adults have iron excess and are at risk of cancer if iron intake is not controlled (Mainous et al., 2005a). It is this subset that any additional iron intake may cause harm. Given the correlations between multivitamin or iron supplements and serum iron levels (Fleming et al., 1998; Kato et al., 2000; Fleming et al., 2002; Liu et al., 2003; Blanck et al., 2005), it is best to enforce the official recommendation of the The World Cancer Research Fund/American Institute for Cancer Research regarding the usage of supplements (The World Cancer Research Fund/American Institute for Cancer Research, 2007) (http://www.dietandcancerreport.org/?p=recommendations). If followed, the recommendation to avoid them will also prevent unnecessary exposure to iron.

Aspirin and protection from cancer: A consensus view has emerged favoring an anticancer effect of long-term aspirin use (Mascitelli et al., 2009). Aspirin-induced loss of stored iron from chronic gastrointestinal bleeding is proposed as a mechanism underlying this beneficial effect. In iron depletion, less iron may be available for carcinogenesis through free-radical mediated mechanisms and for promotion of tumor growth. Low-dose aspirin increases gastrointestinal losses of transfused radiolabeled red cells. Observational studies report lower serum ferritin values with regular aspirin use. Delayed anticancer effects of aspirin are compatible with the proposed mechanism, as continual microbleeding has a gradual cumulative effect on stored iron (Mascitelli et al., 2009). While there is no doubt that the anti-inflammatory effect of aspirin is important in its association with lower cancer incidence, this recently raised hypothesis that it may also work by reducing body iron stores is worth considering in future research.

Birth weight association in childhood leukemia: As discussed in the birth weight chapter, the heavier a baby at birth, the greater the risk for childhood leukemia and certain adult cancers. Recently, experimental evidence has been reported correlating birth weight with iron regulatory gene polymorphisms (Dorak et al., 2009). In this model, increased birth weight is just an epiphenomenon and it is proposed that the same iron regulatory gene polymorphisms increase the cancer risk by causing increased exposure to iron during fetal development, and while increasing the birth weight. Further studies are warranted to explore this possibility further.

Pregnancy and protection from breast cancer: Breast cancer risk is lowered with increasing number of pregnancies. A hormonal effect is obvious but iron loss during pregnancy may contribute to the prevention. In non-pregnant women, there is an inverse relationship between parity and serum ferritin (Milman, 1996) due to a massive amount of iron transfer to developing embryo (Jezerniczky et al., 1976). Estrogen and iron interacts synergistically and some of the estrogen's carcinogenic effects may be mediated by iron (Liehr and Jones, 2001). Likewise duration of estrogen exposure (age-at-menarch, age-at menopause) also correlates with breast cancer risk and this effect may be modified (enhanced) by iron levels in the body.

Blood donors and reduced cancer risk: More than one study has found a protective effect of regular blood donation from cancer (Merk et al., 1990; Edgren et al., 2008). Between the lowest and highest categories of estimated iron loss, there was a trend (P for trend < 0.001) of decreasing risk for cancers of the liver, lung, colon, stomach and esophagus, which are thought to be promoted by iron overload (OR $= 0.70$, 95% CI $= 0.58$–0.84) among men (Edgren et al., 2008). Regular blood donors may have other features like a healthier lifestyle that may lower their cancer risk but given that blood donation correlates with serum ferritin levels (Milman, 1996; Cade et al., 2005; Pedersen and Milman, 2009a), blood loss is a predictor of iron status stronger than either *HFE*-C282Y heterozygosity or diet in men aged 40 years and over (Heath et al., 2008), blood donation reduces levels of markers for oxidative stress (Zheng et al., 2005) and regular phlebotomy drastically decreases cancer incidence in a high risk group of men (Zacharski et al., 2008). It is thus plausible that iron lowering effect of blood donation may contribute to protection from cancer.

17.9 Conclusions

Primary prevention through lifestyle and environmental interventions remains the main way to reduce the burden of cancers. The latest trends that show increasing mortality rates for lung cancer which has now exceeded that of breast cancer in women in USA (Greenwald and Dunn, 2009) document the crucial role played by environment (smoking and lung cancer) in cancer risk and the favorably effect of prevention by screening (mammography and breast cancer). Epidemiological evidence indicates several factors likely to have a major effect on reducing rates of cancer: reduction of smoking, increased consumption of fruits and vegetables, control of infections, avoidance of intense sun exposure, increases in physical activity, reduction of alcohol consumption and possibly red meat (Ames and Gold, 1997; Greenwald and Dunn, 2009). Since reduction in smoking, alcohol and red meat consumption eliminates excessive exposure to iron, eating fruits and vegetables does not expose the body to too much bioavailable iron and perhaps replaces other iron-rich food stuff and avoidance of excess iron levels reduces infections, iron is indirectly involved in the success of these preventive measures. Perhaps it is time to emphasize lower exposure to environmental iron directly as an important factor to reduce the cancer burden in the industrialized world.

References

Acton, R.T., Snively, B.M., Barton, J.C., McLaren, C.E., Adams, P.C., Rich, S.S., Eckfeldt, J.H., Press, R.D., Sholinsky, P., Leiendecker-Foster, C., McLaren, G.D., Speechley, M.R., Harris, E.L., Dawkins, F.W., Gordeuk, V.R., 2007. A genome-wide linkage scan for iron phenotype quantitative trait loci: the HEIRS Family Study. Clin Genet 71, 518–529.

Adams, P.C., 1994. Prevalence of abnormal iron studies in heterozygotes for hereditary hemochromatosis: an analysis of 255 heterozygotes. Am J Hematol 45, 146–149.

Ali, M.A., Akhmedkhanov, A., Zeleniuch-Jaquotte, A., Toniolo, P., Frenkel, K., Huang, X., 2003. Reliability of serum iron, ferritin, nitrite, and association with risk of renal cancer in women. Cancer Detect Prev 27, 116–121.

Ames, B.N., Gold, L.S., 1997. The causes and prevention of cancer: gaining perspective. Environ Health Perspect 105(Suppl 4), 865–873.

Ames, B.N., Wakimoto, P., 2002. Are vitamin and mineral deficiencies a major cancer risk? Nat Rev Cancer 2, 694–704.

Ammann, R.W., Muller, E., Bansky, J., Schuler, G., Hacki, W.H., 1980. High incidence of extrahepatic carcinomas in idiopathic hemochromatosis. Scand J Gastroenterol 15, 733–736.

Andrews, N.C., 2009. Genes determining blood cell traits. Nat Genet 41, 1161–1162.

Balder, H.F., Vogel, J., Jansen, M.C., Weijenberg, M.P., van den Brandt, P.A., Westenbrink, S., van der Meer, R., Goldbohm, R.A., 2006. Heme and chlorophyll intake and risk of colorectal cancer in the Netherlands cohort study. Cancer Epidemiol Biomarkers Prev 15, 717–725.

Barton, J.C., Harmon, L., Rivers, C., Acton, R.T., 1996. Hemochromatosis: association of severity of iron overload with genetic markers. Blood Cells Mol Dis 22, 195–204.

Barton, J.C., Lee, P.L., West, C., Bottomley, S.S., 2006. Iron overload and prolonged ingestion of iron supplements: clinical features and mutation analysis of hemochromatosis-associated genes in four cases. Am J Hematol 81, 760–767.

Barton, J.C., Shih, W.W., Sawada-Hirai, R., Acton, R.T., Harmon, L., Rivers, C., Rothenberg, B.E., 1997. Genetic and clinical description of hemochromatosis probands and heterozygotes: evidence that multiple genes linked to the major histocompatibility complex are responsible for hemochromatosis. Blood Cells Mol Dis 23, 135–145; discussion 145a-b.

Beckman, L.E., Van Landeghem, G.F., Sikstrom, C., Wahlin, A., Markevarn, B., Hallmans, G., Lenner, P., Athlin, L., Stenling, R., Beckman, L., 1999. Interaction between haemochromatosis and transferrin receptor genes in different neoplastic disorders. Carcinogenesis 20, 1231–1233.

Bell, H., Berg, J.P., Undlien, D.E., Distante, S., Raknerud, N., Heier, H.E., Try, K., Thomassen, Y., Haug, E., Raha-Chowdhury, R., Thorsby, E., 2000. The clinical expression of hemochromatosis in Oslo, Norway. Excessive oral iron intake may lead to secondary hemochromatosis even in HFE C282Y mutation negative subjects. Scand J Gastroenterol 35, 1301–1307.

Bensaid, M., Fruchon, S., Mazeres, C., Bahram, S., Roth, M.P., Coppin, H., 2004. Multigenic control of hepatic iron loading in a murine model of hemochromatosis. Gastroenterology 126, 1400–1408.

Benyamin, B., Ferreira, M.A., Willemsen, G., Gordon, S., Middelberg, R.P., McEvoy, B.P., Hottenga, J.J., Henders, A.K., Campbell, M.J., Wallace, L., Frazer, I.H., Heath, A.C., de Geus, E.J., Nyholt, D.R., Visscher, P.M., Penninx, B.W., Boomsma, D.I., Martin, N.G., Montgomery, G.W., Whitfield, J.B., 2009a. Common variants in TMPRSS6 are associated with iron status and erythrocyte volume. Nat Genet 41(11), 1173–1175.

Benyamin, B., McRae, A.F., Zhu, G., Gordon, S., Henders, A.K., Palotie, A., Peltonen, L., Martin, N.G., Montgomery, G.W., Whitfield, J.B., Visscher, P.M., 2009b. Variants in TF and HFE explain approximately 40% of genetic variation in serum-transferrin levels. Am J Hum Genet 84, 60–65.

Beral, V., Bull, D., Doll, R., Peto, R., Reeves, G., 2004. Breast cancer and abortion: collaborative reanalysis of data from 53 epidemiological studies, including 83000 women with breast cancer from 16 countries. Lancet 363, 1007–1016.

Bergeron, R.J., 1986. Iron: a controlling nutrient in proliferative processes. Trends Biochem Sci 11, 133–136.

Blanck, H.M., Cogswell, M.E., Gillespie, C., Reyes, M., 2005. Iron supplement use and iron status among US adults: results from the third National Health and Nutrition Examination Survey. Am J Clin Nutr 82, 1024–1031.

Borgna-Pignatti, C., Castriota-Scanderbeg, A., 1991. Methods for evaluating iron stores and efficacy of chelation in transfusional hemosiderosis. Haematologica 76, 409–413.

Boult, J., Roberts, K., Brookes, M.J., Hughes, S., Bury, J.P., Cross, S.S., Anderson, G.J., Spychal, R., Iqbal, T., Tselepis, C., 2008. Overexpression of cellular iron import proteins is associated with malignant progression of esophageal adenocarcinoma. Clin Cancer Res 14, 379–387.

Bradbear, R.A., Bain, C., Siskind, V., Schofield, F.D., Webb, S., Axelsen, E.M., Halliday, J.W., Bassett, M.L., Powell, L.W., 1985. Cohort study of internal malignancy in genetic hemochromatosis and other chronic nonalcoholic liver diseases. J Natl Cancer Inst 75, 81–84.

Bray, F., McCarron, P., Parkin, D.M., 2004. The changing global patterns of female breast cancer incidence and mortality. Breast Cancer Res 6, 229–239.

Bridle, K., Cheung, T.K., Murphy, T., Walters, M., Anderson, G., Crawford, D.G., Fletcher, L.M., 2006. Hepcidin is down-regulated in alcoholic liver injury: implications for the pathogenesis of alcoholic liver disease. Alcohol Clin Exp Res 30, 106–112.

Brissot, P., Bourel, M., Herry, D., Verger, J.P., Messner, M., Beaumont, C., Regnouard, F., Ferrand, B., Simon, M., 1981. Assessment of liver iron content in 271 patients: a reevaluation of direct and indirect methods. Gastroenterology 80, 557–565.

Brock, J.H., Mulero, V., 2000. Cellular and molecular aspects of iron and immune function. Proc Nutr Soc 59, 537–540.

Bulaj, Z.J., Griffen, L.M., Jorde, L.B., Edwards, C.Q., Kushner, J.P., 1996. Clinical and biochemical abnormalities in people heterozygous for hemochromatosis. N Engl J Med 335, 1799–1805.

Butterworth, J.R., 2006. Another important function for an old friend! The role of iron in colorectal carcinogenesis. Gut 55, 1384–1386.

Cade, J.E., Moreton, J.A., O'Hara, B., Greenwood, D.C., Moor, J., Burley, V.J., Kukalizch, K., Bishop, D.T., Worwood, M., 2005. Diet and genetic factors associated with iron status in middle-aged women. Am J Clin Nutr 82, 813–820.

Cartwright, R.A., Gurney, K.A., Moorman, A.V., 2002. Sex ratios and the risks of haematological malignancies. Br J Haematol 118, 1071–1077.

Cazzola, M., Bergamaschi, G., Dezza, L., Arosio, P., 1990. Manipulations of cellular iron metabolism for modulating normal and malignant cell proliferation: achievements and prospects. Blood 75, 1903–1919.

Chambers, J.C., Zhang, W., Li, Y., Sehmi, J., Wass, M.N., Zabaneh, D., Hoggart, C., Bayele, H., McCarthy, M.I., Peltonen, L., Freimer, N.B., Srai, S.K., Maxwell, P.H., Sternberg, M.J., Ruokonen, A., Abecasis, G., Jarvelin, M.R., Scott, J., Elliott, P., Kooner, J.S., 2009. Genome-wide association study identifies variants in TMPRSS6 associated with hemoglobin levels. Nat Genet 41, 1170–1172.

Chen, G., Fillebeen, C., Wang, J., Pantopoulos, K., 2007. Overexpression of iron regulatory protein 1 suppresses growth of tumor xenografts. Carcinogenesis 28, 785–791.

Chida, Y., Hamer, M., Wardle, J., Steptoe, A., 2008. Do stress-related psychosocial factors contribute to cancer incidence and survival? Nat Clin Pract Oncol 5, 466–475.

Chua, A.C., Herbison, C.E., Drake, S.F., Graham, R.M., Olynyk, J.K., Trinder, D., 2008. The role of Hfe in transferrin-bound iron uptake by hepatocytes. Hepatology 47, 1737–1744.
Cogswell, M.E., Parvanta, I., Ickes, L., Yip, R., Brittenham, G.M., 2003. Iron supplementation during pregnancy, anemia, and birth weight: a randomized controlled trial. Am J Clin Nutr 78, 773–781.
Colditz, G.A., Sellers, T.A., Trapido, E., 2006. Epidemiology – identifying the causes and preventability of cancer? Nat Rev Cancer 6, 75–83.
Conte, D., Narindrasorasak, S., Sarkar, B., 1996. In vivo and in vitro iron-replaced zinc finger generates free radicals and causes DNA damage. J Biol Chem 271, 5125–5130.
Cook, J.D., Watson, S.S., Simpson, K.M., Lipschitz, D.A., Skikne, B.S., 1984. The effect of high ascorbic acid supplementation on body iron stores. Blood 64, 721–726.
Coppin, H., Darnaud, V., Kautz, L., Meynard, D., Aubry, M., Mosser, J., Martinez, M., Roth, M.P., 2007. Gene expression profiling of Hfe-/- liver and duodenum in mouse strains with differing susceptibilities to iron loading: identification of transcriptional regulatory targets of Hfe and potential hemochromatosis modifiers. Genome Biol 8, R221.
Courselaud, B., Troadec, M.B., Fruchon, S., Ilyin, G., Borot, N., Leroyer, P., Coppin, H., Brissot, P., Roth, M.P., Loreal, O., 2004. Strain and gender modulate hepatic hepcidin 1 and 2 mRNA expression in mice. Blood Cells Mol Dis 32, 283–289.
Courville, P., Chaloupka, R., Cellier, M.F., 2006. Recent progress in structure-function analyses of Nramp proton-dependent metal-ion transporters. Biochem Cell Biol 84, 960–978.
Cruz, E., Vieira, J., Almeida, S., Lacerda, R., Gartner, A., Cardoso, C.S., Alves, H., Porto, G., 2006. A study of 82 extended HLA haplotypes in HFE-C282Y homozygous hemochromatosis subjects: relationship to the genetic control of CD8+ T-lymphocyte numbers and severity of iron overload. BMC Med Genet 7, 16.
Dai, J., Huang, C., Wu, J., Yang, C., Frenkel, K., Huang, X., 2004. Iron-induced interleukin-6 gene expression: possible mediation through the extracellular signal-regulated kinase and p38 mitogen-activated protein kinase pathways. Toxicology 203, 199–209.
Danaei, G., Vander Hoorn, S., Lopez, A.D., Murray, C.J., Ezzati, M., 2005. Causes of cancer in the world: comparative risk assessment of nine behavioural and environmental risk factors. Lancet 366, 1784–1793.
Datz, C., Haas, T., Rinner, H., Sandhofer, F., Patsch, W., Paulweber, B., 1998. Heterozygosity for the C282Y mutation in the hemochromatosis gene is associated with increased serum iron, transferrin saturation, and hemoglobin in young women: a protective role against iron deficiency? Clin Chem 44, 2429–2432.
Davis, C.F., Dorak, M.T., 2010. An extensive analysis of the hereditary hemochromatosis gene HFE and neighboring histone genes: associations with childhood leukemia. Ann Hematol 89(4), 375–384.
De Freitas, J.M., Meneghini, R., 2001. Iron and its sensitive balance in the cell. Mutat Res 475, 153–159.
de Lorgeril, M., Salen, P., Martin, J.L., Monjaud, I., Boucher, P., Mamelle, N., 1998. Mediterranean dietary pattern in a randomized trial: prolonged survival and possible reduced cancer rate. Arch Intern Med 158, 1181–1187.
de Sousa, M., 1989. Immune cell functions in iron overload. Clin Exp Immunol 75, 1–6.
de Valk, B., Witlox, R.S., van der Schouw, Y.T., Marx, J.J., 2000. Biochemical expression of heterozygous hereditary hemochromatosis. Eur J Intern Med 11, 317–321.
de Vogel, J., Jonker-Termont, D.S., van Lieshout, E.M., Katan, M.B., van der Meer, R., 2005. Green vegetables, red meat and colon cancer: chlorophyll prevents the cytotoxic and hyperproliferative effects of haem in rat colon. Carcinogenesis 26, 387–393.
Deugnier, Y., Mosser, J., 2008. Modifying factors of the *HFE* hemochromatosis phenotype. Expert Rev Gastroenterol Hepatol 2, 531–540.
Deugnier, Y., Turlin, B., 2001. Iron and hepatocellular carcinoma. J Gastroenterol Hepatol 16, 491–494.
Distante, S., Berg, J.P., Lande, K., Haug, E., Bell, H., 1999. High prevalence of the hemochromatosis-associated Cys282Tyr *HFE* gene mutation in a healthy Norwegian

population in the city of Oslo, and its phenotypic expression. Scand J Gastroenterol 34, 529–534.
Donovan, A., Lima, C.A., Pinkus, J.L., Pinkus, G.S., Zon, L.I., Robine, S., Andrews, N.C., 2005. The iron exporter ferroportin/Slc40a1 is essential for iron homeostasis. Cell Metab 1, 191–200.
Dorak, M.T., 2006. HFE H63D variant and leukemia susceptibility. Leuk Lymphoma 47, 2269–2270.
Dorak, M.T., Burnett, A.K., Worwood, M., 2005. HFE gene mutations in susceptibility to childhood leukemia: HuGE review. Genet Med 7, 159–168.
Dorak, M.T., Mackay, R.K., Relton, C.L., Worwood, M., Parker, L., Hall, A.G., 2009. Hereditary hemochromatosis gene (*HFE*) variants are associated with birth weight and childhood leukemia risk. Pediatr Blood Cancer 53, 1242–1248.
Dorak, M.T., Sproul, A.M., Gibson, B.E., Burnett, A.K., Worwood, M., 1999. The C282Y mutation of *HFE* is another male-specific risk factor for childhood ALL. Blood 94, 3957–3958.
Dunn, G.P., Old, L.J., Schreiber, R.D., 2004. The immunobiology of cancer immunosurveillance and immunoediting. Immunity 21, 137–148.
Dunn, L.L., Rahmanto, Y.S., Richardson, D.R., 2007. Iron uptake and metabolism in the new millennium. Trends Cell Biol 17, 93–100.
Dupic, F., Fruchon, S., Bensaid, M., Borot, N., Radosavljevic, M., Loreal, O., Brissot, P., Gilfillan, S., Bahram, S., Coppin, H., Roth, M.P., 2002. Inactivation of the hemochromatosis gene differentially regulates duodenal expression of iron-related mRNAs between mouse strains. Gastroenterology 122, 745–751.
Eaton, J.W., Qian, M., 2002. Molecular bases of cellular iron toxicity. Free Radic Biol Med 32, 833–840.
Edgren, G., Reilly, M., Hjalgrim, H., Tran, T.N., Rostgaard, K., Adami, J., Titlestad, K., Shanwell, A., Melbye, M., Nyren, O., 2008. Donation frequency, iron loss, and risk of cancer among blood donors. J Natl Cancer Inst 100, 572–579.
Elliott, R.L., Elliott, M.C., Wang, F., Head, J.F., 1993. Breast carcinoma and the role of iron metabolism. A cytochemical, tissue culture, and ultrastructural study. Ann N Y Acad Sci 698, 159–166.
Elmberg, M., Hultcrantz, R., Ekbom, A., Brandt, L., Olsson, S., Olsson, R., Lindgren, S., Loof, L., Stal, P., Wallerstedt, S., Almer, S., Sandberg-Gertzen, H., Askling, J., 2003. Cancer risk in patients with hereditary hemochromatosis and in their first-degree relatives. Gastroenterology 125, 1733–1741.
Ershler, W.B., 1993. The influence of an aging immune system on cancer incidence and progression. J Gerontol 48, B3–B7.
Feder, J.N., Gnirke, A., Thomas, W., Tsuchihashi, Z., Ruddy, D.A., Basava, A., Dormishian, F., Domingo, R., Jr., Ellis, M.C., Fullan, A., Hinton, L.M., Jones, N.L., Kimmel, B.E., Kronmal, G.S., Lauer, P., Lee, V.K., Loeb, D.B., Mapa, F.A., McClelland, E., Meyer, N.C., Mintier, G.A., Moeller, N., Moore, T., Morikang, E., Prass, C.E., Quintana, L., Starnes, S.M., Schatzman, R.C., Brunke, K.J., Drayna, D.T., Risch, N.J., Bacon, B.R., Wolff, R.K., 1996. A novel MHC class I-like gene is mutated in patients with hereditary haemochromatosis. Nat Genet 13, 399–408.
Feng, Z., Hu, W., Teresky, A.K., Hernando, E., Cordon-Cardo, C., Levine, A.J., 2007. Declining p53 function in the aging process: a possible mechanism for the increased tumor incidence in older populations. Proc Natl Acad Sci U S A 104, 16633–16638.
Fleming, D.J., Jacques, P.F., Dallal, G.E., Tucker, K.L., Wilson, P.W., Wood, R.J., 1998. Dietary determinants of iron stores in a free-living elderly population: the Framingham Heart Study. Am J Clin Nutr 67, 722–733.
Fleming, D.J., Jacques, P.F., Massaro, J.M., D'Agostino, R.B., Sr., Wilson, P.W., Wood, R.J., 2001a. Aspirin intake and the use of serum ferritin as a measure of iron status. Am J Clin Nutr 74, 219–226.
Fleming, D.J., Jacques, P.F., Tucker, K.L., Massaro, J.M., D'Agostino, R.B., Sr., Wilson, P.W., Wood, R.J., 2001b. Iron status of the free-living, elderly Framingham Heart Study cohort: an

iron-replete population with a high prevalence of elevated iron stores. Am J Clin Nutr 73, 638–646.

Fleming, D.J., Tucker, K.L., Jacques, P.F., Dallal, G.E., Wilson, P.W., Wood, R.J., 2002. Dietary factors associated with the risk of high iron stores in the elderly Framingham Heart Study cohort. Am J Clin Nutr 76, 1375–1384.

Fleming, R.E., Holden, C.C., Tomatsu, S., Waheed, A., Brunt, E.M., Britton, R.S., Bacon, B.R., Roopenian, D.C., Sly, W.S., 2001c. Mouse strain differences determine severity of iron accumulation in Hfe knockout model of hereditary hemochromatosis. Proc Natl Acad Sci U S A 98, 2707–2711.

Ganesh, S.K., Zakai, N.A., van Rooij, F.J., Soranzo, N., Smith, A.V., Nalls, M.A., Chen, M.H., Kottgen, A., Glazer, N.L., Dehghan, A., Kuhnel, B., Aspelund, T., Yang, Q., Tanaka, T., Jaffe, A., Bis, J.C., Verwoert, G.C., Teumer, A., Fox, C.S., Guralnik, J.M., Ehret, G.B., Rice, K., Felix, J.F., Rendon, A., Eiriksdottir, G., Levy, D., Patel, K.V., Boerwinkle, E., Rotter, J.I., Hofman, A., Sambrook, J.G., Hernandez, D.G., Zheng, G., Bandinelli, S., Singleton, A.B., Coresh, J., Lumley, T., Uitterlinden, A.G., Vangils, J.M., Launer, L.J., Cupples, L.A., Oostra, B.A., Zwaginga, J.J., Ouwehand, W.H., Thein, S.L., Meisinger, C., Deloukas, P., Nauck, M., Spector, T.D., Gieger, C., Gudnason, V., van Duijn, C.M., Psaty, B.M., Ferrucci, L., Chakravarti, A., Greinacher, A., O'Donnell, C.J., Witteman, J.C., Furth, S., Cushman, M., Harris, T.B., Lin, J.P., 2009. Multiple loci influence erythrocyte phenotypes in the CHARGE Consortium. Nat Genet 41, 1191–1198.

Geier, D., Hebert, B., Potti, A., 2002. Risk of primary non-hepatocellular malignancies in hereditary hemochromatosis. Anticancer Res 22, 3797–3799.

Gochee, P.A., Powell, L.W., Cullen, D.J., Du Sart, D., Rossi, E., Olynyk, J.K., 2002. A population-based study of the biochemical and clinical expression of the H63D hemochromatosis mutation. Gastroenterology 122, 646–651.

Good, M.F., Powell, L.W., Halliday, J.W., 1988. Iron status and cellular immune competence. Blood Rev 2, 43–49.

Gordeuk, V., Mukiibi, J., Hasstedt, S.J., Samowitz, W., Edwards, C.Q., West, G., Ndambire, S., Emmanual, J., Nkanza, N., Chapanduka, Z., et al., , 1992. Iron overload in Africa. Interaction between a gene and dietary iron content. N Engl J Med 326, 95–100.

Green, P., Eviatar, J.M., Sirota, P., Avidor, I., 1989. Secondary hemochromatosis due to prolonged iron ingestion. Isr J Med Sci 25, 199–201.

Greenwald, P., Anderson, D., Nelson, S.A., Taylor, P.R., 2007. Clinical trials of vitamin and mineral supplements for cancer prevention. Am J Clin Nutr 85, 314S–317S.

Greenwald, P., Dunn, B.K., 2009. Landmarks in the history of cancer epidemiology. Cancer Res 69, 2151–2162.

Greenwood, D.C., Cade, J.E., Moreton, J.A., O'Hara, B., Burley, V.J., Randerson-Moor, J.A., Kukalizch, K., Thompson, D., Worwood, M., Bishop, D.T., 2005. HFE genotype modifies the influence of heme iron intake on iron status. Epidemiology 16, 802–805.

Hallberg, L., Hulten, L., Gramatkovski, E., 1997. Iron absorption from the whole diet in men: how effective is the regulation of iron absorption? Am J Clin Nutr 66, 347–356.

Hallberg, L., Hulthen, L., 2003. High serum ferritin is not identical to high iron stores. Am J Clin Nutr 78, 1225–1226.

Hann, H.W., Stahlhut, M.W., Blumberg, B.S., 1988. Iron nutrition and tumor growth: decreased tumor growth in iron-deficient mice. Cancer Res 48, 4168–4170.

Hann, H.W., Stahlhut, M.W., Menduke, H., 1991. Iron enhances tumor growth. Observation on spontaneous mammary tumors in mice. Cancer 68, 2407–2410.

Harrison-Findik, D.D., 2007. Role of alcohol in the regulation of iron metabolism. World J Gastroenterol 13, 4925–4930.

Harrison-Findik, D.D., Klein, E., Crist, C., Evans, J., Timchenko, N., Gollan, J., 2007. Iron-mediated regulation of liver hepcidin expression in rats and mice is abolished by alcohol. Hepatology 46, 1979–1985.

Harrison-Findik, D.D., Schafer, D., Klein, E., Timchenko, N.A., Kulaksiz, H., Clemens, D., Fein, E., Andriopoulos, B., Pantopoulos, K., Gollan, J., 2006. Alcohol metabolism-mediated oxidative stress down-regulates hepcidin transcription and leads to increased duodenal iron transporter expression. J Biol Chem 281, 22974–22982.

Heath, A.L., Roe, M.A., Oyston, S.L., Gray, A.R., Williams, S.M., Fairweather-Tait, S.J., 2008. Blood loss is a stronger predictor of iron status in men than C282Y heterozygosity or diet. J Am Coll Nutr 27, 158–167.

Hemminki, K., Lorenzo Bermejo, J., Forsti, A., 2006. The balance between heritable and environmental etiology of human disease. Nat Rev Genet 7, 958–965.

Herbert, V., Jayatilleke, E., Shaw, S., Rosman, A.S., Giardina, P., Grady, R.W., Bowman, B., Gunter, E.W., 1997. Serum ferritin iron, a new test, measures human body iron stores unconfounded by inflammation. Stem Cells 15, 291–296.

Herbert, V., Shaw, S., Jayatilleke, E., Stopler-Kasdan, T., 1994. Most free-radical injury is iron-related: it is promoted by iron, hemin, holoferritin and vitamin C, and inhibited by desferoxamine and apoferritin. Stem Cells 12, 289–303.

Hong, C.C., Ambrosone, C.B., Ahn, J., Choi, J.Y., McCullough, M.L., Stevens, V.L., Rodriguez, C., Thun, M.J., Calle, E.E., 2007. Genetic variability in iron-related oxidative stress pathways (Nrf2, NQ01, NOS3, and HO-1), iron intake, and risk of postmenopausal breast cancer. Cancer Epidemiol Biomarkers Prev 16, 1784–1794.

Hsing, A.W., McLaughlin, J.K., Olsen, J.H., Mellemkjar, L., Wacholder, S., Fraumeni, J.F., Jr., 1995. Cancer risk following primary hemochromatosis: a population-based cohort study in Denmark. Int J Cancer 60, 160–162.

Huang, X., 2003. Iron overload and its association with cancer risk in humans: evidence for iron as a carcinogenic metal. Mutat Res 533, 153–171.

Huang, X., 2008. Does iron have a role in breast cancer? Lancet Oncol 9, 803–807.

Hunt, J.R., Zeng, H., 2004. Iron absorption by heterozygous carriers of the HFE C282Y mutation associated with hemochromatosis. Am J Clin Nutr 80, 924–931.

Hussain, S.P., Hofseth, L.J., Harris, C.C., 2003. Radical causes of cancer. Nat Rev Cancer 3, 276–285.

Jackson, H.A., Carter, K., Darke, C., Guttridge, M.G., Ravine, D., Hutton, R.D., Napier, J.A., Worwood, M., 2001. HFE mutations, iron deficiency and overload in 10,500 blood donors. Br J Haematol 114, 474–484.

Jacolot, S., Le Gac, G., Scotet, V., Quere, I., Mura, C., Ferec, C., 2004. HAMP as a modifier gene that increases the phenotypic expression of the HFE pC282Y homozygous genotype. Blood 103, 2835–2840.

Jalihal, S.S., Barlow, A.M., 1984. Haemochromatosis following prolonged oral iron ingestion. J R Soc Med 77, 690–692.

Jezerniczky, J., Nagy, Z., Dvoracsek, E., Nagy, B., Ilyes, I., Csorba, S., 1976. Trace elements in the serum of mothers and their children. Acta Paediatr Acad Sci Hung 17, 193–197.

Kabat, G.C., Miller, A.B., Jain, M., Rohan, T.E., 2007. Dietary iron and heme iron intake and risk of breast cancer: a prospective cohort study. Cancer Epidemiol Biomarkers Prev 16, 1306–1308.

Kabat, G.C., Rohan, T.E., 2007. Does excess iron play a role in breast carcinogenesis? An unresolved hypothesis. Cancer Causes Control 18, 1047–1053.

Kakhlon, O., Cabantchik, Z.I., 2002. The labile iron pool: characterization, measurement, and participation in cellular processes. Free Radic Biol Med 33, 1037–1046.

Kaltwasser, J.P., Gottschalk, R., Schalk, K.P., Hartl, W., 1990. Non-invasive quantitation of liver iron-overload by magnetic resonance imaging. Br J Haematol 74, 360–363.

Kaltwasser, J.P., Werner, E., Schalk, K., Hansen, C., Gottschalk, R., Seidl, C., 1998. Clinical trial on the effect of regular tea drinking on iron accumulation in genetic haemochromatosis. Gut 43, 699–704.

Kaomongkolgit, R., Cheepsunthorn, P., Pavasant, P., Sanchavanakit, N., 2008. Iron increases MMP-9 expression through activation of AP-1 via ERK/Akt pathway in human head and neck squamous carcinoma cells. Oral Oncol 44, 587–594.

Kato, I., Dnistrian, A.M., Schwartz, M., Toniolo, P., Koenig, K., Shore, R.E., Zeleniuch-Jacquotte, A., Akhmedkhanov, A., Riboli, E., 1999. Iron intake, body iron stores and colorectal cancer risk in women: a nested case-control study. Int J Cancer 80, 693–698.

Kato, I., Dnistrian, A.M., Schwartz, M., Toniolo, P., Koenig, K., Shore, R.E., Zeleniuch-Jacquotte, A., Akhmedkhanov, A., Riboli, E., 2000. Risk of iron overload among middle-aged women. Int J Vitam Nutr Res 70, 119–125.
Kell, D.B., 2009. Iron behaving badly: inappropriate iron chelation as a major contributor to the aetiology of vascular and other progressive inflammatory and degenerative diseases. BMC Med Genomics 2, 2.
Kerenyi, M.A., Grebien, F., Gehart, H., Schifrer, M., Artaker, M., Kovacic, B., Beug, H., Moriggl, R., Mullner, E.W., 2008. Stat5 regulates cellular iron uptake of erythroid cells via IRP-2 and TfR-1. Blood 112, 3878–3888.
Kew, M.C., 2008. Hepatic iron overload and hepatocellular carcinoma. Cancer Lett 286(1), 38–43.
Kew, M.C., Asare, G.A., 2007. Dietary iron overload in the African and hepatocellular carcinoma. Liver Int 27, 735–741.
Kiecolt-Glaser, J.K., Robles, T.F., Heffner, K.L., Loving, T.J., Glaser, R., 2002. Psycho-oncology and cancer: psychoneuroimmunology and cancer. Ann Oncol 13(Suppl 4), 165–169.
Kinlen, L., 2004. Infections and immune factors in cancer: the role of epidemiology. Oncogene 23, 6341–6348.
Knekt, P., Reunanen, A., Takkunen, H., Aromaa, A., Heliovaara, M., Hakulinen, T., 1994. Body iron stores and risk of cancer. Int J Cancer 56, 379–382.
Kohgo, Y., Ikuta, K., Ohtake, T., Torimoto, Y., Kato, J., 2007. Iron overload and cofactors with special reference to alcohol, hepatitis C virus infection and steatosis/insulin resistance. World J Gastroenterol 13, 4699–4706.
Kovacevic, Z., Richardson, D.R., 2006. The metastasis suppressor, Ndrg-1: a new ally in the fight against cancer. Carcinogenesis 27, 2355–2366.
Kowdley, K.V., 2004. Iron, hemochromatosis, and hepatocellular carcinoma. Gastroenterology 127, S79–S86.
Kruszewski, M., 2003. Labile iron pool: the main determinant of cellular response to oxidative stress. Mutat Res 531, 81–92.
Kwok, J.C., Richardson, D.R., 2002. The iron metabolism of neoplastic cells: alterations that facilitate proliferation? Crit Rev Oncol Hematol 42, 65–78.
Lakhal, S., Talbot, N.P., Crosby, A., Stoepker, C., Townsend, A.R., Robbins, P.A., Pugh, C.W., Ratcliffe, P.J., Mole, D.R., 2009. Regulation of growth differentiation factor 15 expression by intracellular iron. Blood 113, 1555–1563.
Larramendy, M., Mello-Filho, A.C., Martins, E.A., Meneghini, R., 1987. Iron-mediated induction of sister-chromatid exchanges by hydrogen peroxide and superoxide anion. Mutat Res 178, 57–63.
Lauffer, R.B., 1991. Exercise as prevention: do the health benefits derive in part from lower iron levels? Med Hypotheses 35, 103–107.
Lawson, K.A., Wright, M.E., Subar, A., Mouw, T., Hollenbeck, A., Schatzkin, A., Leitzmann, M.F., 2007. Multivitamin use and risk of prostate cancer in the National Institutes of Health-AARP Diet and Health Study. J Natl Cancer Inst 99, 754–764.
Le Lan, C., Loreal, O., Cohen, T., Ropert, M., Glickstein, H., Laine, F., Pouchard, M., Deugnier, Y., Le Treut, A., Breuer, W., Cabantchik, Z.I., Brissot, P., 2005. Redox active plasma iron in C282Y/C282Y hemochromatosis. Blood 105, 4527–4531.
Le Marchand, L., 2005. The predominance of the environment over genes in cancer causation: implications for genetic epidemiology. Cancer Epidemiol Biomarkers Prev 14, 1037–1039.
Le, N.T., Richardson, D.R., 2002. The role of iron in cell cycle progression and the proliferation of neoplastic cells. Biochim Biophys Acta 1603, 31–46.
Lecube, A., Hernandez, C., Pelegri, D., Simo, R., 2008. Factors accounting for high ferritin levels in obesity. Int J Obes (Lond) 32, 1665–1669.
Lee, D.H., Anderson, K.E., Folsom, A.R., Jacobs, D.R., Jr., 2005. Heme iron, zinc and upper digestive tract cancer: the Iowa Women's Health Study. Int J Cancer 117, 643–647.
Lee, D.H., Anderson, K.E., Harnack, L.J., Folsom, A.R., Jacobs, D.R., Jr., 2004. Heme iron, zinc, alcohol consumption, and colon cancer: Iowa Women's Health Study. J Natl Cancer Inst 96, 403–407.

Leggett, B.A., Brown, N.N., Bryant, S.J., Duplock, L., Powell, L.W., Halliday, J.W., 1990. Factors affecting the concentrations of ferritin in serum in a healthy Australian population. Clin Chem 36, 1350–1355.
Lehmann, U., Wingen, L.U., Brakensiek, K., Wedemeyer, H., Becker, T., Heim, A., Metzig, K., Hasemeier, B., Kreipe, H., Flemming, P., 2007. Epigenetic defects of hepatocellular carcinoma are already found in non-neoplastic liver cells from patients with hereditary haemochromatosis. Hum Mol Genet 16, 1335–1342.
Lichtenstein, P., Holm, N.V., Verkasalo, P.K., Iliadou, A., Kaprio, J., Koskenvuo, M., Pukkala, E., Skytthe, A., Hemminki, K., 2000. Environmental and heritable factors in the causation of cancer–analyses of cohorts of twins from Sweden, Denmark, and Finland. N Engl J Med 343, 78–85.
Liehr, J.G., Jones, J.S., 2001. Role of iron in estrogen-induced cancer. Curr Med Chem 8, 839–849.
Lipinski, P., Drapier, J.C., Oliveira, L., Retmanska, H., Sochanowicz, B., Kruszewski, M., 2000. Intracellular iron status as a hallmark of mammalian cell susceptibility to oxidative stress: a study of L5178Y mouse lymphoma cell lines differentially sensitive to H(2)O(2). Blood 95, 2960–2966.
Liu, J.M., Hankinson, S.E., Stampfer, M.J., Rifai, N., Willett, W.C., Ma, J., 2003. Body iron stores and their determinants in healthy postmenopausal US women. Am J Clin Nutr 78, 1160–1167.
Madigan, M.P., Ziegler, R.G., Benichou, J., Byrne, C., Hoover, R.N., 1995. Proportion of breast cancer cases in the United States explained by well-established risk factors. J Natl Cancer Inst 87, 1681–1685.
Mainous, A.G., 3rd, Gill, J.M., Carek, P.J., 2004. Elevated serum transferrin saturation and mortality. Ann Fam Med 2, 133–138.
Mainous, A.G., 3rd, Gill, J.M., Everett, C.J., 2005a. Transferrin saturation, dietary iron intake, and risk of cancer. Ann Fam Med 3, 131–137.
Mainous, A.G., 3rd, Wells, B.J., Koopman, R.J., Everett, C.J., Gill, J.M., 2005b. Iron, lipids, and risk of cancer in the Framingham Offspring cohort. Am J Epidemiol 161, 1115–1122.
Mallory, M.A., Kowdley, K.V., 2001. Hereditary hemochromatosis and cancer risk: more fuel to the fire? more fuel to the fire? Gastroenterology 121, 1253–1254.
Martinez di Montemuros, F., Tavazzi, D., Salsano, E., Piepoli, T., Pollo, B., Fiorelli, G., Finocchiaro, G., 2001. High frequency of the H63D mutation of the hemochromatosis gene (HFE) in malignant gliomas. Neurology 57, 1342.
Martins, E.A., Robalinho, R.L., Meneghini, R., 1995. Oxidative stress induces activation of a cytosolic protein responsible for control of iron uptake. Arch Biochem Biophys 316, 128–134.
Mascitelli, L., Pezzetta, F., Sullivan, J.L., 2009. Aspirin-associated iron loss as an anticancer mechanism. Med Hypotheses 74(1), 78–80.
Matsha, T., Brink, L., van Rensburg, S., Hon, D., Lombard, C., Erasmus, R., 2006. Traditional home-brewed beer consumption and iron status in patients with esophageal cancer and healthy control subjects from Transkei, South Africa. Nutr Cancer 56, 67–73.
McCord, J.M., 2004. Iron, free radicals, and oxidative injury. J Nutr 134, 3171S–3172S.
McDermid, J.M., van der Loeff, M.F., Jaye, A., Hennig, B.J., Bates, C., Todd, J., Sirugo, G., Hill, A.V., Whittle, H.C., Prentice, A.M., 2009. Mortality in HIV infection is independently predicted by host iron status and SLC11A1 and HP genotypes, with new evidence of a gene-nutrient interaction. Am J Clin Nutr 90, 225–233.
McGregor, J., McKie, A.T., Simpson, R.J., 2004. Of mice and men: genetic determinants of iron status. Proc Nutr Soc 63, 11–20.
Mello Filho, A.C., Hoffmann, M.E., Meneghini, R., 1984. Cell killing and DNA damage by hydrogen peroxide are mediated by intracellular iron. Biochem J 218, 273–275.
Meneghini, R., 1997. Iron homeostasis, oxidative stress, and DNA damage. Free Radic Biol Med 23, 783–792.
Merk, K., Mattsson, B., Mattsson, A., Holm, G., Gullbring, B., Bjorkholm, M., 1990. The incidence of cancer among blood donors. Int J Epidemiol 19, 505–509.
Merryweather-Clarke, A.T., Pointon, J.J., Jouanolle, A.M., Rochette, J., Robson, K.J., 2000. Geography of HFE C282Y and H63D mutations. Genet Test 4, 183–198.

Meynard, D., Kautz, L., Darnaud, V., Canonne-Hergaux, F., Coppin, H., Roth, M.P., 2009. Lack of the bone morphogenetic protein BMP6 induces massive iron overload. Nat Genet 41, 478–481.

Milet, J., Dehais, V., Bourgain, C., Jouanolle, A.M., Mosser, A., Perrin, M., Morcet, J., Brissot, P., David, V., Deugnier, Y., Mosser, J., 2007. Common variants in the BMP2, BMP4, and HJV genes of the hepcidin regulation pathway modulate HFE hemochromatosis penetrance. Am J Hum Genet 81, 799–807.

Milman, N., 1996. Serum ferritin in Danes: studies of iron status from infancy to old age, during blood donation and pregnancy. Int J Hematol 63, 103–135.

Milman, N., Byg, K.E., Ovesen, L., Kirchhoff, M., Jurgensen, K.S., 2003. Iron status in Danish women, 1984–1994: a cohort comparison of changes in iron stores and the prevalence of iron deficiency and iron overload. Eur J Haematol 71, 51–61.

Milman, N., Kirchhoff, M., Jorgensen, T., 1992. Iron status markers, serum ferritin and hemoglobin in 1359 Danish women in relation to menstruation, hormonal contraception, parity, and postmenopausal hormone treatment. Ann Hematol 65, 96–102.

Milward, E.A., Baines, S.K., Knuiman, M.W., Bartholomew, H.C., Divitini, M.L., Ravine, D.G., Bruce, D.G., Olynyk, J.K., 2008. Noncitrus fruits as novel dietary environmental modifiers of iron stores in people with or without HFE gene mutations. Mayo Clin Proc 83, 543–549.

Miraglia Del Giudice, E., Santoro, N., Amato, A., Brienza, C., Calabro, P., Wiegerinck, E.T., Cirillo, G., Tartaglione, N., Grandone, A., Swinkels, D.W., Perrone, L., 2009. Hepcidin in Obese Children as a Potential Mediator of the Association between Obesity and Iron Deficiency. J Clin Endocrinol Metab 94(12), 5102–5107.

Mura, C., Le Gac, G., Raguenes, O., Mercier, A.Y., Le Guen, A., Ferec, C., 2000. Relation between HFE mutations and mild iron-overload expression. Mol Genet Metab 69, 295–301.

Mura, C., Le Gac, G., Scotet, V., Raguenes, O., Mercier, A.Y., Ferec, C., 2001. Variation of iron loading expression in C282Y homozygous haemochromatosis probands and sib pairs. J Med Genet 38, 632–636.

Mussalo-Rauhamaa, H., Leppanen, A., Salmela, S.S., Pyysalo, H., 1986. Cigarettes as a source of some trace and heavy metals and pesticides in man. Arch Environ Health 41, 49–55.

Nakano, M., Kawanishi, Y., Kamohara, S., Uchida, Y., Shiota, M., Inatomi, Y., Komori, T., Miyazawa, K., Gondo, K., Yamasawa, I., 2003. Oxidative DNA damage (8-hydroxydeoxyguanosine) and body iron status: a study on 2507 healthy people. Free Radic Biol Med 35, 826–832.

Nearman, Z.P., Szpurka, H., Serio, B., Warshawksy, I., Theil, K., Lichtin, A., Sekeres, M.A., Maciejewski, J.P., 2007. Hemochromatosis-associated gene mutations in patients with myelodysplastic syndromes with refractory anemia with ringed sideroblasts. Am J Hematol 82, 1076–1079.

Nelson, R.L., 2001. Iron and colorectal cancer risk: human studies. Nutr Rev 59, 140–148.

Neuhouser, M.L., Wassertheil-Smoller, S., Thomson, C., Aragaki, A., Anderson, G.L., Manson, J.E., Patterson, R.E., Rohan, T.E., van Horn, L., Shikany, J.M., Thomas, A., LaCroix, A., Prentice, R.L., 2009. Multivitamin use and risk of cancer and cardiovascular disease in the Women's Health Initiative cohorts. Arch Intern Med 169, 294–304.

O'Donnell, K.A., Yu, D., Zeller, K.I., Kim, J.W., Racke, F., Thomas-Tikhonenko, A., Dang, C.V., 2006. Activation of transferrin receptor 1 by c-Myc enhances cellular proliferation and tumorigenesis. Mol Cell Biol 26, 2373–2386.

Olsson, K.S., Ritter, B., Hansson, N., 2007. The HLA-A1-B8 haplotype hitchhiking with the hemochromatosis mutation: does it affect the phenotype? Eur J Haematol 79, 429–434.

Olsson, K.S., Vaisanen, M., Konar, J., Bruce, A., 1997. The effect of withdrawal of food iron fortification in Sweden as studied with phlebotomy in subjects with genetic hemochromatosis. Eur J Clin Nutr 51, 782–786.

Olynyk, J.K., Cullen, D.J., Aquilia, S., Rossi, E., Summerville, L., Powell, L.W., 1999. A population-based study of the clinical expression of the hemochromatosis gene. N Engl J Med 341, 718–724.

Osler, M., Milman, N., Heitmann, B.L., 1999. Consequences of removing iron fortification of flour on iron status among Danish adults: some longitudinal observations between 1987 and 1994. Prev Med 29, 32–36.

Palma, S., Perez-Iglesias, R., Prieto, D., Pardo, R., Llorca, J., Delgado-Rodriguez, M., 2008. Iron but not folic acid supplementation reduces the risk of low birthweight in pregnant women without anaemia: a case-control study. J Epidemiol Community Health 62, 120–124.

Papanikolaou, G., Pantopoulos, K., 2005. Iron metabolism and toxicity. Toxicol Appl Pharmacol 202, 199–211.

Pedersen, P., Milman, N., 2009a. Extrinsic factors modifying expressivity of the HFE variant C282Y, H63D, S65C phenotypes in 1,294 Danish men. Ann Hematol 88(10), 957–965.

Pedersen, P., Milman, N., 2009b. Genetic screening for HFE hemochromatosis in 6,020 Danish men: penetrance of C282Y, H63D, and S65C variants. Ann Hematol 88(8), 775–784.

Pietrangelo, A., 2004. Hereditary hemochromatosis–a new look at an old disease. N Engl J Med 350, 2383–2397.

Pinto, J.P., Ramos, P., de Almeida, S.F., Oliveira, S., Breda, L., Michalak, M., Porto, G., Rivella, S., de Sousa, M., 2008. Protective role of calreticulin in HFE hemochromatosis. Free Radic Biol Med 44, 99–108.

Piperno, A., Sampietro, M., Pietrangelo, A., Arosio, C., Lupica, L., Montosi, G., Vergani, A., Fraquelli, M., Girelli, D., Pasquero, P., Roetto, A., Gasparini, P., Fargion, S., Conte, D., Camaschella, C., 1998. Heterogeneity of hemochromatosis in Italy. Gastroenterology 114, 996–1002.

Porto, G., De Sousa, M., 2007. Iron overload and immunity. World J Gastroenterol 13, 4707–4715.

Preziosi, P., Prual, A., Galan, P., Daouda, H., Boureima, H., Hercberg, S., 1997. Effect of iron supplementation on the iron status of pregnant women: consequences for newborns. Am J Clin Nutr 66, 1178–1182.

Raddatz, D., Legler, T., Lynen, R., Addicks, N., Ramadori, G., 2003. HFE genotype and parameters of iron metabolism in German first-time blood donors – evidence for an increased transferrin saturation in C282Y heterozygotes. Z Gastroenterol 41, 1069–1076.

Rochette, J., Pointon, J.J., Fisher, C.A., Perera, G., Arambepola, M., Arichchi, D.S., De Silva, S., Vandwalle, J.L., Monti, J.P., Old, J.M., Merryweather-Clarke, A.T., Weatherall, D.J., Robson, K.J., 1999. Multicentric origin of hemochromatosis gene (HFE) mutations. Am J Hum Genet 64, 1056–1062.

Roe, M.A., Heath, A.L., Oyston, S.L., Macrow, C., Hoogewerff, J.A., Foxall, R., Dainty, J.R., Majsak-Newman, G., Willis, G., Fairweather-Tait, S.J., 2005. Iron absorption in male C282Y heterozygotes. Am J Clin Nutr 81, 814–821.

Rossi, E., Bulsara, M.K., Olynyk, J.K., Cullen, D.J., Summerville, L., Powell, L.W., 2001. Effect of hemochromatosis genotype and lifestyle factors on iron and red cell indices in a community population. Clin Chem 47, 202–208.

Samarasena, J., Winsor, W., Lush, R., Duggan, P., Xie, Y., Borgaonkar, M., 2006. Individuals homozygous for the H63D mutation have significantly elevated iron indexes. Dig Dis Sci 51, 803–807.

Sanchez, M., Galy, B., Dandekar, T., Bengert, P., Vainshtein, Y., Stolte, J., Muckenthaler, M.U., Hentze, M.W., 2006. Iron regulation and the cell cycle: identification of an iron-responsive element in the 3'-untranslated region of human cell division cycle 14A mRNA by a refined microarray-based screening strategy. J Biol Chem 281, 22865–22874.

Schwartz, R.S., 2001. Immunodeficiency, immunosuppression, and susceptibility to neoplasms. J Natl Cancer Inst Monogr, 5–9.

Selby, J.V., Friedman, G.D., 1988. Epidemiologic evidence of an Association between body iron stores and risk of cancer. Int J Cancer 41, 677–682.

Shaheen, N.J., Silverman, L.M., Keku, T., Lawrence, L.B., Rohlfs, E.M., Martin, C.F., Galanko, J., Sandler, R.S., 2003. Association between hemochromatosis (HFE) gene mutation carrier status and the risk of colon cancer. J Natl Cancer Inst 95, 154–159.

Shi, Z., Johnstone, D., Talseth-Palmer, B.A., Evans, T.J., Spigelman, A.D., Groombridge, C., Milward, E.A., Olynyk, J.K., Suchy, J., Kurzawski, G., Lubinski, J., Scott, R.J., 2009. Haemochromatosis HFE gene polymorphisms as potential modifiers of hereditary nonpolyposis colorectal cancer risk and onset age. Int J Cancer 125, 78–83.

Simonart, T., 2006. Role of environmental factors in the pathogenesis of classic and African-endemic Kaposi sarcoma. Cancer Lett 244, 1–7.

Simonart, T., De Dobbeleer, G., Stallenberg, B., 2003. Classic Kaposi's sarcoma of the palm in a metallurgist: role of iron filings in its development? Br J Dermatol 148, 1061–1063.

Simonart, T., Degraef, C., Stordeur, P., Noel, J.C., Mosselmans, R., Van Vooren, J.P., Parent, D., Boelaert, J.R., Heenen, M., Galand, P., 2001. Iron induces Bcl-2 expression in human dermal microvascular endothelial cells. Free Radic Res 34, 221–235.

Simonart, T., Noel, J.C., Andrei, G., Parent, D., Van Vooren, J.P., Hermans, P., Lunardi-Yskandar, Y., Lambert, C., Dieye, T., Farber, C.M., Liesnard, C., Snoeck, R., Heenen, M., Boelaert, J.R., 1998. Iron as a potential co-factor in the pathogenesis of Kaposi's sarcoma? Int J Cancer 78, 720–726.

Sinha, R., Cross, A.J., Graubard, B.I., Leitzmann, M.F., Schatzkin, A., 2009. Meat intake and mortality: a prospective study of over half a million people. Arch Intern Med 169, 562–571.

Sofi, F., Cesari, F., Abbate, R., Gensini, G.F., Casini, A., 2008. Adherence to Mediterranean diet and health status: meta-analysis. BMJ 337, a1344.

Soranzo, N., Spector, T.D., Mangino, M., Kuhnel, B., Rendon, A., Teumer, A., Willenborg, C., Wright, B., Chen, L., Li, M., Salo, P., Voight, B.F., Burns, P., Laskowski, R.A., Xue, Y., Menzel, S., Altshuler, D., Bradley, J.R., Bumpstead, S., Burnett, M.S., Devaney, J., Doring, A., Elosua, R., Epstein, S.E., Erber, W., Falchi, M., Garner, S.F., Ghori, M.J., Goodall, A.H., Gwilliam, R., Hakonarson, H.H., Hall, A.S., Hammond, N., Hengstenberg, C., Illig, T., Konig, I.R., Knouff, C.W., McPherson, R., Melander, O., Mooser, V., Nauck, M., Nieminen, M.S., O'Donnell, C.J., Peltonen, L., Potter, S.C., Prokisch, H., Rader, D.J., Rice, C.M., Roberts, R., Salomaa, V., Sambrook, J., Schreiber, S., Schunkert, H., Schwartz, S.M., Serbanovic-Canic, J., Sinisalo, J., Siscovick, D.S., Stark, K., Surakka, I., Stephens, J., Thompson, J.R., Volker, U., Volzke, H., Watkins, N.A., Wells, G.A., Wichmann, H.E., Van Heel, D.A., Tyler-Smith, C., Thein, S.L., Kathiresan, S., Perola, M., Reilly, M.P., Stewart, A.F., Erdmann, J., Samani, N.J., Meisinger, C., Greinacher, A., Deloukas, P., Ouwehand, W.H., Gieger, C., 2009. A genome-wide meta-analysis identifies 22 loci associated with eight hematological parameters in the HaemGen consortium. Nat Genet 41, 1182–1190.

Stevens, R.G., 2000. Hemochromatosis heterozygotes may constitute a radiation-sensitive subpopulation. Radiat Res 154, 725–726; discussion 726–727.

Stevens, R.G., 2002. Lighting during the day and night: possible impact on risk of breast cancer. Neuro Endocrinol Lett 23(Suppl 2), 57–60.

Stevens, R.G., Kalkwarf, D.R., 1990. Iron, radiation, and cancer. Environ Health Perspect 87, 291–300.

Stevens, R.G., Beasley, R.P., Blumberg, B.S., 1986. Iron-binding proteins and risk of cancer in Taiwan. J Natl Cancer Inst 76, 605–610.

Stevens, R.G., Graubard, B.I., Micozzi, M.S., Neriishi, K., Blumberg, B.S., 1994. Moderate elevation of body iron level and increased risk of cancer occurrence and death. Int J Cancer 56, 364–369.

Stevens, R.G., Jones, D.Y., Micozzi, M.S., Taylor, P.R., 1988. Body iron stores and the risk of cancer. N Engl J Med 319, 1047–1052.

Sullivan, J.L., 2004. Is stored iron safe? J Lab Clin Med 144, 280–284.

Sussman, H.H., 1992. Iron in cancer. Pathobiology 60, 2–9.

Tanaka, T., Roy, C.N., Yao, W., Matteini, A., Semba, R.D., Arking, D., Walston, J.D., Fried, L.P., Singleton, A., Guralnik, J., Abecasis, G.R., Bandinelli, S., Longo, D.L., Ferrucci, L., 2009. A genome-wide association analysis of serum iron concentrations. Blood 115(1), 94–96.

Temme, E.H., Van Hoydonck, P.G., 2002. Tea consumption and iron status. Eur J Clin Nutr 56, 379–386.

The World Cancer Research Fund/American Institute for Cancer Research, 2007. Food, nutrition, physical activity, and the prevention of cancer: a Global Perspective, AICR, Washington, DC.
Thompson, A.B., Bohling, T., Heires, A., Linder, J., Rennard, S.I., 1991. Lower respiratory tract iron burden is increased in association with cigarette smoking. J Lab Clin Med 117, 493–499.
Tiniakos, G., Williams, R., 1988. Cirrhotic process, liver cell carcinoma and extrahepatic malignant tumors in idiopathic haemochromatosis. Study of 71 patients treated with venesection therapy. Appl Pathol 6, 128–138.
Toyokuni, S., 1996. Iron-induced carcinogenesis: the role of redox regulation. Free Radic Biol Med 20, 553–566.
Toyokuni, S., 2002. Iron and carcinogenesis: from Fenton reaction to target genes. Redox Rep 7, 189–197.
Toyokuni, S., 2009. Role of iron in carcinogenesis: cancer as a ferrotoxic disease. Cancer Sci 100, 9–16.
Trowbridge, I.S., Lopez, F., 1982. Monoclonal antibody to transferrin receptor blocks transferrin binding and inhibits human tumor cell growth in vitro. Proc Natl Acad Sci U S A 79, 1175–1179.
Trowbridge, I.S., Omary, M.B., 1981. Human cell surface glycoprotein related to cell proliferation is the receptor for transferrin. Proc Natl Acad Sci U S A 78, 3039–3043.
Tuomainen, T.P., Loft, S., Nyyssonen, K., Punnonen, K., Salonen, J.T., Poulsen, H.E., 2007. Body iron is a contributor to oxidative damage of DNA. Free Radic Res 41, 324–328.
Tussing-Humphreys, L.M., Liang, H., Nemeth, E., Freels, S., Braunschweig, C.A., 2009. Excess adiposity, inflammation, and iron-deficiency in female adolescents. J Am Diet Assoc 109, 297–302.
Valko, M., Morris, H., Cronin, M.T., 2005. Metals, toxicity and oxidative stress. Curr Med Chem 12, 1161–1208.
van Asperen, I.A., Feskens, E.J., Bowles, C.H., Kromhout, D., 1995. Body iron stores and mortality due to cancer and ischaemic heart disease: a 17-year follow-up study of elderly men and women. Int J Epidemiol 24, 665–670.
Varkonyi, J., Tarkovacs, G., Karadi, I., Andrikovics, H., Varga, F., Demeter, J., Tordai, A., 2003. High incidence of hemochromatosis gene mutations in the myelodysplastic syndrome: the Budapest Study on 50 patients. Acta Haematol 109, 64–67.
Waladkhani, A.R., Clemens, M.R., 1998. Effect of dietary phytochemicals on cancer development (review). Int J Mol Med 1, 747–753.
Walker, E.M., Jr., Walker, S.M., 2000. Effects of iron overload on the immune system. Ann Clin Lab Sci 30, 354–365.
Ward, P.P., Conneely, O.M., 2004. Lactoferrin: role in iron homeostasis and host defense against microbial infection. Biometals 17, 203–208.
Weinberg, E.D., 1984. Iron withholding: a defense against infection and neoplasia. Physiol Rev 64, 65–102.
Weinberg, E.D., 1996. The role of iron in cancer. Eur J Cancer Prev 5, 19–36.
Weinberg, E.D., 1999. The development of awareness of the carcinogenic hazard of inhaled iron. Oncol Res 11, 109–113.
Weinberg, E.D., 2009. Tobacco smoke iron: an initiator/promoter of multiple diseases. Biometals 22, 207–210.
Weizer-Stern, O., Adamsky, K., Margalit, O., Ashur-Fabian, O., Givol, D., Amariglio, N., Rechavi, G., 2007. Hepcidin, a key regulator of iron metabolism, is transcriptionally activated by p53. Br J Haematol 138, 253–262.
Whitfield, J.B., Cullen, L.M., Jazwinska, E.C., Powell, L.W., Heath, A.C., Zhu, G., Duffy, D.L., Martin, N.G., 2000. Effects of HFE C282Y and H63D polymorphisms and polygenic background on iron stores in a large community sample of twins. Am J Hum Genet 66, 1246–1258.
Whitfield, J.B., Treloar, S., Zhu, G., Powell, L.W., Martin, N.G., 2003. Relative importance of female-specific and non-female-specific effects on variation in iron stores between women. Br J Haematol 120, 860–866.

Wild, P., Bourgkard, E., Paris, C., 2009. Lung cancer and exposure to metals: the epidemiological evidence. Methods Mol Biol 472, 139–167.

Wish, J.B., 2006. Assessing iron status: beyond serum ferritin and transferrin saturation. Clin J Am Soc Nephrol 1(Suppl 1), S4–S8.

Worwood, M., 1997. The laboratory assessment of iron status–an update. Clinica Chimica Acta 259, 3–23.

Wu, K.J., Polack, A., Dalla-Favera, R., 1999. Coordinated regulation of iron-controlling genes, H-ferritin and IRP2, by c-MYC. Science 283, 676–679.

Wu, T., Sempos, C.T., Freudenheim, J.L., Muti, P., Smit, E., 2004a. Serum iron, copper and zinc concentrations and risk of cancer mortality in US adults. Ann Epidemiol 14, 195–201.

Wu, X., Zhao, H., Suk, R., Christiani, D.C., 2004b. Genetic susceptibility to tobacco-related cancer. Oncogene 23, 6500–6523.

Wurzelmann, J.I., Silver, A., Schreinemachers, D.M., Sandler, R.S., Everson, R.B., 1996. Iron intake and the risk of colorectal cancer. Cancer Epidemiol Biomarkers Prev 5, 503–507.

Xu, Z., Pan, G.W., Liu, L.M., Brown, L.M., Guan, D.X., Xiu, Q., Sheng, J.H., Stone, B.J., Dosemeci, M., Fraumeni, J.F., Jr., Blot, W.J., 1996. Cancer risks among iron and steel workers in Anshan, China, Part I: Proportional mortality ratio analysis. Am J Ind Med 30, 1–6.

Yu, Y., Kovacevic, Z., Richardson, D.R., 2007. Tuning cell cycle regulation with an iron key. Cell Cycle 6, 1982–1994.

Zacharski, L.R., Chow, B.K., Howes, P.S., Shamayeva, G., Baron, J.A., Dalman, R.L., Malenka, D.J., Ozaki, C.K., Lavori, P.W., 2008. Decreased cancer risk after iron reduction in patients with peripheral arterial disease: results from a randomized trial. J Natl Cancer Inst 100, 996–1002.

Zacharski, L.R., Ornstein, D.L., Woloshin, S., Schwartz, L.M., 2000. Association of age, sex, and race with body iron stores in adults: analysis of NHANES III data. Am Heart J 140, 98–104.

Zafon, C., Lecube, A., Simo, R., 2009. Iron in obesity. An ancient micronutrient for a modern disease. Obes Rev 11(4), 322–328.

Zhang, K.H., Tian, H.Y., Gao, X., Lei, W.W., Hu, Y., Wang, D.M., Pan, X.C., Yu, M.L., Xu, G.J., Zhao, F.K., Song, J.G., 2009. Ferritin heavy chain-mediated iron homeostasis and subsequent increased reactive oxygen species production are essential for epithelial-mesenchymal transition. Cancer Res 69, 5340–5348.

Zheng, H., Cable, R., Spencer, B., Votto, N., Katz, S.D., 2005. Iron stores and vascular function in voluntary blood donors. Arterioscler Thromb Vasc Biol 25, 1577–1583.

Zhou, W., Park, S., Liu, G., Miller, D.P., Wang, L.I., Pothier, L., Wain, J.C., Lynch, T.J., Giovannucci, E., Christiani, D.C., 2005. Dietary iron, zinc, and calcium and the risk of lung cancer. Epidemiology 16, 772–779.

Glossary

Biostatistic, Epidemiologic and Genetic Terms Used in Genetic and Environmental Epidemiology of Cancer

Following are the description of terms used in genetic environmental epidemiology of cancer or other chronic diseases to indicate hazard/risk and statistical parameter of measures and test.

This glossary has been compiled from online sources at http://www.dorak.info/glosssary

by M. Tevfik Dorak.

Absolute risk Probability of an event over a period of time; expressed as a cumulative incidence like 10-year risk of 10% (meaning 10% of individuals in the group of interest will develop the condition in the next 10 year period). It shows the actual likelihood of contracting the disease and provides more realistic and comprehensible risk than relative risk/odds ratio.

Addition rule The probability of any of one of several mutually exclusive events occurring is equal to the sum of their individual probabilities. A typical example is the probability of a baby to be homozygous or heterozygous for a Mendelian recessive disorder when both parents are carriers. This equals to $1/4 + 1/2 = 3/4$. A baby can be either homozygous or heterozygous but not both of them at the same time; thus, these are mutually exclusive events.

Additive genetic model In a disease association study, if the risk conferred by an allele is increased r-fold for heterozygotes and 2r-fold for homozygotes, this corresponds to additive model. These data are best analyzed using Armitage trend test for genotype frequencies or by logistic regression.

Adjusted odds ratio In a multiple logistic regression model where the response variable is the presence or absence of a disease, an odds ratio for a binomial exposure variable is an adjusted odds ratio for the levels of all other risk factors included in a multivariable model. It is also possible to calculate the adjusted odds ratio for a continuous exposure variable. An adjusted odds ratio results from the comparison

D. Roy, M.T. Dorak (eds.), *Environmental Factors, Genes, and the Development of Human Cancers*, DOI 10.1007/978-1-4419-6752-7,

of two strata similar at all variables except exposure (or the marker of interest). It can be calculated when stratified data are available as contingency tables by Mantel-Haenszel test.

Adoption studies A design for assessing the proportion of variance due to genetic and environmental sources. The assumptions are that the resemblance between an adopted child and biological parent is due only to genetic effects, while that between the adopted child and the adoptive parent is only environmental in origin.

Affected Family-Based Controls (AFBAC) Method One of several family-based association study designs. This one uses affected siblings as controls and examines the sharing between two affected family members. The parental marker alleles not transmitted to an affected child or never transmitted to an affected sib pair form the so-called affected family-based controls (AFBAC) population.

Age-standardized rate An age-standardized rate is a weighted average of the age-specific rates, where the weights are the proportions of a standard population in the corresponding age groups. The potential confounding effect of age is removed when comparing age-standardized rates computed using the same standard population.

Allele Alternative form of a genetic locus; a single allele at each locus is inherited from each parent.

Alternative hypothesis In practice, this is the hypothesis that is being tested in an experiment. It is the conclusion that is reached when a null hypothesis is rejected. It is the opposite of null hypothesis, which states that there is a difference between the groups or something to that effect.

ANOVA (analysis of variance) A test for significant differences between multiple means by comparing variances. It concerns a normally distributed response (outcome) variable and a categorical explanatory (predictor) variable, which represents treatments or groups. Major assumptions of ANOVA are the homogeneity of variances (it is assumed that the variances in the different groups of the design are similar) and normal distribution of the data within each treatment group. When the assumptions of ANOVA are not met, its non-parametric equivalent Kruskal-Wallis test may be used.

Arithmetic mean $M = (x_1 + x_2 + \ldots x_n)/n$ (n = sample size).

Association A statistically significant correlation between an environmental exposure or a biochemical/genetic marker and a disease or condition. An association may be an artifact (random error-chance, bias, confounding) or a real one but never implies causation. A significant association should be presented together with a measure of the strength of association (odds ratio, relative risk or relative hazard and its 95% confidence interval) and when appropriate a measure of potential impact (attributable risk, prevented fraction, attributable fraction/etiologic fraction).

Asymptotic Refers to a curve that continually approaches either the x or y axis but does not actually reach it until x or y equals infinity. The axis so approached is the asymptote. An example is the normal distribution curve.

Asymptotically unbiased In point estimation, the property that the bias approaches zero as the sample size (N) increases. Therefore, estimators with this property improve as N increases.

Attributable risk (AR) Also called excess risk or risk difference. A measure of potential impact of an association. It quantifies the additional risk of disease following exposure over and above that experienced by individuals who are not exposed. It shows how much of the disease is eliminated if no one had the risk factor (unrealistic). The information contained in AR combines the *relative risk* and the risk factor prevalence. The larger the AR, the greater the effect of the risk factor on the exposed group.

Attributable fraction (etiologic fraction) It shows what proportion of disease in the exposed individuals is due to the exposure.

Balanced design An experimental design in which the same number of observations is taken for each combination of the experimental factors.

Bayesian inference An inference method radically different from the classical frequentist approach which takes into account the prior probability for an event. Established as a new method by Reverend Thomas Bayes.

Bernoulli distribution Models the behavior of data taking just two distinct values (0 and 1).

Bias An estimator for a parameter is unbiased if its expected value is the true value of the parameter. Otherwise, the estimator is biased. If bias tends to decrease as n gets larger, this is called asymptotic unbiasedness.

Binary (dichotomous) variable A discrete random variable that can only take two possible values (success or failure).

Binomial distribution The binomial distribution gives the probability of obtaining exactly *r* successes in *n* independent trials, where there are two possible outcomes one of which is conventionally called success.

Bioavailability The degree and rate at which a substance is made available at the site of physiological activity.

Biologic plausibility One of the criteria used in the assessment of whether an association is casual.

Biomarker A molecular marker of a biological function or external exposure.

Bonferroni Correction A conservative technique to adjust the statistical analysis results for multiple comparisons.

Bootstrap An application of resampling statistics. It is a data-based simulation method used to estimate variance and bias of an estimator and provide confidence intervals for parameters where it would be difficult to do so in the usual way.

Candidate gene study A study of specifically selected genes in which variation might influence the risk of a specific disease, usually because the gene is part of a biological pathway that is plausibly related to the disease.

Caretakers Products of genes involved in DNA repair to stabilize genome as a tumor suppressor mechanism.

Case-control study A design preferred over cohort studies for relatively rare diseases in which cases with a disease or exposure are compared with controls randomly selected from the same study base. This design yields odds ratio as opposed to relative risk from cohort studies.

Case-only design A study design that is used to assess deviations from purely multiplicative interactions. The case-only design has been shown to be more efficient for detecting gene and environment interaction than traditional designs in detection of gene-gene and gene-environment interactions. It estimates departure from multiplicative risk ratios (if genotype and environmental exposure are not associated in the population) as opposed to odds or rate ratio. The method cannot be used as a substitute for traditional case-control studies since it is limited to the detection of interactions only.

Causal relationship It does not matter how small it is, a *P* value does not signify causality. To establish a causal relationship, the following non-statistical evidence is required (Hills's criteria of causality): consistency (reproducibility), biological plausibility, dose-response, temporality (when applicable) and strength of the relationship (as measured by odds ratio/relative risk/hazard ratio). The original reference for Hill's criteria is Hill AB: The environment and disease: association or causation. Proc R Soc Med 1965;58:295–300.

Categorical (nominal) variable A variable that can be assigned to categories. A non-numerical (*qualitative*) variable measured on a (discrete) nominal scale such as gender, drug treatments, disease subtypes; or on an ordinal scale such as low, median or high dosage. A variable may alternatively be quantitative (continuous or discrete).

Censored observation Observations that survived to a certain point in time before dropping out from the study for a reason other than having the outcome of interest (lost to follow up or not enough time to have the event). Thus, censoring is simply an incomplete observation that has ended before time-to-event. These observations are still useful in survival analysis.

Central limit theorem The means of a relatively large (>30) number of random samples from any population (not necessarily a normal distribution) will be approximately normally distributed with the population mean being their mean and variance being the (population variance/n). This approximation will improve as the sample size (the number of samples) increases.

Chi-squared distribution A distribution derived from the normal distribution. Chi-squared (X^2) is distributed with v degrees of freedom with mean = v and variance = 2v.

Chi-squared test The most commonly used test for frequency data and goodness-of-fit. In theory, it is nonparametric but because it has no parametric equivalent, it is not classified as such. It is not an exact test and with the current level of computing facilities, there is not much excuse not to use Fisher's exact test for 2×2 contingency table analysis instead of Chi-squared test. Also for larger contingency tables, the G-test (log-likelihood ratio test) may be a better choice. The Chi-square value is obtained by summing up the values (residual^2/fit) for each cell in a contingency. In this formula, residual is the difference between the observed value and its expected counterpart and fit is the expected value.

Cochran's Q Test A nonparametric test examining change in a dichotomous variable across more than two observations. If there are two observations, McNemar's test should be used.

Coefficient of variation It is a measure of spread for a set of data. It is a measure of variation in relation to the mean. Calculated as standard deviation divided by the mean ($\times100$).

Cohort effect The tendency for persons born in certain years to carry a relatively higher or lower risk of a given disease. This may have to be taken into account in case-control studies.

Complex disease The term complex trait/disease refers to any phenotype that does not exhibit classic Mendelian inheritance attributable to a single gene; although they may exhibit familial clustering. A complex trait is the result of interactions between multiple genes and environmental exposures. Hallmarks of complex diseases include known or suspected environmental risk factors; seasonal, birth order, and cohort effects; late or variable age of onset; and variable disease progression.

Conditional logistic regression The conditional logistic regression (CLR) model is used in studies where cases and controls can be matched (as pairs) with regard to variables believed to be associated with the outcome of interest. The model creates a likelihood that conditions on the matching variable. It is the preferred method for the analysis of nested case-control studies when matching is done at the individual level (there may be more than one control per case).

Confounding variable A variable that is associated with both the outcome and the exposure variable. A classic example is the relationship between heavy drinking and lung cancer. Here, the data should be controlled for smoking as it is related to both drinking and lung cancer. The data should be stratified before analyzing it if there is a confounding effect. Mantel-Haenszel test is designed to analyze stratified data to control for a confounding variable. Alternatively, a multivariable regression model can be used to adjust for the effects of potential confounders.

Congenital Any trait present at birth, whether the result of a genetic or nongenetic factor.

Conservative test A test where the chance of type I error (false positive) is reduced and type II error risk is increased. Thus, these tests tend to give larger *P* values compared to non-conservative (liberal) tests for the same comparison.

Convenience sample A sample that has not been specifically and randomly collected for the purpose of a specific study. Such already existing samples may make running a study easier but may suffer from serious bias.

Copy number variation (CNV) Gains and losses of genomic segments resulting in variation in the number of copies of a genomic region or gene per diploid genome. Most genes show this variation and study of disease associations with CNV is becoming common. Reference gene in CNV studies is commonly RNAse P (RPPH1), which invariably exists in two copies in human diploid genome.

Cox proportional hazards model A regression method described by D.R. Cox for modeling survival times. It is also called proportional hazards model because it estimates the ratio of the risks (hazard ratio or relative hazard). As in any regression model, there are multiple predictor variables (such as prognostic markers whose individual contribution to the outcome is being assessed in the presence of the others) and the outcome variable (e.g., whether the patients survived 5 years, or died during follow-up, etc). Cox's regression model has been the most widely used method in survival data analysis regardless of whether the survival time is discrete or continuous and whether there is censoring.

Covariate Generally used to mean explanatory variable, less generally an additional explanatory variable is of no interest but included in the model. More specifically, it denotes a 'continuous' explanatory variable which is unaffected by treatments and has a linear relationship to the response. The intention is to produce more precise estimates of the effect of the explanatory variable of main interest. In the analysis, a model is first fitted using the covariate (and the blocking factor, if any). Then the main explanatory variable is added and its additional effect is assessed statistically. Whether the use of a covariate is wise can be judged by checking its effect on the residual (error) mean square (variance). If the addition of covariate reduces it remarkably, it will improve the analysis.

Cramer's coefficient of association (C) Also known as contingency coefficient. While Chi-squared is used to determine significance of an association (and varies by sample size for the same association), Cramer's C is a measure of association varying from 0 (no association) to 1 (perfect association) that is independent of the sample size. However, it seldom reaches its upper limit. It allows direct comparison of the degree of association between different contingency tables. It is calculated directly from the Chi-squared value and the total sample size as $(X^2/X^2+N)^{1/2}$.

Cramer's V A measure of the strength association for any size of contingency tables. It can be seen as a correction of the Chi-squared value for sample size. The transformation of the chi-squared value provides a value between 0 and 1 for relative comparison of the strength of the association. For a 2×2 table, Cramer's V is equal to the *Phi coefficient*. Cramer's V is most useful for large contingency tables. It can also be used as a global linkage disequilibrium value for multiallelic loci.

Crossover design A clinical trial design during which each subject crosses over from receiving one treatment to another one.

Cross-sectional data Data collected at one point in time (as opposed to longitudinal/cohort data for example).

Discrete variable A variable of countable number of integer outcomes. Examples include -ordinal multinomial- several prognostic outcomes (such as poor, median and good) as a function of treatment modalities, stage of the disease, age etc., or -multinomial- people's choices of hospitals (hospital A, B or C) as a function of their income level, age, education etc. A discrete variable may be binomial: diseased or non-diseased in a cohort or case-control study. The nature of the outcome variable as discrete or continuous is crucial in the choice of a regression model.

Dominant A phenotype that is expressed even when only one copy of the causative allele is present.

Dominant-negative mutation A (heterozygous) dominant mutation on one allele blocking the activity of wild-type protein still encoded by the normal allele (often by dimerizing with it) causing a loss-of-function phenotype. The phenotype is indistinguishable from that of homozygous dominant mutation.

Dose-response relationship The correlation between the amount of an exposure and the response such as changes in health. One of the criteria in the assessment of whether an association is causal.

Dummy variables A binary variable that is used to represent a given level of a categorical variable. In genetic data analysis, for example, it is created for each allele at a multiallelic locus. The most common choices as dummy variables are 0 and 1. For each level of the variable, 1 denotes having the feature and 0 denotes all other levels. Also called indicator variables. If an indicator variable is used, the regression coefficient gives the change per unit compared to the reference value.

Dunn's Test This test is used when a difference between the groups is found in a non-parametric ANOVA test. Dunn's test is a post hoc test that makes pairwise (multiple) comparisons to identify the different group.

Dunnett's test When ANOVA shows a significant difference between groups, if one of the groups is a control (reference) group, Dunnett's Test is used as a post hoc test. This multiple comparison test can be used to determine the significant differences between a single control group mean and the remaining treatment group means in an analysis of variance setting. It is one of the least conservative post hoc tests.

Ecological study Analyses based on data grouped to the municipal, provincial or national level.

Ecological fallacy The aggregation bias, which is the unfortunate consequence of making inferences for individuals from aggregate data. It results from thinking that relationships observed for groups necessarily hold for individuals. The problem is that it is not valid to apply group statistics to an individual member of the same group.

Effect modification The situation in which a measure of effect changes over values of another variable (the association estimates are different in different subpopulations of the sample). The relative risk or odds ratio associated with exposure will be different depending on the value of the effect modifier. For example if in a disease association study, the odds ratios are different in different age groups or in different sexes, age or sex are effect modifiers. Effect modification is highly related to statistical interaction in regression models. If where an exposure decreases risk for one value of the effect modifier and increases risk for another value of effect modifier, this is called crossover. Effect modification can be detected by stratified analysis and cannot be controlled by adjustment in statistical analysis (which adjusts for potential confounders not effect modifiers).

Empirical *P* value A *P* value obtained by a simulation program such as Monte Carlo statistics (permutation test). This is less likely to be affected by multiple comparisons.

Empirical rule In variables normally distributed, 68% of the data values are within 1SD of the mean; 95% are within 2SD of the mean; and 99.7% (nearly all) are within 3SD of the mean.

Environment Almost anything that is not genetic. Environmental factors include diet (food, preservatives, coloring, composition of diet and amount); air (clean air, smog, pollution, tobacco, workplace chemical fumes, dust, humidity, temperature); radiation (sunlight, tanning lights, X rays, microwaves, radio waves); infectious agents (bacteria, viruses, fungi, parasites), hormonal exposures and in utero environment.

Epidemiology A discipline that seeks to explain the extent to which factors that people are exposed to (environmental or genetic) influence their risk of disease, by means of population-based investigations.

Epigenetics The study of heritable changes in gene expression that occur without a change in DNA sequence. Epigenetic phenomena violate Mendelian principles of heredity. Epigenetic studies link genotype to phenotype working out the chain of processes.

Epialleles Alleles at genetic loci that are similar in DNA sequence but different in their epigenetic properties (methylation, histone modifications and RNA-mediated silencing).

Epistasis Original meaning was related to the genetic interaction of two or more genes that encode enzymes catalyzing steps in a common pathway. It has come to be synonymous with almost any type of gene interaction. The most extreme form of epistasis (interaction) results in a multiplicative model in which the total risk is the product of the individual risks at each locus (or allele).

Epistatic interaction In genetic epidemiology, an epistatic effect is the modification of the risk conferred by one marker by the presence of a marker from an unrelated gene (unlinked gene-gene interaction).

Exploratory data analysis An initial look at the data with minimal use of formal mathematics or statistical methods, but more with an informal graphical approach. Scatter plots, correlation matrices and contingency tables (for binary data) can be used to get an initial idea for relationships between explanatory variables (for collinearity) or between an explanatory variable(s) and a response variable(s) (correlation). In ANOVA, normality can be checked by box-plots. It gives some indication of which variables should be in the model and which one of them should be put into the model first, and whether linear relationship is adequate.

Exposure In an epidemiologic study, exposure may represent an environmental exposure, an intervention or the presence of a marker (biomarker/genetic marker).

Expressivity The range of phenotypes resulting from a given genotype (cystic fibrosis, for example, may have a variable degree of severity).

Fisher's exact test An exact significance test to analyze 2×2 tables for any sample size. It is a misconception that it is suitable only for small sample sizes. This arises from the demanding computational procedure for large samples, which is no longer an issue. It is the only test for a 2×2 table when an expected number in any cell is smaller than 5.

Framingham Heart Study The objective of the Framingham Heart Study was to identify the common factors or characteristics that contribute to cardiovascular disease by following its development over a long period of time in a large group of participants who had not yet developed overt symptoms of cardiovascular disease or suffered a heart attack or stroke. The study has expanded to three generations of related participants

Friedman test This non-parametric test is an extension of Wilcoxon matched pairs signed ranks test which is concerned with more than two time periods of data collection or conditions, and groups of three or more matched subjects.

Gatekeepers Genes whose products play a role in prevention of growth of cancer cells and accumulation of mutations that lead to increased cellular proliferation.

Genetic epidemiology Genetic epidemiology is the epidemiological evaluation of the role of inherited causes of disease in families and in populations; it aims to detect the inheritance pattern of a particular disease, localize the gene and find a marker associated with disease susceptibility. Gene-gene and gene-environment interactions are also studied in genetic epidemiology of a disease. In its broad context, genetic epidemiology includes family studies, molecular epidemiologic studies with genetic components, and more traditional cohort and case-control studies with family history components.

Genetic heterogeneity Distinct alleles at the same or different loci that give rise independently to the same genetic disease. In clinical settings genetic heterogeneity refers to the presence of a variety of genetic defects which cause the same disease, which may be the mutations at different positions on the same gene, a finding common to many human diseases (including Alzheimer disease, cystic fibrosis, lipoprotein lipase and polycystic kidney disease).

Genome All the genetic material in the chromosomes of a particular organism. Its size is generally given as its total number of base pairs.

Genome-wide association study (GWAS) Simultaneous investigation of up to one million genetic variants covering the whole genome in complex genetic diseases using microarray chips. Variants included in these chips are generally common haplotype tagging SNPs with low penetrance and not all genes are represented.

Genotype The genetic constitution of an individual at specific loci. A genotype consists of alleles in a locus and maybe homozygous or heterozygous.

Genotype-environment (GxE) interaction (GEI) This term refers to both the modification of genetic risk factors by environmental risk and protective factors, and the role of specific genetic risk factors in determining individual differences in vulnerability to environmental risk factors. When GxE interaction is present, a specific environmental change influences the outcome in different ways depending on the genotype.

Geometric mean $G = (x_1.x_2 \ldots x_n)^{1/n}$ where n is the sample size. This can also be expressed as antilog ((1/n) $\sum$ log x), which means the antilog of the mean of the logs of each value.

Half-normal plot A diagnostic test for model inadequacy or revealing the presence of outliers. It compares the ordered residuals from the data to the expected values of ordered observations from a normal distribution. While the full-normal plots use the signed residuals, half-normal plots use the absolute values of the residuals. Outliers appear at the top right of the plot as distinct points, and departures from a straight line mean that the model is not satisfactory. It is appropriate to use a half-normal plot only when the distribution is symmetrical about zero because any information on symmetry will be lost.

Haplotype A set of variants on a chromosome that are inherited together in a "block". Any particular SNP that characterizes the haplotype is referred to as a "haplotype tagging SNP."

HapMap (International Haplotype Mapping Project) A major international effort designed to obtain a map of haplotype blocks, the specific SNPs that identify the haplotypes (htSNPs) and linkage disequilibrium patterns in multiple populations.

Hardy-Weinberg equilibrium (HWE) In an infinitely large population, gene and genotype frequencies remain stable as long as there is no selection, mutation, or migration. For a bi-allelic locus where the gene frequencies are p and q: $p^2+2pq+q^2 = 1$. HWE should be assessed in controls in a case-control study and any deviation from HWE should alert for genotyping errors. Relying only on HWE tests to detect genotyping errors is not recommended as this is a low power test

Harmonic mean Of a set of numbers (y_1 to y_n), the harmonic mean is the reciprocal of the arithmetic mean of the reciprocal of the numbers [$H = N/(1/(y_1 + y_2 +\ldots y_n))$]. The harmonic mean is either smaller than or equal to the arithmetic mean. It is a measure of position.

Hazard function (instantaneous failure rate, conditional failure, intensity, or force of mortality function) The function that describes the probability of failure during a very small time increment (assuming that no failures have occurred prior to that time). Hazard is the slope of the survival curve – a measure of how rapidly subjects are having the event (dying, developing an outcome etc).

Hazard Rate It is a time-to-failure function used in survival analysis. It is defined as the probability per time unit that a case that has survived to the beginning of the respective interval will fail in that interval. Specifically, it is computed as the number of failures per time units in the respective interval, divided by the average number of surviving cases at the mid-point of the interval.

Hazard Ratio (Relative Hazard) Hazard ratio compares two groups differing in treatments or prognostic variables etc. If the hazard ratio is 2.0, then the rate of failure in one group is twice the rate in the other group. The computation of the hazard ratio assumes that the ratio is consistent over time, and that any differences are due to random sampling. Before performing any tests of hypotheses to compare survival curves, the proportionality of hazards assumption should be checked (and should hold for the validity of Cox's proportional hazard models).

Healthy People A set of health objectives for the Nation to achieve over the prescribed decade. Healthy People 2010 outlined the objectives for the decade 2000–2010; Healthy People 2020 will outline the objectives for the decade 2010–2020. It can be used by many different people, States, communities, professional organizations, and others to help them develop programs to improve health.

Heritability (h^2) The proportion of the phenotypic variability due to genetic variance. A high h^2 does not mean that the trait cannot be influenced by environment. In a different environment the same h^2 may not be that high. Heritability does not indicate the degree to which a trait is genetic; it measures the proportion of phenotypic variance that is the result of genetic factors.

Interaction If the effect of one factor depends on the level of another factor, the two factors involved are said to interact. Interaction is closely linked with effect modification in epidemiology.

Interpolation Making deductions from a model for values that lie between data points. Deductions for values beyond the data points are called extrapolation and the results are not valid.

Interval variable A quantitative variable measured on a scale with constant intervals (like days, milliliters, kilograms, miles so that equal-sized differences on different parts of the scale are equivalent) where the zero point and unit of measurement are arbitrary.

Kin-cohort study A study design for estimation of penetrance of a disease mutation. Individuals with and without family histories are included in the study sample and the family histories of the mutation carriers are compared with the family histories of the non-carriers. This design works only when the carrier frequency is more than 1% and when a founder effect is present (i.e, no genetic heterogeneity).

Kolmogorov-Smirnov two-sample test A non-parametric test applicable to continuous frequency distributions. It is considered to be the equivalent of the X^2-test for quantitative data and has greater power than the G-statistics or X^2-test for goodness of fit especially when the sample size is small. It can be used to compare two independent groups.

Kruskal-Wallis test (One-way ANOVA by ranks) It is one of the non-parametric tests equivalent to one-way ANOVA that are used to compare multiple independent samples. The interpretation of the Kruskal-Wallis test is identical to that of one-way ANOVA, but is based on ranks rather than means.

Large sample effect In large samples, even small or trivial differences can become statistically significant. This should be distinguished from biological/clinical importance.

Linkage The proximity of two or more markers on a chromosome; the closer the markers, the lower the probability that they will be separated during DNA repair or replication processes, hence the greater the probability that they will be inherited together.

Linkage disequilibrium (gametic association) Increased probability for two or more alleles to be on the same chromosome. When there is linkage disequilibrium, the observed haplotype frequency is different from the expected frequency. Linkage disequilibrium can derive from selection, population admixture, tight linkage or elapse of insufficient time for the population to reach equilibrium.

Log transformation This transformation pulls smaller data values apart and brings the larger data values together and closer to the smaller data values (shrinkage effect). Thus, it is mostly used to shrink highly positively skewed data.

Longitudinal data Data collected over a period of time as in cohort studies. These data are usually analyzed by using survival analysis techniques.

Loss of Heterozygosity (LOH) When one copy of a tumor suppressor gene has a mutation, it is masked by the normal (wildtype) allele on the other chromosome. The loss of heterozygosity events are genomic deletions that discard the normal copies of tumor suppressor genes and uncover the existing mutations. Inherited abnormalities of tumor suppressor genes are associated with familial cancer syndromes that cause a variety of cancers at an early age.

Mann-Whitney (U) test A non-parametric test for comparing the distribution of a continuous variable between two independent groups. It is analogous to the independent two-sample t-test, so that it can be used when the data are ordinal or not normally distributed. The Wilcoxon signed ranks T-test for independent samples is another non-parametric alternative to the t-test in this context (for paired samples, Wilcoxon matched pairs signed rank test should be used).

Mantel-Haenszel X^2 test A test for a null hypothesis of no overall relationship in a series of 2×2 tables for stratified data derived either from a cohort or a case-control study. It allows analysis of confounding and gives an adjusted odds ratio or relative risk.

Median test This is a crude version of the Kruskal-Wallis ANOVA in that it assesses the difference in samples in terms of a contingency table. The median test is particularly useful when the scale contains artificial limits, and many cases fall at either extreme of the scale.

Mendelian randomization A natural randomization process that occurs at conception to determine a person's genotype. According to the second law of Mendel (random assignment of genes), the inheritance of one trait is independent of the inheritance of other traits. The distribution of genetic polymorphisms is largely unrelated to the confounders (socioeconomic or behavioral) that distort interpretations of observational epidemiological studies. Mendelian randomization concept can be used as a tool for epidemiological inference on environmental risk factors by examining the genetic counterpart of a suspected environmental exposure association. The basis of Mendelian randomization is best seen in parent–offspring designs that study the way phenotype and alleles co-segregate during transmission from parents to offspring. This study design is closely analogous to that of randomized clinical trials as by Mendelian principles there should be an equal probability of either allele being randomly transmitted to the offspring.

Meta-analysis A systematic approach yielding an overall answer by analyzing a set of studies that address a related question. This approach is best suited to questions, which remain unanswered after a series of studies. Meta-analysis provides a weighted average of the measure of effect (such as odds ratio). The rationale is to increase the power by analyzing the sets of data.

Microsatellite A DNA variant due to tandem repetition of a short DNA sequence (usually two to four nucleotides). Also called short tandem repeat (STR). As multilallelic markers, they provide higher polymorphism information content (PIC) than SNPs.

Microsatellite instability (MSI) Changes in a microsatellite size in the tumor tissue compared with normal tissue. It is a hallmark of DNA mismatch repair defect and a marker for neoplastic transformation.

Migrant studies Studies on migrants based on the assumption that in migrants genetic components remain the same but environment has changed. If the rates of disease among migrants change in the new environment, this is taken as evidence for environmental influence. Considerations in the interpretation of migrant studies include the following: migrants are a highly selected group (usually younger, healthier and of higher socioeconomic status), age at migration varies (exposure to relevant environmental factor may have already occurred) and most migrants may retain their lifestyle (environmental) factors.

Misclassification Errors in the classification of individuals by phenotype, exposures or genotype that can lead to errors in results. The probability of misclassification can be the same across all groups in a study (nondifferential) or vary among groups (differential).

Modifier genes Not all genes that influence the appearance of a trait contribute equally to the phenotype: major genes have a large influence, while modifier genes have a more subtle, secondary effect. Modifier genes alter the phenotypes produced by the alleles of other genes.

Monte Carlo trial Studying a complex relationship difficult to solve by mathematical analysis by means of computer simulations. Frequently used in the analysis of association studies to obtain empirical *P* values.

Multicolinearity In multiple regression, two or more X variables are colinear if they show strong linear relationships. Multicolinearity may make the determination of the main predictor variable having an effect on the outcome difficult.

Multiple regression A regression analysis used to quantify the relationship between several independent (explanatory) variables and a normally distributed dependent (outcome) variable.

Multiple regression correlation coefficient (R^2 – R-squared) R^2 is a measure of the proportion of variability explained by, or due to the regression (linear relationship) in a sample of data (equal to the percentage of variance accounted for). The square root of the R^2 is the correlation coefficient (r) and has the same sign (minus or plus) as the slope.

Multivariable analysis As opposed to univariable analysis, statistical analysis performed in the presence of more than one explanatory variable to determine the relative contributions of each to a single event is called multivariable analysis (in practice, however, it is called univariate and multivariate analysis more frequently).

Multivariate analysis Methods to deal with more than one related 'outcome/dependent variable' (like two outcome measures from the same individual) simultaneously with adjustment for multiple confounding variables (covariates). Unfortunately, the word 'multivariate' is most frequently used instead of 'multivariable' analysis.

Mutation Any heritable change (not only point mutation) brought about by an alteration in the genetic material. Besides, point mutations, insertion, deletion, duplication and other changes in the sequence also cause mutations. Mutation is preferred to polymorphism to describe a disease-causing gene variation.

Nonparametric methods Statistical methods that do not assume a particular population distribution. For small sample sizes, non-parametric tests have greater statistical power than parametric tests. In general, parametric tests are more robust, more complicated to compute and have greater power. In large (e.g., $n > 100$) data sets, it makes little sense to use nonparametric statistics.

Normal distribution (Gaussian distribution) is a model for values on a continuous scale. A normal distribution can be completely described by two parameters: mean (μ) and variance (σ^2).

Observational study A study in which subjects select themselves into groups (such as cases and controls) and the investigator is a passive observer (no intervention). An observational study may be descriptive or analytic.

Odds The odds of a success is defined as the ratio of the probability of a success to the probability of a failure ($p/(1-p)$).

Odds ratio (OR) Also known as relative odds and approximate relative risk. It is the ratio of the odds of the risk factor in a diseased group and in a non-diseased (control) group (the ratio of the frequency of presence/absence of the marker in cases to the frequency of presence/absence of the marker in controls). An odds ratio $= 1$ indicates no risk; an odds ratio $< 1 =$ a protective factor; an odds ratio $> 1 =$ a risk factor. When the confidence interval includes 1, the odds ration is considered "not statistically significant". OR is used in retrospective case-control studies.

Omnibus test If the chi-square test has more than one degree of freedom (larger than 2×2 table), it is called an 'omnibus' test, which evaluates the significance of an overall hypothesis containing multiple sub-hypotheses (these multiple sub-hypotheses then need to be tested using follow up tests).

Oncogene A gene that normally directs cell growth. When mutated, an oncogene can promote and/or allow the uncontrolled growth of cancer. Genetic or epigenetic mutations in oncogenes occur via environmental exposures or hereditary factors.

One-way ANOVA A comparison of several groups of observations, all of which are independent and subjected to different levels of a single treatment (such as cells exposed to different dosage of a growth factor). It may be that different groups were exposed to the same treatment (different cell types exposed to a new agent). The main interest focuses on the differences among the means of groups.

Ordinal variable An ordered (ranked) qualitative/categorical variable. When two groups are compared for an ordinal variable, it is inappropriate to use ordinary Chi-squared test but the trend test or its equivalents must be used.

Outcome (response, dependent) variable The observed variable, which is shown on y axis. A statistical model shows this as a function of predictor variable(s).

Overfitting In a multivariable model, having more variables than can be justified from sample size. The statistical rule of thumb is to have at least ten events for each variable investigated.

Overmatching When cases and controls are matched by an unnecessary non-confounding variable, this is called overmatching and causes underestimation of an association.

Pearson's correlation coefficient (r) A measure of the strength of the 'linear' relationship between two quantitative variables. A major assumption is the normal distribution of variables. If this is not met, the non-parametric equivalent Spearman's rank correlation should be used.

Pedigree A family tree diagram that shows how a particular genetic trait has been transmitted through generations.

Penetrance The proportion of individuals with a given genotype who express an expected trait at any degree of clinical severity.

Phase I enzymes Enzymes that convert carcinogen molecules to metabolites easier to excrete. The metabolite may be more reactive than the original molecule.

Phase II enzymes Enzymes that detoxify the active metabolites of carcinogens by conjugation leading to their breakdown or excretion.

Phenocopy A non-genetic condition resembling a genetically determined one. Such conditions confound the interpretation of pedigrees and therefore genetic counseling. Some teratogens may cause congenital anomalies mimicking genetically caused anomalies (thalidomide syndrome vs phocomegalia). Deafness is another example of phenocopy which may be genetic (autosomal or sex-linked) or non-genetic (rubella embryopathy).

Phenotype The observed properties of an organism that are the product of the interactions between genotypes and environmental factors.

Polycyclic aromatic hydrocarbons Chemicals that are formed during the incomplete burning of organic substances such as charbroiled meat, tobacco or coal.

Polymorphism The existence of two or more variants at a locus. Conventionally, the frequency in the population should be above 1% to be referred to as a polymorphism. Because of the confusion between polymorphism and mutation, the Human Genome Variation Society recommends the use of 'sequence variant', 'alteration' or 'allelic variant' for any genomic change regardless of their frequency or phenotypic effects.

Polytomous variable A variable with more than two levels. If there are two levels it is called dichotomous (as in the most common form of *logistic regression*).

Population The population is the universe of all the objects from which a sample could be drawn for an experiment.

Population attributable risk The proportion of a disease in a specified population attributable to a specific factor (such as a genetic risk factor).

Population stratification (cryptic substructure) An example of 'confounding by ethnicity' in which the co-existence of different disease rates and allele frequencies within population sub-sections lead to a spurious association between the two at a whole population level. Case-control association studies can still be conducted by using genomic controls to adjust for population stratification.

Post hoc test A test following another one. The most common example is performing multiple comparisons between groups when the overall comparison between groups shows a significant difference.

Predictor (explanatory, independent) variable The variable already in hand in the beginning of an experiment or observation and whose effect on an outcome variable is being modeled.

Prevented fraction The amount of a health problem that actually has been prevented by a prevention strategy in real world.

Prior probability An attempt to distinguish between more likely and less likely interactions on the basis of knowledge of biological mechanisms, before an association or interaction is observed.

***P* value (SP = significance probability)** The *P* value gives the probability that the null hypothesis is correct; therefore, if it is a small value (like <0.05), null hypothesis is rejected. In an association study, the *P* value represents the probability of error in accepting the alternative hypothesis (or rejecting the null hypothesis) for the presence of an association. For example, the *P* level of 0.05 (i.e., 1/20) indicates that assuming there was no relation between those variables whatsoever (the null hypothesis is correct), and we were repeating experiments like ours one after another, we could expect that approximately in every 20 replications of the same experiment, there may be one in which the relation between the variables in question would be equal to or more extreme than what has been found due to sampling error. A *P* value does not indicate the size of an effect. A *P* value >0.05 does not necessarily mean lack of association if statistical power is insufficient.

Qualitative Qualitative (categorical) variables define different categories or classes of an attribute. Examples are gender, blood groups or disease states. A qualitative (categorical) variable may be *nominal* or *ordinal*. When there are only two categories, it is termed binary (like sex, dead or alive).

Quantitative Quantitative variables are variables for which a numeric value representing an amount is measured. They may be discrete (for example, taking values of integers) or continuous (such as weight, height, blood pressure). If a quantitative variable is categorized, it becomes an ordinal variable.

Random error A nonsystematic type of error that occurs by chance such as sampling error.

Ratio variable A quantitative variable that has a zero point as its origin (like 0 cm = 0 inch) so that ratios between values are meaningfully defined. Unlike the interval variables, which do not have a true zero point, the ratio of any two values in the scales is independent of the unit of measurement.

Recessive A phenotype that is expressed only two copies of the (autosomal) causative alleles are present.

Relative risk (RR) Also known as risk ratio. The RR shows how many times more or less the individuals with the risk factor are likely to get the disease relative to those who do not have the risk factor.

Resampling statistics Data-based simulation procedures that sample (with replacement) repeatedly from observed data to generate empirical estimates of results that would be expected by chance. Examples include bootstrapping and permutation tests.

Reverse causation The possibility that an observed association may actually reflect the relationship in the opposite direction. Childhood infections are believed to reduce the risk for asthma but 'reverse causation' meaning that asthma may cause increased risk for infections to result in the observed association is a distinct possibility. Increased cancer risk associated with low lipid levels and the relationship between sleeping less and obesity may be examples of reverse causation.

Sample size determination Mathematical process of deciding how many subjects should be studied. Among the factors to consider are the incidence or prevalence of the condition, the magnitude of difference expected between cases and controls, the power that is desired and the allowable magnitude of type I error (pre-determined significance probability).

Scales of measurement The type of data is always one of the following four scales of measurement: nominal, ordinal, interval, or ratio. Each of these can be discrete or continuous.

Sensitivity Sensitivity is the proportion of true positives that are correctly identified by a diagnostic test. Those that produce few false negatives have higher sensitivity.

Simple linear regression model The linear regression model for a normally distributed outcome (response) variable and a single predictor (explanatory) variable. The null hypothesis stating that the explanatory variable has no effect on the response (in other words, the slope of the fitted line is zero) can be tested statistically. The two main aims of regression analysis are to predict the response and to understand the relationships between variables.

Single nucleotide polymorphism (SNP) A single nucleotide variation in the DNA sequence. It is the most common type of stable genetic variation and usually biallelic. The effects of SNPs, if any, are generally on gene expression or protein structure. Functional changes that may be caused by SNPs are gene transcription changes (promoter and intronic enhancer SNPs), truncated protein (nonsense coding region SNPs), structural changes (coding region SNPs), alternative splicing (intronic splice site SNPs), and mRNA stability changes (3' untranslated region SNPs).

Skewness The degree of (lack of) asymmetry about a central value of a distribution. A distribution with many small values and few large values is positively (right) skewed (long tail in the distribution curve or stemplot is to the right); the opposite (left tail) is negatively (left) skewed. The measures of location median, midinterquartile range (midQ) and midrange decrease in this order for a left-skewed distribution.

Somatic mutations Mutations that occur in somatic (non-germline) cells as happens during carcinogenesis.

Spearman's rank correlation A non-parametric correlation coefficient (rho) that is calculated by computing the Pearson's correlation coefficient (r) for the association between the ranks given to the values of the variables involved. It is used for ordinal data and interval/ratio data.

Specificity Specificity is the proportion of true negatives that are correctly identified by the test. Those that produce few false positives have higher specificity.

Square root transformation Usually used for highly positively skewed data, but especially in transforming Poisson counts to normality.

Standard deviation Like variance, the standard deviation (SD) is a measure of spread (scatter) of a set of data. Unlike variance, which is expressed in squared units of measurement, the SD is expressed in the same units as the measurements of the original data. It is the square root of the variance. If a distribution's SD is greater than its mean, the mean is inadequate as a representative measure of central tendency. SD should not be confused with the standard error of the mean (SEM).

Standard error The standard error (SE) or as commonly called the standard error of the mean (SEM) is a measure of the extent to which the sample mean deviates from the true but unknown population mean. It is the standard deviation (SD) of the random sampling distribution of means (i.e., means of multiple samples from the same population). As such, it measures the precision of the statistic as an estimate of a population. When the sample size is relatively large ($N \geq 100$), the sample SD provides a reliable estimate of the SE.

Statistical Power The probability that in the presence of a real difference, a statistical test will produce a significant difference at a given significance level is called the power of the test. This is equal to the probability of rejecting the null hypothesis when it is untrue, i.e., making the correct decision. It is 1 minus the probability of a type II error. Ideally, power should be at least 0.80 to detect a reasonable departure from the null hypothesis.

Stepwise regression model A method in multiple regression studies aimed to find the best model. This method seeks a model that balances a relatively small number of variables with a good fit to the data by seeking a model with high $R^2{}_a$ (the most parsimonious model with the highest percentage accounted for).

Student's t-test A parametric test for the significance between means (two independent sample t-test or paired samples t-test) or between a mean and a hypothesized value (one-sample t-test). One assumption is that the observations must be normally distributed, and the ratio of variances in two samples should not be more than three.

Synergism A joint effect of two treatments being greater than the sum of their effects when administered separately (positive synergism) or the opposite (negative synergism).

Transformations (ladder of powers) Transformation deals with non-normality of the data points and non-homogeneous variance. The power transformations form the following ladder:. . ., x^{-2}, x^{-1}, $x^{-1/2}$, $\log x$, $x^{1/2}$; x^1, x^2, x^3,. . .. Provided $x > 1$, powers below 1 (such as $x^{1/2}$ or $\log x$) reduce the high values relative to the low values as in positively skewed data, whereas, powers above 1 (such as x^2) have the opposite effect of stretching out high values relative to low ones, as in negatively skewed data. All power transformations are monotonic when applied to positive data (they are either increasing or decreasing, but not first increasing and then decreasing, or vice versa).

Trend test for counts and proportions A special application of the Chi-squared test for ordinal data tabulated as a $2 \times k$ table. It should be used when the intention is not just to compare the differences between the two groups but to whether there is a consistent trend towards decrease or increase in the difference between the groups. A frequent application is the analysis of dose-response relationships. The trend test for counts and proportions is called Cochrane-Armitage trend test.

Tumor suppressor gene (also known as anti-oncogene) Genes whose products control cell growth. When mutated, aberrant cell growth and subsequently cancer may occur. As with oncogenes, mutations in tumor suppressor genes can occur via environmental exposures or hereditary factors.

Variance The major measure of variability for a data set. To calculate the variance, all data values, their mean, and the number of data values are required. It is expressed in the squared unit of measurement. Its square root is the standard deviation. It is symbolized by σ^2 for a population and S^2 for a sample.

Women's Health Initiative (WHI) A long-term national health study that focuses on strategies for preventing heart disease, breast and colorectal cancer and fracture in postmenopausal women. This 15-year project involves over 161,000 women ages 50–79, and is one of the most definitive, far reaching programs of research on women's health ever undertaken in the U.S.

Xenobiotic A potentially harmful compound that is normally present in the body.

See also National Cancer Institute Dictionary: http://www.nci.nih.gov/dictionary

Index

D

P

FSC
www.fsc.org
MIX
Papier aus verantwortungsvollen Quellen
Paper from responsible sources
FSC® C105338

If you have any concerns about our products,
you can contact us on
ProductSafety@springernature.com

In case Publisher is established outside the EU,
the EU authorized representative is:
Springer Nature Customer Service Center GmbH
Europaplatz 3, 69115 Heidelberg, Germany

Printed by Libri Plureos GmbH
in Hamburg, Germany